Patient Reported Outcome Measures in Rheumatic Diseases

Yasser El Miedany
Editor

Patient Reported Outcome Measures in Rheumatic Diseases

Springer

Editor
Yasser El Miedany, MD, FRCP
Honorary Senior Clinical Lecturer
King's College London
London, UK

Professor of Rheumatology and Rehabilitation
Ain Shams University
Cairo, Egypt

Department of Rheumatology
Darent Valley Hospital
Dartford, Kent, UK

ISBN 978-3-319-32849-2 ISBN 978-3-319-32851-5 (eBook)
DOI 10.1007/978-3-319-32851-5

Library of Congress Control Number: 2016944141

Printed on acid-free paper

This Springer imprint is published by Springer Nature
The registered company is Springer International Publishing AG Switzerland

Preface

The recently introduced patient-centered approach mandated a shift of the rheumatologist's understanding toward placing the inflammatory arthritic conditions themselves, their associated comorbidities, and the possible interactions at equal distance. Patient-reported outcomes (PROs) are defined as measures of a patient's health status or health-related quality of life reported directly by the patient, whereas patient-reported outcome measures (PROMs) are the tools used to measure the patient-reported outcomes. PROs represent "the patient's voice" in both standard clinical practice and clinical trials. PROMs not only provide clinicians with timely information on the patient's symptoms as well as functional and emotional status, but it also enhances the patient-clinician communication and facilitates the recently introduced concept of patient activation-physician activation. In parallel with the patient-reported outcomes, this book also presents the newly developed Physician RheuMetric measures, designed to enable the treating clinician to record the patient's disease activity and impact from the physician's own perspective.

Integrating patient-reported outcome measures into standard clinical practice and sharing its aggregated data with the patient have a disease-modifying potential and globally offer the prospective to help transform healthcare. In addition to helping the patients and clinicians make better decisions, PROMs enable comparative-effectiveness research. Comparing providers' performances helps to stimulate improvements in services and encourages change in the standard practice. The recent move toward integrating electronic patient-reported outcome measures (e-PROMs) into a global electronic health record format, together with clinician alerts for the concerning symptoms and disease flare-ups, forms a major step forward toward the ideal health service where the patient and clinician speak the same language. There have been several ongoing initiatives to develop standards and clinical practice tools in this area both in America and Europe.

The main purpose of this book is to deliver a very practical and reader-friendly guide. On one hand, it delivers the evidence and advanced knowledge base of PROMs in different rheumatic diseases. On the other, it provides examples of PROM tools, which readers/researchers can use for their standard practice/trials. The PROM questionnaires included in the book were meticulously selected to give the reader a clear guide toward implementation in real-life practice. Focusing on the major values of "meaningful outcomes" in rheumatic diseases, this book with its 18 chapters fills an important void in the current literature. It represents what can be considered to be the best current thinking on the role of PROMs in the management of different rheumatic diseases. Therefore, this book can serve as both an excellent introduction and a very good reference resource for implementation in standard clinical practice and future reading.

This work has been the outcome of cooperative effort of a large international group of leaders in PROMs. They have done a superb job in producing authoritative chapters that include vast amounts of scientific and clinical data and provide state-of-the-art descriptions of outcome measures encompassed in different rheumatic diseases. Special thanks to my colleagues and family for their support throughout the whole project, which helped to make this book complete.

Personally, I feel privileged to have compiled this work and am enthusiastic about all that it offers our readers. I hope you too will find this edition a uniquely valuable educational resource.

London, UK Yasser El Miedany, MD, FRCP

Contents

Contributors

Xenofon Baraliakos, MD Rheumazentrum Ruhrgebiet, Herne, Germany

Ruhr-University Bochum, Herne, Germany

Martin J. Bergman, MD Arthritis and Rheumatology, Taylor Hospital, Ridley Park, PA, USA

Jürgen Braun, MD Rheumazentrum Ruhrgebiet, Herne, Germany

Marwan Bukhari, MBBS, MSc, PhD, FRCP Department of Rheumatology, Royal Lancaster Infirmary, Lancaster, Lancashire, UK

Loreto Carmona, MD, PhD Instituto de Salud Musculoesquelética, Madrid, Spain

Isabel Castrejon, MD, PhD Division of Rheumatology, Rush University Medical Center, Chicago, IL, USA

Jacquelin Chua, MD Division of Rheumatology, Department of Internal Medicine, Rush University Medical Center, Chicago, IL, USA

Natalie J. Collins, PhD, MSports Physio, BPhty(Hons) School of Health and Rehabilitation Sciences, The University of Queensland, St. Lucia, QLD, Australia

Alessandro Consolaro, MD, PhD Universita degli studi di Genova, Genoa, Italy

Pediatria 2, Reumatologia, Istituto Giannina Gaslini, Genoa, Italy

Rafael J. Curbelo, MSc, PhD Instituto de Salud Musculoesquelética, Calle Conde de la Cimera, Madrid, Spain

Maha El Gaafary, MD Community and Public Health Department, Ain Shams University, Cairo, Egypt

Kathryn A. Gibson, MD, PhD Department of Rheumatology, Liverpool Hospital, Liverpool, NSW, Australia

Laure Gossec, MD, PhD Department of Rheumatology, AP-HP, Pitié Salpêtrière Hospital, UPMC, Sorbonne Universitées, Paris, France

Brian Bekker Hansen, MSc Global Market Access, Novo Nordisk A/S, Søborg, Denmark

Mohamed Osama Hegazi, MRCP (UK) Medical Department, Al Adan Hospital, Hadiya, Kuwait

Lise Højbjerre, MSc, PhD Global Market Access, Novo Nordisk A/S, Søborg, Denmark

Concepción González Isabel, PhD Instituto de Salud Osteoarticular, Madrid, Spain

Christina Kampling, MD Policlinic for Rheumatology and Hiller Research Centre for Rheumatology, University Clinic Duesseldorf, Heinrich-Heine-University Duesseldorf, Duesseldorf, Germany

Uta Kiltz, MD Rheumazentrum Ruhrgebiet, Herne, Germany

Mart A.F.J. van de Laar, MD, PhD Department of Rheumatology and Clinical Immunology, University of Twente, Enschede, The Netherlands

Stefano Lanni, MD Pediatria 2, Reumatologia, Istituto Giannina Gaslini, Genoa, Italy

Yasser El Miedany, MD, FRCP Honorary Senior Clinical Lecturer, King's College London, London, UK

Professor of Rheumatology and Rehabilitation, Ain Shams University, Cairo, Egypt

Department of Rheumatology, Darent Valley Hospital, Gravesend, Kent, UK

Mwidimi Ndosi, PhD, MSc, BSc (Hons), RN School of Healthcare, University of Leeds, Baines Wing, Leeds, West Yorkshire, UK

Deborah Palmer, Diploma Rheumatology Nursing Department of Rheumatology, North Middlesex University Hospital, London, UK

Russell E. Pellar, BESc Schulich School of Medicine and Dentistry, University of Western Ontario, London, ON, Canada

Theodore Pincus, MD Division of Rheumatology, Department of Internal Medicine, Rush University Medical Center, Chicago, IL, USA

Janet E. Pope, MD, MPH, FRCPC Division of Rheumatology, Schulich School of Medicine and Dentistry, University of Western Ontario, London, ON, Canada

Division of Rheumatology, Department of Medicine, St. Joseph's Health Care, London, ON, Canada

Angelo Ravelli, MD Universita degli studi di Genova, Genoa, Italy

Pediatria 2, Reumatologia, Istituto Giannina Gaslini, Genoa, Italy

Jutta Richter, MD Policlinic for Rheumatology and Hiller Research Centre for Rheumatology, University Clinic Duesseldorf, Medical Faculty, Heinrich-Heine-University Duesseldorf, Duesseldorf, Germany

Ewa M. Roos, PhD Department of Sports and Clinical Biomechanics, University of Southern Denmark, Odense, Denmark

Nicolino Ruperto, MD, MPH Pediatria 2, Reumatologia, Istituto Giannina Gaslini, Genoa, Italy

Matthias Schneider, MD Policlinic for Rheumatology and Hiller Research Centre for Rheumatology, University Clinic Duesseldorf, Medical Faculty, Heinrich-Heine-University Duesseldorf, Duesseldorf, Germany

Nipam Shah, MBBS, MPH Department of Medicine, University of Alabama at Birmingham, Birmingham, AL, USA

Jasvinder Singh, MBBS, MPH Department of Medicine, University of Alabama at Birmingham, Birmingham, AL, USA

Theresa M. Tingey, BArtsSc Schulich School of Medicine and Dentistry, University of Western Ontario, London, ON, Canada

Jacqueline Uson, MD Department of Rheumatology, Hospital Universitario de Móstoles, Madrid, Spain

Martijn A.H. Oude Voshaar, MSc, PhD Department of Psychology, Health & Technology, University of Twente, Enschede, The Netherlands

Yusuf Yazici, MD Division of Rheumatology, Department of Internal Medicine, NYU Hospital for Joint Diseases, New York, NY, USA

Sally Youssef, MD Rheumatology and Rehabilitation Department, Ain Shams University, Cairo, Egypt

Chapter 1
PROMs and Quality of Care

Martijn A.H. Oude Voshaar and Mart A.F.J. van de Laar

Concepts and Definitions

Patient-reported outcomes (PROs) are standardized measures directly reported by the patient that characterize the patient's perception of the impact of disease and treatment on health and functioning. As defined by the US Food and Drug Administration (FDA), PRO is "a measurement based on a report that comes directly from the patient about the status of a patient's condition without amendment or interpretation of the patient's response by a clinician or anyone else." PRO instruments are useful when measuring concepts that are best known to the patient or best measured from the patient's perspective [1]. For an increasing number of outcome domains in rheumatology, PROs are standard and a large literature exists that supports the measurement properties of PROs in rheumatology [2, 3]. Frequently, PROs provide information that would otherwise be difficult to quantify, such as in the cases of symptom burden, social participation, and pain. However, even in cases where it would in principle be possible to use objective tests, PROs offer a number of advantages. For example, PROs are usually more feasible to implement and associated with lower costs since less health professional time is required and no specific training ususally needed for them to be implemented. Finally, PROs reflect the values and priorities of patients. Ultimately, most people seek treatmentbecasue of functional disability, pain, fatigue, or restrictions in social participation, which

M.A.H.O. Voshaar (✉)
Department of Psychology, Health & Technology, University of Twente,
Drienerlolaan 5, Enschede 7522 NB, The Netherlands
e-mail: a.h.oudevoshaar@utwente.nl

M.A.F.J. van de Laar
Department of Rheumatology and Clinical Immunology, University of Twente,
Ariensplein 1, Cubicus, Room B125, Enschede 7500 KA, The Netherlands
e-mail: M.vandeLaar@mst.nl

Y. El Miedany (ed.), *Patient Reported Outcome Measures in Rheumatic Diseases*,
DOI 10.1007/978-3-319-32851-5_1

provides a strong rationale to systematically monitor these outcomes besides traditional clinical outcome measurese [4].

PROs can be used to measure health concepts that cover the full spectrum of human functioning. Individual PRO domains can be considered to exist on a continuum of increasing social complexity [5]. On one end of this continuum are biological and psychological factors and on the other end are complex, integrated domains such as social role participation and work disability [5]. A conceptual framework or structured representation of PRO outcome concepts is provided by the International Classification of Impairments, Disabilities, and Handicaps (ICIDH) [6]. ICIDH was published by the World Health Organization (WHO) in 1980 as a tool for the classification of the consequences of disease and implications for the lives of individuals. This framework is based on a multidimensional perspective of health as physical, psychological, and social functioning and well-being, in accordance with the WHO definition of health: a "state of complete physical, mental, and social well-being and not merely the absence of disease and infirmity" [7]. Because of its comprehensive scope, ICIDH and particularly its recent revision—the International Classification of Functioning, Disability, and Health (ICF)—is increasingly used as a standard to judge the relevance and comprehensiveness of PROs in rheumatology [8, 9]. This general framework describes the direct and indirect ways that (rheumatic) disease may impact patients' lives in terms of impairments, disabilities, and handicaps, which are considered hierarchical concepts that refer to different levels of consequences of disease.

Patient-Reported Outcomes of Impairments

Within ICIDH, the most fundamental determinants of subjective health status are biological factors. In ICIDH any loss or abnormality of psychological, physiological, or anatomical structure or function are referred to as impairments. Impairments can be further classified into signs, which are manifestations of impairments that can be objectively observed, and symptoms, which are manifestations of impairments that are experienced by and might be reported by patients. Symptoms, particularly pain and fatigue, are key domains for PRO measures since they are by definition subjective and can therefore be best assessed from the perspective of the patient. Moreover, in survey and qualitative studies among patients with rheumatic diseases it has been a consistent finding that PRO domains reflecting symptoms, particularly pain, are considered the most important priorities for improvement, compared with PRO domains reflecting disability and impairment, throughout the various stages of disease [10].

Patient-Reported Outcomes of Disability

Disability was defined in the ICIDH framework as "any restriction or lack of ability to perform an activity in the manner or within the range considered normal for a human being" [6]. In the ICIDH conceptual framework, impairments are determinants of disability. This means that the ability of individuals to engage in everyday activities might be impacted by the presence of symptoms. For instance, in many rheumatic diseases, impairments such as pain and joint damage may prevent patients from engaging in everyday activities. Health concepts in the disability domain focus on essential components of everyday life. Activity limitations of particular relevance to rheumatology are those directly associated with musculoskeletal function; i.e., health concepts related to self-care, mobility, and domestic life (household, work, and chores). The negative impact of signs and symptoms of rheumatic disease on physical function is well established. Therefore physical function has always been considered a key outcome of many rheumatic diseases and a variety of physical function PROs have been proposed and validated over time [2]. However, in earlier times clinicians as well as researchers preferred to use performance based measures off physical function, such as, for example, standardized assessments of grip strength or walking or buttoning time [8]. In contemporary settings, these tests have mostly been abandoned in the field of RA since PROs are cheaper and easier to implement, provide a more comprehensive assessment of physical function (i.e., greater content validity), have been found to be better predictors of relevant outcomes such as mortality and work disability compared with more objective measures, and recognize the patients' own perspective on their disease as a valued treatment endpoint [4].

Patient-Reported Outcomes of Participation Restrictions

Finally, handicaps are defined in ICIDH as "a disadvantage for an individual, resulting from an impairment or a disability that limits or prevents the fulfillment of a role that is normal for that individual considering the age, sex, and social and cultural factor for that individual [6]." Handicap considers the person's participation in social roles. In ICF, the term "handicap" was replaced by the term "participation restrictions." Participation restrictions describe areas of human functioning that may indirectly be affected by disease due to the presence of disease-related impairments or disability. In the ICF framework, participation restrictions may involve major life areas (education or work), community, social, or civic life (e.g., engaging in leisure activities) and interpersonal interactions and relationships (e.g., maintaining family relationships). Since participation restrictions are indirect consequences of rheumatic disease, the interest in PRO domains at this level of the hierarchy, such as social role participation and work productivity losses, has evolved only relatively recently in rheumatology. Increased attention for economic aspects of rheumatology care results from increased pressure for efficient use of available economic resources, particularly in light of the ageing general population and increased use of expensive biological monoclonal antibodies. However, increased attention for the measurement of participation restrictions in rheumatology also reflects the realization that disease outcomes should be assessed in those outcome domains that matter most to the everyday lives of patients [11]. Despite rheumatic disease, individuals want to engage in social roles that are important to them. The increased attention for participation restrictions as a valued outcome domain therefore also reflects a general shift from a purely pathophysiological model of health toward a biopsychosocial model where health is seen as an interaction of individual, social, and environmental factors [12].

Health-Related Quality of Life

The foregoing intends to make clear that rheumatic disease may affect the quality of life of patients either through direct suffering caused by impairments or indirectly through activity limitations imposed by impairments and participation restrictions resulting from impairments and/or disability and that PROs may focus on any of these consequences. Collectively, all the ways in which rheumatic disease may affect subjective experience of health and well-being is referred to as health-related quality of life (HRQOL). While no comprehensive definition of HRQOL presently exists, a consensus among health researchers is that it is a multidimensional construct composed of at least the dimensions of physical and psychologic function (i.e., disability), social role function (i.e., handicaps), and disease or treatment symptoms (i.e., impairments). Fig. 1.1 presents the HRQOL profile of patients with early rheumatoid arthritis enrolled in a tight control study, compared with the health profile of similar age in the Dutch general population [13, 14]. It can be seen that the

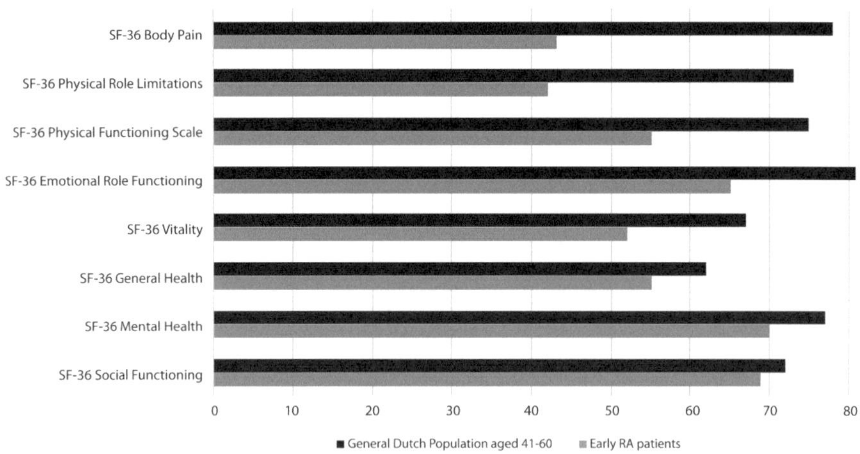

Fig. 1.1 Health profile of patients with active early rheumatoid arthritis compared with the general population of similar age. *Bars* represent Short Form-36 Health Survey subscale scores, range 0–100 with higher values indicating better health. Dutch general population data were adapted from Aaronson et al. [13]. Data for Early RA patients are unpublished observations from data collected as part of the DREAM remission induction study by Vermeer et al. [14]

HRQOL of patients with early rheumatoid arthritis is below typical levels and that in particular the physical aspects of HRQOL are significantly impaired compared to the general population. PRO instruments can be designed to comprehensively assess the overall HRQOL. Such instruments are commonly referred to as *generic* instruments. Alternatively, PROs may be designed with a specific focus on a particular disease, population, or aspect of HRQOL. These PROs are called *specific* instruments [15].

Generic Instruments

Two types of generic instruments are commonly distinguished. *Health profiles* are multidimensional tools with separate scales and scoring rules to assess individual aspects of HRQOL. Health profiles aim to provide comprehensive information regarding aspects of HRQOL that are relevant across types and severities of disease, medical treatments, and across demographic and cultural subgroups [15, 16]. Becasue of this, they tend to focus on nonspecific aspects of HRQOL. Probably the most commonly used health profile across rheumatic diseases is the Short Form-36 Health Survey (SF-36), which assesses HRQOL in the domains of general health, physical functioning, bodily pain, physical role functioning, emotional role functioning, social role functioning, vitality, and mental health. Other health profiles that have, particularly in earlier times, been used in rheumatology are: (1) the Nottingham Health Profile, which assesses the domains: energy level, pain, emotional reaction, sleep, social isolation, and physical abilities; and (2) the Sickness Impact Profile, which assesses the domains of somatic autonomy, mobility control and range, social behavior, emotional stability, and psychological autonomy. As is typical for health profiles, all three of these instruments assess domains referring to impairments, disability, and participation restrictions. A commonly cited drawback of health profiles and generic measures in general is that they might be less responsive to change due to their focus on general aspects of HRQOL. However, this phenomenon seems to apply in particular to the assessment of HRQOL aspects at the participation level in rheumatology [17–21].

The other types of generic instrument, *utility measures* of quality of life, are grounded in health economics and reflect the preferences of patients for treatment process and health outcome [15]. Preference-based or indirect utility measures can be utilized to calculate quality-adjusted life years (QALYs) to be used in cost–utility analyses. Such instruments express HRQOL as a single number along a continuum that usually ranges fromdeath (0.0) to full health (1.0). Utility scores reflect both the health status and the value of that health status to the patient. Utility measures are of interest in economic analysis to justify the resources devoted to treatment. However, they provide no information on the domains in which improvement or deterioration occur [15].

Specific Instruments

PROs may also be specific to an area of primary interest [15]. These instruments are more limited in scope but are supposed to have favorable measurement properties and content validity due to their focus on clinically significant aspects of HRQOL. Because of this, *disease-specific* PROs are believed to be able to discriminate more finely between levels of severity of the measured trait, and of being more sensitive to change. The arthritis impact measurement scales and the gout assessment questionnaire are health profiles that intend to provide information on overall HRQOL with particular focus on aspects of those respective diseases [22, 23]. Measures may also be *condition*-specific (e.g., depression), or *population*-specific, as is the case for many PROs developed for use with juveniles or the elderly. *Domain*-specific instruments focus on particular components of health-related quality of life. Such instruments are typically used when the area covered is of particular clinical relevance. For instance the Health Assessment Questionnaire Disability index is a PRO that focuses on physical function alone [24].

Application of Patient-Reported Outcomes in Different Settings in Rheumatology

PROs are used in a variety of settings and for different reasons in rheumatology. For the sake of comparability across studies, researchers and clinicians usually favor the use of a single patient-reported outcome measure (PROM) in order to facilitate the comparability across studies. However, because different PRO characteristics and foci are relevant in different settings, a substantial number of PROs for similar outcome domains have nonetheless been proposed over time.

Clinical Trials

It is increasingly recognized across all fields of medicine that PROs should be included as endpoints of clinical trials [25]. In rheumatology, one of the main reasons for this is that no cure is currently available for most rheumatic diseases and consequently the primary aim of treatment often is to suppress disease activity in order to preserve function and structural integrity of the body and/or to manage symptoms. Many relevant outcomes of rheumatologic care such as pain relief or effect on mood are known only to the patient. Another motivation for the use of PROs as (secondary) trial endpoints is that improvements in clinical measures of a condition may not necessarily correspond to improvements on how the patient functions or feels [1]. The FDA has stated that "findings measured by a well-defined and reliable PRO instrument in appropriately designed investigations can be used to support a claim in medical product labeling if the claim is consistent with the instrument's documented measurement capability." [1] In fact, several new biologics for treatment of RA have an approved PRO label claim. However, in rheumatology, interest in PROs preceded these recent developments and PROs have had a prominent role in clinical trials for several decades. For many years the primary application of PROs was in this setting. For instance, 3 out of 7 endorsed outcome domains for clinical trials in rheumatoid arthritis are PROs. Physical function, pain, and patient global assessment of disease activity have been respectively used as outcome measures in 90, 70, and 70 % of contemporary clinical trials [26]. In some rheumatic diseases, such as acute gout and osteoarthritis, patient-reported pain frequently is the primary outcome of clinical trials [27]. Like for any application, PROs to be used in clinical trials should be valid and feasible. However, the primary aim of clinical trials is to assess the within-subject change over time. The ability to detect clinically relevant change, responsiveness, is therefore another key property of PROs to be used in trials that may affect achieved statistical power of a trial (in case it is the primary outcome [16]. The Outcome Measures in Rheumatology (OMERACT) group has summarized relevant measurement properties of PROs to be used in clinical trials in their OMERACT filter as respectively: truth, feasibility, and discrimination [28].

Comparative Effectiveness Research

Comparative effectiveness studies involve evaluating costs and health outcomes between competing treatment alternatives. Typically, cost–utility analyses are employed in such studies, which involve calculating incremental (direct and indirect) costs associated with incremental quality-adjusted life years gained. In these studies, evidence is first needed for the overall effect of an intervention on perceived health-related quality of life. However, this evidence should be presented in a way that permits comparisons with other interventions within or across treatment areas and patient populations. The most common way this is achieved is by tobtaining Quality-Adjusted Life Years (QALY). Within the QALY methodology, the quality and quantity of life gains are expressed as a single index that can be used to inform decision-making relating to the allocation of healthcare resources. Specifically, it is assumed that a year of life lived in perfect health is worth 1 QALY, while a year lived in less than perfect health is worth less than 1. Different techniques are used to obtain QALYs, including the time-trade-off (asking patients how many years of their life they would be willing to give in order to be restored to full health) or by visual analogue scale (VAS). However the most popular method is probably using multi-item PROs such as the EuroQOL 5d or SF-6D questionnaires. Quality-adjusted life years associated with an intervention are simply obtained by multiplying the utility value associated with a health state (QALY) by the time spent in that health state. The most important advantages of the QALY approach to health economics are that it allows comparison across different settings by using a common unit of measurement (i.e., cost per QALY). However, different preference elicitation techniques lead to different QALY estimates.

Direct and indirect costs associated with health interventions can also be assessed using PROs. While patient records, databases from insurance companies, hospital, or provider databases are ideally used to quantify direct costs, this is often infeasible in practical settings. Moreover, no information about direct, non-medical costs incurred by patients can be gathered through these data sources. Therefore various standardized, validated questionnaires or diaries exist that can be used by patients to record the direct and indirect medical costs that they make while participating in a clinical trial [29]. Indirect non-medical costs associated with work productivity can also be assessed using various PROs. Most of these PROs can be used to assess work productivity loss, absenteeism, and presentism. However, it has been found that the agreement between different questionnaires is often low, which might be explained by differing recall periods and operationalization of concepts [30]. Finally, PROs can be used to assess the side effects of treatment [31].

Individual Patient Care

The use of PRO as supplemental information to clinical outcome measures in clinical practice in rheumatology has long been advocated by various authors [4, 32]. PROs may be used in clinical practice for a variety of purposes [33]. PROs have long been used as *screening tools* to facilitate detection of physical or psychological problems that might otherwise not be adressed during clinic visits [34]. Disease-related distress or psychiatric comorbidity is often overlooked in clinical practice [35]. Consequently, most screening tools for use in the clinic, such as the Patient Health Questionnaire, focus on assessing these issues [36]. However, generic HRQOL or symptom PROs instruments can also be used to identify particularly bothersome issues to the patient that would otherwise remain undetected, such as sleep disturbance, pain, participation restrictions, and work disability.

PROs can also be used to *monitor* disease over time and to provide information about the impact of prescribed treatment in terms of outcomes that matter to patients. In clinical care settings, electronic health records increasingly integrate patient portals that can be used to store and give insight to patients regarding the progression of their HRQOL outcomes since treatment has started. This feedback may direct patient–physician interactions and informing clinical decision-making [35, 37]. According to Greenhalgh, the use of PROs in clinical practice may also serve to facilitate patient-centered care by bringing the patient's desired outcomes to the clinical agenda [33]. Integration into routine clinic visits of PROs reflecting issues of importance to the patient provide a means for them to communicate effectively with their physicians about their priorities for care. This might be beneficial since patients and doctors may not always agree on which outcomes are most important.

Greenhalgh hypothesizes that effective communication between physician and patient may lead to initiation of a treatment regime that optimally corresponds with the patient's treatment goals and therefore facilitate treatment adherence.

It has been suggested that PROs designed for standard care should first and foremost be feasible in view of scarce time in busy clinics. Specifically this means that PROs designed for use in the clinic should be amenable to being scored and reviewed easily during standard clinical care and patients should be able to complete them in a few minutes [4]. Consequently many PROs that have been developed for use in the clinic, such as the Modified Health Assessment Questionnaire are short (8 items), and easy to complete and score [39]. However, these have been frequently associated with unfavorable measurement properties such as floor or ceiling effects and low reliability, which is easily explained by a limited number of items. These particular shortcomings seriously undermine the utility of such measures for monitoring individual level outcomes over time on the one hand because patients at the ceiling of a scale cannot improve further (and vice versa) and on the other hand because measurement error has a larger attenuating effect on individual scores compared with aggregated scores. Consequently measurement instruments for use at the individual levels actually need higher reliability compared with measurement instruments for use at the group level.

Quality Assurance

Recently there is also increased interest in the use of PROs in the assessment and documentation of quality of care. PROs are expected to playa prominent role in assessing performance, particularly because of this growing emphasis on patient-centered care and value-based payment approaches. The central tenets of value-based healthcare are that value can be defined as health outcome per unit of costs expended and that if all healthcare system participants have to compete on value, value will improve [40]. According to Porter and Teisberg, competition for resources should take place on the level of specific conditions and over the full cycle of care, rather than the level of specific interventions [40]. Furthermore, competition should focus on results—that is, patient outcomes achieved per unit of cost expended. This requires that results are measured and made widely available. Healthcare providers are increasingly expected to provide evidence that the care they have delivered produced value for the patient—as reported by the patient. To this end the performance of healthcare providers in terms of HRQOL benefits are frequently benchmarked, potentially allowing payers to link reimbursement to evidence of the effectiveness of their treatment. The international consortium for health outcomes measurement is one initiative that aims to "unlock the potential for value-based healthcare by defining consensus-based global standard sets of outcome measures that really matter to patients for the most relevant medical conditions and by driving adoption and reporting of these measures worldwide" to be used across healthcare providers for a given medical condition. In the value-based healthcare framework hierarchy of outcome domains, patient health status achieved is the highest tier. Consequently, PROs will play an important role in the assessment of delivered quality of care.

Population Studies

Finally, PROs are frequently used in population studies to describe the burden of illness faced in a certain condition and to provide information about the health profile and healthcare needs of the population. The objective of this type of studies is frequently to compare the burden of illness between populations. Generic instruments are typically most suitable for this. Comparisons across different diseases, population groups, or interventions require instruments that are reliable.

Single- and Multi-Item Scales

Single-Item Scales

PROs can be either single-item scales or multi-item instruments. Single-item instruments are typically used for the assessment of specific symptoms/impairments (i.e., pain or stiffness) or otherwise simple concepts that require patients to report on information that is readily retrieved from memory and requires relatively little cognitive processing [41]. For instance, most people can give sufficiently accurate reports regarding their disease duration or employment status and therefore such variables are typically assessed in a single-item format. The most commonly employed single-item instruments in rheumatology are numerical rating scales (NRS) and visual analogue scales (VAS). A VAS is comprised of a line, 100 mm in length, anchored by 2 verbal descriptorsre presenting the domain extremes. The NRS is a numeric version of the visual analogue scale in which patients are asked to select the integer (typically 0–10) that best reflects their standing on the measured trait. Measurement properties of NRS and VAS are generally similar [11]. Less frequently used single-item instruments are Likert scales. These are dissimilar to NRS in that they typically contain fewer response options (usually 5) and are characterized by an equal numbers of positive and negative positions around a neutral response option. Although it has been said that patients might prefer the clarity provided by Likert scales, they provide less statistical information than NRS/VAS and have consistently been shown to be inferior in comparative studies [42]. General advantages of single-item scales over multi-item instruments are that they are easy to implement and to interpret, are least burdensome to patients, and in many cases provide relevant information for monitoring outcomes over time. However, limitations of single-item instruments are that they provide less statistical information compared with more elaborate tools, which undermines their reliability. Moreover, it is frequently difficult to fully characterize a domain using single-item instruments.

Multi-Item Scales

Multi-item PROs are typically applied to assess constructs that require the patient to reconstruct, interpret, judge, compare, or otherwise evaluate complex or abstract information. Under such circumstances multiple items may better capture the essence of the phenomenon of interest [41]. Another important advantage of multi-item scales is that more statistical information is provided so that scores are less affected by measurement error. As a result multi-item questionnaires are usually more reliable instruments. Although all multi-item PROs have in common that their constituent items are combined to produce a total score, different measurement models can be distinguished based on how individual items relate to the overarching concept that the measure pertains to assess. That is, the items making up the scale may either be hypothesized to be indicators of the measured trait, in which case the individual items are referred to as effect indicators and the instrument is a *scale* or the items together define the measured trait, in which case the items are referred to as causal indicators and instrument an *index* [43]. For example, the Bath Ankylosing Spondylitis Disease Activity Index (BASDAI) [44] is a patient-reported *index* of disease severity that comprises 6 items pertaining to the five major symptoms of AS: fatigue, spinal pain, joint pain/swelling, enthesitis, morning stiffness duration, and morning stiffness severity. The total BASDAI score is obtained by averaging the six individual items. The overarching, multidimensional concept of disease activity is defined by, or emerges from, these individual constituting measures. If any one of the five core symptoms of AS would be omitted from the BASDAI then this would result in a less comprehensive assessment of disease activity. Disease indices typically, but not exclusively, focus on PROs on the impairment level. By contrast, the SF-36 physical functioning scale is a commonly used physical function PRO that assesses disability across ten items that assess various aspects of physical function [45]. Although a total score is similarly obtained by combining the individual items, the individual items are considered more or less interchangeable examples or realizations of the underlying construct of physical function. Hypothetically, different specific indicators of physical function could have been used, without changing the conceptual meaning of the trait that is assessed with the scale. The reason that the same items have to be administered time and again relates to the fact that total scores would not be comparable if patients would fill out different items at different times. Items in a scale typically, but not exclusively, focus on PROs at the disability or handicap level.

The measurement model that has been adopted has some implications for the development or analysis of the respective PRO. Effect indicators are considered to be more or less interchangeable realizations of the latent variable. Consequently many statistical procedures that aim to evaluate the quality of individual items with respect to measuring the desired outcome focus on the intercorrelation among items. By contrast, causal indicators do not necessarily need to be correlated and when developing an index, researchers tend to pay most attention to the ability of individual indicators to discriminate between clinical relevant states [46]. Generally speaking, items are considered to have high quality in a scale if they are substantially

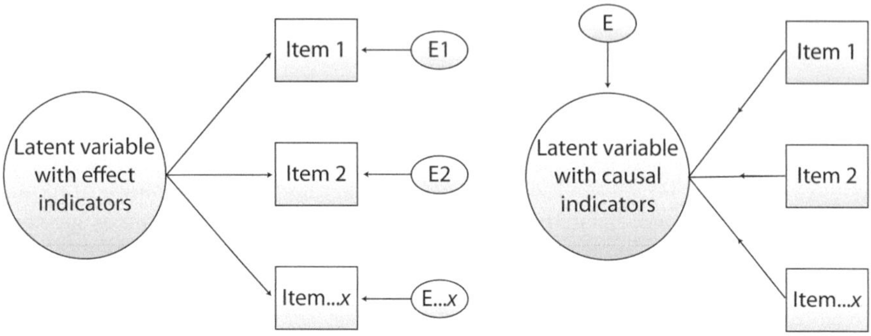

- Latent variable explains variability of item scores
- Item scores are presumed to be correlated
- Items are more or less interchangeable realizations of the construct that may be omitted from the instrument without altering the construct in a substantial way
- Measurement error occurs at the item level

- Item scores explain variability in latent variable
- No specific assumptions are made with respect to the intercorrelation of item scores
- Meaning of the construct may change depending on the items of the instrument
- Measurement error occurs at the construct level

Fig. 1.2 Graphical representation of latent variables with effect indicators and latent variables with causal indicators

intercorrelated, whereas in the case of an index, items that intercorrelate to the smallest extent possible are usually favored in the interest of parsimony. Similarities and differences between these approaches to PRO measurement models are illustrated in more detail in Fig. 1.2.

Measurement Theory and Models

PROs typically focus on subjective and nonobservable or "latent" phenomena, such as the amount of pain a patient experiences or the amount of difficulty faced by the patient in participating in their normal social roles. Measurement theories provide a general framework for linking observable variables, such as test or item scores, to latent variables, such as pain and physical disability [47].

Classical Test Theory

Classical test theory (CTT) is a theory that can be applied to PRO (total) scores revolving around the concepts: observed score, true score, and error score. Classical test theory is concerned with the relations between these concepts in order to evaluate to what extent the total score of *a*(*n*) (PRO) instrument is affected by the random measurement error. It may also provide instrument developers with a framework that they can use to help develop more reliable tests. It is a desirable quality of any measurement instrument to be as free as possible from measurement error because measurement error adds variability to the data, which makes it more difficult to measure change over time or to identify differences between groups. Most frequently, the observed score (*O*) is defined as the sum of 2 unobservable, or latent variables: the true score (*T*) and the error score (*E*); i.e.,

$$X = T + E$$

The associated variances are similarly related:

$$\sigma_x^2 = \sigma_t^2 + \sigma_e^2$$

Since *T* and *E* are unknown, it has to be further assumed that (1) *T* and *E* are uncorrelated, (2) measurement errors occur at random, and (3) error scores on parallel tests are uncorrelated. As demonstrated by Lord, however, these assumptions more or less follow from the definition of *T* and *E* [48]. Because of the assumption that the expected value of *E* equals 0, the presence of measurement error will not systematically distort the expected value of *O* away from the expected value of *T*. Consequently, *O* is an unbiased estimate of *T*. More problematic is the relationship between the variances of *X*, *T*, and *E* of which only σ_x^2 is known. Many CTT models are concerned with obtaining information regarding σ_t^2. Various ways to obtain reliability coefficients have been proposed over time that expresses the ratio of true score variance to the total variance of test scores:

$$R = \frac{\sigma_t^2}{\sigma_x^2} = \frac{\sigma_t^2}{\sigma_t^2 + \sigma_e^2}$$

The most principled way to obtain the reliability coefficient would be to calculate the correlation coefficient between two parallel forms of an instrument, which would involve the availability of parallel versions of a PRO instrument that is a PRO on which patients have the same true score and with equal errors of measurement across instruments. Of course, the construction of parallel forms is a requirement that can never be exactly met. A lot of work has therefore been directed at developing methods that can be used not only to evaluate reliability without parallel forms, such as generalizability theory but also to the practice of test–retest reliability [49].

The CTT framework is very useful from a theoretical and practical point of view because it provides an explanation for various statistical phenomena related to measurement errors, such as regression toward the mean. CTT-based reliability coefficients can also be applied, for example, to identify, from a set of PRO instruments for a given outcome domain, the instrument that would be least affected by distortion due to measurement error. Finally, in the development of PRO instruments the theory provides means for scale developers to ensure the reliability of their instrument. An advantage of CTT over more complicated approaches is that CTT is based on relatively weak assumptions that are likely to be met under practical situations and that these approaches are generally well-known in the field of rheumatology. Consequently, the majority of papers on measurement properties of PROs in rheumatology utilize CTT approaches to reliability.

Key shortcomings of CTT as a test theory for PROs are that CTT scores are instrument-dependent and apply only to the total score of a specific measure. For instance, if we would be interested in measuring physical disability in a certain population of patients, we may choose from a number of available PROs for this purpose. However, each individual PRO is associated with its own true score, since individual PROs tend to have idiosyncratic items, response options, and scoring procedures. Consequently, scores can only be compared between studies or over time if the exact same instrument is administered. This has led to the situation that only limited different PROs are typically used for a given purpose in a field and that it is difficult to deal with the phenomenon of floor and ceiling effects. Similarly, many item and person parameters derived from CTT are also instrument-dependent. For instance, it is easy to see that the reliability coefficient defined previously would change as a function of the true score variance if measurement error remains constant.

Item Response Theory

Item response theory (IRT) is a statistical framework that allows a more flexible approach to assigning PRO scores. IRT was developed to overcome measurement problems with CTT and is increasingly utilized in the development of new instruments or to facilitate the comparability between existing ones. In IRT, the focus moves from the scale level to the level of individual items. Individual items are described by item characteristic functions, which give the probability that a patient will give a certain response to a PRO item as a monotonically increasing function of a patient's overall level of the measured trait. Most typically, the logistic function is used as an elemental unit to trace the conditional probability that a patient will respond in category x, rather than $x-1$, given that the response was in x or $x-1$. The main advantage of IRT over the classical approach is that its item level models provide item and person parameters that are invariant with respect to the population that was used to obtain them. This means that the parameters that characterize the item do not depend on the ability distribution of the sample that was used to estimate them and conversely that the parameter(s) that characterize(s) a patient do(es) not depend on the specific set of items that were used to estimate them. Therefore, once the item parameters of a set of items have been estimated, an estimate of the location of a responding patient on the underlying distribution of the measured trait may be obtained from any subset of the calibrated items, and researchers are no longer bound to static questionnaires in order to obtain information regarding a PRO domain. It should be noted though that the latent scale in IRT models itself is arbitrary, so that item parameters of unequated item banks are invariant only up to a set of linear transformations [50]. Calibrated item banks can be used to create more efficient measures by administering only the most relevant questions for specific research needs, either by manually selecting items that are believed to closely match the levels of the measured trait of interest in the target population or by computerized adaptive testing (CAT) algorithms. CAT algorithms sequentially statistically optimize estimated trait levels by presenting only items that match the trait level of the respondent, as estimated from previously responded to items or other prior information [51]. By tailoring the assessment to the level of the measured trait of individual patients, trait levels can be estimated with an optimal, prespecified level of precision, while using a lower number of items compared with traditional instruments. This is achieved by capitalizing on the fact that reliability is locally defined in IRT. That is, item response models can be used to construct the so-called information functions, which describe the measurement precision of individual items at each of the different levels of the measured trait. Information functions also provide researchers with more detailed information regarding the influence of measurement error on the information that is provided by the PRO instrument and its items, compared with the CTT-based reliability indices. Consequently IRT-based analysis is also ideally suited for scale construction and refinement. This information can be utilized to develop measures that are optimally relevant to the disability levels of the studied population, while response burden can be managed. Another application of IRT-based item banking is the establishment of a common IRT-based metric between existing outcome measures that are used for the same purpose in a setting. Once established, such metrics facilitate the comparability and interpretability of outcomes by the development of IRT-based scoring procedures that allow study results to be expressed on 1 standardized metric, irrespective of the questionnaire that was used in a specific study. This would allow results obtained in different settings to be compared despite that different individual measures were used in individual studies.

Future Directions

Over the last few decades, a variety of PROs have become available for use in various settings in rheumatology. While traditionally PROs have been used primarily to assess beneficial effects of treatment in clinical trials in this field, the increasing attention for the patient as the center of healthcare has led to the proliferation of PROs in other settings, such a clinical practice, comparative effectiveness research and in the assessment of quality of care. Different settings require a different focus and different measurement attributes of a PRO instrument. For instance, feasibility issues are often considered key in clinical practice, whereas reliability is more important in clinical trials. To accommodate the needs of specific settings, a host of new PRO measures have been developed over the last decade. Unfortunately, individual instruments are frequently only used within a single disease population and/or specific setting. For example, the HAQ-DI (Health Assessment Questionnaire Disability Index) and WOMAC (Western Ontario and McMaster Universities Arthritis Index) are both measures of disability primarily used in respectively rheumatoid arthritis and osteoarthritis. Since most of the current generation of measures were developed according to the principles of classical test theory with a fixed number of items and a scoring rule based on combining individual items, results can only be compared across studies that used the same PRO. One of the challenges facing the field of PRO outcome research in rheumatology is therefore to facilitate the comparability of outcomes across settings and diseases. As was demonstrated in this chapter, PROs can assess health-related concepts reflecting different levels of consequences of rheumatic diseases. At the most fundamental level are impairments or symptoms of disease. In some cases this may require disease-specific instruments. However, disability and particularly participation restrictions are universally relevant outcomes across all rheumatic diseases, and indeed across all diseases. Because of their indirect association with the disease process, these outcomes typically do not require disease- or population-specific measures. Particularly for these higher level outcome domains, IRT-based concurrent calibration of existing measures may facilitate the development of a common currency of domain outcomes across rheumatic diseases. For instance, a common metric of physical function may be built in which all physical function instruments that are used across rheumatic diseases are calibrated in one IRT-based item bank. Once this has been achieved, fully comparable physical function estimates may be obtained from any subset of calibrated items. This system can then be used to compare results across (completed) studies and across diseases, irrespective of which instrument has been used. Furthermore, it would allow researchers to select the most relevant questionnaire or even to construct study-specific forms based on what is known about the disability levels of the target population. Another useful feature of IRT-based item banking is that various linking procedures exist that can be used to add new items to the item bank, without altering the item characteristics of preexisting items. This can be utilized to improve the information richness of the item bank in poorly represented areas of the measured trait. Finally, due to the fact that PROs are increasingly collected in electronic format, we foresee an increasing role for computerized adaptive testing as a means to resolve the trade-off between feasibility and reliability that is associated with the use of traditional fixed-length questionnaires.

References

1. US Department of Health and Human Services, Food and Drug Administration, Center for Drug Evaluation and Research (CDER), Center for Biologics Evaluation and Research (CBER), Center for Devices and Radiological Health (CDRH). Guidance for industry: patient-reported outcome measures: use in medical product development to support labeling claims: draft guidance. Rockville, MD: Food and Drug Administration. 2006. http://www.fda.gov/ohrms/dockets/98fr/06d-0044-gdl0001.pdf.
2. van Tuyl LHD, Boers M. Patient-reported outcomes in core domain sets for rheumatic diseases. Nat Rev Rheumatol. 2015;11:705–12.
3. Garratt A, Schmidt L, Mackintosh A, Fitzpatrick R. Quality of life measurement: bibliographic study of patient assessed health outcome measures. BMJ. 2002;324:1417.

4. Wolfe F, Pincus T. Listening to the patient: a practical guide to self-report questionnaires in clinical care. Arthritis Rheum. 1999;42:1797–808.
5. Wilson IB, Cleary PD. Linking clinical variables with health-related quality of life. A conceptual model of patient outcomes. JAMA. 1995;273:59–65.
6. World Health Organization (WHO). International classification of impairments, disabilities, and handicaps: a manual of classification relating to the consequences of disease, published in accordance. 1980. http://apps.who.int/iris/handle/10665/41003.
7. World Health Organization (WHO). World health organization constitution. *Basic Doc* 1948. http://www.who.int/governance/eb/who_constitution_en.pdf.
8. Boonen A, Stucki G, Maksymowych W, Rat AC, Escorpizo R, Boers M. The OMERACT-ICF reference group: integrating the ICF into the OMERACT process: opportunities and challenges. J Rheumatol. 2009;36:2057–60.
9. Stucki G, Cieza A. The international classification of functioning, disability and health (ICF) core sets for rheumatoid arthritis: a way to specify functioning. Ann Rheum Dis. 2004;63 Suppl 2:ii40–5.
10. ten Klooster PM, Veehof MM, Taal E, van Riel PLCM, van de Laar MAFJ. Changes in priorities for improvement in patients with rheumatoid arthritis during 1 year of anti-tumour necrosis factor treatment. Ann Rheum Dis. 2007;66:1485–90.
11. Bartlett SJ, Bykerk VP, Cooksey R, Choy EH, Alten R, Christensen R, et al. Feasibility and domain validation of rheumatoid arthritis (RA) flare core domain set: report of the OMERACT 2014 RA flare group plenary. J Rheumatol. 2015;42(11):2185–9.
12. Gignac MAM, Backman CL, Davis AM, Lacaille D, Mattison CA, Montie P, et al. Understanding social role participation: what matters to people with arthritis? J Rheumatol. 2008;35:1655–63.
13. Aaronson NK, Muller M, Cohen PD, Essink-Bot ML, Fekkes M, Sanderman R, et al. Translation, validation, and norming of the Dutch language version of the SF-36 health survey in community and chronic disease populations. J Clin Epidemiol. 1998;51:1055–68.
14. Vermeer M, Kuper HH, Hoekstra M, Haagsma CJ, Posthumus MD, Brus HLM, et al. Implementation of a treat-to-target strategy in very early rheumatoid arthritis: results of the Dutch Rheumatoid Arthritis Monitoring remission induction cohort study. Arthritis Rheum. 2011;63:2865–72.
15. Guyatt GH, Feeny DH, Patrick DL. Measuring health-related quality of life. Ann Intern Med. 1993;118:622–9.
16. Patrick DL, Deyo RA. Generic and disease-specific measures in assessing health status and quality of life. Med Care. 1989;27:S217–32.
17. Linde L, Sørensen J, Ostergaard M, Hørslev-Petersen K, Hetland ML. Health-related quality of life: validity, reliability, and responsiveness of SF-36, 15D, EQ-5D [corrected] RAQoL, and HAQ in patients with rheumatoid arthritis. J Rheumatol. 2008;35:1528–37.
18. Hagen KB, Smedstad LM, Uhlig T, Kvien TK. The responsiveness of health status measures in patients with rheumatoid arthritis: comparison of disease-specific and generic instruments. J Rheumatol. 1999;26:1474–80.
19. Russell AS, Conner-Spady B, Mintz A, Maksymowych WP. The responsiveness of generic health status measures as assessed in patients with rheumatoid arthritis receiving infliximab. J Rheumatol. 2003;30:941–7.
20. Buchbinder R, Bombardier C, Yeung M, Tugwell P. Which outcome measures should be used in rheumatoid arthritis clinical trials? Clinical and quality-of-life measures' responsiveness to treatment in a randomized controlled trial. Arthritis Rheum. 1995;38:1568–80.
21. Verhoeven AC, Boers M, van Der Linden S. Responsiveness of the core set, response criteria, and utilities in early rheumatoid arthritis. Ann Rheum Dis. 2000;59:966–74.
22. Colwell HH, Hunt BJ, Pasta DJ, Palo WA, Mathias SD, Joseph-Ridge N. Gout assessment questionnaire: Initial results of reliability, validity and responsiveness. Int J Clin Pract. 2006;60:1210–7.
23. Meenan RF, Gertman PM, Mason JH. Measuring health status in arthritis. The arthritis impact measurement scales. Arthritis Rheum. 1980;23:146–52.

24. Fries JF, Spitz P, Kraines RG, Holman HR. Measurement of patient outcome in arthritis. Arthritis Rheum. 1980;23:137–45.
25. Calvert M, Blazeby J, Altman DG, Revicki DA, Moher D, Brundage MD. Reporting of patient-reported outcomes in randomized trials: the CONSORT PRO extension. JAMA. 2013; 309:814–22.
26. Kalyoncu U, Dougados M, Daures J-P, Gossec L. Reporting of patient-reported outcomes in recent trials in rheumatoid arthritis: a systematic literature review. Ann Rheum Dis. 2009;68:183–90.
27. Schumacher HR, Taylor W, Edwards L, Grainger R, Schlesinger N, Dalbeth N, et al. Outcome domains for studies of acute and chronic gout. J Rheumatol. 2009;36:2342–5.
28. Boers M, Brooks P, Strand CV, Tugwell P. The OMERACT filter for outcome measures in rheumatology. J Rheumatol. 1998;25:198–9.
29. Goossens ME, Rutten-van Mölken MP, Vlaeyen JW, van der Linden SM. The cost diary: a method to measure direct and indirect costs in cost-effectiveness research. J Clin Epidemiol. 2000;53:688–95.
30. Braakman-Jansen LMA, Taal E, Kuper IH, van de Laar MAFJ. Productivity loss due to absenteeism and presenteeism by different instruments in patients with RA and subjects without RA. Rheumatology (Oxford). 2012;51:354–61.
31. Basch E, Reeve BB, Mitchell SA, Clauser SB, Minasian LM, Dueck AC, et al. Development of the National Cancer Institute's patient-reported outcomes version of the common terminology criteria for adverse events (PRO-CTCAE). J Natl Cancer Inst. 2014;29:106(9).
32. Pincus T, Yazici Y, Sokka T. Quantitative measures of rheumatic diseases for clinical research versus standard clinical care: differences, advantages and limitations. Best Pract Res Clin Rheumatol. 2007;21:601–28.
33. Greenhalgh J. The applications of PROs in clinical practice: what are they, do they work, and why? Qual Life Res. 2009;18:115–23.
34. Hilarius D. Patient-reported outcomes in daily clinical oncology practice: a tool for patient monitoring and quality of care assessment. FMG: Psychology Research Institute. 2011. http://dare.uva.nl/document/2/91414.
35. Greenhalgh J, Meadows K. The effectiveness of the use of patient-based measures of health in routine practice in improving the process and outcomes of patient care: a literature review. J Eval Clin Pract. 1999;5:401–16.
36. Kroenke K, Spitzer RL, Williams JBW. The patient health questionnaire-2: validity of a two-item depression screener. Med Care. 2003;41:1284–92.
37. Ahmed S, Berzon RA, Revicki DA, Lenderking WR, Moinpour CM, Basch E, et al. The use of patient-reported outcomes (PRO) within comparative effectiveness research: implications for clinical practice and health care policy. Med Care. 2012;50:1060–70.
38. Valderas JM, Kotzeva A, Espallargues M, Guyatt G, Ferrans CE, Halyard MY, et al. The impact of measuring patient-reported outcomes in clinical practice: a systematic review of the literature. Qual Life Res. 2008;17:179–93.
39. Pincus T, Summey JA, Soraci SA, Wallston KA, Hummon NP. Assessment of patient satisfaction in activities of daily living using a modified Stanford health assessment questionnaire. Arthritis Rheum. 1983;26:1346–53.
40. Porter M, Teisberg EO. Redefining health care: creating value-based competition on results. Boston: Harvard Business Review Press; 2006.
41. DeVellis R. Scale development: theory and applications. Newbury Park: Sage; 2012.
42. Hjermstad MJ, Fayers PM, Haugen DF, Caraceni A, Hanks GW, Loge JH, et al. Studies comparing numerical rating scales, verbal rating scales, and visual analogue scales for assessment of pain intensity in adults: a systematic literature review. J Pain Symptom Manage. 2011;41: 1073–93.
43. Bollen K, Lennox R. Conventional wisdom on measurement: a structural equation perspective. Psychol Bull. 1991;110(2):305–14.
44. Garrett S, Jenkinson T, Kennedy LG, Whitelock H, Gaisford P, Calin A. A new approach to defining disease status in ankylosing spondylitis: the bath ankylosing spondylitis disease activity index. J Rheumatol. 1994;21:2286–91.

45. Ware JE, Sherbourne CD. The MOS 36-item short-form health survey (SF-36). I. Conceptual framework and item selection. Med Care. 1992;30:473–83.
46. Feinstein AR. An additional basic science for clinical medicine: IV. The development of clinimetrics. Ann Intern Med. 1983;99:843–8.
47. Hambleton R, Van der Linden W. Advances in item response theory and applications: an introduction. Appl Psychol Meas. 1982;6(4):373–8.
48. Lord FM. Applications of item response theory to practical testing problems. Hillsdale: Erlbaum; 1980.
49. Brennan RL. Generalizability theory. Educ Meas Issues Pract. 1992;11(4):27–34.
50. Rupp A, Zumbo B. Understanding parameter invariance in unidimensional IRT models. Educ Psychol. 2006;66(1):63–84.
51. van der Linden W, Glas CAW. Computerized adaptive testing: theory and practice. Boston: Springer; 2000.

Chapter 2
A Guide to PROMs Methodology and Selection Criteria

Maha El Gaafary

Introduction

In general, medical management outcomes can be classified into clinical (e.g., cure, survival), personal (e.g., emotional status, self-helplessness, ability to carry out activities of daily living), and economical (e.g., expenses, cost effectiveness). In a clinical scenario, the outcomes can be clinician reported (e.g., progression of the case in response to therapy), physiologic (e.g., tumor size assessed by ultrasound [US] or magnetic resonance imaging [MRI]), caregiver reported (e.g., functional disability), or patient reported (e.g., symptoms or quality of life) [1, 2]. If the patient is monitored for the outcomes by clinician, caregiver, or researcher, then the outcomes become observer reported outcomes (OROs). On the other hand, if the patient is revealing how he/she feels about their medical problem and its impact on their lives, it becomes patient reported outcome (PRO). Proxy reported outcome is different from a PRO or ORO, as it is a measurement based on the report given by someone else on behalf of the patient or as if he or she is the patient.

As the patient is considered "the center" for any healthcare system, "patient-centered care" got to center stage in discussions of the modern healthcare system [3]. Patient-centered care is considered the best approach able to reflect the quality of personal, professional, and organizational relationships. According to the US Food and Drug Administration (FDA), a patient reported outcome is any report of the status of a patient's health condition that comes directly from the patient, without interpretation of the patient's response by a clinician or anyone else [4, 5]. No wonder PRO has been used as effectiveness end points in clinical trials as well as in standard clinical practice.

M. El Gaafary (✉)
Community and Public Health Department, Ain Shams University, Cairo, Egypt
e-mail: maha_gafary@yahoo.com

Y. El Miedany (ed.), *Patient Reported Outcome Measures in Rheumatic Diseases*,
DOI 10.1007/978-3-319-32851-5_2

Importance of Patient Reported Outcome Measures

Though medical technology has enabled the treating healthcare professionals to measure the patients' physical, physiological, or biochemical parameters, it is not able to calibrate the treatment outcomes or the disease progression/regression from the patients' perspectives. Further, some data can only be obtained from the patient. This includes [2]:

- Various symptoms
- Symptoms not obvious to observers; e.g., fatigue, headache
- Psychological symptoms; e.g., depression, anxiety
- Symptoms in absence of observer; e.g., sleep disturbances
- Frequency of symptoms; e.g., Does the headache occur daily or weekly or monthly?
- Severity of symptoms; e.g., Headache is severe or moderate or mild?
- Nature and severity of disability of the patient; e.g., How severe is the breathlessness?
- The impact of disease or condition on daily life of the patient; e.g., Does rheumatoid arthritis interfere with the activities of daily living of the patient? If yes, how much is the impact?
- Perception or feeling of the patient toward the disease or the treatment given; e.g., Is the patient satisfied with the treatment given?

Such important symptoms can only be reported by the patient. Patient reported outcome measures (PROMs) represent a formal tool able to make the clinician "treat the patient not just the source of bleeding."

However, the PROMs role goes beyond simple assessment of the patients' symptomatology. Various types of outcomes measured by PROMs include social well-being, cognitive functioning, role activities, personal constructs, satisfaction with care [6], health related quality of life (HRQOL) [7], adherence to medical regimens [8], and clinical trial outcomes [6]. Furthermore, PROMs can be helpful in the determination of the patient's eligibility for certain clinical trials; e.g., inclusion criterion for the trial is female patients with hot flushes. It can be used also for confirmation of the measures; e.g., patients with morning stiffness are most likely to be suffering from rheumatoid disease. In other cases, PROMs can help to interpret the patient's symptoms or eliminate other possibilities; e.g., if the patient has breathlessness and the patient is a smoker then chronic obstructive pulmonary disease (COPD) can be expected rather than anemia. In addition, PROMs are useful for the assessment of patients' compliance or reasons for nonadherence to therapy; for example, are the side effects so severe? Also, PROMs have been used as study end points; e.g., efficacy of analgesic drug by determining pain levels [2]. On the other hand, PROMs play an important role to monitor the case progression and determine its impact on the patient's quality of life. In diseases such as cancer, as a result of the cancer progression patients experience multiple symptoms, economical burden, home management problems, and lack of emotional well-being, all of which can adversely affect quality of life [9]. The role of QOL/PROMs in cancer care can be considered in the following conditions such as [10]:

- Comparison of two standard therapies having similar survival outcomes
- Identification of negative effects of the therapy when survival time is long
- To find out whether a new therapy is preferable to standard therapy
- To determine whether a therapeutic regimen is better than supportive care only, when survival time is short
  - Identification of the needs for the supportive care
  - Determination of negative effects of the adjuvant therapy
- Targeting problems and making communication easier in clinical practice

PROM Instrument Types

Before selecting a PROMs instrument, clinicians should consider the different tools available and how they meet the requirements of the proposed objectives [6]. Review of the literature revealed seven major types of instruments available. They differ in content as well as their intended purpose or application. In view of the growing interest in the PROMs subject, this classification should not be interpreted too rigidly and is not mutually exclusive:

- *Disease-specific*: e.g., PROMs-Arthritis/Spondyloarthritis/Fibromyalgia, Asthma Quality of Life Questionnaire
- *Population-specific*: e.g., Child health assessment questionnaire, Child Health and Illness Profile-Child Edition/CHIP-CE
- *Dimension-specific*: e.g., Beck Depression Inventory
- *Generic*: e.g., Short-Form Health Survey (SF-36)
- *Individualized*: e.g., Patient Generated Index
- *Summary items*: e.g., UK General Household Survey questions about long-standing illness
- *Utility measures*: e.g., EuroQol, EQ-5D

Disease-Specific/Condition-Specific

These instruments have been developed to measure the patient's perceptions of a specific disease or health problem. The Patient Reported Outcome Measures for Rheumatoid Arthritis consists of eight items that produce four dimension scores relating to activity limitations, quality of life, disease activity measures (pain score, patient global assessment, fatigue, duration of morning stiffness), self-reported joint tenderness, and comorbidity as well as self-helplessness assessment [11].

Being disease-specific, this makes these instruments clinically relevant. On the other side, it is not generally possible to administer disease-specific instruments to individuals without the relevant health problem. This means that health status scores cannot be compared with those for the general population, which is a common approach for assessing the impact of a particular disease on health status. Similarly, it is not possible to make comparisons across treatments for different diseases, which limits the application of disease-specific instruments in economic evaluation where different lines of management for the same condition could be compared.

Population-Specific

In the literature, the term "population-specific" may be used to describe both disease-specific/condition-specific instruments and those specific to particular demographic groups or populations, such as children or elderly people or even culturally specific groups (e.g., Asian, White British).

The Childhood Health Assessment Questionnaire (CHAQ) consists of eight subscales: dressing and grooming, arising, eating, walking, hygiene, reach, grip, and activities in addition to visual analog scale (VAS) for pain and global assessment. There are 30 items in the Disability Index, one item each in the Discomfort Index and Health Status Index. Separate questions are included to assess for aids or devices that the child usually uses for any of the aforementioned activities [12]. The population target is children with juvenile arthritis, 1–19 years of age. CHAQ has been validated for use in children with juvenile idiopathic inflammatory and myopathies. The World Health Organization (WHO) International Classification of Functioning, Disability and Health (ICF) components include impairment (pain), activity limitation (ADLs), and participation restriction-overall health status.

The domains and items of population-specific instruments are mostly more relevant to the group in question; e.g., in the case of young children, a school performance domain is included. A specifically tailored format, such as the use of cartoon and clipart illustrations, is used to convey instructions rather than text. This can make these measures more acceptable and comprehensible—enabling individuals who are often not consulted directly to report on their own health and preferences. However, using population-specific measures carries the same disadvantages as disease-specific measures, ruling out comparisons with the general population, and being difficult to be used to compare the efficacy of particular treatments across population groups.

Dimension-Specific

Dimension-specific instruments assess one particular aspect of health status. Those aspects are summarized as [6]:

- *I—Physical function*: mobility, dexterity, range of movement, physical activity; activities of daily living: ability to eat, wash, dress
- *II—Symptoms*: pain; nausea; appetite; energy, vitality, fatigue; sleep and rest
- *III—Global judgments of health*
- *IV—Psychological well-being*: psychological illness, anxiety, depression; coping, positive well-being and adjustment, sense of control, self-esteem
- *V—Social well-being*: family and intimate relations; social contact, integration, and social opportunities; leisure activities; sexual activity and satisfaction
- *VI—Cognitive functioning*: cognition, alertness, concentration, memory, confusion, ability to communicate.
- *VII—Role activities*: employment, household management, financial concerns
- *VIII—Personal constructs*: satisfaction with bodily appearance, stigma and stigmatizing conditions, life satisfaction, spirituality
- *IX—Satisfaction with care*: The most common types are those that measure psychological well-being.

The Beck Depression Inventory contains 21 items that address symptoms of depression [13]. The instrument was originally developed for use with psychiatric patients but it is increasingly used to assess depression in the physically ill. They provide an assessment of a particular dimension of health that is often more detailed than that provided by disease-specific or generic instruments. There is a wide range of data available for comparing and interpreting results. However, measures of psychological well-being in particular were often developed with a primary objective of discrimination in diagnosis and needs assessment. Therefore, the outcome measures appropriateness of such instruments should be tested carefully before use.

Generic

Generic instruments are designed to measure very broad aspects of health and are therefore potentially suitable for a wide range of patient groups and the general population. The Short-Form Health Survey (SF-36) is one of the most widely used generic instruments [14–16]. It is a 36-item instrument that measures health across eight dimensions of physical functioning, social functioning, role limitations due to physical problems, and role limitations due to emotional problems, mental health, vitality, pain, and general health perceptions. The dimension scores form physical and mental component summary scores [16, 17].

The main advantage of generic instruments is that they are suitable for use across a broad range of health problems. They can be used for comparisons between treatments for different patient groups to assess comparative effectiveness. They can also be used with healthy populations to generate normative data that can be used to compare different patient groups. Their broad scope means that they have potential to capture the influence of comorbidity on health, as well as unexpected positive or negative effects of an intervention. This makes them useful for assessing the impact of new healthcare technologies when the therapeutic effects are uncertain. However, some level of detail has to be sacrificed, which may limit the relevance of generic instruments when applied to a specific patient population. Generic instruments are also potentially less responsive to clinically important changes in health.

Individualized

Individualized instruments allow respondents to select the content of items and/or rate the importance of individual items. The Patient Generated Index asks respondents to list the five most important areas of their lives affected by a disease or health problem and then to rate how badly affected they are in each area, and in the rest of their lives [18, 19]. They then give a number of "points" to the areas in which they would most value an improvement. The individual area ratings are weighted by the "points" given and summed to produce a single index designed to measure the extent to which a patient's actual situation falls short of their hopes and expectations in those areas of life in which they most value an improvement.

Individualized instruments address the concerns of the individual patient rather than impose an external standard that may be less relevant. Therefore individualized instruments can have high content validity. However, individualized instruments have to be administered by interview in order to produce response rates similar to those for standardized instruments. This has implications on the feasibility of individualized instruments when compared to standardized instruments that can be self-administered.

Summary Items

Summary items ask respondents to summarize diverse aspects of their health status using a single item or a very small number of items. Since 1974 the General Household Survey for England and Wales has used two questions relating to chronic illness and disability: "Do you have any long-standing illness or disability?" and "Does this illness or disability limit your activities in any way?" Transition items are a form of summary item that ask the respondent to assess their current health compared with a specific point in the past, such as their last clinic visit. The SF-36 contains a transition item that asks: "Compared to one year ago, how would you rate your health in general now: excellent, very good, good, fair, and poor?"

Summary items are brief and make the least demands on respondents' time. Despite their obvious simplicity, there is some short evidence for the measurement properties of summary items including reliability and validity. Summary items that relate to global health also offer a potential means of exploring apparently contradictory trends in different dimensions of health, for example, an improvement in physical function that coincides with a deterioration in psychological well-being. However, the brevity of summary items limits the specific inferences that can be made about particular aspects of health. Responses to transition items may suffer from recall bias and may be unduly influenced by current health status.

Utility Measures

Utility measures incorporate preferences or values attached to individual health states and express health states as a single index. This type of instrument produces evidence for the overall value of health states to society and can be used in cost-utility analysis. The EuroQol EQ-5D consists of five items relating to mobility, self-care, main activity, pain/discomfort, and anxiety/depression [20, 21]. On the basis of their responses to the five items, patients are classified into a health state with a preference weight attached. Preferences for health states are derived from general population surveys using techniques such as the rating scale, standard gamble, and time trade-off. These techniques are sometimes used to obtain direct health state values from patients.

Being a single index, this facilitates comparisons between treatments for different health problems and is useful for economic evaluation including cost-utility analysis. Utility measures are usually broad in their focus and are therefore subject to the same criticisms as generic instruments. Some respondents have difficulty understanding the nature of the experimental tasks they are required to perform.

Selecting a PROMs Instrument

Several types of instrument are available in the literature. In selecting an instrument, users must consider the different types of tools that are available and how they meet the requirements of the proposed aim. There are several ways to stratify the PROMs instruments:

- *Type*—The simplest and most useful distinctive approach is to classify them into generic, which can be widely applicable, and those specific to particular health problems or populations. These instruments can be used in a number of applications including clinical trials, economic evaluation, and routine patient care.
- *Mode*—Different modes of instrument administration are presented, the main forms being self-administered and interviewer-administered.
- *Properties*—Instrument selection should be based on a number of criteria including certain psychometric properties such as reliability and validity, as well as more general issues such as the appropriateness of an instrument for a specific application.

- *Evidence*—Instrument selection should consider expert recommendations that are based on comprehensive reviews and professional consensus. The PROMs Bibliography can be searched for reviews and recommendations that relate to specific health problems. However, they are not available for all health problems and often need updating.

Selection Criteria

Following the identification of literature pertaining to instruments it is important that users revise the necessary criteria required to select the most suitable instrument(s). There are eight criteria that should be considered in the selection of patient reported outcome measures. These criteria are not uniformly described in the literature; they are also not prioritized in terms of importance, rather they should be considered in relation to the proposed application and objective.

Appropriateness

Appropriateness is the extent to which instrument content is appropriate to the particular application. "Is the instrument content appropriate to the questions that the application seeks to address?" Is it appropriate or not—this ultimately depends on the users' specific questions and the content of instruments. Instrument selection is often dominated by **psychometric considerations** of reliability and validity, with insufficient attention given to the content of instruments. The names of instruments and constituent scales or dimensions should not be taken at face value [22]. Users should consider the content of individual items within instruments.

PROMs have three broad measurement objectives: discrimination, evaluation, and prediction [23]:

- *Discrimination* is concerned with the measurement of differences between patients when there is no external criterion available to validate the instrument. For example, measures of psychological well-being have been developed to identify individuals suffering from anxiety and depression.
- *Evaluation* is concerned with the measurement of changes over time. For example, PROMs administered before and after treatment are used as outcome measures in clinical trials.
- *Prediction* is concerned with classifying patients when a criterion is available to determine whether the classification is correct. For example, PROMs may be used in diagnosis and screening as a means of identifying individuals for suitable forms of treatment.

The three measurement objectives are not necessarily mutually exclusive. Discrimination and evaluation may be complementary if both are concerned with the measurement of differences that are clinically important, be they cross-sectional or longitudinal. However, an item that asks about family history of a particular disease or previous environmental exposure may be useful for determining which patients have the disease (prediction) but will be inappropriate for evaluation.

It is also important to consider how broad a measure of health is required. Specific instruments can have a very restricted focus on symptoms and signs of disease, but may also take account of the impact of disease on quality of life. Generic instruments measure provides broader aspects of health and quality of life that are of general importance. Where feasible, it is recommended that both specific and generic instruments be used to measure health outcomes [24, 25].

Acceptability

Acceptability is the extent to which an instrument is accepted by the patients. Indicators of acceptability include "administration time, response rates, and extent of missing data" [6]. There are a number of factors that can influence acceptability, including the mode of administration, questionnaire design (user friendly), and the health status of respondents. Layout, appearance, and legibility have their effect on whether a responder will either complete or refuse filling out the questionnaire. The format of patient-reported instruments can also influence acceptability. For example, the task faced by respondents completing individualized instruments is usually more difficult than that for instruments based on summated rating scales [19].

The instrument must be presented in a language that is familiar to respondents. Guidelines are available that are designed to ensure a high standard of translation [26, 27]. These guidelines recommend the comparison of several independent translations, back translation, and the testing of acceptability of new translations. Issues of acceptability should be considered at the design stage of instrument and questionnaire development. Patients' views about a new instrument should be obtained at the pretesting phase, prior to formal tests of instrument measurement properties including reliability [28]. Patients can be asked by means of additional questions or semi-structured interview whether they found any questions difficult or distressing.

Feasibility

Feasibility concerns the ease of administration and processing of an instrument. These are important considerations for staff and researchers who collect and process the information produced by patient-reported instruments [9, 29].

Is the instrument easy to administer and process? Instruments that are difficult to administer and process may impede the conduct of research and disrupt clinical care. The complexity and length of an instrument will have implications on the mode of administration. The mode of administration of the instrument may either complicate or facilitate data collection from the patient. Additional resources are required for interviewer administration over self-administration. Staff training needs must be considered before undertaking interviewer administration. Staff may also have to be available within the clinic to help patients who have difficulty with self-administration. Finally, staff attitudes and acceptance of patient-reported instruments can make a substantial difference to respondent acceptability.

Interpretability

Interpretability concerns the meaningfulness of scores produced by an instrument. To some extent, the lack of familiarity in the use of instruments may be an obstacle to interpretation. Three approaches to interpretation have been proposed:

1. First, changes in instrument scores have been compared to previously documented change scores produced by the same instrument at, for example, major life events such as loss of a job or with modification in the line of management or lifestyle [10].
2. Secondly, attempts have been made to identify the minimal clinically important difference (MCID), which is equal to the smallest change in instrument scores that is perceived as beneficial by patients [30, 31]. External judgments, including summary items such as health transition questions, are used to determine the MCID.
3. Thirdly, normative data from the general population can be used to interpret scores from generic instruments [32, 33].

The standardization of instrument scores is an extension of this form of interpretation that allows score changes to be expressed in terms of the score distribution for the general population and the deviation in this score with particular types of patients or in particular situations [33].

Precision

How close to the actual patient experience is the instrument measure or score? It relates to methods of scaling and scoring items, and the distribution of items over the range of the construct being measured.

The scaling of items within instruments has important implications for precision. The binary/dichotomous or "yes" or "no" is the simplest form of response category, but it does not allow respondents to report different degrees of difficulty or severity.

The majority of instruments use adjectival or Likert type scales such as strongly agree, agree, uncertain, disagree, and strongly disagree. Visual analog scales appear to offer greater precision but there is insufficient evidence to support this and they may be less acceptable to respondents.

There are a number of instruments that incorporate weighting systems, the most widely used being preferences or values derived from the general public for utility measures such as the EuroQol EQ-5D [20] and the Health Utilities Index [34].

Weighting schemes have also been applied to instruments based on summated rating scales, including the Nottingham Health Profile [35] and the Sickness Impact Profile [36]. Such weighting schemes may seem deceptively precise and should be examined for evidence of reliability and validity.

The items and scores of different instruments may vary in how well they capture the full range of the underlying construct being measured. End effects occur when a large proportion of respondents score at the floor or ceiling of the score distribution. If a large proportion of items have end effects then instrument scores will be similarly affected. End effects are evidence that an instrument may be measuring a restricted range of a construct and may limit both discriminatory power and responsiveness [37, 38].

The application of Item Response Theory (IRT) can further help determine the precision of an instrument. IRT assumes that a measurement construct, such as physical disability, can be represented by a hierarchy that ranges from the minimum to maximum level of disability [39]. IRT has shown that a number of instruments have items concentrated around the middle of the hierarchy with relatively fewer items positioned at the ends [39–41].

The scores produced by such instruments are not only a function of the health status of patients but also the precision of measurement.

Reliability

Reliability refers to whether an instrument is internally consistent or reproducible, and it assesses the extent to which an instrument is free from measurement error. As the measurement error of an instrument increases, this would necessitate an increase in the sample size to obtain precise estimates of the effects of an intervention [6].

Internal consistency is measured with a single administration of an instrument and assesses how well items within a scale measure a single underlying dimension. Internal consistency is usually assessed using Cronbach's alpha, which measures the overall correlation between items within a scale [42].

Caution should be exercised in the interpretation of alpha because its size is dependent on the number of items as well as the level of correlation between items [43].

Reproducibility assesses whether an instrument produces the same results on repeated administrations when respondents have not changed. This is assessed by test-retest reliability. There is no exact agreement about the length of time between administrations, but in practice it tends to be between 2 and 14 days [43].

The reliability coefficient is normally calculated by correlating instrument scores for the two administrations. It is recommended that the intra-class correlation coefficient be used in preference to Pearson's correlation coefficient, which fails to take sufficient account of systematic error [6]. Reliability is not a fixed property and must be assessed in relation to the specific population and context [43].

Validity

Validity is the extent to which an instrument measures what is intended. Validity can be assessed qualitatively through an examination of instrument content, and quantitatively through factor analysis and comparisons with related variables. As with reliability, validity should not be seen as a fixed property and must be assessed in relation to the specific population and measurement objectives.

Content and face validity assess whether items adequately address the domain of interest [6]. They are qualitative matters of judging whether an instrument is suitable for its proposed application. Face validity is concerned with whether an instrument appears to be measuring the domain of interest. Content validity is a judgment about whether instrument content adequately covers the domain of interest.

There is increasing evidence that items within instruments tend to be concentrated around the middle of the scale hierarchy, with relatively fewer items at the extremes representing lower and higher levels of health. Instrument content should be examined for relevance to the application and for adequate coverage of the domain of interest.

Further evidence can be obtained from considering how the instrument was developed. This includes the extent of involvement in instrument development of experts with relevant clinical or health status measurement experience [44].

Validity testing should also involve some quantitative assessment. *Criterion* validity is assessed when an instrument correlates with another instrument or measure that is regarded as a more accurate or criterion variable. Within the field of patient-reported health measurement it is rarely the case that a criterion or "gold standard" measure exists that can be used to test the validity of an instrument. There are two exceptions. The first is when an instrument is reduced in length, with the longer version used as the "gold standard" to develop the short version [16]. Scores for short and long versions of the instrument are compared, the objective being a very high level of correlation. Secondly, instruments that have the measurement objective of prediction have a gold standard available either concurrently or in the future. For example, the criterion validity of an instrument designed to predict the presence of a particular disease (screening) can be assessed through a comparison with the results of diagnosis or a prospective outcome like length of hospital stay or mortality.

In the absence of a criterion variable, validity testing takes the form of *construct* validation. PROMs are developed to measure some underlying construct such as physical functioning or pain. On the basis of current understanding, such constructs can be expected to have a set of quantitative relationships with other constructs. For example, patients experiencing more severe pain may be expected to take more analgesics. Construct validity is assessed by comparing the scores produced by an instrument with sets of variables. Expected levels of correlation should be specified at the outset of studies [45].

Many instruments are multidimensional and measure several constructs, including physical functioning, mental health, and social functioning. These constructs should be considered when assessing construct validity as should the expected relationships with sets of variables. Furthermore, the internal structure of such instruments can be assessed by methods of construct validation. Factor analysis and principal component analysis provide empirical support for the dimensionality or internal construct validity of an instrument [46]. These statistical techniques can pick up separate health domains within an instrument [47].

Responsiveness

Responsiveness is concerned with the measurement of *important changes* in health and is therefore relevant when instruments are to be used in an evaluative context for the measurement of health outcomes. Does the instrument detect changes over time that matter to patients?

Just as with reliability and validity, estimates of responsiveness are related to applications within specific populations and are not an inherent or fixed property of an instrument.

Responsiveness is usually assessed by examining changes in instrument scores for groups of patients whose health is known to have changed. This may follow an intervention of known efficacy or a specific life event that is known to affect the health aspect measured. Alternatively, patients may be asked how their current health compares to some previous point in time by means of a health transition question. There is no single agreed upon method of assessing responsiveness and a number of statistical techniques are used for quantifying responsiveness.

The effect size statistic is equal to the mean change in instrument scores divided by the baseline standard deviation [48]. The standardized response mean is equal to the mean change in scores divided by the standard deviation of the change in scores [49]. The modified standardized response mean, sometimes referred to as the index of responsiveness, is equal to the mean change in scores divided by the standard deviation of change scores in stable subjects [50]. The denominator for the latter can be derived from the test-retest method of reliability testing.

Ideal Properties of PROMs Instrument

Ideal properties of a PROMs instrument can be summarized as follows [3, 51]:

- It should be specific to the *concept* being measured.
- It should be based on *end-point model.*
- It should have *conceptual equivalence* (equivalence in relevance and meaning across languages and cultures).
- It should be based on the *conceptual framework.*
- It should contain *optimum number of items.*
- It should have *easy and specific measurement properties*; i.e., use of the scale that is the easiest for the intended population to understand.
- It should maintain the *confidentiality* of the patient.
- It should be *reproducible.*

Types of Responses to PROM Items

Responses to a certain PROM item may vary between dichotomous and polytomous scale of measurement. Some item responses are expressed as yes/no, present/absent, and true/false. This is referred to as binary or dichotomous response scale of measurement. However, many tests, questionnaires, and inventories in the behavioral sciences include more than 2 response options. It is a set of answer choices that fall into an order, e.g., from highest to lowest. For example, many personality questionnaires include self-relevant statements (e.g., "I enjoy having conversation with friends"), and respondents are given 3 or more response options (e.g., strongly disagree, disagree, neutral, agree, strongly agree). Such items are known as a *polytomous items*, and they require IRT models that are different from those required by binary items.

A scale may be composed of pictures, numbers, or categories [2]. Recording of events is also one of the methods to determine the response that can be included by the patient, e.g., diary maintain. The following types of response scales or options may be used in a PRO instrument [3].

Types of Rating Scales

Likert Scale

The most frequently used rating scale is the Likert scale. Respondents are offered the choice of selecting 1 of 7 pre-defined or even 9 pre-coded responses, with a neutral point being equivocal along the continuum of the scale. Likert scales may evaluate:

- Agreement (strongly agree, agree, undecided, disagree, strongly disagree),
- Frequency (very frequently, frequently, occasionally, rarely, never),
- Importance (very important, important, moderately important, of little importance, unimportant),
- Likelihood (almost always true, usually true, occasionally true, usually not true, almost never true), or
- Other different attitudes (Fig. 2.1).

Fig. 2.1 Likert scale. Example showing agreement response category options

Strongly Disagree	Disagree	Undecided	Agree	Strongly Agree
(1)	(2)	(3)	(4)	(5)

Pictorial Scale

Drawing pictures or clipart can be used to express feelings and emotions items in a PROM instrument. They illustrate the rating scale in a more approachable way, especially within a population with a low level of literacy (Fig. 2.2).

Visual Analog Scale

A psychometric tool measuring that can be used to assess a rather subjective outcome such as feeling pain, happiness, or any characteristic or attitude that cannot be measured in a direct way (Fig. 2.3).

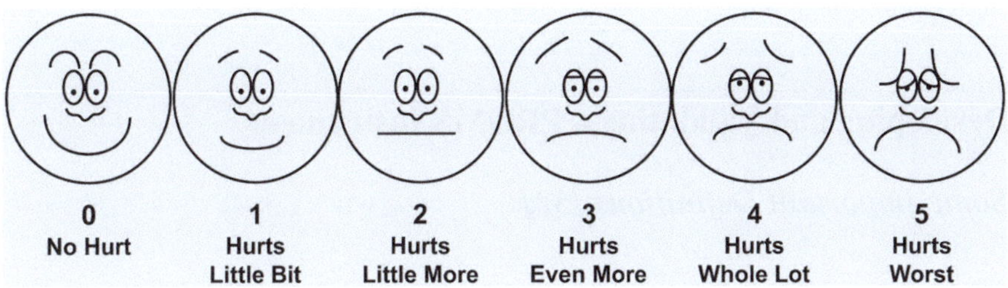

Fig. 2.2 Pictorial scale illustrating different levels of pain as clipart facial expressions

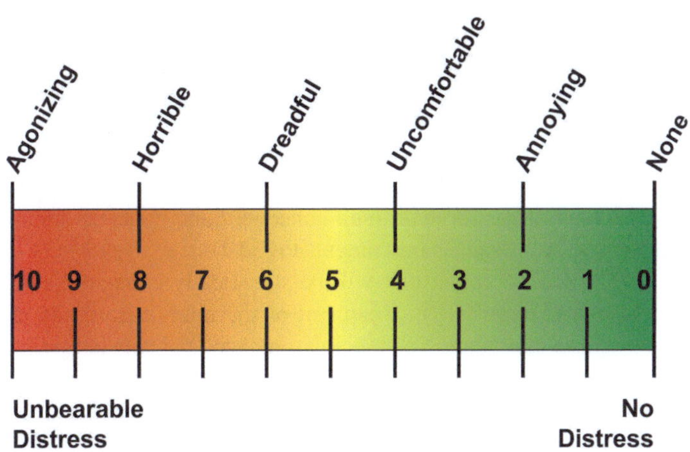

Fig. 2.3 Visual analog scale displaying, on a 10-point scale, the state of distress exerted by a respondent

Rating Scale

A grading continuum is provided for respondents to express the frequency of a particular health event or attack. For example, how many times did you express blue status during the last week? □ Once □ Twice □ Thrice □ More than 3

Checklist

Items presented in a PROM using a checklist are usually binary or dichotomous outcome items. Respondents are asked to check in a box the occurrence of certain events or symptoms. There is no response grading or continuum in this case and the item is analyzed as a dichotomous item. Example: Please place a check (√) in the box in front of the symptoms you expressed more during the last month. □ Insomnia □ Dyspnea □ Body aches □ Fatigue

Developing and Validating a PROMS Instrument

Some Important Definitions [52]

PRO Concept—It is the event intended to be measured by the tool. It can be called as the specific measurable goal of the instrument; e.g., symptom or group of symptoms.

PRO Domain—A sub-concept represented by a score of an instrument that measures a larger concept comprised of multiple domains; e.g., depression sometimes referred as scale.

PRO Item—An individual question, statement, or task (and its standardized response options) that should be answered by the patient and it addresses a particular concept; e.g., Are you feeling depressed?

Conceptual Framework—The conceptual framework explicitly defines the concepts measured by the instrument in a diagram that presents a description of the relationships between items, domain (sub-concepts), and concepts measured and the scores produced by a PROMs instrument (Fig. 2.4).

End Point—The measurement that will be statistically compared among treatment groups to assess the effect of treatment or the intervention, and that corresponds again with the intervention's objectives, design, and data analysis.

End-Point Model—A diagram of the hierarchy of relationships among all end points, both PRO and non-PRO, that corresponds to the clinical trial's objectives, design, and data analysis plan (Fig. 2.5).

Conceptual Equivalence—It is the equivalence in relevance and meaning of the concepts being measured in different languages and/or cultures [53].

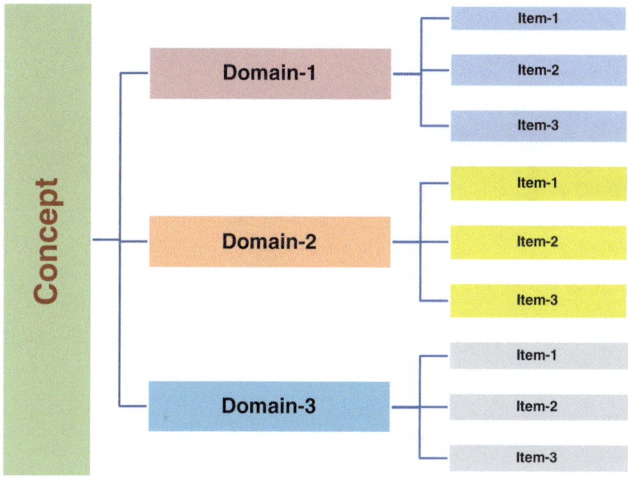

Fig. 2.4 Conceptual framework for a PROM instrument development displaying three domains and corresponding items

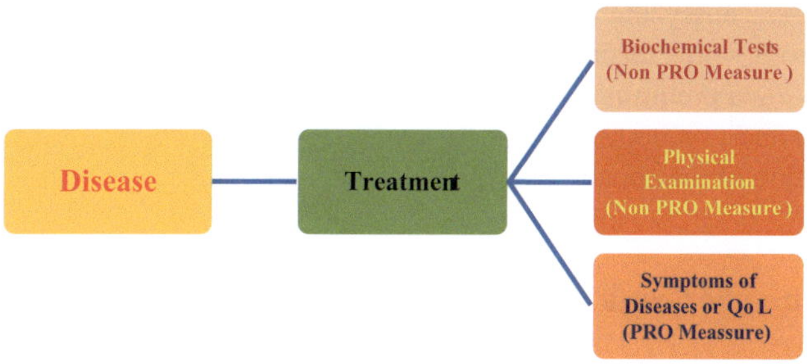

Fig. 2.5 End-point model diagram displaying different outcome measures in response to a specific treatment including PROM

Development of PROMs Instrument

Figure 2.6 illustrates different steps in development of a PROM instrument. The proposed steps are generated from different resources.

Steps in Developing a PROM Instrument

Step I: Conceptual Framework Construction

1. Establishing the need for a new measure by reviewing previous literature.
2. Defining the targeted population in terms of characteristics and accessibility.

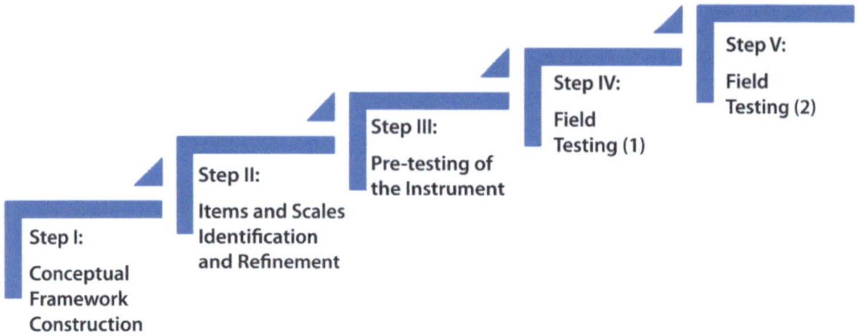

Fig. 2.6 Major steps in developing a PROM instrument as conceptualized from different sources

3. Generating a literature-review domains or scales.
4. Defining the end-point models.
5. Assorting the recall period.
6. Formulating the conceptual framework using clinical expert opinion.
7. Qualitatively interviewing a limited number of people from the concerned population for revision of the preliminary framework.
8. Qualitative analyzing interview transcripts to produce an exhaustive list of items from words taken from people.
9. Generating a preliminary items list.
10. Clinical and psychometric experts review.
11. Production of the conceptual framework of outcomes.

Step II: Items and Scales Identification and Refinement

1. Operationalization and content analysis to classify different items on different domains/scales of measurement.
2. Setting different response options and format.
3. Psychometric analysis with reduction of PROM items using different item selection statistical processes.
4. Clinical and psychometric expert review.
5. Production of the preliminary version of the instrument and its content validity.

Step III: Pretesting of the Instrument

1. Semi-structured cognitive interviews with individuals from the target population—a relatively larger number of respondents are required than step I.
2. Identification of problems with items: ambiguity, confusion, layout and format of the instrument, and the proper mode of administration.
3. Psychometric analysis and revision of the instrument on the base of respondents' recommendations.

4. Rephrasing of items, population response options and mode of administration, translation and cultural adaptation of the instrument, evaluation and documentation of the changes.
5. Clinical and psychometric experts review.
6. Production of the first draft of the version.

Step IV: Field Testing (1)

1. Administration of the instrument to a larger sample of the targeted population—sample size is calculated considering the number of items.
2. Psychometric analysis and modification of the tool according to responses.
3. Testing the effect of mode of administration on differential item functioning (DIF).
4. Rephrasing of items, population response options, and cultural adaptation of the instrument; evaluation and documentation of the changes.
5. Clinical and psychometric experts review.
6. Production of the modified first draft version.

Step V: Field Testing (2)

1. Proper administration of the instrument to a calculated sample of the target population—a control group could be added to test discrimination
2. Final psychometric analysis—traditional and Rash methods could be used.
3. Minimal modification in rephrasing of items, population response options, and cultural adaptation of the instrument; evaluation and documentation of the changes.
4. Clinical and psychometric experts review.
5. Production of the final version.

Scoring of Items and Domains

For each item, numerical scores should be assigned to each answer category based on the most appropriate scale of measurement for the item (e.g., nominal, ordinal, interval, or ratio scales). Reviewing the distribution of item responses is essential to ensure that response choices represent appropriate intervals. A scoring algorithm creates a single score from multiple items. Equally weighted scores for each item are appropriate when the responses to the items are independent. If two items are dependent, their collected information is less than two independent items and they are over-weighted when they are treated as two equally weighted items. Over-weighting also may be a concern when the number of response options or the values associated with response options vary by item.

Investigators should justify the method chosen to combine items to create a score or to combine domain scores to create a general score using qualitative research or defined statistical techniques.

Total scores combining multiple domains should be supported by evidence that the total score represents a single complex concept. Conceptual framework of a PRO instrument: The instrument's final conceptual framework documents the concept represented by each score [3].

Validation of a PROM Instrument

Validation of different criteria of a PROM instrument requires the use of different psychometric tests and setting off specific criteria would make the instrument ready to be used for a certain objective fulfillment [54].

Acceptability and Data Quality—Completeness of item-level and scale-level data.

- Score distributions: a relatively low number of persons at extreme (i.e., floor/ceiling) ends of the measurement continuum and skewness testing
- Even distribution of endorsement frequencies across response categories (>80 %)
- Percentage of item-level missing data (<10 %)
- Percentage of computable scale scores (>50 % completed items)
- Items in scales rated "not relevant" <35 %

Scaling Assumptions—Legitimacy of summing a set of items (items should measure a common underlying construct).

- Similar items' mean scores and SDs
- Positive residual "*r*" between items (<0.30) to assess model prediction.
- Items have adequate corrected Item to Total Correlation (ITC ≥ 0.3).
- High negative residual "*r*" (>0.60) suggests redundancy.
- Items have similar ITCs.
- Items sharing common variance suggest unidimensionality.
- Items do not measure at the same point on the scale.
- Evenly spaced items spanning whole measurement range.

Item Response Categories—Categories are set in a logical hierarchy.

- Ordered set of response thresholds for each scale item.

Targeting—Extent to which the range of the variable measured by the scale matches the range of that variable in the study sample.

- Scale scores spanning entire scale range
- Person-item threshold distribution: person locations should be covered by items.

- Item locations covered by persons when both calibrated on the same metric scale.
- Floor and ceiling (proportion sample at minimum and maximum scale score) effects should be low (<15 %).
- Skewness statistics should range from −1 to +1.
- Good targeting demonstrated by the mean location of items and persons around zero.

Reliability

Internal Consistency—Extent to which items comprising a scale measure the same construct (e.g., homogeneity of the scale).

- Cronbach's alphas for summary scores (adequate scale internal consistency is ≥0.70. Cronbach's α(alpha) is calculated using the following equation [42]:

$$\alpha = \frac{K}{K-1}\left(1-\frac{\sum_{i=1}^{K}\sigma_{Y_i}^2}{\sigma_X^2}\right)$$

where K = the number of items
σ(sigma)$_x$ = the variance of the observed total test scores
$\sigma(\text{sigma})_{Y_i}$ = the variance of component i for the current sample of persons.

- High person separation index >0.7; quantifies how reliably person measurements are separated by items.
- Item-total r (ITC) between +0.4 and +0.6 indicates items are moderately correlated with scale scores; higher values indicate well-correlated items with scale scores.
- Power-of-tests indicate the power in detecting the extent to which the data do not fit the model.
- Items with ordered thresholds.

Test-Retest Reliability—Stability of a measuring instrument.

- Intra-class r coefficient (ICC) > 0.70 between test and retest scores
- Statistical stability across time points (no uniform or non-uniform item DIF [p = >0.05 or Bonferroni adjusted value])
- Pearson r: >0.7 indicates reliable scale stability

Validity

It involves accumulating evidence from different forms.

Content Validity—Extent to which the content (items) of a scale is representative of the conceptual construct it is intended to measure.

- Consideration of item sufficiency and the target population.
- Clearly defined construct.
- Qualitative evidence from individuals for whom the measure is targeted, expert opinion and literature review (e.g., theoretical and/or conceptual definitions).
- Validity comes from careful item construction and consideration of what each item is meant to measure, then testing against model expectations.

The content validity index (CVI) is widely used for quantifying content validity for scales. Item-level CVI (I-CVI) is calculated by having experts to rate the relevance of each item to its own subdomain (1 = not relevant, 2 = somewhat relevant, 3 = quite relevant, 4 = highly relevant). The I-CVI of each item is defined as the number of experts offering a rating of 3 or 4, divided by the total number of experts.

As an adjustment for chance agreements, the multi-rater kappa statistic (K^*) was adopted and is described as follows:

$$p_c = \left[\frac{n!}{A!(n-A)!}\right] \times 0.5^n$$

where *Pc* is the probability of chance agreement, *n* is the number of experts, and *A* is the number approving with good relevance. K^* was calculated using the I-CVI and the probability of chance agreement as follows:

$$K^* = \frac{\text{I-CVI} - P_c}{1 - P_c}$$

Each item on the scale was then rated as "fair," "good," or "excellent," based on the following rating criteria: fair, $K^* = 0.40–0.59$; good, $K^* = 0.60–0.74$; excellent, $K^* > 0.74$. Any item that received a "fair" rating was deleted [52].

Construct Validity

1. Within-scale analyses

   Extent to which a distinct construct is being measured and that items can be combined to form a scale score.

   - Cronbach alpha for scale scores >0.70
   - Fit residuals (item-person interaction) within given range +/−2.5
   - ITC>0.30
   - Homogeneity coefficient (IIC mean and range >0.3).

- Nonsignificant chi-square (item-trait interaction) values.
- Scaling success.
- No under- or over-discriminating ICC.
- Mean fit residual close to 0.0; SD approaching 1.0.
- Person fit residuals within given range +/−2.5.

Measurement Continuum—extent to which scale items mark out the construct as a continuum on which people can be measured.

- Individual scale items located across a continuum in the same way locations of people are spread across the continuum.
- Items spread evenly over a reasonable measurement range. Items with similar locations may indicate item redundancy.
- Response dependency—response to one item determines response to another.
- Response dependency is indicated by residual "*r*" >0.3 for pairs of items.

2. Between scale analysis

Criterion Validity—hypotheses based on criterion or "gold standard" measure.

- In the majority of cases, there is no true gold standard test for criterion validation of the PROM instrument.

Convergent Validity—scale correlated with other measures of the same/similar constructs.

- Moderate to high "*r*" predicted for similar scales; criteria used as guides to the magnitude of "*r*," as opposed to pass/fail benchmarks (high $r>0.7$; moderate $r=0.3$–0.7; low $r<0.3$).

Discriminant Validity—scale not correlated with measures of different constructs

- Low *r* (<0.3) predicted between scale scores and measures of different constructs (e.g., age, gender).

Known Groups Differences—ability of a scale to differentiate known groups.

- Generate hypotheses (based on subgroups known to differ on construct measured) and compare mean scores (e.g., predict a stepwise change across severity of illness)
- Hypothesis testing (e.g., clinical questions are formulated and the empirical testing comes from whether or not data fit the Rasch model)
- Statistically significant differences in mean scores (ANOVA)

Differential Item Functioning (Item Bias)—The extent of any conditional relationships between item response and group membership.

- Persons with similar ability should respond in similar ways to individual items regardless of group membership (e.g., age).
- Uniform Differential Item Functioning (DIF)—uniformity amongst differences between groups.
- Non-uniform DIF—non-uniformity amongst differences between groups; can be considered at 1 % (Bonferroni adjusted) and 5 % CIs.

Item Reduction Process

The item-reduction processes of the preliminary scale are resorted to when some items are found to be not relevant or difficult by the qualitative analysis recommendations. They are based on both classical test theory (CTT) (e.g., discrete trend, factor analysis, correlation coefficient, Cronbach's α(alpha) if item deleted [CAID] values, and corrected item-total correlation [CITC]) and item response theory (IRT) [55]. It involves five steps:

1. *Step 1*: Items with low standard deviation indicates low degree of differentiation and should be removed. SD of <0.96 is recommended as a cutoff point.
2. *Step 2*: Principal component factor analysis with varimax rotation to identify the contribution of items to different scales. Sampling adequacy is tested by Kaiser–Meyer–Olkin measure; it should be >0.5. Items with low factor loading (<0.4) or with factor loading close to other items should be considered for removal.
3. *Step 3*: Item to scale Pearson correlation <0.6 is described as *not* representing the domain or scale.
4. *Step 4*: Internal consistency is evaluated using corrected item to total correlation (CITC) and Cronbach's alpha if item deleted (CAID). CITC>0.45 indicates high contribution of the item to scale, while increased CAID indicates low contribution of the item to scale.
5. *Step 5*: Item Response Theory (IRT) is used in terms of discrimination (α[alpha]) and difficulty (b). Items with α(alpha) <0.4 should be deleted. Items' difficulties are scored on a standardized metric. A range of −3 to +3 is allowed. Values for items outside this range are considered for removal.

Both statistical and clinical relevance of items should be taken in account before item removal decision.

IRT and Rash Models

Item Response Theory is a psychometric approach emphasizing the fact that an individual's response to a particular test item is influenced by qualities of the *individual* and by qualities of the *item*. IRT provides procedures for obtaining information about individuals, items, and tests. Various forms of IRT exist, representing different degrees of complexity or different applicability to various kinds of tests.

The basic form of IRT states that an individual's response to an item is affected by the individual's trait level and the item's difficulty level. More complex forms of IRT include additional factors (or parameters) affecting an individual's responses to items.

Determinants of an Item Response

Respondent Trait Level

One factor affecting an individual's probability of responding in a particular way to an item is the individual's level on the psychological trait being assessed by the item. An individual who has a high level of mathematical ability will be more likely to respond correctly to a math item than will an individual who has a low level of mathematical ability. Similarly, an individual who has a high level of extraversion will be more likely to endorse or agree with an item that measures extraversion than will an individual who has a low level of extraversion. An employee who has a high level of job satisfaction will be more likely to endorse an item that measures job satisfaction than will an employee with a low level of job satisfaction.

Item Difficulty

An item's level of difficulty is another factor affecting an individual's probability of responding in a particular way. A math item that has a high level of difficulty will be less likely to be answered correctly than a math item that has a low level of difficulty (i.e., an easy item).

Similarly, an extraversion measuring item that has a high level of difficulty will be less likely to be endorsed than an extraversion item that has a low level of difficulty. At first, the notion of "difficulty" might not be intuitive in the case of a personality trait such as extraversion, but consider these two hypothetical items: "I enjoy having conversations with friends" and "I enjoy speaking before large audiences." Assuming that these two items are validly interpreted as measures of extraversion, the first item is, in a sense, easier to undertake than the second item. In another way, it is likely that more people would agree with the statement about having a conversation with friends than with the statement about speaking in front of a large audience.

In the context of job satisfaction, the statement "My job is OK" is likely an easier item to agree with than is the statement "My job is the best thing in my life."

Although they are separate issues in an IRT analysis, trait level and item difficulty are intrinsically connected. In fact, item difficulty is conceived in terms of trait level. Specifically, a difficult item requires a relatively high trait level in order to be answered correctly, but an easy item requires only a low trait level to be answered correctly.

In an IRT analysis, trait levels and item difficulties are usually scored on a standardized metric, so that their means are 0 and the standard deviations are 1. Therefore, an individual who has a trait level of 0 has an average level of that trait, and an individual who has a trait level of 1.5 has a trait level that is 1.5 standard deviations above the mean. Similarly, an item with a difficulty level of 0 is an average item, and an item with a difficulty level of 1.5 is a relatively difficult item.

In IRT, item difficulty is expressed in terms of trait level. Specifically, an item's difficulty is defined as the trait level required for participants to have a 0.50 probability of answering the item correctly. If an item has a difficulty of 0, then an individual with an average trait level (i.e., an individual with a trait level of 0) will have a 50/50 chance of correctly answering the item. For an item with a difficulty of 0, an individual with a high trait level (i.e., a trait level greater than 0) will have a higher chance of answering the item correctly, and an individual with a low trait level (i.e., a trait level less than 0) will have a lower chance of answering the item correctly.

Item Discrimination

Just as the items on a test might differ in terms of their difficulties (some items are more difficult than others), the items on a test might also differ in terms of the degree by which they can differentiate individuals who have high trait levels from individuals who have low trait levels. This item characteristic is called item discrimination, and it is analogous to an item–total correlation from classical test theory (CTT) perspectives [56].

An item's discrimination value indicates the relevance of the item to the trait being measured by the test. An item with a positive discrimination value is at least somewhat consistent with the underlying trait being measured, and a relatively large discrimination value (e.g., 3.5 vs. 0.5) indicates a relatively strong consistency between the item and the underlying trait. In contrast, an item with a discrimination value of 0 is unrelated to the underlying trait supposedly being measured, and an item with a negative discrimination value is inversely related to the underlying trait (i.e., high trait scores make it *less* likely that the item will be answered correctly). Thus, it is generally desirable for items to have a large positive discrimination value.

IRT Measurement Models

From an IRT perspective, we can specify the components affecting the probability that an individual will respond in a particular way to a particular item. A *measurement model* expresses the mathematical links between an outcome (e.g., a respondent's score on a particular item) and the components that affect the outcome (e.g., qualities of the respondent and/or qualities of the item).

A variety of models have been developed from the IRT perspective (Table 2.1), and these models differ from each other in at least two important ways. One is in terms of the item characteristics, or *parameters*, that are included in the models. A second is in terms of the response option format.

The simplest IRT model is often called the *Rasch model* or the *one-parameter logistic model* (1PL). According to the Rasch model, an individual's response to a

Table 2.1 Commonly used item response theory (IRT) models

IRT model	Item response format	Model characteristics
Rash/one parameter logistic model	Dichotomous	Discrimination power equal across all items. Threshold varies across items
Two parameters logistic model	Dichotomous	Discrimination and threshold parameters vary across items
Graded response model	Polytomous	Ordered responses. Discrimination varies across items
Nominal model	Polytomous	No pre-specified item response order. Discrimination varies across items
Partial credit model	Polytomous	Discrimination power constrained to be equal across items
Rating scale model	Polytomous	Discrimination equal across items. Distance between item threshold steps equal across items
Generalized partial credit model	Polytomous	Generalization of the partial credit model that allows discrimination to vary across items

binary item (i.e., right/wrong, true/false, agree/disagree) is determined by the individual's trait level and the difficulty of the item. One way of expressing the Rasch model is in terms of the probability that an individual with a particular trait level will correctly answer an item that has a particular difficulty. This is often presented as [56]:

$$P\left(X_{\text{is}} = 1 \mid \theta_{\text{s}}, \beta_{\text{i}}\right) = \frac{e^{(\theta_{\text{s}} - \beta_{\text{i}})}}{1 + e^{(\theta_{\text{s}} - \beta_{\text{i}})}}$$

where:

X_{is} refers to response (X) made by subject s to item i.

θ(theta)$_{\text{s}}$ refers to the trait level of subject s.

β(beta)$_{\text{i}}$ refers to the difficulty of item i.

$X_{\text{is}} = 1$ refers to a "correct" response or an endorsement of the item.

e is the base of the natural logarithm (i.e., $e = 2.7182818$ …), found on many calculators.

So, $P(X_{\text{is}} = 1 | \theta[\text{theta}]_{\text{s}}, \beta[\text{beta}]_{\text{i}})$ refers to the probability (P) that subject s will respond to item i correctly or in a particular way. The vertical bar in this statement indicates that this is a "conditional" probability. The probability that the subject will correctly respond to the item depends on (i.e., is conditional upon) the subject's trait level ($\theta[\text{theta}]_{\text{s}}$) and the item's difficulty ($\beta[\text{beta}]_{\text{i}}$). In an IRT analysis, trait levels and item difficulties are usually scaled on a standardized metric, so that their means are 0 and the standard deviations are 1.

A slightly more complex IRT model is called the *two-parameter logistic model* (2PL) because it includes 2 item parameters. The difference between the 2PL and the Rasch model is the inclusion of the item discrimination parameter. This can be presented as [56]:

$$P\left(X_{\text{is}} = 1 \mid \theta_{\text{s}}, \beta_{\text{i}}, \alpha_{\text{i}}\right) = \frac{e^{\left(\alpha_{\text{i}}\left(\theta_{\text{s}} - \beta_{\text{i}}\right)\right)}}{1 + e^{\left(\alpha_{\text{i}}\left(\theta_{\text{s}} - \beta_{\text{i}}\right)\right)}}$$

where α(alpha)$_{\text{i}}$ refers to the discrimination of item *i*, with higher values representing more discriminating items. The 2PL model states that the probability of a respondent answering an item correctly is conditional upon the respondent's trait level (θ[theta]$_{\text{s}}$), the item's difficulty (β[beta]$_{\text{i}}$), and the item's discrimination (α[alpha]$_{\text{i}}$).

Just as the 2PL model is an extension of the Rasch model (i.e., the 1PL model), there are other models that are extensions of the 2PL model. The *three-parameter logistic model* (3PL) adds yet another item parameter. The third parameter here is an adjustment for guessing. In sum, the 1PL, 2PL, and 3PL models represent IRT measurement models that differ with respect to the number of item parameters that are included in the models.

A second way in which IRT models differ is in terms of the response option format. So far, the 1PL, 2PL, and 3PL models are designed to be used for binary outcomes as the response option. However, many tests, questionnaires, and inventories in the behavioral sciences include more than two response options. For example, many personality questionnaires include self-relevant statements (e.g., "I enjoy having conversation with friends"), and respondents are given three or more response options (e.g., strongly disagree, disagree, neutral, agree, strongly agree). Such items are known as *polytomous items*, and they require IRT models that are different from those required by binary items. Although these models differ in terms of the response options that they can accommodate, they rely on the same general principles as the models designed for binary items. That is, they reflect the idea that an individual's response to an item is determined by the individual's trait level and by item properties, such as difficulty and discrimination.

IRT Models Assumptions [57]:

1. Unidimensionality
2. Local independence
3. IRT model fits the data

It is important that these assumptions be evaluated. However, IRT models are robust to minor violations and no real data ever meet the assumptions perfectly. Unidimensionality requires that the set of items measure a single continuous latent construct θ(theta). Scale dimensionality can be evaluated by factor analysis of item responses. If multi-dimensionality is indicated by factor analysis and supported clinical theory, it may be appropriate to divide the scale into subscales.

Local independence means that if θ(theta) is held constant, there should be no association among the item responses. Violation of this assumption may result in biased parameter estimated leading to erroneous decisions when selecting items for scale construction. Local independence can be evaluated by examining the residual correlation matrices for systematic error among item clusters that may indicate violation of the assumption.

Model fit can be examined at both the item and person level to determine whether the estimated item and person parameters can reproduce the observed item responses. Since IRT is probabilistic in nature, most fit indices measure deviations between predicted and observed response frequencies. Many types of residual analysis can be used to evaluate model fit.

$$\text{Rasch Model}\left(\text{the 1 PL} = \text{One Parameter Logistic Model}\right)$$

The Rasch model includes two determinants of an item response—the respondent's trait level and the items' difficulty level.

The initial estimates of trait levels can be seen as a two-step process. First, we determine the proportion of items that each respondent answered correctly. For a respondent, the proportion correct is simply the number of items answered correctly, divided by the total number of items that were answered. To obtain estimates of trait levels, we next take the natural log of a ratio of proportion correct to proportion incorrect:

$$\theta_5 = \text{LN}\left(\frac{P_s}{1-P_s}\right)$$

where P_s is the proportion of items answered correctly by Respondent 5 (a specific respondent).

The initial estimates of item difficulties also can be seen as a two-step process. First, we determine the proportion of correct responses for each item. For an item, the proportion of correct responses is the number of respondents who answered the item correctly, divided by the total number of respondents who answered the item. To obtain estimates of item difficulty, we compute the natural log of the ratio of the proportion of incorrect responses to the proportion of correct responses:

$$\beta_i = \text{LN}\left(\frac{1-P_i}{P_i}\right)$$

where P_i is the proportion of correct responses for item i.

Item and Test Information

As a psychometric approach, IRT provides information about items and about tests. In an IRT analysis, item characteristics are combined in order to reflect characteristics of the test as a whole. In this way, item characteristics such as difficulty and

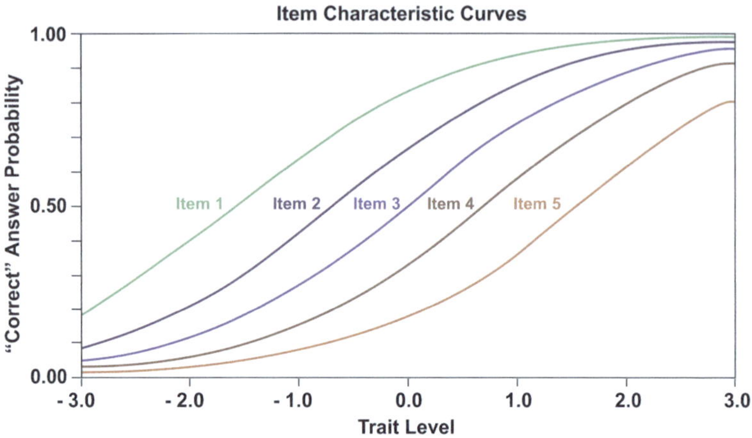

Fig. 2.7 Item characteristic curve for 5 dichotomous items showing different probabilities of a correct answer at different trait levels of respondents [58]

discrimination can be used to evaluate the items and to maximize the overall quality of a test.

Item characteristic curves, such as those presented in Fig. 2.7 [58], reflect the probabilities with which individuals across a range of trait levels are likely to answer each item correctly.

The item characteristic curves in Fig. 2.7 are based on the five items from the hypothetical mathematics test analyzed [58]. For item characteristic curves, the *X*-axis reflects a wide range of trait levels, and the *Y*-axis reflects probabilities ranging from 0 to 1.0. Each item has a curve, and we can examine an item's curve to find the likelihood that an individual with a particular trait level will answer the item correctly.

For Item 1, what is the probability that an individual with an average level of mathematical ability will answer the item correctly? We find the point on the Item 1 curve that is directly above the "0" point on the *X*-axis (recall that the trait level is in *z* score units, so zero is the average trait level), and we see that this point lies between 0.80 and 0.90 on the *Y*-axis. Looking at the other curves, we see that an individual with an average level of mathematical ability has about a 0.65 probability of answering Item 2 correctly, a 0.50 chance of answering Item 3 correctly, and a 0.17 probability of answering Item 5 correctly.

By entering an item's difficulty and a particular trait level (say, –3.0) into the model, we obtain the probability with which an individual with that particular trait level will answer that item correctly. We can then enter a different trait level into the model (say, –2.9) and obtain the probability with which an individual with the different trait level will answer the item correctly. After conducting this procedure for

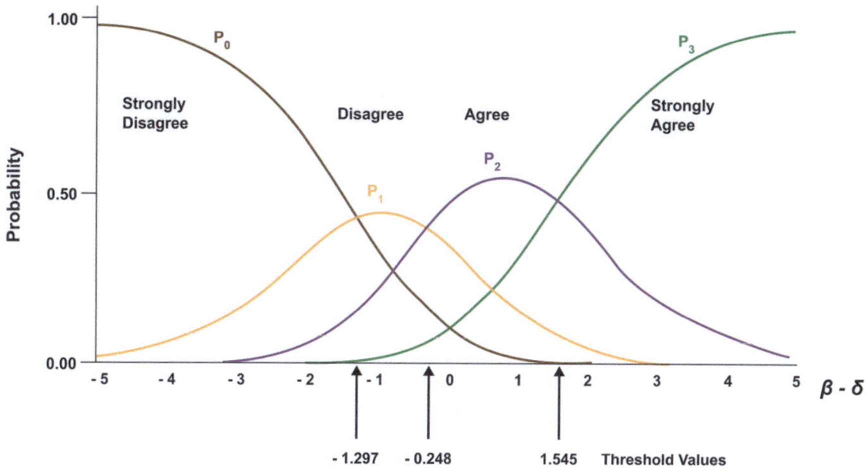

Fig. 2.8 Item characteristic curve for a polytomous item showing the probability of different responses according to different trait levels

many different trait levels, we simply plot the probabilities that we have obtained. The line connecting these probabilities reflects the item's characteristic curve.

Figure 2.8 displays an item characteristic curve for a polytomous item. It shows the highest probability of answering P0 (Strongly Disagree) is associated with the lowest trait level. While P3 (Strongly Agree) corresponds with the highest trait level.

Item information function can identify items that perform well or poorly. Low information for one item may indicate that the item:

1. Measures something different from other items in the scale
2. Is poorly worded and need to be rewritten
3. Too complex for the respondents
4. Placed out of context in the questionnaire

Test Information

From the perspective of CTT, reliability was an important psychometric consideration for a test. For example, we might compute coefficient alpha as an estimate of the test's reliability. An important point to note is that we would compute only 1 reliability estimate for a test, and that estimate would indicate the degree to which observed test scores are correlated with true scores.

The idea that there is a single reliability for a particular test is an important way in which CTT differs from IRT.

From the perspective of IRT, a test does not have a single "reliability." Instead, a test might have stronger psychometric quality for some people than for others. That is, a test might provide better information at some trait levels than at other trait levels.

How could a test provide information that differs by trait level? Why would a test be able to discriminate between people who have relatively high trait levels but not between people who have relatively low trait levels?

We can use IRT to pinpoint the psychometric quality of a test across a wide range of trait levels. This can be seen as a 2-step process. First, we evaluate the psychometric quality of each item across a range of trait levels. Just as we can compute the probability of a correct answer for an item at a wide range of trait levels (as illustrated in item characteristic curves), we use the probabilities to compute information at the same range of trait levels. For the Rasch model, item information can be computed as follows [56]:

$$I(\theta) = P_i(\theta)(1 - P_i(\theta))$$

where $I(\theta$[theta]) is the item's information value at a particular trait level (θ[theta]), and $P_i(\theta$[theta]) is the probability that a respondent with a particular trait level will answer the item correctly. If we compute information values at many more trait levels, we could display the results in a graph called an *item information curve (IIC)*.

Figure 2.9 illustrates item information characteristics for a 5-item test [58]. It illustrates the spanning of different item information along the trait level of participants in the test.

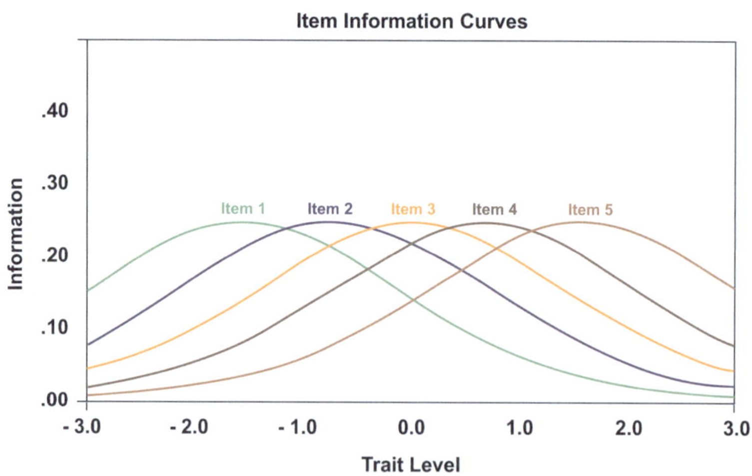

Fig. 2.9 Item Information Curves (IIC) for different items of a test showing different maximum information levels for different items [58]

Higher information values indicate greater psychometric quality. Item 1 has higher psychometric quality at relatively low trait levels than at relatively high trait levels. That is, it is more capable of discriminating among people with low trait levels than among high trait levels (presumably because most people with high trait levels will answer the item correctly).

The height of the curve indicates the amount of information that the item provides. The highest point on a curve represents the trait level at which the item provides the most information. In fact, an item provides the most information at a trait level that corresponds with its difficulty level, estimated earlier. Note that the items differ in the points at which they provide good information. Item 1 provides good information at relatively low trait levels, Item 3 provides good information at average trait levels, and Item 5 provides good information at relatively high trait levels.

Of course, when we actually use a psychological test, we are concerned with the quality of the test as a whole more than the qualities of individual items. Therefore, we can combine item information values to obtain test information values (Fig. 2.10).

Specifically, item information values at a particular trait level can be added together to obtain a test information value at that trait level.

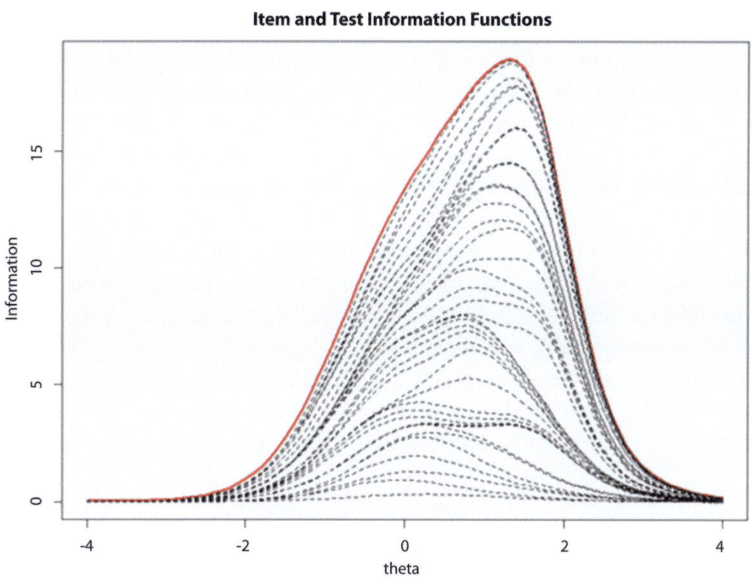

Fig. 2.10 Item and Test Information Function where theta denotes the different ability or trait levels of the respondents

From an IRT perspective, a test's psychometric quality can vary across trait levels. This is an important but perhaps underappreciated difference between the CCT and IRT approaches to test theory.

Differential Item Functioning

From an IRT perspective, analyses can be conducted to evaluate the presence and nature of differential item functioning (DIF). Differential item functioning occurs when an item's properties in one group are different from the item's properties in another group. For example, DIF exists when a particular item has one difficulty level for males and a different difficulty level for females. In another way, the presence of differential item functioning means that a male and a female who have the same trait level have different probabilities of answering the item correctly. The existence of DIF between groups indicates that the groups cannot be meaningfully compared on the item.

For example, Smith and Reise (1998) [59] used IRT to examine the presence and nature of DIF for males and females on the Stress Reaction scale of the Multidimensional Personality Questionnaire. The Stress Reaction scale assesses the tendency to experience negative emotions such as guilt and anxiety, and previous research had shown that males and females often have different means on such scales. Smith and Reise [59] argued that this difference could reflect a true gender difference in such traits or that it could be produced by differential item functioning on such scales. Their analysis indicated that, although females do appear to have higher trait levels of stress reaction, DIF does exist for several items. Furthermore, their analyses revealed interesting psychological meaning for the items that did show DIF. Smith and Reise [59] state that items related to "emotional vulnerability and sensitivity in situations that involve self-evaluation" were easier for females to endorse, but items related to "the general experience of nervous tensions, unexplainable moodiness, irritation, frustration, and being on-edge" were easier for males to endorse. Smith and Reise [59] concluded that inventories designed to measure negative emotionality will show a large gender difference when "female DIF-type items" are overrepresented and that such inventories will show a small gender difference when "male DIF-type items" are overrepresented. Such insights can inform the development and interpretation of important psychological measures.

Person Fit

Another interesting application of IRT is a phenomenon called *person fit* [60]. When we administer a psychological test, we might find an individual whose pattern of responses seems strange compared to typical responses.

Consider 2 items that might be found on a measure of friendliness:

1. I like my friends.
2. I am willing to lend my friends as much money as they might ever want.

Most people would probably agree with the first statement (i.e., it is an "easy" item). In contrast, fewer people might agree with the second statement. Although most of us like our friends and would be willing to help them, not all of us would be willing to lend our friends "as much money as they might ever want." It would be quite odd to find someone who would be willing to lend any amount of money to her friends if she does not like her friends.

The analysis of person fit is an attempt to identify individuals whose response pattern does not seem to fit any of the expected patterns of responses to a set of items. Although there are several approaches to the analysis of person fit [60], the general idea is that IRT can be used to estimate item characteristics and then to identify individuals whose responses to items do not adhere to those parameters.

The identification of individuals with poor person fit to a set of items has several possible implications. In a personality assessment context, poor person fit might reveal that an individual's personality is unique in that it produces responses that do not fit the "typically expected" pattern of responses generated from the tested population.

Conclusion

Despite the conceptual and computational challenges and difficulties, the many potential advantages of IRT models should not be ignored. Knowledge of IRT is spreading within the academic disciplines of psychology, education, and public health. More books and tutorials are being written on this subject, and user friendly software is being developed. Research that applies IRT models is appearing more frequently in health outcomes literature. A better understanding of the models and applications of IRT is emerging and this will result in health outcome instruments that are shorter, more reliable, and better at targeting the population of interest.

References

1. Singh DP. Quality of life in cancer patients receiving palliative care. Indian J Palliat Care. 2010;16:36–43.
2. Kozma CM, Reeder CE, Schulz RM. Economic, clinical, and humanistic outcomes: a planning model for pharmacoeconomic research. Clin Ther. 1993;15:1121–32. Discussion 1120.
3. International Alliance of Patients' Organizations. What is patient centred health care? A review of definitions and principles. 2nd ed. London: IAPO; 2007. p. 1–34.
4. Chin R, Lee BY. Economics and patient reported outcomes, principles and practice of clinical trial medicine. London: Elsevier; 2008. p. 145–66.
5. U.S. Department of Health and Human Services Food and Drug Administration Guidance for Industry: Patient-Reported Outcome Measures: Use in Medical Product Development to Support Labeling Claims. U.S. FDA, Clinical/Medical. 2009. [http://www.fda.gov/downloads/Drugs/GuidanceComplianceRegulatoryInformation/Guidances/UCM193282.pdf]. Accessed 17 Aug 2015.

6. Fitzpatrick R, Davey C, Buxton MJ, Jones DR. Evaluating patient-based outcome measures for use in clinical trials. Health Technol Assess. 1998;2:1–74.
7. Chen H, Taichman DB, Doyle RL. Health-related quality of life and patient-reported outcomes in pulmonary arterial hypertension. Proc Am Thorac Soc. 2008;5:623–30.
8. Chao J, Nau DP, Aikens JE. Patient-reported perceptions of side effects of antihyperglycemic medication and adherence to medication regimens in persons with diabetes mellitus. Clin Ther. 2007;29:177–80.
9. Erickson P, Taeuber RC, Scott J. Operational aspects of quality-of-life assessment: choosing the right instrument: review article. PharmacoEconomics. 1995;7:39–48.
10. Testa MA, Simonson DC. Assessment of quality-of-life outcomes. N Engl J Med. 1996;334:835–40.
11. El Miedany Y, El Gaafary M, Youssef S, Palmer D. Incorporating patient reported outcome measures in clinical practice: development and validation of a questionnaire for inflammatory arthritis. Clin Exp Rheumatol. 2010;28:734–44.
12. Singh G, Athreya B, Fries J, Goldsmith D. Measurement of health status in children with juvenile rheumatoid arthritis. Arthritis Rheum. 1994;37(12):1761–9.
13. Beck A, Ward C, Medelson M, Mock J, Erbaugh J. An inventory for measuring depression. Arch Gen Psychiatry. 1961;4:561–71.
14. Ware JE, Sherbourne CD. The MOS 36-item short-form health survey (SF-36): i. Conceptual framework and item selection. Med Care. 1992;30:473–83.
15. Garratt AM, Ruta DA, Abdalla MI, Buckingham JK, Russell IT. The SF-36 health survey questionnaire: an outcome measure suitable for routine use within the NHS? Br Med J. 1993;306:1440–3.
16. Ware JE, Kosinski M, Bayliss MS, McHorney C, Rogers WH, Raczek A. Comparison of methods for scoring and statistical analysis of the SF-36 health profile and summary measures: summary of results from the medical outcomes study. Med Care. 1995;33:S264–79.
17. Ware JE, Kosinski M, Keller SD. A 12-item short-form health survey. Construction of scales and preliminary tests of validity and reliability. Med Care. 1995;34:220–33.
18. Ruta DA, Garratt AM, Leng M, Russell IT, Macdonald LM. A new approach to the measurement of quality of life: the patient-generated index. Med Care. 1994;11:1109–26. 8.
19. Ruta DA, Garratt AM, Russell IT. Patient centred assessment of quality of life for patients with four common conditions. Qual Health Care. 1999;8:22–9.
20. Group EQ. EuroQol—a new facility for the measurement of health related quality of life. Health Policy. 1990;16:199–208.
21. Brooks R with the EuroQol Group. EuroQol: the current state of play. Health Policy. 1996;37:53–72.
22. Ware JE. Standards for validating health measures: definition and content. J Chronic Dis. 1987;40:473–80.
23. Kirshner B, Guyatt G. A methodological framework for assessing health indices. J Chronic Dis. 1985;38:27–36.
24. Cox DR, Fitzpatrick R, Fletcher AE, Gore SM, Spiegelhalter DJ, Jones DR. Quality of life measurement: can we keep it simple? J R Stat Soc. 1992;155:353–93.
25. Garratt AM, Ruta DA, Abdalla MI, Russell IT. Responsiveness of the SF-36 and a condition-specific measure of health for patients with varicose veins. Qual Life Res. 1996;5:223–34.
26. Bullinger M. Ensuring international equivalence of quality of life measures. In: Orley J, Kuykken W, editors. Quality of life assessment: international perspectives. Berlin: Springer; 1994. p. 33–40.
27. Leplege A, Verdier A. The adaptation of health status measures: methodological aspects of the translation procedure. In: Shumaker S, Berzon R, editors. The international assessment of health-related quality of life: theory, translation, measurement and analysis. Oxford: Rapid Communications of Oxford; 1995. p. 93–101.
28. Sprangers MA, Cull A, Bjordal K, Groenvold M, Aaronson NK. The European organization for research and treatment of cancer. Approach to quality of life assessment: guidelines for

developing questionnaire modules. EORTC study group on quality of life. Qual Life Res. 1993;2:287–95.
29. Aarsonson NK. Assessing the quality of life of patients in cancer clinical trials: common problems and common sense solutions. Eur J Cancer. 1992;28A:1304–7.
30. Jaeschke R, Singer J, Guyatt GH. Measurement of health status. Ascertaining the minimal clinically important difference. Control Clin Trials. 1989;10:407–15.
31. Juniper EF, Guyatt GH, Willan A, Griffith LE. Determining a minimal important change in a disease-specific quality of life questionnaire. J Clin Epidemiol. 1994;47:81–7.
32. Stewart AL, Greenfield S, Hays RD, Wells K, Rogers WH, Berry SD, McGlynn EA, Ware JE. Functional status and well-being of patients with chronic conditions: results from the medical outcomes study. J Am Med Assoc. 1989;262:907–13.
33. Garratt AM, Ruta DA, Abdalla MI, Russell IT. The SF-36 health survey questionnaire: ii responsiveness to changes in health status in four common clinical conditions. Qual Health Care. 1994;3:186–92.
34. Feeny DH, Furlong W, Boyle M, Torrance GW. Multi-attribute health status classification systems: Health Utilities Index. PharmacoEconomics. 1995;7:490–502.
35. Hunt SM, McEwen J, McKenna SP. Measuring health status: a new tool for clinicians and epidemiologists. J R Coll Gen Pract. 1985;35:185–8.
36. Bergner M, Bobbitt RA, Carter WB, Gilson BS. The sickness impact profile: development and final revision of a health status measure. Med Care. 1981;19:787–805.
37. Bindman AB, Keane D, Lurie N. Measuring health changes among severely ill patients: the floor phenomenon. Med Care. 1990;28:1142–52.
38. Gardiner PV, Sykes HR, Hassey GA, Walker DJ. An evaluation of the health assessment questionnaire in long-term follow-up of disability in rheumatoid arthritis. Br J Rheumatol. 1993;32:724–8.
39. Stucki G, Daltroy L, Katz JN, Johannesson M, Liang MH. Interpretation of change scores in ordinal clinical scale and health status measures: the whole may not equal the sum of the parts. J Clin Epidemiol. 1996;49:711–7.
40. Tennant A, Hillman M, Fear J, Pickering A, Chamberlain MA. Are we making the most of the Stanford health assessment questionnaire. Br J Rheumatol. 1996;35:574–8.
41. Garratt AM in collaboration with UKBEAM. Rasch analysis of the Roland disability questionnaire. Spine. 2003;28:79–84.
42. Cronbach LJ. Coefficient alpha and the internal structure of tests. Psychometrika. 1951;16:297–334.
43. Streiner GL, Norman RD. Health measurement scales: a practical guide to their development and use. 2nd ed. Oxford: Oxford University Press; 1995.
44. Guyatt GH, Cook DJ. Health status, quality of life and the individual. J Am Med Assoc. 1994;272:630–1.
45. McDowell I, Jenkinson C. Development standards for health measures. J Health Serv Res Policy. 1996;1:238–46.
46. Jolliffe IT, Morgan BJT. Principal component analysis and exploratory factor analysis. Stat Methods Med Res. 1992;1:69–95.
47. Garratt AM, Hutchinson A, Russell IT. The UK version of the Seattle Angina Questionnaire (SAQ-UK): reliability, validity and responsiveness. J Clin Epidemiol. 2001;54:907–15.
48. Kazis LE, Anderson JJ, Meenan RF. Effect sizes for interpreting changes in health status. Med Care. 1989;27:MS178–89.
49. Liang MH, Fossel AH, Larson MG. Comparisons of five health status instruments for orthopedic evaluation. Med Care. 1990;28:632–42.
50. Guyatt G, Walter S, Norman G. Measuring change over time: assessing the usefulness of evaluative instruments. J Chronic Dis. 1987;40:171–8.
51. Acquadro C, Berzon R, Dubois D, Leidy NK, Marquis P, Revicki D, et al. Incorporating the patient's perspective into drug development and communication: an ad hoc task force report of

the patient-reported outcomes (PRO) harmonization group meeting at the food and drug administration, February 16, 2001. Value Health. 2003;6:522–31.
52. Deshpande PR, Rajan S, Lakshmi Sudeepthi B, Abdul Nazir CP. Patient-reported outcomes: a new era in clinical research. Perspect Clin Res. 2011;2(4):137–44.
53. Pashos CL, Klein EG, Wanke LA, editors. ISPOR Lexicon™. Princeton: International Society for Pharmacoeconomics and Outcomes Research; 1998.
54. Goreck C, Brown JM, Cano S, Lamping DL, Briggs M, Coleman S, Dealey C, McGinnis E, Nelson AE, Stubbs N, Wilson L, Nixon J. Development and validation of a new patient-reported outcome measure for patients with pressure ulcers: the PU-QOL instrument. Health Qual Life Outcomes. 2013;11:95.
55. Luo Y, Yang J, Zhang Y. Development and validation of a patient-reported outcome measure for stroke patients. Health Qual Life Outcomes. 2015;13:53.
56. Embretson SE, Reise S. Item response theory for psychologists. Mahwah: Lawrence Erlbaum; 2000.
57. Reeve BB, Fayers P. Applying item response theory modeling for evaluating questionnaire item and scale properties. In: Fayers P, Hays RD, editors. Assessing quality of life in clinical trials: methods of practice. 2nd ed. New York: Oxford University Press; 2005. p. 53–73.
58. Furr M, Bacharach VR. Chapter 13. Item response theory and Rasch models, Psychometrics: an introduction. New York: Sage; 2007.
59. Smith LL, Reise SP. Gender differences on negative affectivity: an IRT study of differential item functioning on the multi-dimensional personality questionnaire stress reaction scale. J Pers Soc Psychol. 1998;75:1350–62.
60. Meijer RR, Sijtsma K. Methodology review: evaluating person fit. Appl Psychol Meas. 2001;25(2):107–35.

Chapter 3
PROMs (MDHAQ/RAPID3) and Physician RheuMetric Measures

Theodore Pincus, Jacquelin Chua, Martin J. Bergman, Yusuf Yazici, and Kathryn A. Gibson

Introduction

Many important advances in medical care have resulted from assessment and monitoring of patient status in terms of quantitative data rather than only as narrative descriptions. Most such advances classically have resulted from laboratory tests and other high-technology sources, according to a "biomedical model" [1] (Table 3.1). A classical report in 1977 introduced the concept of limitations of a biomedical model, and possible advantages of a complementary "biopsychosocial model" [1], in which physicians and health professionals often learn as much about diagnosis, management, prognosis, and outcomes from patients as from high-technology sources.

T. Pincus (✉) • J. Chua
Division of Rheumatology, Department of Internal Medicine, Rush University Medical Center, 1611 West Harrison Street, Suite 510, Chicago 60612, IL, USA
e-mail: tedpincus@gmail.com; jacquelin_r_chua@rush.edu

M.J. Bergman
Arthritis and Rheumatology, Taylor Hospital,
8 Morton Avenue, Suite 204, Ridley Park 19078, PA, USA
e-mail: mjbergman@prodigy.net

Y. Yazici
Division of Rheumatology, Department of Internal Medicine, NYU Hospital for Joint Diseases, 10016 New York, NY, USA
e-mail: Yusuf.Yazici@nyumc.org

K.A. Gibson
Department of Rheumatology, Liverpool Hospital,
Elizabeth St and Goulburn Street, Liverpool 2170, NSW, Australia
e-mail: kathy.gibson@slhd.nsw.gov.au

Y. El Miedany (ed.), *Patient Reported Outcome Measures in Rheumatic Diseases*,
DOI 10.1007/978-3-319-32851-5_3

Table 3.1 Comparison of a "biomedical model" and a "biopsychosocial model" of disease

	Biomedical model	Biopsychosocial model
Cause	Each disease has a single "cause"	Disease etiology is multifactorial: external pathogens, toxins, and internal host milieu, genes, behavior, social support
Diagnosis	Identified primarily through laboratory tests, radiographs, scans; information from patients of value primarily (or only) to suggest appropriate tests	A patient medical history provides 50–90 % of the information needed to make many, perhaps most, diagnoses
Prognosis	Also established most accurately on the basis of information from high technology sources, rather than from a patient	Information provided by a patient often is the most valuable data to establish a prognosis
Treatment	Involves only actions of health professionals; e.g., medications, surgery	Must involve patient, family, social structure
Role of health professionals and patients in general health and disease outcomes	Health and disease outcomes are determined primarily by decisions and actions of health professionals	Health and outcomes of chronic diseases are determined as much by actions of individual patient as by health professionals

A Biopsychosocial Model to Supplement a Biomedical Model in Rheumatology

Recognition of limitations of a biomedical model and of the value of a biopsychosocial model is particularly prominent in rheumatic diseases, supported by at least three types of evidence:

1. A survey of 313 physicians, 154 rheumatologists and 159 non-rheumatologists, indicated that medical history data are far more prominent in diagnosis and management decisions in RA than laboratory tests or ancillary studies, in contrast to seven other prevalent chronic diseases [2] (Fig. 3.1). As expected, vital signs dominated hypertension, laboratory tests diabetes and hyperlipidemia, and ancillary studies were most prominent in lymphoma, pulmonary fibrosis, ulcerative colitis, and congestive heart failure. RA was the only one of the eight chronic conditions physicians reported in which a patient history accounted for more than 50 % of the information required for diagnosis and management [2].
2. Physical function scores on a patient self-report questionnaire generally are considerably more significant than laboratory tests or other high-technology data to predict most severe long-term outcomes of RA, including work disability [3–7], costs [8, 9], joint replacement surgery [10], and premature death [4, 11–13]. Severe RA according to a quantitative patient questionnaire was documented to be associated with premature mortality in RA, comparable to Stage IV Hodgkin's

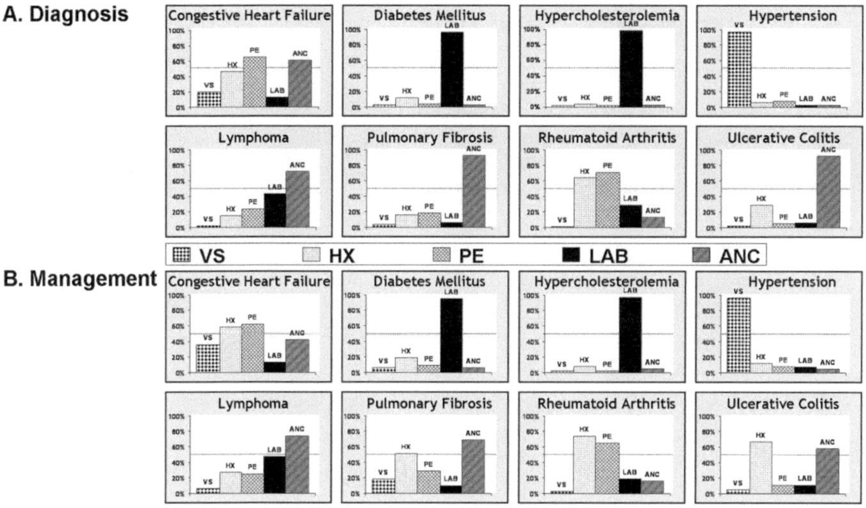

Fig. 3.1 Levels of 5 sources of information for (**a**) diagnosis and (**b**) management of 8 chronic diseases (congestive heart failure, diabetes mellitus, hypercholesterolemia, hypertension, lymphoma, pulmonary fibrosis, rheumatoid arthritis, and ulcerative colitis), according to survey of 313 physicians (154 rheumatologists and 159 non-rheumatologists). *VS* vital signs, *HX* patient history, *PE* physical examination, *LAB* laboratory tests, *ANC* ancillary studies

disease or three-vessel atherosclerotic cardiovascular disease 30 years ago (Fig. 3.2) [14]. This observation has been extended in many subsequent studies; a review of all 53 reports (as of 2008) in which clinical markers as possible prognostic variables for RA mortality were included indicated that self-report of physical function (and comorbidities) were more likely significant to predict mortality in univariate and multivariate analyses than laboratory tests, joint counts, and/or hand radiographic scores (Fig. 3.3) [15].

Laboratory tests, including rheumatoid factor, elevated ESR, elevated CRP, the shared epitope based on the major histocompatibility locus [16], etc., are associated with a higher level of radiographic progression [17], but physical function scores are far more significant than laboratory tests (or radiographic progression) in prognosis of other severe RA outcomes. Although not as extensively documented as in RA, similar findings appear in other rheumatic diseases. In one study in a general, non-diseased normal elderly cohort, poor physical function on a patient questionnaire was as significant in the prediction of 5-year survival as smoking [18].

3. Long-term outcomes of rheumatic diseases (and many chronic diseases) appear determined as much by actions of individual patients as by actions of health professionals and medications [16, 19–21]. A valuable surrogate for patient actions is formal education level; low education is associated with high incidence, prevalence, morbidity, and mortality of many chronic diseases. For example, education level also is often more significant than poor laboratory tests, joint counts, and/or

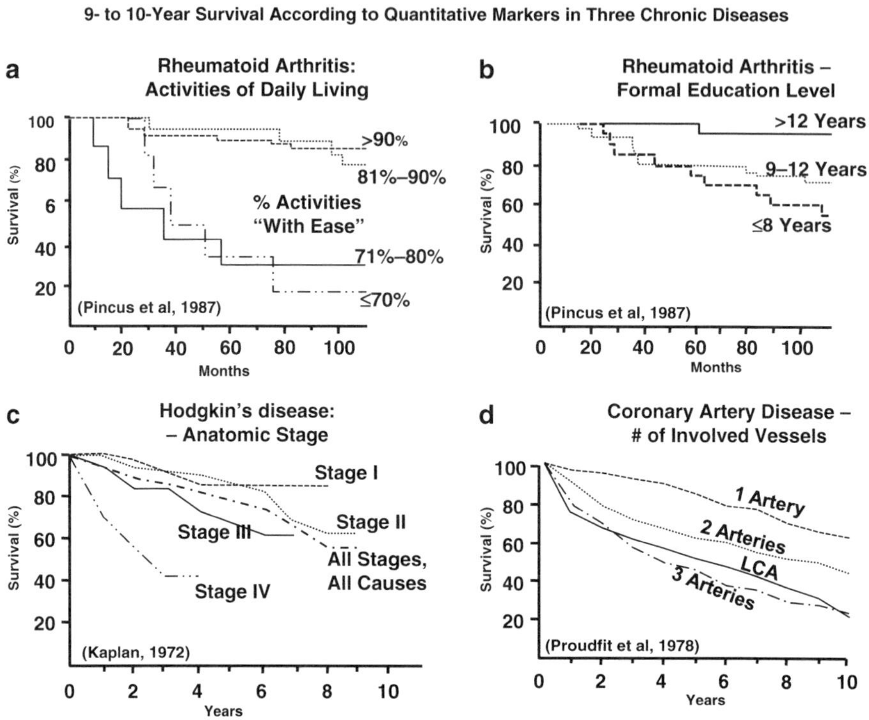

Fig. 3.2 9- to 10-year survival according to quantitative markers in 3 chronic diseases: (**a**, **b**) rheumatoid arthritis, (**c**) Hodgkin's Disease, and (**d**) coronary artery disease

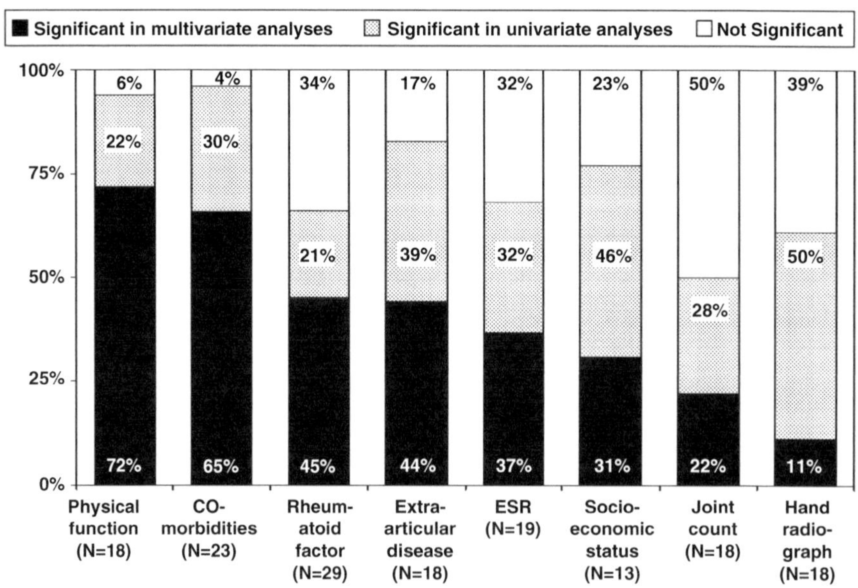

Fig. 3.3 Significance of 8 variables as predictors of mortality, in a review of 84 reports concerning mortality in RA, 53 cohorts presented predictors of mortality. For each variable, n = the number of reports that included the variable, and *bars* indicate the percentage of those reports in which the variable was a significant predictor of mortality in multivariate analyses (*black*), in univariate analyses (*dotted*), or not significant (*white*)

hand radiographic scores to predict mortality in RA [14, 19, 22, 23]. Figures 3.2 and 3.3 Poor RA status according to a joint examination, laboratory measures, and patient questionnaire measures is more likely to be identified according to low education level than high age or long duration of disease [24, 25]. Low socioeconomic status is associated with a higher likelihood of premature mortality in the general population, including RA [26]. Socioeconomic status may be regarded as a surrogate for the importance of patient actions, in addition to actions of health professionals, in the course and outcomes of rheumatic and other chronic diseases.

Limitations of Laboratory Test Biomarkers in Rheumatic Diseases

The discovery in 1948 of rheumatoid factor [27] and the LE cell [28] raised hopes that diagnosis and management of rheumatic diseases could be approached with "gold standard" biomarkers, analogous to blood pressure in hypertension or serum glucose in diabetes. Rheumatoid factor and other laboratory discoveries have been indispensable to understanding of pathogenesis and development of new treatments. For example, biological therapies, which have added considerably to the capacity to treat rheumatic diseases, would likely not be available without the discovery of of rheumatoid factor, leading to subsequent recognition of likely cytokines, immunoactive cells, and other biomarkers.

In contrast to their immense value for research to understand pathogenesis and develop new treatments, biomarkers remain of limited value in *clinical* diagnosis and management of rheumatic diseases. For example, in RA, rheumatoid factor, anticitrullinated protein antibodies (ACPA), elevated ESR and CRP are found in more than half of patients with RA at presentation. However, each of these four biomarker tests is not abnormal in 30–40 % of new patients—a substantial minority.

A meta-analysis of all available studies indicated that rheumatoid factor is found in only 69 % of patients with RA in 50 studies (similar to the initial 1948 report [27]) and ACPA (reported in 1998 [29]) in only 67 % of patients in 37 studies; furthermore, 5 % of normal individuals have a (false) positive test [30]. Of course, an individual who has a positive test for rheumatoid factor or ACPA has a considerably higher likelihood to have RA compared to individuals in the general population. However, the prevalence of RA is 0.5 %. In other words, 5 in 1000 people have RA, while formal studies suggest that 50 among 1000 individuals in the general population have a positive rheumatoid factor test [30]. Therefore, only 1 in 10 with rheumatoid factor has RA, and most people in the general population who have a positive test for rheumatoid factor (or ACPA) do not have RA.

Most people do not have a positive rheumatoid factor test, but the high prevalence of musculoskeletal symptoms [31] leads to many "false-positive" tests. Since the medical history and physical examination dominate clinical decisions in the management of RA, (unlike many chronic diseases) [2], one could argue that the *clinical* approach to RA need not include a test for rheumatoid factor or ACPA, although most rheumatologists would not agree.

ESR and CRP may be useful to monitor clinical activity in certain patients with RA [32]; however, at least 40 % of new patients with RA identified from clinical settings over the last 20 years have normal values for each of these tests at presentation [33–36]. Furthermore, improvement in clinical status may be accompanied by continued abnormal, and often unchanged, ESR, as well as CRP [37]. A larger proportion of patients had abnormal values for ESR in earlier periods [38], and a decline in the likelihood of an abnormal ESR or CRP may reflect improved status of RA patients over the last few decades [39]. One might suggest that the purpose of monitoring ESR and/or CRP is as much to recognize a possible infection or malignancy in an individual patient with RA as to recognize a flare of disease activity.

In SLE, laboratory evidence does appear required, as no characteristic clinical finding such as joint swelling in RA is seen in all patients. However, while the initial screening test for antinuclear antibodies (ANA) is positive in >99 % of patients with SLE (perhaps ANA-negative SLE exists, perhaps not), it also is positive in at least 10–15 % of women in the general population [40]. SLE occurs in about 0.05 % of the population; therefore, about 1 in 100 people with a positive ANA has SLE, an important problem when a non-rheumatologist (and sometimes a rheumatologist) orders an ANA as a "screening test" [41, 42] for individuals with any specific or nonspecific musculoskeletal problem. A "positive ANA" is a frequent basis for a referral to a rheumatologist, usually with no clinical findings to support a diagnosis of SLE. Nonetheless, many erroneous "diagnoses" of SLE are made in people who have musculoskeletal symptoms and a positive ANA test.

A positive test for DNA antibodies was found in 75 % of SLE patients in 1969, and reduction of levels of these antibodies (and ESR), along with increases in serum complement, were recognized in association with clinical improvement [43]. However, even in the initial report, 25 % of SLE patients had negative tests for DNA antibodies [43], a pattern that continues to this day [40, 44]. This phenomenon is similar to findings with rheumatoid factor and ACPA, and has been overlooked in expectation that better methods would unearth these antibodies in all patients or other "diagnostic" biomarkers might be discovered, but that has not been the case over more than five decades.

A number of ANA subsets have been described to be associated with different features of SLE, such as associations of anti-Smith (Sm) with renal disease and anti-ribonucleoprotein (RNP) with mixed connective tissue disease (MCTD) [45]. However, none of these tests are more than 70 % specific to any clinical findings or particular diagnosis to affect clinical decisions, which are made on the basis of clinical findings [46]. Indeed, a follow-up study indicated that almost half of the initial MCTD patients appeared to have different diagnoses, including RA or systemic sclerosis, on subsequent evaluation years later [47]. This phenomenon is seen in most rheumatic disease databases over a decade or longer, in which at least 5 % of patients have a different primary diagnosis. Tests of ANA subsets have important value for research concerning pathogenesis and treatment, as seen for rheumatoid factor in RA, but appear to add expense without value in routine clinical care.

One reason that biomarkers such as laboratory tests and radiographs are emphasized in diagnosis and monitoring involves the biomedical model paradigm, as noted previously, which is highly effective in many diseases [1]. However, a more pragmatic reason is that changes in laboratory values are seen over days and are the most significant predictor of radiographic progression [17], which could be recognized over 6–12 months in patient groups in clinical trials [48]. By contrast, outcomes of work disability and premature mortality require 5–15 years for analyses [49]. Observation of long-term outcomes is outside the time frame of clinical trials and requires maintenance of long-term databases, which remain unavailable in most rheumatology clinical settings. Therefore, more attention concerning outcomes of RA has been directed to radiographic progression than to work disability and premature mortality, for which biomarkers are not nearly as significant in prognosis as physical function on a patient questionnaire.

Patient Questionnaires for Research Versus Clinical Care

The experience of most physicians with patient questionnaires has been in clinical trials and other clinical research, and/or in many clinical care using an "intake" questionnaire for new patients (Table 3.2). Patient questionnaires for many clinical trials and clinical research studies frequently are long, and not amenable to easy completion by patients or review by physicians in busy clinical settings. Indeed, in clinical trials, a clinician generally is directed *not* to review the questionnaire, other than for completeness (often the responsibility of a study coordinator), which is forwarded to a "data center" for analysis. The questionnaire is not designed to have any impact on clinical care (Table 3.2).

Patient "intake" questionnaires for initial clinical care visits are used to facilitate compilation of a patient's medical history and demographic data. Information on an intake questionnaire generally is not recorded in a *standard*, "scientific," protocol-driven format. Furthermore, most intake questionnaires do not include quantitative scores (for pain, function, fatigue, etc.), analogous to laboratory tests. Therefore, most intake questionnaires remain "subjective" and "nonscientific" (Table 3.2). The information is entered into a medical record by a physician or assistant through typing, dictation, or handwriting. Patients who see a new doctor, particularly in a different locale from a previous doctor (but sometimes in the same locale), usually must complete a new intake questionnaire, as the information from previous intake questionnaires has not been recorded in an easily retrievable format.

By contrast, patient questionnaires designed to guide clinical care, such as a health assessment questionnaire (HAQ) (see Appendix chapter) [50], derivative multidimensional HAQ (MDHAQ) [51, 52], HAQii [53], and others, are short—generally two sides of a single sheet of paper (Table 3.2). The emphasis is on feasibility and clinical utility, although psychometric criteria (see Appendix chapter A) for validity and reliability required for all questionnaires must be met. A 4-page format of the MDHAQ facilitates a more advanced intake questionnaire, as described later. The MDHAQ (see Appendix chapter B) and similar questionnaires are standardized and meet criteria for "scientific" measures, involving protocol-driven (same format) quantitative scores, analogous to laboratory tests, to help guide clinical decisions (Table 3.2).

Table 3.2 Patient questionnaire measures for clinical research versus clinical care

Feature	Clinical research	New patient intake	Clinical care
Design considerations	Complete, long	Provide medical history	Patient friendly, short, completed by patient within 5–10 min
Effect on patient visit	Adds time, interferes with flow	*Saves* time for MD and patient	*Saves* time for MD and patient
Type of questionnaire	May be "generic," "disease specific," other research goals	Applicable to patients with all rheumatic diseases	Applicable to patients with all rheumatic diseases
Scoring	Complex, requires computer	Simple, may "eyeball" results in ~30 s	Simple, may "eyeball" results; scored in 10–15 s
Goal of data	Add to research database	Add to clinical care	Add to clinical care
Focus of analysis	Groups of patients in clinical trials or observational databases	Individual patients cared for by individual physicians	Individual patients cared for by individual physicians
Data management	Send to data center	May enter into office database to initiate patient record	Review for patient care; may enter into flow-sheet to compare to previous visits
Quantitative scores	Yes	No	Yes
Entry into structured database	Yes	Usually not	Yes
Major criteria for use	Validity, reliability; assess minimal clinically important significant difference (MCID)	New patient history	Document status, medical and medico-legal rationale for aggressive therapies
Disposition of questionnaire	Central study data center enters into computer	Physician enters into computer	Enter into flow sheet in medical record

Despite their value in assessment, monitoring, prognosis, and outcomes, patient questionnaires are not implemented at this time in most rheumatology care settings [54]. Changes in status of most patients with rheumatic diseases continue to be recorded at most busy rheumatology sites only as narrative descriptions without quantitative patient data. The only quantitative data in the medical records of most patients of rheumatologists are laboratory tests, the limitations of which led to recognition of a need for indices [42, 55].

Emphasis on laboratory tests, without quantitative patient or physician scores to monitor patient status, may continue to result in a situation described more than 30 years ago in which "clinicians may easily write 'doing well' in the notes of the patient who has become progressively crippled before their eyes" [56]. It is ironic that pharmaceutical companies collect self-report questionnaires to document improvement in patient status for registration of new therapies, but most rheumatologists have not adopted this practice in usual clinical care. The issue of feasibility is important, as expressed in an editorial that queried, "Is it better to have 80 % of the information in 100 % of patients or 100 % of the information in 5 % of patients?" [57]. Much of this chapter is concerned with documenting the value of a feasible "80 % measure" that will contribute to patient welfare, in contrast to a possibly preferable "100 % measure" that may be more informative in clinical research, but generally not feasible in routine clinical care and therefore not used at all.

Development of MDHAQ as a Clinical Tool for Continuous Quality Improvement in Usual Care, Rather Than as a Research Tool

A major milestone for rheumatology was seen in 1980 with publication of the health assessment questionnaire (HAQ) [50] and arthritis impact measurement scales (AIMS) [58]. These reports introduced the concept that rheumatic diseases could be viewed quantitatively from a patient's perspective, consistent with a "biopsychosocial model" that is complementary to a biomedical model [1]. Patient self-report questionnaires can be used to record patient history information as quantitative, standard scores, which meet criteria for "scientific" data, analogous to laboratory tests, to supplement and substitute for narrative descriptions.

Over the ensuing 36 years, patient self-report questionnaires have advanced knowledge concerning the prognosis, course, and outcomes of rheumatic diseases, much of which was unavailable previously prior to availability of patient self-report data.

Soon after publication in 1980, the HAQ and AIMS were introduced to usual clinical care in one clinical setting at Vanderbilt University [59, 60]. Although the psychometric properties of the AIMS were well established, it became apparent that the HAQ was more patient-friendly. Furthermore, it was far more feasible to ask *each* patient with *any* diagnosis to complete the *same* simple questionnaire than to attempt to select different patients to compete different (or no) questionnaires [60].

Experience over the years emphasizing feasibility and clinical relevance led to many changes to facilitate the value of completion of questionnaire each at visit to both patients and doctors in clinical care and outcomes research. These changes over more than 25 years to develop an MDHAQ are viewed primarily as a continuous quality improvement (CQI) activity with the primary aim of improving patient care, rather than as a research activity [59, 60], although quantitative data from the MDHAQ have provided valuable clinical research results [39, 61–66]. As noted, the emphasis was on feasibility, clinical value, saving time for the physician, and relevance to predict an outcome, as seen with a laboratory test, although it was also regarded as necessary and important to meet psychometric criteria for validity and reliability required in all questionnaires.

The CQI approach differs from traditional clinical research and clinical trials in seeking to account for *all* patients rather than a few *selected* patients, as in most clinical trials, and to implement findings in actual care. CQI involves a series of

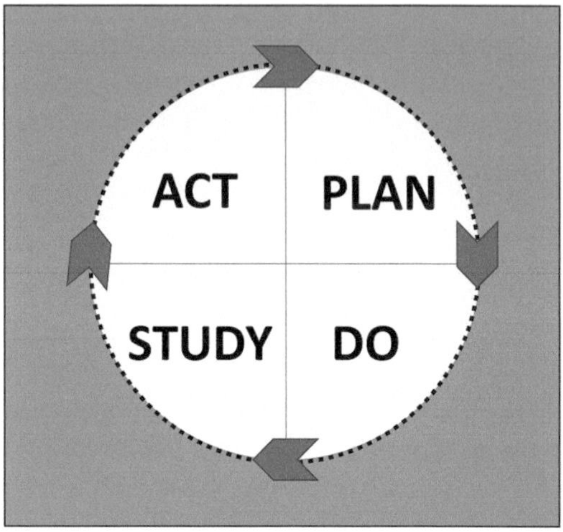

Fig. 3.4 Four stages of Continuous Quality Improvement (CQI) cycles: plan, do, study, act

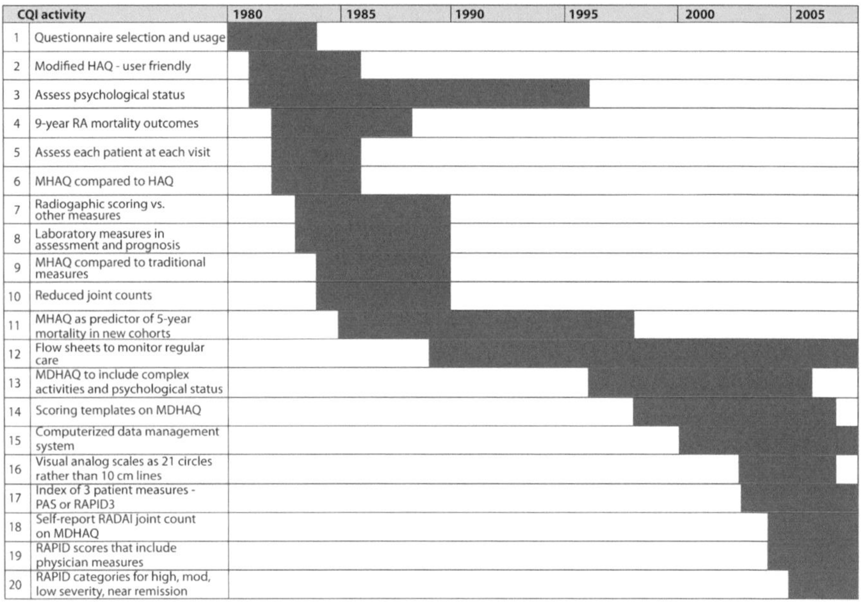

Fig. 3.5 Development of multidimensional health assessment questionnaire (MDHAQ) over 25 years as a continuous quality improvement (CQI) activity: *HAQ* Health Assessment Questionnaire, *MHAQ* modified HAQ, *RAPID* Routine Assessment of Patient Index

small "plan-do-study-act" cycles (Fig. 3.4), rather than a grand "definitive" research design. At least 20 cycles of changes in the HAQ, initially as a modified HAQ (MHAQ) reported in 1983 [67], and ultimately as a multidimensional HAQ (MDHAQ) reported in 1999 [51] and 2005 [52], can be identified (Fig. 3.5).

The MDHAQ Compared to the HAQ

Both the HAQ (see Appendix Chapter) and MDHAQ (see Appendix A) for "return" patients (Table 3.3) are 2-page questionnaires (both sides of a single sheet of paper) completed by a patient in 5–10 min, and both have templates for a composite quantitative score. Both include a score for physical function by patient self-report on a 0–3 scale (0 = without any difficulty, 1 = with some difficulty, 2 = with much difficulty, 3 = unable to do). Both include scores for pain and patient global estimate on a 0–10 visual analog scale (VAS). Quantitative scores for physical function, pain, and patient global estimate are the three self-report measures in an RA core data set of seven measures [68].

Primary differences between the HAQ and MDHAQ, developed to enhance feasibility, provide clinical information in a busy setting, save time for the physician and patient, and improve documentation, include (Table 3.3):

1. *Activities*: The HAQ includes 20 activities grouped into 8 categories of 2 or 3 activities each, while the MDHAQ includes 10 activities, 8 verbatim from the HAQ (1 from each of the 8 HAQ categories), and 2 additional complex activities, added in the 1990s, when patient status was much improved from 2 decades earlier [39]. By the 1980's, many patients had scores of "zero" on the simple HAQ activities, suggesting "normal" physical function, despite experiencing ongoing limitations to perform more difficult physical activities [51]. A scoring template is available to convert the sum of ten 0–3 scores (range 0–30) to a 0–10 physical function score through division by 3.

Table 3.3 Comparison of health assessment questionnaire (HAQ) and multidimensional health assessment questionnaire (MDHAQ)

	HAQ	MDHAQ
First report	1980	1999
Patient completion	5–10 min	5–10 min
# Activities of daily living	20	10
Pain VAS	10 cm line	21 circles
Patient global VAS	10 cm line	21 circles
Fatigue	No	21 circles
Psychological variables: sleep, anxiety, depression	No	3-HAQ format
Review of systems	No	60 symptoms
Medical history	No	Yes
Demographic data	No	Yes
Social history	No	Yes
Scoring templates	No	Yes
MD scan ("eyeball")	30 s	5 s
Time to score	41.8 s	4.5 s
Time to score index of 3 measures	Not available	9.5 s

2. *Psychological queries in HAQ format*: Many patients also reported problems with sleep, anxiety, and depression, which appeared relevant to document. Therefore, three new queries were introduced in the patient-friendly HAQ format concerning sleep quality and capacity to deal with anxiety and depression.
3. *Visual analog scales (VAS) for pain and patient global estimate* on the MDHAQ are in a 21-circle format, rather than a 10-cm line as on the HAQ [69], which facilitates scoring for patients, doctors, and staff. A ruler is not needed, and boxes are available to enter scores for these individual measures, to calculate RAPID3 (routine assessment of patient index data).
4. *RAPID3 (routine assessment of patient index data)*—a 0–30 composite index of 3 0–10 scales for physical function, pain, and patient global estimate [70, 71].
5. *Self-report joint count*, as a rheumatoid arthritis disease activity index (RADAI) [52], is positioned on the MDHAQ between two 0–10 VAS for pain and global status in order to reduce the likelihood of patients giving the same answer on both VAS (although scores are similar in most patients, as level of pain is related to global well-being). RADAI scores are correlated significantly with tender joint count ($r=0.55$) and swollen joint count ($r=0.42$), in the same range as ESR with CRP ($r=0.50$) in the same database [71].
6. *Symptom checklist:* The MDHAQ includes a symptom checklist not found on the HAQ, introduced initially to serve as a review of systems. Over the years, it has been found that patients who check more than 20 of 60 symptoms generally have non-inflammatory problems of distress, such as fibromyalgia or depression, although they may also meet formal criteria for RA, systemic lupus erythematosus (SLE), or other rheumatic disease [61, 63]. Fibromyalgia is seen in 15–30% of patients with RA [72] or SLE [73], and a clue from a symptom checklist can be quite helpful clinically in these patients.
7. *Fatigue VAS*: The MDHAQ also includes a 0–10 VAS for fatigue, not found on the HAQ. Fatigue is an important problem for many patients with rheumatic diseases [74].
8. *Exercise status*: The MDHAQ includes queries about exercise status. Lack of exercise is an important prognostic indicator for mortality in the general elderly population, as significant as smoking in the prognosis of 5-year survival [18].
9. *Medical history information*: The MDHAQ includes 12 queries concerning recent medical history: surgeries, illnesses, hospitalization, etc. A series of "no" responses saves a physician at least 2 min, whereas a "yes" response indicates a matter that should be characterized at the visit.
10. *Demographic data*: Date of birth, gender, ethnic group, marital status, occupation, and formal education level are queried, so a database can be developed directly from the questionnaire.

As noted, the most effective strategy for collection of an MDHAQ in standard clinical care is to distribute the questionnaire to each patient with any diagnosis upon registration at the reception desk in any clinical setting [75]. Completion in the waiting area helps prepare the patient for the visit, improves doctor–patient communication, and saves time for both doctor and patient. The MDHAQ allows a health professional to obtain information in 5–10 s that otherwise would require 10–15 min of conversation. Nonetheless, self-report of a medical history *always* requires *interpretation* by a knowledgeable health professional, as is the case with a laboratory test such as ESR or CRP, or ancillary study such as ultrasound, as discussed later in the section on the RheuMetric checklist [76].

Routine Assessment of Patient Index Data (RAPID3): An Index of Only Patient Self-Report Measures

RAPID3 is an index of only the 3 RA Core Data Set patient self-report measures [77, 78]. The MDHAQ (Appendix A) includes small boxes to enter scores for physical function (FN), pain (PN), patient global estimate of status (PATGL) (each scored 0–10), as well as a composite RAPID3 score (0–30), in "For Office Use Only" sections. RAPID3 on an MDHAQ is scored in about 5 s, versus almost 2 min for Disease Activity Score (DAS28) or Clinical Disease Activity Index (CDAI) [71] (Fig. 3.6). RAPID3 appears feasible to implement a treat-to-target strategy in usual clinical care [79]. Four categories of RAPID3 scores—for high, moderate, and low severity, and remission—are correlated significantly with similar categories using DAS28 and CDAI [71, 78, 80]. RAPID3 offers many scientific and pragmatic advantages to patients and doctors [81] as discussed below.

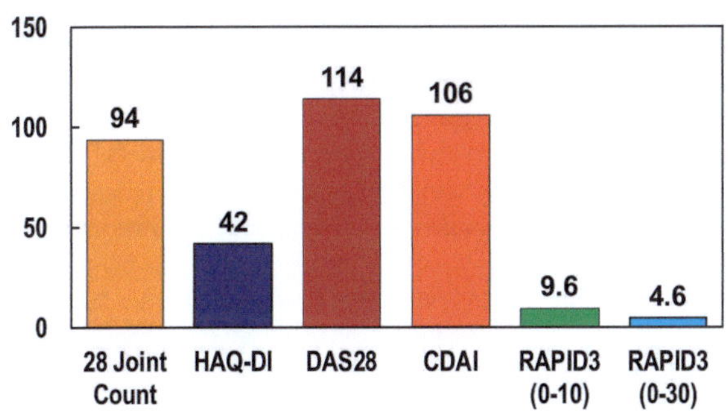

Fig. 3.6 Time to score various rheumatoid arthritis indices in seconds, including 28 joint count, health assessment questionnaire-disability index (HAQ-DI), disease activity score 28 (DAS28), clinical disease activity index (CDAI), routine assessment of patient index data (RAPID3) scores 0–10, RAPID3 scored 0–30

Scientific Advantages of MDHAQ/RAPID3

The "scientific" value of MDHAQ/RAPID3 scores is supported by extensive evidence (Table 3.4) [4–6, 8, 10–13, 25, 77, 81–110]. As noted, physical function scores on a patient self-report questionnaire are more significant than laboratory tests, radiographs, or other high-technology data to predict premature death [4, 11–13], confirmed in a review of all 53 RA cohorts, which included prognostic variables for RA mortality [15] (Fig. 3.3). Physical function scores on a patient self-report questionnaire generally also are more significant than laboratory tests or radiographs to predict most other severe long-term outcomes of rheumatoid arthritis (RA), including work disability [3–7], costs [8, 9], and joint replacement surgery [10]. Radiographic progression is the only major RA outcome predicted by laboratory tests, including rheumatoid factor, elevated ESR, elevated CRP, and the shared epitope of the major histocompatibility locus [17]. However, physical function scores are far more significant than laboratory tests (or radiographic progression) in prognosis of other severe RA outcomes.

Patient questionnaire scores are more reproducible than formal joint counts [82–88] (Table 3.5 [111]) in large part because a single observer (in this case the patient) is likely more consistent than two observers (a joint count has input from both doctor and patient) [88]. RAPID3 is correlated significantly with DAS28 and CDAI in clinical trials [77, 93–95] and clinical care [71, 78] (Fig. 3.7), including categories for high, moderate, low disease severity, and remission [71, 78, 80, 95]. Individual patient self-report measures of physical function, pain, and patient global estimate of status are as efficient as joint counts and laboratory tests to distinguish active from control treatments in clinical trials [89–92] (Fig. 3.8). RAPID3 gives

Table 3.4 Scientific advantages of MDHAQ/RAPID3

	Scientific foundation of MDHAQ/RAPID3
1	MDHAQ scores are more reproducible than formal joint counts by physicians [82–88]
2	Individual patient self-report measures of physical function, pain, and patient global estimate of status, and RAPID3, are as efficient as joint counts, laboratory tests, DAS28 or CDAI to distinguish active from control treatments in clinical trials [89–92]
3	RAPID3 is correlated significantly with DAS28 and CDAI in clinical trials [77, 93–95] and clinical care [71, 78], including categories for high, moderate, low severity and remission [71, 78, 80, 95]
4	Physical function scores on MDHAQ and other questionnaires are far more significant than radiographs or laboratory tests in the prognosis of severe outcomes in RA, including work disability, costs, joint replacement surgery and premature death [4–6, 8, 10–13, 25, 96–100]
5	More likely to be abnormal in RA than laboratory tests [81]
6	More likely to be document incomplete response to methotrexate and initiation of biological agent in RA than ESR [101]
7	RAPID3 provides criteria for remission in RA comparable to Boolean and SDAI criteria [102]
8	RAPID3 is informative in most, if not all, rheumatic diseases[103–110]

Table 3.5 Correlations and test-retest reliability of RA measures and indices at 2 time points [111]

Measure/index	Spearman rho	ICC
TJC28	0.76	0.83
SJC28	0.74	0.78
Physician global	0.69	0.79
Patient global	0.80	0.78
Function	0.98	0.96
Pain	0.83	0.88
ESR	0.84	0.95
CRP	0.71	0.97
DAS28	0.85	0.85
SDAI	0.87	0.88
CDAI	0.89	0.89
RAPID3	0.88	0.90
RADAI	0.89	0.92

similar results to DAS28 and CDAI to distinguish active from control treatments in clinical trials of leflunomide [93], methotrexate [93], adalimumab [94], abatacept [77], and certolizumab [95].

RAPID3 is more likely to be abnormal in new patients with RA than laboratory tests [81], and more likely than ESR to document incomplete responses to methotrexate and initiation of a biological agent in RA [101] (Table 3.6). RAPID3 also provides criteria for remission in RA, documented in a recent report concerning the ESPOIR usual care cohort in France [102]. MDHAQ/RAPID3 is informative to assess improvement or worsening of patient status over time in many rheumatic diseases [104] (Fig. 3.9, Table 3.7 [61, 63, 103–108, 110, 112]), including systemic lupus erythematosus [103, 104], osteoarthritis [104], ankylosing spondylitis [104–108], psoriatic arthritis [104], gout [104], vasculitis [109], and others [104, 110]. These data indicate that patient self-report scores can be as "scientific" as laboratory tests.

Pragmatic Advantages of MDHAQ/RAPID3

MDHAQ/RAPID3 presents many pragmatic advantages to both patients and doctors for rheumatology care (Table 3.8) [81, 113]. Advantages to the patient include: The patient prepares for the encounter by focusing on concerns to discuss with the doctor. The MDHAQ empowers the patient as a partner in care, and improves doctor/patient communication, with an "agenda" or "road map" available *before* the encounter for both patient and doctor [113].

Pragmatic advantages to the rheumatologist include (Table 3.8): The patient does almost all the work. MDHAQ/RAPID3 does not disrupt office flow or require any time and effort from the doctor to collect the data, when presented to each patient

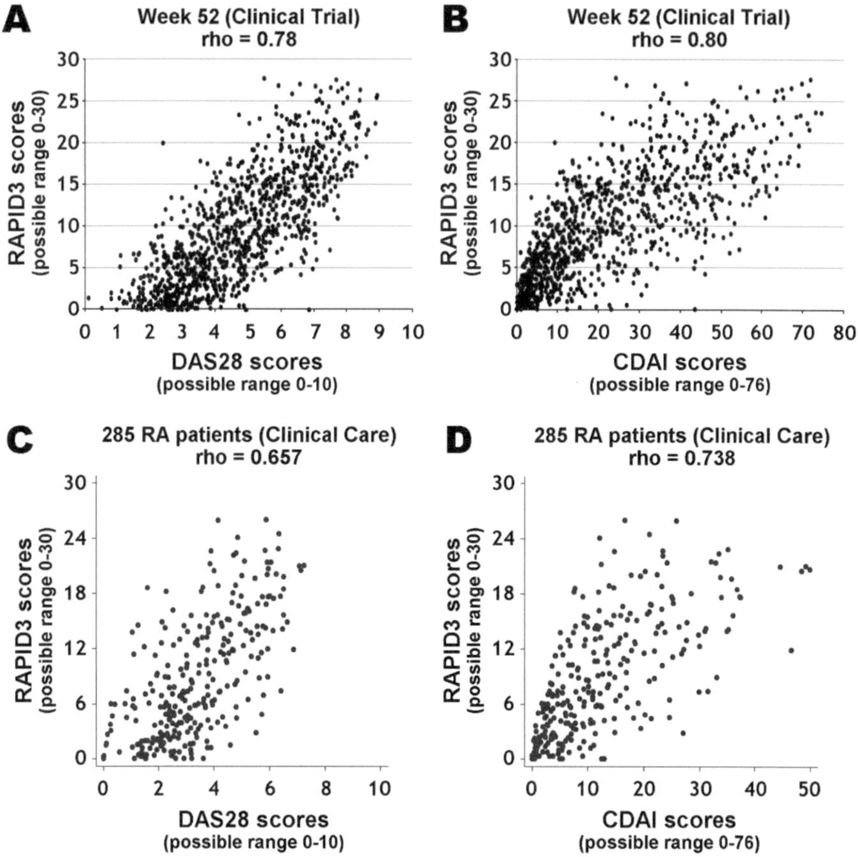

Fig. 3.7 Spearman correlations of RAPID3 (routine assessment of patient index data 3) scores with (**a**, **c**) the Disease Activity Score (DAS28) and (B, D) Clinical Disease Activity Index (CDAI) in (**a**, **b**) the rheumatoid arthritis prevention of structural damage (RAPID1) clinical trial of certolizumab pegol in 982 patients at 52 weeks and (**c**, **d**) in 285 patients with RA seen in usual clinical care

for completion at each visit as part of the infrastructure of care. Indeed, MDHAQ saves time for the doctor by providing a 10–15 s overview of medical history data that would otherwise require about 10–15 min of conversation, including the self-report joint count, fatigue VAS, improvement scale, symptom checklist, and recent medical history.

RAPID3 is scored in 5 s, as noted previously, compared to about 40 s for a HAQ, 90–95 s for a formal joint count, 104 s for a CDAI, and 116 s for a DAS28 [71] (Fig. 3.6). RAPID3 levels for high, moderate, low disease severity and remission can be used effectively for “treat-to-target” in RA. Unlike a formal joint count, MDHAQ/RAPID3 does not require the same examiner at each assessment, as a

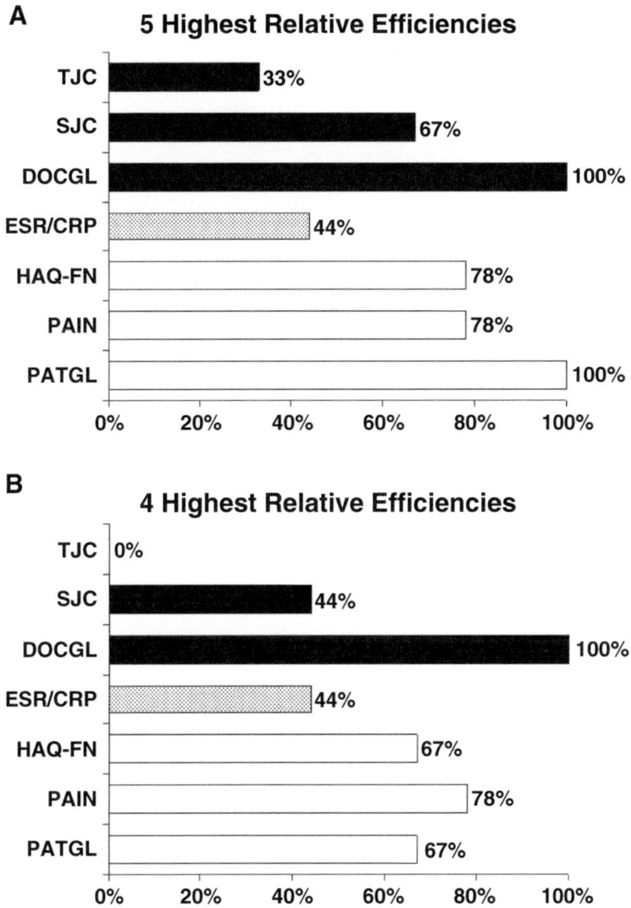

Fig. 3.8 (**a–d**) Relative efficiencies of seven rheumatoid arthritis (RA) Core Data Set measures to distinguish active from control treatments in 9 clinical trials, involving methotrexate, leflunomide, placebo, infliximab, adalimumab, and abatacept according to arithmetic and percentage changes

single observer (the patient) provides the data for clinical interpretation by the physician. Monitoring of a patient according to, say, DAS28 or CDAI may not be possible at the time of a patient contact or visit, due to: insufficient time to perform a formal joint count, absence of a laboratory test (for DAS28), the patient has traveled to another locale, and/or others. Collection of an MDHAQ/RAPID3 assures that *some* quantitative data concerning patient status is recorded at every visit, and certainly does not preclude scoring a DAS28, CDAI, or any other quantitative measure or index that is regarded as informative by the treating physician.

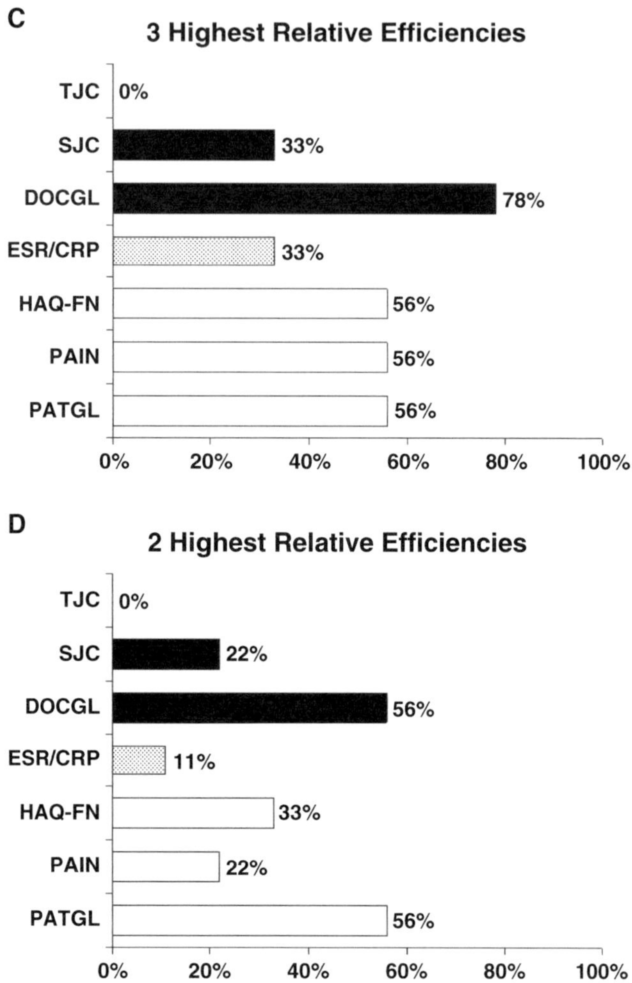

Fig. 3.8 (continued)

Table 3.6 Median levels of all patients for erythrocyte sedimentation rate (ESR), 3 (0–10) MDHAQ scores for physical function, pain, and patient global estimate and composite routine assessment of patient index data (RAPID3) scores at initiation of methotrexate 1996–2001 and mean of 2.6 years later in (A) *30 incomplete responders* initiating biologic agent, and (B) *63 "control" adequate responders* continuing Methotrexate [101]

	A. 30 Incomplete responders		B. 63 Adequate responders ("Controls")	
	MTX start	Biologic start	MTX start	Follow-up (NO biologic)
ESR (mm/h)	28	18	24	16
MDHAQ-function (0–10)	3.2	3.3	2.3	1.0
Pain (0–10)	5.2	6.8	4.1	1.4
Patient global (0–10)	5.5	5.5	4.2	0.9
RAPID3 (0–30)	14.9	16.2	10.6	3.6

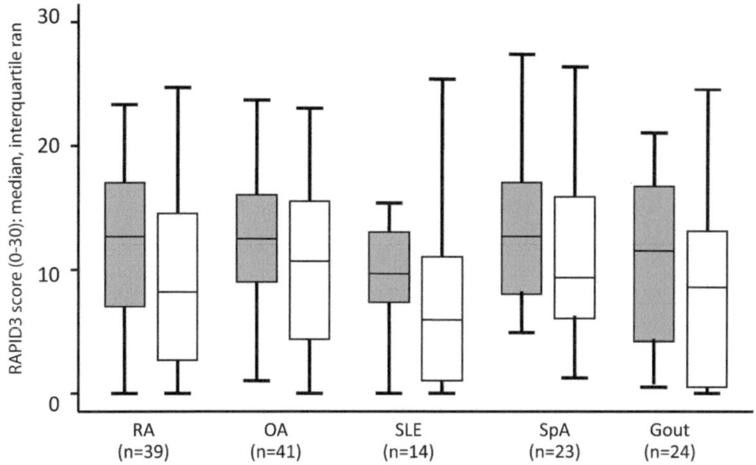

Fig. 3.9 Improvement in RAPID3 (routine assessment of patient index data 3) scores over 2 months in patients with 5 rheumatic diseases: rheumatoid arthritis (RA), osteoarthritis (OA), systemic lupus erythematosus (SLE), spondyloarthritis (SpA), gout

Table 3.7 Rheumatic diseases in which RAPID3 has been reported to be informative about patient status and/or change in status

Rheumatic disease(s)	References
Systemic lupus erythematosus	Askanase et al. [103]
	Castrejon et al. [104]
Osteoarthritis	Castrejon et al. [104]
Ankylosing spondylitis	Castrejon et al. [104]
	Danve et al. [105]
	Cinar et al. [106]
	Michelsen et al. [107]
	Park et al. [108]
Psoriatic arthritis	Castrejon et al. [104]
Gout	Castrejon et al. [104]
Vasculitis	Annapureddy et al. [109]
Fibromyalgia	Callahan et al. [112]
	DeWalt et al. [61]
	Pincus et al. [63]
Other	Castrejon et al. [104]
	Pincus et al. [110]

A 4-Page MDHAQ: Patient Questionnaires to Provide a Standard, "Scientific" Medical History for Updating by Patients and Doctors, Rather Than Narrative Descriptions

As noted earlier, many physicians include an "intake" patient questionnaire at initial visits. However, few intake questionnaires include quantitative scores analogous to laboratory tests, or record narrative information in a *standard*, "scientific,"

Table 3.8 Pragmatic advantages of MDHAQ/RAPID3

A	*Pragmatic advantages of MDHAQ/RAPID3 to the patient*
1	Helps prepare the patient for encounter by focusing on concerns to discuss with the doctor
2	Empowers patient as partner in care
3	Improves doctor–patient communication—"agenda" or "road map" available for both *before* encounter
B	*Pragmatic advantages of MDHAQ/RAPID3 to the doctor*
1	The patient does almost all the work
2	Does not disrupt office flow or require any time and effort from the doctor, when presented to each patient for completion at each visit as part of the infrastructure of care
3	MDHAQ saves time for the doctor, providing a 10–15 s overview of medical history data that would otherwise require about 10–15 min of conversation, including a self-report joint count, review of systems, recent medical history
4	RAPID3 is scored in 5 s, compared to 40 s for a HAQ, 90–95 s for a formal joint count, 104 s for a CDAI, and 116 s for a DAS28
5	RAPID3 levels for high, moderate, and low severity, and remission, can be used effectively for treat-to-target in RA
6	More reproducible than joint counts or radiographic scores, as there is only one observer (the patient): does not require the same examiner at each assessment, unlike joint count or radiographic score
7	Ensures that quantitative data concerning patient status is recorded at every visit, even if joint count or physician global not preformed and/or lab test is not available
8	Informative in most, if not all, rheumatic diseases—also included in scientific advantages

protocol-driven format. Therefore, most intake questionnaires remain "subjective" and "nonscientific" (Table 3.2). A patient who is seen by different health professionals often is asked to complete new intake questionnaires, although 50 % or more of the information is redundant with previously completed questionnaires.

The 4-page version of the MDHAQ (Appendix B) for an initial patient visit (or initial entry into a database) includes medical history information for entry into a medical database for a medical record. This version includes scales for physical function, pain, global status, RAPID3, fatigue, self-report joint count, review of systems, exercise, change in status, morning stiffness, recent medical history, and demographic data found on the 2-page MDHAQ (Appendix A). In addition, a 4-page (2 sheets of paper) version includes elements of a standard medical history: previous illnesses, surgeries, hospitalizations, allergies to medications and other substances, family history, social history, and current medications.

The 4-page MDHAQ also includes a request for two patient consents, in addition to usual consents asked of new patients:

1. to share de-identified data beyond the patient's physician with a few selected research colleagues designated by the attending physician, for possible collab-

orative analyses of data at other locations in multicenter databases, while maintaining strict confidentiality of patient data.

2. to be contacted up to every 6 months by a data center in the future, if the patient is no longer seen at the same initial clinical setting (a much more frequent occurrence than recognized by most clinicians), to monitor patient status indefinitely in longitudinal observations of long-term outcomes.

Most patients have been pleased to learn of an interest by health professionals in long-term outcomes, and offer consent; although a few do not consent—a phenomenon that unfortunately may be increasing with incidents of breaching of security and privacy.

An electronic patient history may be summarized in two reports, one for the physician and one for the patient. The report for the physician presents a listing of past history, including illnesses, surgeries, hospitalizations, allergies, family history, and social history in a medical record format, for direct entry into an electronic medical record (EMR) after review by the physician if desired. The attending physician must add a "chief complaint," present illness narrative (which can be quite brief), physical examination, and management plan. This capacity requires a design to interface with an EMR, with a design to overcome the problem of multiple incompatible EMRs through an HL7 interface and SMART on FHIR [114–116], which is incorporated into development of the electronic 2- and 4-page MDHAQ. Implementation of an interface with the EMR does require initial collaboration with the EMR vendor. However, the possible complexity of this collaboration for an interface could reduce considerably the burden of typing or dictation by the physician or assistant with each individual patient.

The second report of 4-page MDHAQ data to the patient is designed for the patient to amend and/or correct errors in her/his medical history. Of course, a medical record is a legal document that cannot be altered. However, a medical history database could be amended by the patient for future visits, to review for accuracy and completeness, and amend with new developments over the patient's lifetime. The electronic history also could be made available by the patient to other practitioners involved in the patient's care, or through the EMR with patient consent, for capacity for review and endorsement within the record by the physician, and the possibility of extracting the data for subsequent clinical research. Again an HL7 interface and SMART on FHIR appears required to overcome the problem of multiple incompatible EMRs.

Availability of electronic MDHAQ data in a single database could facilitate analyses of research questions; e.g., how many patients in a particular practice are taking methotrexate or a specific biological agent, how many people being treated for RA have a history of pneumonia, or joint replacement surgery. A database in the infrastructure of all rheumatology care could obviate a need for specific registries and greatly reduce costs of assessing outcomes in patients with rheumatic diseases. Readers and EMR developers are invited to inquire about use of an electronic MDHAQ by contacting the senior author at tedpincus@gmail.com.

A Quantitative RheuMetric Physician Checklist to Assess Patient Status

The importance of expressing clinical phenomena as quantitative data beyond narrative descriptions has been a basis for extensive attention to patient self-report questionnaires, as noted in this chapter and most of the entire book. It is curious that relatively little attention has been directed to advance more physician information from narrative descriptions to quantitative scores. To be sure, 3 of the 7 RA Core data set measures used in all clinical trials are swollen joint count, tender joint count, and physician/assessor global estimate of patient status (DOCGL) [68]. (The abbreviation "DOCGL" rather than "PGA" is used to avoid confusion, as "PGA" appears in the rheumatology literature to represent either patient and physician estimates of disease activity in different reports.) At the same time, important limitations are seen of both formal joint counts and DOCGL as quantitative measures.

Limitations of the joint count include: (1) poor reproducibility [82–88], with a requirement to be performed by the same observer at each visit; (2) likelihood to improve with placebo treatment more than the other 5 RA Core Data Set measures [91]; (3) similar or lower relative efficiencies than global or patient measures to document differences between active and control treatments in clinical trials [117] (Fig. 3.8); (4) improvement over 5 years while joint damage and functional disability may progress [118, 119]; (5) lower sensitivity to detect inflammatory activity than ultrasound and magnetic resonance imaging (MRI) [120]; (6) most visits to a rheumatologist in routine care do not include a formal quantitative joint count [54, 121], unless required to provide a biological therapy.

DOCGL has the highest relative efficiency of all RA Core Data Set measures to distinguish active from control treatment in more clinical trials than joint counts, laboratory tests, and patient self-report measures [117]. In a clinical trial, the physician global estimate often meets its initial purpose to assess disease activity. However, a DOCGL may be sensitive not only to disease activity or reversible signs and symptoms, but also organ damage (e.g., to joints in RA, kidneys in SLE, and muscles in polymyositis) or irreversible symptoms, and/or distress (e.g., fibromyalgia and depression) in which patients may have high levels of pain, fatigue, and other symptoms, which remain unexplained by reversible or irreversible physical findings or laboratory values.

This matter appears more prominent when applied in routine clinical practice, in which patients have not been selected for high levels of inflammatory activity, as seen in clinical trials [122, 123].

These considerations have led to development of a RheuMetric (formerly called RHEUMDOC, but name changed to avoid possible confusion with an electronic medical record of the same name) checklist (Appendix C) to record quantitative physician scores [76, 124]. RheuMetric includes DOCGL score, supplemented by 3 separate (0–10) physician global estimate subscales for inflammation or reversible findings (DOCINF), damage or irreversible findings (DOCDAM), and distress (DOCSTR) (previously termed DOCNON) [76]. A rationale for these subscales includes:

1. A survey of 313 physicians, 154 rheumatologists and 159 non-rheumatologists, as noted previously, indicated that medical history and physical examination data are far more prominent in diagnosis and management decisions in RA than laboratory tests or ancillary studies, in contrast to 7 other prevalent chronic diseases [2]. RA was the only one of the eight chronic conditions in which a patient history and physical examination data accounted for more than 50 % of the information required for diagnosis and management [2] (Fig. 3.1).
2. A formal joint count has many limitations, as noted earlier, and is not performed by most rheumatologists at most visits [54, 121]. It may be suggested that it is very important to recognize whether an RA patient has 2 or 12 (or 1 or 11) swollen joints, but it is less important to determine whether the patient has 2 or 1 (or 12 or 11) swollen joints. Only about 10–15 s are required to perform a careful joint examination without recording each specific joint for swelling or tenderness, while 90 s or more are required to perform a formal joint count [71]. A 0–10 DOCINF estimate may summarize findings of a formal joint count in a much more feasible manner, and, hence, be more likely to be available, although formal studies of this possibility remain ongoing. It has been recognized that remission criteria without a formal joint count on the basis of 0 or 1 swollen joints give virtually identical results to formal Boolean and SDAI remission criteria [102].
3. Since no "gold standard measure" is available to assess and monitor *all* individual patients with most rheumatic diseases, pooled indices of multiple measures are needed [55]. Pooled indices have been developed for patients with rheumatoid arthritis (RA) [93, 125–129], psoriatic arthritis [130, 131], systemic lupus erythematosus (SLE) [132–139], ankylosing spondylitis [140–144], vasculitis [145–148], osteoarthritis [149], fibromyalgia [150], and other diseases (Table 3.9) [50–53, 68, 77, 78, 125–127, 129, 130, 132–138, 141, 142, 144–166]. These indices generally include a patient self-report measure, reflecting the importance of the patient history in decisions concerning diagnosis and management in rheumatic diseases [2].

   A patient with distress may have a high score on rheumatic disease index, which includes a patient self-report. The high score may reflect fibromyalgia, depression, or other chronic pain or somatization syndromes, rather than high disease activity. Moreover, some patients who meet criteria for RA or SLE may have high disease activity, as well as significant distress [72, 73]. This information may not be captured quantitatively by a physician global score. For example, a patient with fibromyalgia might have no swollen joints at all, an ESR of 20, but 28 tender joints and PATGL of 10; this patient, would have a RAPID3 score of up to 20, DAS28 of 6.1, and a CDAI of 38, all suggesting high disease activity, although there are no swollen joints and DOCGL may be 0 (Table 3.10) [76]. Even a patient with 14 tender joints and PATGL of 10, but no swollen joints and an ESR of 10 would have a DAS28 of 5.1 and CDAI of 27, suggesting high disease activity (Table 3.10). High scores in patients with fibromyalgia on DAS28, CDAI, and RAPID3 all might be interpreted (inapropriately) as indicating high

Table 3.9 Measures and indices of activity or damage, or both, used to assess and monitor patients with different rheumatic diseases

Disease	Indices/measures
All rheumatic diseases	Health assessment questionnaire (HAQ) [50] HAQII [53] Multidimensional HAQ (MDHAQ) [51, 52]
Rheumatoid arthritis	ACR Core Data Set [68, 151, 152]
	Disease activity score (DAS) [125, 126]
	Clinical disease activity index (CDAI); simplified disease activity index (SDAI) [127]
	Routine assessment of patient index data 3 (RAPID3), based on 3 RA Core Data Set measures from self-report on the MDHAQ: physical function, pain, patient estimate of global status [77, 78]
	Patient activity scale (PAS/PAS-II) [129]
	OMERACT criteria for minimal disease activity [153]
	Sharp score [154–156]
	van der Heijde modified sharp score [157, 158]
	Larsen score [159, 160]
	Rantigen score [161]
Psoriatic arthritis	ACR Core Data Set [68, 151, 152]
	Disease activity score (DAS) [125, 126]
	Psoriatic arthritis response criteria (PsARC) [162]
	Psoriasis area and severity index (PASI) [130]
Systemic lupus erythematosus	SLE disease activity index (SLEDAI) [132]
	British Isles Lupus Assessment Group (BILAG) index [133]
	Systemic lupus activity measure (SLAM) [134]
	Lupus activity index (LAI) [135]
	European consensus lupus activity measurement (ECLAM) [136, 137]
	Systemic Lupus International Collaborating Clinics (SLICC)/ACR damage index [138]
Ankylosing spondylitis	Bath ankylosing spondylitis disease activity index (BASDAI) [163]
	Modified Stoke ankylosing spondylitis spin score (mSASSS) [164]
	Bath ankylosing spondylitis radiology index (BASRI) [165]
	Bath ankylosing spondylitis functional index (BASFI) [141]
	Bath ankylosing spondylitis metrology index [142]
	Dougados functional index (DFI) [144]
Vasculitis	Birmingham vasculitis activity score (BVAS) [145]
	Vasculitis activity index (VAI) [166]
	Birmingham vasculitis damage index [146]
Wegener granulomatosis	BVAS-derived Wegener granulomatosis activity index [147]
	Wegener granulomatosis damage index [148]
Osteoarthritis	Western Ontario McMaster osteoarthritis index (WOMAC) [149]
Fibromyalgia	Fibromyalgia impact questionnaire (FIQ) [150]

Table 3.10 Scores for three indices in two patients with fibromyalgia, with no swollen joint and normal ESR, illustrating high scores of DAS28 (disease activity score 28), CDAI (clinical disease activity index), and RAPID3 (Routine Assessment of Patient Index Data) indices not due to inflammatory activity

	TJC28	SJC28	DOC GL	ESR	FN	PN	PATGL	Index score
Patient #1	**28**	**0**	**0**	**20**	**1**	**10**	**10**	
DAS28	**28**	**0**	NI	**20**	NI	NI	**10**	**6.45H**
CDAI	**28**	**0**	**0**	NI	NI	NI	**10**	**38H**
RAPID3	NI	NI	NI	NI	**1**	**10**	**10**	**21H**
Patient #2	**14**	**0**	**3**	**10**	**1**	**10**	**10**	
DAS28	**14**	**0**	NI	**10**	NI	NI	**10**	**5.11H**
CDAI	**14**	**0**	**3**	NI	NI	NI	**10**	**27H**
RAPID3	NI	NI	NI	NI	**1**	**10**	**10**	**21H**

activity and a need for intensification of therapy. Specific estimates for DOCSTR might help to recognize this interpretation as not appropriate.

4. Many patients often have inflammatory diseases may also have significant damage, as well as distress, which often affects clinical management. A study of why a recommended treat-to-target strategy to intensify therapy in RA patients who have index scores indicating high disease activity [167] was not implemented by Australian rheumatologists indicated that 2 of the primary reasons were joint damage and fibromyalgia, which caused elevated DAS28 scores that suggested moderate or high disease activity [42]. It appears that damage may be as much of a consideration in management of RA at this time as inflammation (unpublished data).
5. It may be suggested that the expertise of a rheumatologist in both diagnosis and management involves not only quantitation of the level of pain, fatigue, or other problems in each patient, but also the extent to which the etiology of these problems may result from inflammation or reversible problems, damage or irreversible problems, or distress. Availability of separate scales for inflammation and distress provides an opportunity to clarify this matter.

Analyses of new patients with many diagnoses by two rheumatologist (Table 3.11) indicated that mean overall DOCGL scores were highest for patients with fibromyalgia, followed by RA, spondyloarthropathies, osteoarthritis, gout, and systemic lupus erythematosus. Among the three subscales, mean DOCINF scores were highest in RA, spondyloarthropathies, gout, and systemic lupus erythematosus, mean DOCDAM highest in osteoarthritis, and mean DOCSTR in fibromyalgia [76] (Table 3.11). In patients with RA, mean DOCDAM and DOCSTR scores indicated coexistence of clinically important damage and/or fibromyalgia in some patients [76]. These data indicate face validity of the three physician global estimates on subscales for inflammation, damage, and symptoms due to neither inflammation nor damage. Further analyses are ongoing—development of RheuMetric at this time may be regarded as analogous to development of MDHAQ 15–25 years ago.

Table 3.11 Mean scores assigned by two rheumatologists in six diagnosis categories: rheumatoid arthritis (RA), osteoarthritis (OA), fibromyalgia (Fibro), systemic lupus erythematosus (SLE), spondyloarthropathy (SPA), and gout (43). All physician scores ≥5 are indicated in **bold** font

Rheumatologist A	RA (n=174)	OA (n=32)	Fibro (n=196)	SLE (n=34)	SPA (n=30)	Gout (n=12)
Overall global	**6.3**	**6.3**	**6.3**	**5.0**	**6.3**	**5.0**
Inflammation	**7.0**	3.3	2.3	3.6	**7.7**	**6.0**
Damage	**5.0**	**6.0**	1.7	2.3	4.3	3.0
Distress	4.0	3.7	**9.0**	**6.3**	4.0	2.3
Rheumatologist B	RA (n=48)	OA (n=67)	Fibro (n=15)	SLE (n=13)	SPA (n=23)	Gout (n=31)
Overall global	3.90	3.28	4.53	2.23	3.61	2.36
Inflammation	**4.35**	0.79	0.94	**2.28**	**4.35**	**2.64**
Damage	2.18	**3.56**	1.65	0.76	1.65	0.44
Distress	0.91	0.97	**6.13**	1.02	1.35	0.77

Adapted from [76]
Rheumatologist A: 478 new patients seen from 1996 to 2007
Rheumatologist B: 197 new patients seen between 2008 and 2012

Conclusion

This chapter has summarized evidence that scores on a patient MDHAQ self-report questionnaire and RheuMetric physician checklist may be regarded as meeting criteria for "scientific" evidence from a patient history and physical examination, with standardized, quantitative measures according to a protocol. Data from a patient history and physical examination are more important for clinical decisions in RA than laboratory tests, unlike many common chronic diseases. The MDHAQ also provides pragmatic advantages of helping the patient prepare for the visit, improving doctor/patient communication, and saving time for the doctor with RAPID3 scores, self-report joint count, review of systems, and recent medical history. Scoring RAPID3 on an MDHAQ requires 5 s, compared to almost 2 min for a DAS28 or CDAI, while distinguishing active from control treatment in clinical trials as effectively as these indices. RAPID3 scores are valuable in all rheumatic diseases. Physical function according to patient questionnaire scores is the most significant predictor of severe clinical outcomes in RA, including work disability and death. A Rheumatic checklist provides the clinical to document levels of inflammation, damage, and/or distress, in formulating a clinical decision concerning diagnosis and management. It is suggested that MDHAQ/RAPID3 and RheuMetric be considered in all routine rheumatology care in all settings, to improve assessment, monitoring, documentation, and outcomes.

Appendix A: 2-Page version of the MDHAQ. © Health Report Services. Reprinted with permission

Multi-Dimensional Health Assessment Questionnaire (MDHAQ™)(R923-NP2R)

This questionnaire includes information not available from blood tests, X-rays, or any source other than you. Please try to answer each question, even if you do not think it is related to you at this time. Try to complete as much as you can yourself, but if you need help, please ask. <u>There are no right or wrong answers.</u> Please answer exactly as you think or feel. Thank you.

1. Please check (√) the ONE best answer for your abilities at this time:

OVER THE PAST WEEK, were you able to:	Without **ANY** difficulty	With **SOME** difficulty	With **MUCH** difficulty	**UNABLE** to do
a. Dress yourself, including tying shoelaces and doing buttons?	☐ 0	☐ 1	☐ 2	☐ 3
b. Get in and out of bed?	☐ 0	☐ 1	☐ 2	☐ 3
c. Lift a full cup or glass to your mouth?	☐ 0	☐ 1	☐ 2	☐ 3
d. Walk outdoors on flat ground?	☐ 0	☐ 1	☐ 2	☐ 3
e. Wash and dry your entire body?	☐ 0	☐ 1	☐ 2	☐ 3
f. Bend down to pick up clothing from the floor?	☐ 0	☐ 1	☐ 2	☐ 3
g. Turn regular faucets on and off?	☐ 0	☐ 1	☐ 2	☐ 3
h. Get in and out of a car, bus, train, or airplane?	☐ 0	☐ 1	☐ 2	☐ 3
i. Walk two miles or three kilometers, if you wish?	☐ 0	☐ 1	☐ 2	☐ 3
j. Participate in recreational activities and sports as you wish?	☐ 0	☐ 1	☐ 2	☐ 3
k. Get a good night's sleep?	☐ 0	☐ 1.1	☐ 2.2	☐ 3.3
l. Deal with feelings of anxiety or being nervous?	☐ 0	☐ 1.1	☐ 2.2	☐ 3.3
m. Deal with feelings of depression or feeling blue?	☐ 0	☐ 1.1	☐ 2.2	☐ 3.3

2. How much pain have you had because of your condition OVER THE PAST WEEK? Please indicate below how severe your pain has been:

NO PAIN ○ 0 ○ 0.5 ○ 1.0 ○ 1.5 ○ 2.0 ○ 2.5 ○ 3.0 ○ 3.5 ○ 4.0 ○ 4.5 ○ 5.0 ○ 5.5 ○ 6.0 ○ 6.5 ○ 7.0 ○ 7.5 ○ 8.0 ○ 8.5 ○ 9.0 ○ 9.5 ○ 10 PAIN AS BAD AS IT COULD BE

3. Please place a check (√) in the appropriate spot to indicate the amount of pain you are having today in each of the joint areas listed below:

<u>LEFT SIDE:</u>	None	Mild	Moderate	Severe	<u>RIGHT SIDE:</u>	None	Mild	Moderate	Severe
a. <u>LEFT FINGERS</u>	☐ 0	☐ 1	☐ 2	☐ 3	i. <u>RIGHT FINGERS</u>	☐ 0	☐ 1	☐ 2	☐ 3
b. <u>LEFT WRIST</u>	☐ 0	☐ 1	☐ 2	☐ 3	j. <u>RIGHT WRIST</u>	☐ 0	☐ 1	☐ 2	☐ 3
c. <u>LEFT ELBOW</u>	☐ 0	☐ 1	☐ 2	☐ 3	k. <u>RIGHT ELBOW</u>	☐ 0	☐ 1	☐ 2	☐ 3
d. <u>LEFT SHOULDER</u>	☐ 0	☐ 1	☐ 2	☐ 3	l. <u>RIGHT SHOULDER</u>	☐ 0	☐ 1	☐ 2	☐ 3
e. <u>LEFT HIP</u>	☐ 0	☐ 1	☐ 2	☐ 3	m. <u>RIGHT HIP</u>	☐ 0	☐ 1	☐ 2	☐ 3
f. <u>LEFT KNEE</u>	☐ 0	☐ 1	☐ 2	☐ 3	n. <u>RIGHT KNEE</u>	☐ 0	☐ 1	☐ 2	☐ 3
g. <u>LEFT ANKLE</u>	☐ 0	☐ 1	☐ 2	☐ 3	o. <u>RIGHT ANKLE</u>	☐ 0	☐ 1	☐ 2	☐ 3
h. <u>LEFT TOES</u>	☐ 0	☐ 1	☐ 2	☐ 3	p. <u>RIGHT TOES</u>	☐ 0	☐ 1	☐ 2	☐ 3
q. <u>YOUR NECK</u>	☐ 0	☐ 1	☐ 2	☐ 3	r. <u>YOUR BACK</u>	☐ 0	☐ 1	☐ 2	☐ 3

4. Considering all the ways in which illness and health conditions may affect you at this time, please indicate below how you are doing:

VERY WELL ○ 0 ○ 0.5 ○ 1.0 ○ 1.5 ○ 2.0 ○ 2.5 ○ 3.0 ○ 3.5 ○ 4.0 ○ 4.5 ○ 5.0 ○ 5.5 ○ 6.0 ○ 6.5 ○ 7.0 ○ 7.5 ○ 8.0 ○ 8.5 ○ 9.0 ○ 9.5 ○ 10 VERY POORLY

FOR OFFICE USE ONLY

1.a-j FN (0-10): ☐

1=0.3	16=5.3
2=0.7	17=5.7
3=1.0	18=6.0
4=1.3	19=6.3
5=1.7	20=6.7
6=2.0	21=7.0
7=2.3	22=7.3
8=2.7	23=7.7
9=3.0	24=8.0
10=3.3	25=8.3
11=3.7	26=8.7
12=4.0	27=9.0
13=4.3	28=9.3
14=4.7	29=9.7
15=5.0	30=10

2.PN (0-10): ☐

4.PTGL (0-10): ☐

RAPID 3™ (0-30) ☐

Cat:
HS = >12
MS = 6.1-12
LS = 3.1-6
R = ≤3

Page 1 of 2 **PLEASE TURN TO THE OTHER SIDE** **R923NP2R**

5. Please check (√) if you have experienced any of the following over the last month:

__Fever	__Lump in your throat	__Paralysis of arms or legs	**FOR OFFICE USE ONLY**
__Weight gain (>10 lbs)	__Cough	__Numbness or tingling of arms or legs	5. ROS: ☐
__Weight loss (>10 lbs)	__Shortness of breath	__Fainting spells	
__Feeling sickly	__Wheezing	__Swelling of hands	
__Headaches	__Pain in the chest	__Swelling of ankles	
__Unusual fatigue	__Heart pounding (palpitations)	__Swelling in other joints	
__Swollen glands	__Trouble swallowing	__Joint pain	
__Loss of appetite	__Heartburn or stomach gas	__Back pain	
__Skin rash or hives	__Stomach pain or cramps	__Neck pain	
__Unusual bruising or bleeding	__Nausea	__Use of drugs not sold in stores	
__Other skin problems	__Vomiting	__Smoking cigarettes	
__Loss of hair	__Constipation	__More than 2 alcoholic drinks per day	
__Dry eyes	__Diarrhea	__Depression - feeling blue	
__Other eye problems	__Dark or bloody stools	__Anxiety - feeling nervous	
__Problems with hearing	__Problems with urination	__Problems with thinking	
__Ringing in the ears	__Gynecological (female) problems	__Problems with memory	
__Stuffy nose	__Dizziness	__Problems with sleeping	
__Sores in the mouth	__Losing your balance	__Sexual problems	
__Dry mouth	__Muscle pain, aches, or cramps	__Burning in sex organs	
__Problems with smell or taste	__Muscle weakness	__Problems with social activities	

Please check (√) here if you have had none of the above over the last month: ______.

6. When you awakened in the morning OVER THE LAST WEEK, did you feel stiff? ☐ No ☐ Yes
If "No," please go to Item 7. If **"Yes," please indicate the number of minutes______, or hours ______** until you are as limber as you will be for the day.

7. How do you feel TODAY compared to ONE WEEK AGO? Please check (✓) only one.
Much **B**etter ☐ (1), **B**etter ☐ (2), the **S**ame ☐ (3), **W**orse ☐ (4), **M**uch **W**orse ☐ (5) than one week ago

8. How often do you exercise aerobically (sweating, increased heart rate, shortness of breath) **for at least one-half hour** (30 minutes)**? Please check (✓) only one.**
☐ 3 or more times a week (3) ☐ 1-2 times per month (1)
☐ 1-2 times per week (2) ☐ Do not exercise regularly (0) ☐ Cannot exercise due to disability/ handicap (9)

9. How much of a problem has UNUSUAL fatigue or tiredness been for you OVER THE PAST WEEK?

FATIGUE IS NO PROBLEM	○ 0	○ 0.5	○ 1.0	○ 1.5	○ 2.0	○ 2.5	○ 3.0	○ 3.5	○ 4.0	○ 4.5	○ 5.0	○ 5.5	○ 6.0	○ 6.5	○ 7.0	○ 7.5	○ 8.0	○ 8.5	○ 9.0	○ 9.5	○ 10	FATIGUE IS A MAJOR PROBLEM

10. Over the last 6 months have you had: [Please check (√)]

☐No ☐Yes An operation or new illness	☐No ☐Yes Change(s) of arthritis or other medication
☐No ☐Yes Medical emergency or stay overnight in hospital	☐No ☐Yes Change(s) of address
☐No ☐Yes A fall, broken bone, or other accident or trauma	☐No ☐Yes Change(s) of marital status
☐No ☐Yes An important new symptom or medical problem	☐No ☐Yes Change job or work duties, quit work, retired
☐No ☐Yes Side effect(s) of any medication or drug	☐No ☐Yes Change of medical insurance, Medicare, etc.
☐No ☐Yes Smoke cigarettes regularly	☐No ☐Yes Change of primary care or other doctor

Please explain any "Yes" answer below, or indicate any other health matter that affects you:

____

____

SEX: ☐ Female, ☐ Male **ETHNIC GROUP:** ☐ Asian, ☐ Black, ☐ Hispanic, ☐ White, ☐ Other________________

Your Occupation ______________________ **Please circle the number of years of school you have completed:**
Work Status: ☐ Full-time, ☐ Part-time, ☐ Disabled 1 2 3 4 5 6 7 8 9 10
☐ Homemaker, ☐ Self-Employed, ☐Retired, 11 12 13 14 15 16 17 18 19 20
☐ Seeking work, ☐ Other________________ **Please write your weight:** _____ **pounds** or **kg** **height:** _____ **inches** or **cm**

Your Name______________________________ **Date of Birth** ___________ **Today's Date** ____________

Page 2 of 2 Thank you for completing this questionnaire to help keep track of your medical care. R923NP2R

FOR OFFICE USE ONLY: I have reviewed and recorded relevant questionnaire responses.
Date: ______________________ Signature______________________________

Appendix B: 4-Page version of the MDHAQ. © Health Report Services. Reprinted with permission

Multi-Dimensional Health Assessment Questionnaire (MDHAQ™)(R923-NP2R)

This questionnaire includes information not available from blood tests, X-rays, or any source other than you. Please try to answer each question, even if you do not think it is related to you at this time. Try to complete as much as you can yourself, but if you need help, please ask. There are no right or wrong answers. Please answer exactly as you think or feel. Thank you.

1. Please check (√) the ONE best answer for your abilities at this time:

OVER THE PAST WEEK, were you able to:	Without **ANY** difficulty	With **SOME** difficulty	With **MUCH** difficulty	**UNABLE** to do
a. Dress yourself, including tying shoelaces and doing buttons?	☐ 0	☐ 1	☐ 2	☐ 3
b. Get in and out of bed?	☐ 0	☐ 1	☐ 2	☐ 3
c. Lift a full cup or glass to your mouth?	☐ 0	☐ 1	☐ 2	☐ 3
d. Walk outdoors on flat ground?	☐ 0	☐ 1	☐ 2	☐ 3
e. Wash and dry your entire body?	☐ 0	☐ 1	☐ 2	☐ 3
f. Bend down to pick up clothing from the floor?	☐ 0	☐ 1	☐ 2	☐ 3
g. Turn regular faucets on and off?	☐ 0	☐ 1	☐ 2	☐ 3
h. Get in and out of a car, bus, train, or airplane?	☐ 0	☐ 1	☐ 2	☐ 3
i. Walk two miles or three kilometers, if you wish?	☐ 0	☐ 1	☐ 2	☐ 3
j. Participate in recreational activities and sports as you wish?	☐ 0	☐ 1	☐ 2	☐ 3
k. Get a good night's sleep?	☐ 0	☐ 1.1	☐ 2.2	☐ 3.3
l. Deal with feelings of anxiety or being nervous?	☐ 0	☐ 1.1	☐ 2.2	☐ 3.3
m. Deal with feelings of depression or feeling blue?	☐ 0	☐ 1.1	☐ 2.2	☐ 3.3

2. How much pain have you had because of your condition OVER THE PAST WEEK? Please indicate below how severe your pain has been:

NO PAIN ○ 0 ○ 0.5 ○ 1.0 ○ 1.5 ○ 2.0 ○ 2.5 ○ 3.0 ○ 3.5 ○ 4.0 ○ 4.5 ○ 5.0 ○ 5.5 ○ 6.0 ○ 6.5 ○ 7.0 ○ 7.5 ○ 8.0 ○ 8.5 ○ 9.0 ○ 9.5 ○ 10 PAIN AS BAD AS IT COULD BE

3. Please place a check (√) in the appropriate spot to indicate the amount of pain you are having today in each of the joint areas listed below:

LEFT SIDE:	None	Mild	Moderate	Severe	RIGHT SIDE:	None	Mild	Moderate	Severe
a. LEFT FINGERS	☐ 0	☐ 1	☐ 2	☐ 3	i. RIGHT FINGERS	☐ 0	☐ 1	☐ 2	☐ 3
b. LEFT WRIST	☐ 0	☐ 1	☐ 2	☐ 3	j. RIGHT WRIST	☐ 0	☐ 1	☐ 2	☐ 3
c. LEFT ELBOW	☐ 0	☐ 1	☐ 2	☐ 3	k. RIGHT ELBOW	☐ 0	☐ 1	☐ 2	☐ 3
d. LEFT SHOULDER	☐ 0	☐ 1	☐ 2	☐ 3	l. RIGHT SHOULDER	☐ 0	☐ 1	☐ 2	☐ 3
e. LEFT HIP	☐ 0	☐ 1	☐ 2	☐ 3	m. RIGHT HIP	☐ 0	☐ 1	☐ 2	☐ 3
f. LEFT KNEE	☐ 0	☐ 1	☐ 2	☐ 3	n. RIGHT KNEE	☐ 0	☐ 1	☐ 2	☐ 3
g. LEFT ANKLE	☐ 0	☐ 1	☐ 2	☐ 3	o. RIGHT ANKLE	☐ 0	☐ 1	☐ 2	☐ 3
h. LEFT TOES	☐ 0	☐ 1	☐ 2	☐ 3	p. RIGHT TOES	☐ 0	☐ 1	☐ 2	☐ 3
q. YOUR NECK	☐ 0	☐ 1	☐ 2	☐ 3	r. YOUR BACK	☐ 0	☐ 1	☐ 2	☐ 3

4. Considering all the ways in which illness and health conditions may affect you at this time, please indicate below how you are doing:

VERY **WELL** ○ **0** ○ **0.5** ○ **1.0** ○ **1.5** ○ **2.0** ○ **2.5** ○ **3.0** ○ **3.5** ○ **4.0** ○ **4.5** ○ **5.0** ○ **5.5** ○ **6.0** ○ **6.5** ○ **7.0** ○ **7.5** ○ **8.0** ○ **8.5** ○ **9.0** ○ **9.5** ○ **10** VERY **POORLY**

FOR OFFICE USE ONLY

1.a-j FN (0-10): ☐

1=0.3	16=5.3
2=0.7	17=5.7
3=1.0	18=6.0
4=1.3	19=6.3
5=1.7	20=6.7
6=2.0	21=7.0
7=2.3	22=7.3
8=2.7	23=7.7
9=3.0	24=8.0
10=3.3	25=8.3
11=3.7	26=8.7
12=4.0	27=9.0
13=4.3	28=9.3
14=4.7	29=9.7
15=5.0	30=10

2.PN (0-10): ☐

4.PTGL (0-10): ☐

RAPID 3™ (0-30) ☐

Cat:

HS = >12

MS = 6.1-12

LS = 3.1-6

R = ≤3

Page 1 of 2 **PLEASE TURN TO THE OTHER SIDE** **R923NP2R**

5. Please check (√) if you have experienced any of the following over the last month:

__Fever	__Lump in your throat	__Paralysis of arms or legs
__Weight gain (>10 lbs)	__Cough	__Numbness or tingling of arms or legs
__Weight loss (>10 lbs)	__Shortness of breath	__Fainting spells
__Feeling sickly	__Wheezing	__Swelling of hands
__Headaches	__Pain in the chest	__Swelling of ankles
__Unusual fatigue	__Heart pounding (palpitations)	__Swelling in other joints
__Swollen glands	__Trouble swallowing	__Joint pain
__Loss of appetite	__Heartburn or stomach gas	__Back pain
__Skin rash or hives	__Stomach pain or cramps	__Neck pain
__Unusual bruising or bleeding	__Nausea	__Use of drugs not sold in stores
__Other skin problems	__Vomiting	__Smoking cigarettes
__Loss of hair	__Constipation	__More than 2 alcoholic drinks per day
__Dry eyes	__Diarrhea	__Depression - feeling blue
__Other eye problems	__Dark or bloody stools	__Anxiety - feeling nervous
__Problems with hearing	__Problems with urination	__Problems with thinking
__Ringing in the ears	__Gynecological (female) problems	__Problems with memory
__Stuffy nose	__Dizziness	__Problems with sleeping
__Sores in the mouth	__Losing your balance	__Sexual problems
__Dry mouth	__Muscle pain, aches, or cramps	__Burning in sex organs
__Problems with smell or taste	__Muscle weakness	__Problems with social activities

FOR OFFICE USE ONLY
5. ROS: ☐

Please check (√) here if you have had none of the above over the last month: ______.

6. When you awakened in the morning OVER THE LAST WEEK, did you feel stiff? ☐ No ☐ Yes
If "No," please go to Item 7. If **"Yes," please indicate the number of minutes______, or hours _____** until you are as limber as you will be for the day.

7. How do you feel TODAY compared to ONE WEEK AGO? Please check (✓) only one.
Much **B**etter ☐ (1), **B**etter ☐ (2), the **S**ame ☐ (3), **W**orse ☐ (4), **M**uch **W**orse ☐ (5) than one week ago

8. How often do you exercise aerobically (sweating, increased heart rate, shortness of breath) **for at least one-half hour** (30 minutes)**? Please check (✓) only one.**
☐ 3 or more times a week (3) ☐ 1-2 times per month (1)
☐ 1-2 times per week (2) ☐ Do not exercise regularly (0) ☐ Cannot exercise due to disability/ handicap (9)

9. How much of a problem has UNUSUAL fatigue or tiredness been for you OVER THE PAST WEEK?

FATIGUE IS NO PROBLEM	○	○	○	○	○	○	○	○	○	○	○	○	○	○	○	○	○	○	○	○	○	FATIGUE IS A MAJOR PROBLEM
	0	0.5	1.0	1.5	2.0	2.5	3.0	3.5	4.0	4.5	5.0	5.5	6.0	6.5	7.0	7.5	8.0	8.5	9.0	9.5	10	

10. Over the last 6 months have you had: [Please check (√)]

☐No ☐Yes An operation or new illness
☐No ☐Yes Medical emergency or stay overnight in hospital
☐No ☐Yes A fall, broken bone, or other accident or trauma
☐No ☐Yes An important new symptom or medical problem
☐No ☐Yes Side effect(s) of any medication or drug
☐No ☐Yes Smoke cigarettes regularly
☐No ☐Yes Change(s) of arthritis or other medication
☐No ☐Yes Change(s) of address
☐No ☐Yes Change(s) of marital status
☐No ☐Yes Change job or work duties, quit work, retired
☐No ☐Yes Change of medical insurance, Medicare, etc.
☐No ☐Yes Change of primary care or other doctor

Please explain any "Yes" answer below, or indicate any other health matter that affects you:

____
____

SEX: ☐ Female, ☐ Male **ETHNIC GROUP:** ☐ Asian, ☐ Black, ☐ Hispanic, ☐ White, ☐ Other________________

Your Occupation ________________________
Work Status: ☐ Full-time, ☐ Part-time, ☐ Disabled
☐ Homemaker, ☐ Self-Employed, ☐Retired,
☐ Seeking work, ☐ Other________________

Please circle the number of years of school you have completed:
1 2 3 4 5 6 7 8 9 10
11 12 13 14 15 16 17 18 19 20

Please write your weight: _____ **pounds** or **kg** **height:** _____ **inches** or **cm**

Your Name_______________________________ **Date of Birth** ___________ **Today's Date** ___________

Page 2 of 2 Thank you for completing this questionnaire to help keep track of your medical care. R923NP2R

FOR OFFICE USE ONLY: I have reviewed and recorded relevant questionnaire responses.
Date: ___________________________ Signature________________________________

Appendix C: RheuMetric. © Health Report Services. Reprinted with permission

R928 RheuMetric:™ PATIENT ________________, MR #___________, DATE ________, P 1

PHYSICIAN INITIALS _______ Check if new Pt ☐, If not: ______ Yr of 1st visit to this doctor
______ Yr of 1st visit to this site

1. a. PHYSICIAN GLOBAL ASSESSMENT (DOCGL) at this visit:

EXCELLENT ○○○○○○○○○○○○○○○○○○○○○ VERY POOR
0 0.5 1 1.5 2 2.5 3 3.5 4 4.5 5 5.5 6 6.5 7 7.5 8 8.5 9 9.5 10

2. DISEASE ACTIVITY, DAMAGE and DISTRESS:

b. Degree of INFLAMMATION or REVERSIBLE DISEASE (DOCINF) at this visit:

NONE ○○○○○○○○○○○○○○○○○○○○○ MOST SEVERE
0 0.5 1 1.5 2 2.5 3 3.5 4 4.5 5 5.5 6 6.5 7 7.5 8 8.5 9 9.5 10

c. Degree of joint or organ STRUCTURAL DAMAGE or IRREVERSIBLE DISEASE (DOCDAM) at this visit:

NONE ○○○○○○○○○○○○○○○○○○○○○ MOST SEVERE
0 0.5 1 1.5 2 2.5 3 3.5 4 4.5 5 5.5 6 6.5 7 7.5 8 8.5 9 9.5 10

d. Degree of DISTRESS (findings due to neither inflammation nor damage, eg, fibromyalgia)(DOCSTR):

NONE ○○○○○○○○○○○○○○○○○○○○○ MOST SEVERE
0 0.5 1 1.5 2 2.5 3 3.5 4 4.5 5 5.5 6 6.5 7 7.5 8 8.5 9 9.5 10

e. If DOCGL>2, % of clinical decision based on (total=100%): _____ inflammation,
_____ damage
_____ distress

f. If DOCGL>2, proportion of clinical decision due to _(total=100%): ______rheumatic disease(s)
______non-RD(s)

g. OVERALL CHANGE in clinical status compared to one week ago (DOCCHG) (please √ one):

☐ Much Better (1), ☐ Better (2), ☐ the Same (3), ☐ Worse (4), ☐ Much Worse (5)

3. PROGNOSIS

i. WITHOUT therapy (√ one): ☐ Excellent (1), ☐ Very Good (2), ☐ Good (3), ☐ Fair (4), ☐ Poor (5)

j. WITH therapy (√ one): ☐ Excellent (1), ☐ Very Good (2), ☐ Good (3), ☐ Fair (4), ☐ Poor (5)

4. DIAGNOSIS k. Primary (1°) Rheumatic diagnosis: (May be provisional): ____________________

l. Year of 1st symptoms:______, Month, if <2 years:________ Year of Diagnosis:________________

m. Diagnostic certainty - 1° Rheumatic diagnosis: ☐ High (1), ☐ Moderate (2), ☐ Low (3), ☐ None (4).

PATIENT ETHNICITY: ☐ Asian, ☐ Black, ☐ Hispanic, ☐ Indian, ☐ White, ☐ Other______________
(Please specify)

PLEASE TURN TO OTHER SIDE FOR JOINT COUNT

References

1. Engel GL. The need for a new medical model: a challenge for biomedicine. Science. 1977;196(4286):129–36.
2. Castrejon I, McCollum L, Tanriover MD, Pincus T. Importance of patient history and physical examination in rheumatoid arthritis compared to other chronic diseases: results of a physician survey. Arthritis Care Res. 2012;64(8):1250–5.
3. Yelin E, Meenan R, Nevitt M, Epstein W. Work disability in rheumatoid arthritis: effects of disease, social, and work factors. Ann Intern Med. 1980;93(4):551–6.
4. Pincus T, Callahan LF, Sale WG, Brooks AL, Payne LE, Vaughn WK. Severe functional declines, work disability, and increased mortality in seventy-five rheumatoid arthritis patients studied over nine years. Arthritis Rheum. 1984;27(8):864–72.
5. Callahan LF, Bloch DA, Pincus T. Identification of work disability in rheumatoid arthritis: physical, radiographic and laboratory variables do not add explanatory power to demographic and functional variables. J Clin Epidemiol. 1992;45(2):127–38.
6. Wolfe F, Hawley DJ. The longterm outcomes of rheumatoid arthritis: work disability: a prospective 18 year study of 823 patients. J Rheumatol. 1998;25(11):2108–17.
7. Puolakka K, Kautiainen H, Mottonen T, Hannonen P, Hakala M, Korpela M, et al. Predictors of productivity loss in early rheumatoid arthritis: a 5 year follow up study. Ann Rheum Dis. 2005;64(1):130–3.
8. Lubeck DP, Spitz PW, Fries JF, Wolfe F, Mitchell DM, Roth SH. A multicenter study of annual health service utilization and costs in rheumatoid arthritis. Arthritis Rheum. 1986;29(4):488–93.
9. Michaud K, Messer J, Choi HK, Wolfe F. Direct medical costs and their predictors in patients with rheumatoid arthritis: a three-year study of 7,527 patients. Arthritis Rheum. 2003;48(10):2750–62.
10. Wolfe F, Zwillich SH. The long-term outcomes of rheumatoid arthritis: a 23-year prospective, longitudinal study of total joint replacement and its predictors in 1,600 patients with rheumatoid arthritis. Arthritis Rheum. 1998;41(6):1072–82.
11. Leigh JP, Fries JF. Mortality predictors among 263 patients with rheumatoid arthritis. J Rheumatol. 1991;18(9):1307–12.
12. Wolfe F, Kleinheksel SM, Cathey MA, Hawley DJ, Spitz PW, Fries JF. The clinical value of the Stanford Health Assessment Questionnaire Functional Disability Index in patients with rheumatoid arthritis. J Rheumatol. 1988;15(10):1480–8.
13. Soderlin MK, Nieminen P, Hakala M. Functional status predicts mortality in a community based rheumatoid arthritis population. J Rheumatol. 1998;25(10):1895–9.
14. Pincus T, Callahan LF. Taking mortality in rheumatoid arthritis seriously—predictive markers, socioeconomic status and comorbidity. J Rheumatol. 1986;13(5):841–5.
15. Sokka T, Abelson B, Pincus T. Mortality in rheumatoid arthritis: 2008 update. Clin Exp Rheumatol. 2008;26(5 Suppl 51):S35–61.
16. Olsen NJ, Callahan LF, Brooks RH, Nance EP, Kaye JJ, Stastny P, et al. Associations of HLA-DR4 with rheumatoid factor and radiographic severity in rheumatoid arthritis. Am J Med. 1988;84(2):257–64.
17. Sokka T, Pincus T. Poor physical function, pain and limited exercise: risk factors for premature mortality in the range of smoking or hypertension, identified on a simple patient self-report questionnaire for usual care. BMJ Open. 2011;1(1), e000070.
18. Pincus T, Callahan LF. Associations of low formal education level and poor health status: behavioral, in addition to demographic and medical, explanations? J Clin Epidemiol. 1994;47(4):355–61.
19. Pincus T, Esther R, DeWalt DA, Callahan LF. Social conditions and self-management are more powerful determinants of health than access to care. Ann Intern Med. 1998; 129(5):406–11.

20. Sokka T, Kautiainen H, Pincus T, Toloza S, da Rocha Castelar Pinheiro G, Lazovskis J, et al. Disparities in rheumatoid arthritis disease activity according to gross domestic product in 25 countries in the QUEST-RA database. Ann Rheum Dis. 2009;68(11):1666–72.
21. Wolfe F, Michaud K. Severe rheumatoid arthritis (RA), worse outcomes, comorbid illness, and sociodemographic disadvantage characterize RA patients with fibromyalgia. J Rheumatol. 2004;31(4):695–700.
22. Pincus T. Formal educational level—a marker for the importance of behavioral variables in the pathogenesis, morbidity, and mortality of most diseases? J Rheumatol. 1988;15(10):1457–60.
23. Maiden N, Capell HA, Madhok R, Hampson R, Thomson EA. Does social disadvantage contribute to the excess mortality in rheumatoid arthritis patients? Ann Rheum Dis. 1999;58(9):525–9.
24. Callahan LF, Pincus T. Formal education level as a significant marker of clinical status in rheumatoid arthritis. Arthritis Rheum. 1988;31(11):1346–57.
25. Callahan LF, Pincus T, Huston 3rd JW, Brooks RH, Nance Jr EP, Kaye JJ. Measures of activity and damage in rheumatoid arthritis: depiction of changes and prediction of mortality over five years. Arthritis Care Res. 1997;10(6):381–94.
26. Ruberman W, Weinblatt E, Goldberg JD, Chaudhary BS. Psychosocial influences on mortality after myocardial infarction. N Engl J Med. 1984;311(9):552–9.
27. Rose HM, Ragan C, et al. Differential agglutination of normal and sensitized sheep erythrocytes by sera of patients with rheumatoid arthritis. Proc Soc Exp Biol Med. 1948;68(1):1–6.
28. Hargraves MM, Richmond H, Morton R. Presentation of two bone marrow elements; the tart cell and the L.E. cell. Proc Staff Meet Mayo Clin. 1948;23(2):25–8.
29. Schellekens GA, de Jong BA, van den Hoogen FH, van de Putte LB, van Venrooij WJ. Citrulline is an essential constituent of antigenic determinants recognized by rheumatoid arthritis-specific autoantibodies. J Clin Invest. 1998;101(1):273–81.
30. Nishimura K, Sugiyama D, Kogata Y, Tsuji G, Nakazawa T, Kawano S, et al. Meta-analysis: diagnostic accuracy of anti-cyclic citrullinated peptide antibody and rheumatoid factor for rheumatoid arthritis. Ann Intern Med. 2007;146(11):797–808.
31. Lawrence RC, Felson DT, Helmick CG, Arnold LM, Choi H, Deyo RA, et al. Estimates of the prevalence of arthritis and other rheumatic conditions in the united states. Part II. Arthritis Rheum. 2008;58(1):26–35.
32. Shovman O, Gilburd B, Zandman-Goddard G, Sherer Y, Orbach H, Gerli R, et al. The diagnostic utility of anti-cyclic citrullinated peptide antibodies, matrix metalloproteinase-3, rheumatoid factor, erythrocyte sedimentation rate, and c-reactive protein in patients with erosive and non-erosive rheumatoid arthritis. Clin Dev Immunol. 2005;12(3):197–202.
33. Wolfe F, Michaud K. The clinical and research significance of the erythrocyte sedimentation rate. J Rheumatol. 1994;21(7):1227–37.
34. Wolfe F. The many myths of erythrocyte sedimentation rate and c-reactive protein. J Rheumatol. 2009;36(8):1568–9.
35. Smedstad LM, Moum T, Guillemin F, Kvien TK, Finch MB, Suurmeijer TP, et al. Correlates of functional disability in early rheumatoid arthritis: a cross-sectional study of 706 patients in four European countries. Br J Rheumatol. 1996;35(8):746–51.
36. Sokka T, Pincus T. Erythrocyte sedimentation rate, c-reactive protein, or rheumatoid factor are normal at presentation in 35–45% of patients with rheumatoid arthritis seen between 1980 and 2004: analyses from Finland and the united states. J Rheumatol. 2009;36(7):1387–90.
37. Wolfe F, Pincus T. The level of inflammation in rheumatoid arthritis is determined early and remains stable over the longterm course of the illness. J Rheumatol. 2001;28(8):1817–24.
38. Abelson B, Sokka T, Pincus T. Declines in erythrocyte sedimentation rates in patients with rheumatoid arthritis over the second half of the 20th century. J Rheumatol. 2009; 36(8):1596–9.
39. Pincus T, Sokka T, Kautiainen H. Patients seen for standard rheumatoid arthritis care have significantly better articular, radiographic, laboratory, and functional status in 2000 than in 1985. Arthritis Rheum. 2005;52(4):1009–19.

40. Slater CA, Davis RB, Shmerling RH. Antinuclear antibody testing. A study of clinical utility. Arch Intern Med. 1996;156(13):1421–5.
41. Pincus T. A pragmatic approach to cost-effective use of laboratory tests and imaging procedures in patients with musculoskeletal symptoms. Prim Care. 1993;20(4):795–814.
42. Pincus T, Sokka T. Laboratory tests to assess patients with rheumatoid arthritis: advantages and limitations. Rheum Dis Clin North Am. 2009;35(4):731–4. vi–vii.
43. Pincus T, Schur PH, Rose JA, Decker JL, Talal N. Measurement of serum DNA-binding activity in systemic lupus erythematosus. N Engl J Med. 1969;281(13):701–5.
44. Pincus T, Gibson KA, Shmerling RH. An evidence-based approach to laboratory tests in usual care of patients with rheumatoid arthritis. Clin Exp Rheumatol. 2014;32(5 Suppl 85):S-23–8.
45. Sharp GC, Irvin WS, Tan EM, Gould RG, Holman HR. Mixed connective tissue disease—an apparently distinct rheumatic disease syndrome associated with a specific antibody to an extractable nuclear antigen (ENA). Am J Med. 1972;52(2):148–59.
46. Munves EF, Schur PH. Antibodies to Sm and RNP. Prognosticators of disease involvement. Arthritis Rheum. 1983;26(7):848–53.
47. Nimelstein SH, Brody S, McShane D, Holman HR. Mixed connective tissue disease: a subsequent evaluation of the original 25 patients. Medicine. 1980;59(4):239–48.
48. van der Heijde D, Landewe R, Klareskog L, Rodriguez-Valverde V, Settas L, Pedersen R, et al. Presentation and analysis of data on radiographic outcome in clinical trials: experience from the tempo study. Arthritis Rheum. 2005;52(1):49–60.
49. Pincus T. Assessment of long-term outcomes of rheumatoid arthritis. How choices of measures and study designs may lead to apparently different conclusions. Rheum Dis Clin North Am. 1995;21(3):619–54.
50. Fries JF, Spitz P, Kraines RG, Holman HR. Measurement of patient outcome in arthritis. Arthritis Rheum. 1980;23(2):137–45.
51. Pincus T, Swearingen C, Wolfe F. Toward a multidimensional health assessment questionnaire (MDHAQ): assessment of advanced activities of daily living and psychological status in the patient-friendly health assessment questionnaire format. Arthritis Rheum. 1999;42(10):2220–30.
52. Pincus T, Sokka T, Kautiainen H. Further development of a physical function scale on a MDHAQ [corrected] for standard care of patients with rheumatic diseases. J Rheumatol. 2005;32(8):1432–9.
53. Wolfe F, Michaud K, Pincus T. Development and validation of the health assessment questionnaire ii: a revised version of the health assessment questionnaire. Arthritis Rheum. 2004;50(10):3296–305.
54. Anderson J, Caplan L, Yazdany J, Robbins ML, Neogi T, Michaud K, et al. Rheumatoid arthritis disease activity measures: American college of rheumatology recommendations for use in clinical practice. Arthritis Care Res. 2012;64(5):640–7.
55. Goldsmith CH, Smythe HA, Helewa A. Interpretation and power of a pooled index. J Rheumatol. 1993;20(3):575–8.
56. Smith T. Questions on clinical trials. Br Med J. 1983;287(6392):569.
57. Pincus T, Wolfe F. Patient questionnaires for clinical research and improved standard patient care: is it better to have 80% of the information in 100% of patients or 100% of the information in 5% of patients? J Rheumatol. 2005;32(4):575–7.
58. Meenan RF, Gertman PM, Mason JH. Measuring health status in arthritis. The arthritis impact measurement scales. Arthritis Rheum. 1980;23(2):146–52.
59. Pincus T, Yazici Y, Bergman M, Maclean R, Harrington T. A proposed continuous quality improvement approach to assessment and management of patients with rheumatoid arthritis without formal joint counts, based on quantitative routine assessment of patient index data (RAPID) scores on a multidimensional health assessment questionnaire (MDHAQ). Best Pract Res Clin Rheumatol. 2007;21(4):789–804.

60. Pincus T, Maclean R, Yazici Y, Harrington JT. Quantitative measurement of patient status in the regular care of patients with rheumatic diseases over 25 years as a continuous quality improvement activity, rather than traditional research. Clin Exp Rheumatol. 2007;25(6 Suppl 47):69–81.
61. DeWalt DA, Reed GW, Pincus T. Further clues to recognition of patients with fibromyalgia from a simple 2-page patient multidimensional health assessment questionnaire (MDHAQ). Clin Exp Rheumatol. 2004;22(4):453–61.
62. Yazici Y, Pincus T, Kautiainen H, Sokka T. Morning stiffness in patients with early rheumatoid arthritis is associated more strongly with functional disability than with joint swelling and erythrocyte sedimentation rate. J Rheumatol. 2004;31(9):1723–6.
63. Pincus T, Hassett AL, Callahan LF. Clues on the MDHAQ to identify patients with fibromyalgia and similar chronic pain conditions. Rheum Dis Clin North Am. 2009;35(4):865–9. xii.
64. Singh H, Gupta V, Ray S, Kumar H, Talapatra P, Kaur M, et al. Evaluation of disease activity in rheumatoid arthritis by routine assessment of patient index data 3 (RAPID3) and its correlation to disease activity score 28 (DAS28) and clinical disease activity index (CDAI): an Indian experience. Clin Rheumatol. 2012.
65. Pincus T, Sokka T, Castrejon I, Cutolo M. Decline of mean initial prednisone dosage from 10.3 to 3.6 mg/day to treat rheumatoid arthritis between 1980 and 2004 in one clinical setting, with long-term effectiveness of dosages less than 5 mg/day. Arthritis Care Res. 2013;65(5):729–36.
66. Sokka T, Pincus T. Ascendancy of weekly low-dose methotrexate in usual care of rheumatoid arthritis from 1980 to 2004 at two sites in Finland and the united states. Rheumatology (Oxford). 2008;47(10):1543–7.
67. Pincus T, Summey JA, Soraci Jr SA, Wallston KA, Hummon NP. Assessment of patient satisfaction in activities of daily living using a modified Stanford Health Assessment Questionnaire. Arthritis Rheum. 1983;26(11):1346–53.
68. Boers M, Tugwell P, Felson DT, van Riel PL, Kirwan JR, Edmonds JP, et al. World Health Organization and International League of Associations for Rheumatology core endpoints for symptom modifying antirheumatic drugs in rheumatoid arthritis clinical trials. J Rheumatol Suppl. 1994;41:86–9.
69. Pincus T, Bergman M, Sokka T, Roth J, Swearingen C, Yazici Y. Visual analog scales in formats other than a 10 centimeter horizontal line to assess pain and other clinical data. J Rheumatol. 2008;35(8):1550–8.
70. Pincus T, Bergman MJ, Yazici Y. RAPID3-an index of physical function, pain, and global status as "vital signs" to improve care for people with chronic rheumatic diseases. Bull NYU Hosp Jt Dis. 2009;67(2):211–25.
71. Pincus T, Swearingen CJ, Bergman MJ, Colglazier CL, Kaell AT, Kunath AM, et al. RAPID3 (routine assessment of patient index data) on an MDHAQ (multidimensional health assessment questionnaire): agreement with DAS28 (disease activity score) and CDAI (clinical disease activity index) activity categories, scored in five versus more than ninety seconds. Arthritis Care Res. 2010;62(2):181–9.
72. Wolfe F, Cathey MA, Kleinheksel SM. Fibrositis (fibromyalgia) in rheumatoid arthritis. J Rheumatol. 1984;11(6):814–8.
73. Wolfe F, Petri M, Alarcon GS, Goldman J, Chakravarty EF, Katz RS, et al. Fibromyalgia, systemic lupus erythematosus (SLE), and evaluation of SLE activity. J Rheumatol. 2009;36(1):82–8.
74. Kirwan JR, Minnock P, Adebajo A, Bresnihan B, Choy E, de Wit M, et al. Patient perspective: fatigue as a recommended patient centered outcome measure in rheumatoid arthritis. J Rheumatol. 2007;34(5):1174–7.
75. Pincus T, Oliver AM, Bergman MJ. How to collect an MDHAQ to provide rheumatology vital signs (function, pain, global status, and RAPID3 scores) in the infrastructure of rheumatology care, including some misconceptions regarding the MDHAQ. Rheum Dis Clin North Am. 2009;35(4):799–812.

76. Bergman MJ, Castrejon I, Pincus T. RHEUMDOC: a one-page rheumatology doctor form with four physician global estimates for overall status, inflammation, damage, and symptoms based on neither inflammation nor damage. Bull Hosp Jt Dis. 2014;72(2):142–7.
77. Pincus T, Bergman MJ, Yazici Y, Hines P, Raghupathi K, Maclean R. An index of only patient-reported outcome measures, routine assessment of patient index data 3 (RAPID3), in two abatacept clinical trials: similar results to disease activity score (DAS28) and other rapid indices that include physician-reported measures. Rheumatology (Oxford). 2008;47(3):345–9.
78. Pincus T, Swearingen CJ, Bergman M, Yazici Y. RAPID3 (routine assessment of patient index data 3), a rheumatoid arthritis index without formal joint counts for routine care: proposed severity categories compared to disease activity score and clinical disease activity index categories. J Rheumatol. 2008;35(11):2136–47.
79. Pincus T. Can RAPID3, an index without formal joint counts or laboratory tests, serve to guide rheumatologists in tight control of rheumatoid arthritis in usual clinical care? Bull NYU Hosp Jt Dis. 2009;67(3):254–66.
80. Pincus T, Hines P, Bergman MJ, Yazici Y, Rosenblatt LC, MacLean R. Proposed severity and response criteria for routine assessment of patient index data (RAPID3): results for categories of disease activity and response criteria in abatacept clinical trials. J Rheumatol. 2011;38(12):2565–71.
81. Pincus T, Yazici Y, Castrejon I. Pragmatic and scientific advantages of MDHAQ/RAPID3 completion by all patients at all visits in routine clinical care. Bull NYU Hosp Jt Dis. 2012;70 Suppl 1:30–6.
82. Sokka T, Pincus T. Joint counts to assess rheumatoid arthritis for clinical research and usual clinical care: advantages and limitations. Rheum Dis Clin North Am. 2009;35(4):713–22. v–vi.
83. Hart LE, Tugwell P, Buchanan WW, Norman GR, Grace EM, Southwell D. Grading of tenderness as a source of interrater error in the Ritchie articular index. J Rheumatol. 1985;12(4):716–7.
84. Lewis PA, O'Sullivan MM, Rumfeld WR, Coles EC, Jessop JD. Significant changes in Ritchie scores. Br J Rheumatol. 1988;27(1):32–6.
85. Klinkhoff AV, Bellamy N, Bombardier C, Carette S, Chalmers A, Esdaile JM, et al. An experiment in reducing interobserver variability of the examination for joint tenderness. J Rheumatol. 1988;15(3):492–4.
86. Thompson PW, Hart LE, Goldsmith CH, Spector TD, Bell MJ, Ramsden MF. Comparison of four articular indices for use in clinical trials in rheumatoid arthritis: patient, order and observer variation. J Rheumatol. 1991;18(5):661–5.
87. Scott DL, Choy EH, Greeves A, Isenberg D, Kassinor D, Rankin E, et al. Standardising joint assessment in rheumatoid arthritis. Clin Rheumatol. 1996;15(6):579–82.
88. Uhlig TKT, Pincus T. Test-retest reliability of disease activity core set measures and indices in rheumatoid arthritis. Ann Rheum Dis. 2009;68:972–5.
89. Wells G, Li T, Maxwell L, Maclean R, Tugwell P. Responsiveness of patient reported outcomes including fatigue, sleep quality, activity limitation, and quality of life following treatment with abatacept for rheumatoid arthritis. Ann Rheum Dis. 2008;67(2):260–5.
90. Pincus T, Amara I, Segurado OG, Bergman M, Koch GG. Relative efficiencies of physician/assessor global estimates and patient questionnaire measures are similar to or greater than joint counts to distinguish adalimumab from control treatments in rheumatoid arthritis clinical trials. J Rheumatol. 2008;35(2):201–5.
91. Strand V, Cohen S, Crawford B, Smolen JS, Scott DL, Leflunomide Investigators G. Patient-reported outcomes better discriminate active treatment from placebo in randomized controlled trials in rheumatoid arthritis. Rheumatology (Oxford). 2004;43(5):640–7.
92. Pincus T, Richardson B, Strand V, Bergman MJ. Relative efficiencies of the 7 rheumatoid arthritis core data set measures to distinguish active from control treatments in 9 comparisons from clinical trials of 5 agents. Clin Exp Rheumatol. 2014;32(5 Suppl 85):47–54.

93. Pincus T, Strand V, Koch G, Amara I, Crawford B, Wolfe F, et al. An index of the three core data set patient questionnaire measures distinguishes efficacy of active treatment from that of placebo as effectively as the American College of Rheumatology 20% response criteria (ACR20) or the disease activity score (DAS) in a rheumatoid arthritis clinical trial. Arthritis Rheum. 2003;48(3):625–30.
94. Pincus T, Chung C, Segurado OG, Amara I, Koch GG. An index of patient reported outcomes (pro-index) discriminates effectively between active and control treatment in 4 clinical trials of adalimumab in rheumatoid arthritis. J Rheumatol. 2006;33(11):2146–52.
95. Pincus T, Furer V, Keystone E, Yazici Y, Bergman MJ, Luijtens K. RAPID3 (routine assessment of patient index data 3) severity categories and response criteria: similar results to DAS28 (disease activity score) and CDAI (clinical disease activity index) in the RAPID1 (rheumatoid arthritis prevention of structural damage) clinical trial of certolizumab pegol. Arthritis Care Res. 2011;63(8):1142–9.
96. Wolfe F, Cathey MA. The assessment and prediction of functional disability in rheumatoid arthritis. J Rheumatol. 1991;18(9):1298–306.
97. Sokka T, Kautiainen H, Mottonen T, Hannonen P. Work disability in rheumatoid arthritis 10 years after the diagnosis. J Rheumatol. 1999;26(8):1681–5.
98. Pincus T, Brooks RH, Callahan LF. Prediction of long-term mortality in patients with rheumatoid arthritis according to simple questionnaire and joint count measures. Ann Intern Med. 1994;120(1):26–34.
99. Callahan LF, Cordray DS, Wells G, Pincus T. Formal education and five-year mortality in rheumatoid arthritis: mediation by helplessness scale score. Arthritis Care Res. 1996;9(6):463–72.
100. Sokka T, Hakkinen A, Krishnan E, Hannonen P. Similar prediction of mortality by the health assessment questionnaire in patients with rheumatoid arthritis and the general population. Ann Rheum Dis. 2004;63(5):494–7.
101. Pincus T. RAPID3, an index of only 3 patient self-report core data set measures, but not ESR, recognizes incomplete responses to methotrexate in usual care of patients with rheumatoid arthritis. Bull Hosp Jt Dis. 2013;71(2):117–20.
102. Castrejon I, Dougados M, Combe B, Guillemin F, Fautrel B, Pincus T. Can remission in rheumatoid arthritis be assessed without laboratory tests or a formal joint count? Possible remission criteria based on a self-report RAPID3 score and careful joint examination in the ESPOIR cohort. J Rheumatol. 2013;40(4):386–93.
103. Askanase AD, Castrejon I, Pincus T. Quantitative data for care of patients with systemic lupus erythematosus in usual clinical settings: a patient multidimensional health assessment questionnaire and physician estimate of noninflammatory symptoms. J Rheumatol. 2011;38(7):1309–16.
104. Castrejon I, Bergman MJ, Pincus T. MDHAQ/RAPID3 to recognize improvement over 2 months in usual care of patients with osteoarthritis, systemic lupus erythematosus, spondyloarthropathy, and gout, as well as rheumatoid arthritis. J Clin Rheumatol. 2013;19(4):169–74.
105. Danve A, Reddy A, Vakil-Gilani K, Garg N, Dinno A, Deodhar A. Routine assessment of patient index data 3 score (RAPID3) correlates well with bath ankylosing spondylitis disease activity index (BASDAI) in the assessment of disease activity and monitoring progression of axial spondyloarthritis. Clin Rheumatol. 2015;34(1):117–24.
106. Cinar M, Yilmaz S, Cinar FI, Koca SS, Erdem H, Pay S, et al. A patient-reported outcome measures-based composite index (RAPID3) for the assessment of disease activity in ankylosing spondylitis. Rheumatol Int. 2015;35(9):1575–80.
107. Michelsen B, Fiane R, Diamantopoulos AP, Soldal DM, Hansen IJ, Sokka T, et al. A comparison of disease burden in rheumatoid arthritis, psoriatic arthritis and axial spondyloarthritis. PLoS One. 2015;10(4), e0123582.

108. Park SH, Choe JY, Kim SK, Lee H, Castrejon I, Pincus T. Routine assessment of patient index data (RAPID3) and bath ankylosing spondylitis disease activity index (BASDAI) scores yield similar information in 85 Korean patients with ankylosing spondylitis seen in usual clinical care. J Clin Rheumatol. 2015;21(6):300–4.
109. Annapureddy N, Elsallabi O, Baker J, Sreih AG. Patient-reported outcomes in ANCA-associated vasculitis. A comparison between Birmingham Vasculitis Activity Score and routine assessment of patient index data 3. Clin Rheumatol. 2015;35(2):395–400.
110. Pincus T, Askanase AD, Swearingen CJ. A multi-dimensional health assessment questionnaire (MDHAQ) and routine assessment of patient index data (RAPID3) scores are informative in patients with all rheumatic diseases. Rheum Dis Clin North Am. 2009;35(4):819–27. x.
111. Kvien TK, Mowinckel P, Heiberg T, Dammann KL, Dale O, Aanerud GJ, et al. Performance of health status measures with a pen based personal digital assistant. Ann Rheum Dis. 2005;64(10):1480–4.
112. Callahan LF, Pincus T. A clue from a self-report questionnaire to distinguish rheumatoid arthritis from noninflammatory diffuse musculoskeletal pain. The P-VAS:D-ADL ratio. Arthritis Rheum. 1990;33(9):1317–22.
113. Pincus T, Skummer PT, Grisanti MT, Castrejon I, Yazici Y. MDHAQ/RAPID3 can provide a roadmap or agenda for all rheumatology visits when the entire MDHAQ is completed at all patient visits and reviewed by the doctor before the encounter. Bull NYU Hosp Jt Dis. 2012;70(3):177–86.
114. Mandl KD, Mandel JC, Murphy SN, Bernstam EV, Ramoni RL, Kreda DA, et al. The smart platform: early experience enabling substitutable applications for electronic health records. J Am Med Inform Assoc. 2012;19(4):597–603.
115. Mandl KD, Mandel JC, Kohane IS. Driving innovation in health systems through an apps-based information economy. Cell Syst. 2015;1(1):8–13.
116. Franz B, Schuler A, Krauss O. Applying FHIR in an integrated health monitoring system. EJBI. 2015;11(2):en51–6.
117. Cohen SB, Strand V, Aguilar D, Ofman JJ. Patient- versus physician-reported outcomes in rheumatoid arthritis patients treated with recombinant interleukin-1 receptor antagonist (anakinra) therapy. Rheumatology (Oxford). 2004;43(6):704–11.
118. Scott DL, Coulton BL, Chapman JH, Bacon PA, Popert AJ. The long-term effects of treating rheumatoid arthritis. J R Coll Physicians Lond. 1983;17(1):79–85.
119. Scott DL, Grindulis KA, Struthers GR, Coulton BL, Popert AJ, Bacon PA. Progression of radiological changes in rheumatoid arthritis. Ann Rheum Dis. 1984;43(1):8–17.
120. Mulherin D, Fitzgerald O, Bresnihan B. Clinical improvement and radiological deterioration in rheumatoid arthritis: evidence that the pathogenesis of synovial inflammation and articular erosion may differ. Br J Rheumatol. 1996;35(12):1263–8.
121. Pincus T, Segurado OG. Most visits of most patients with rheumatoid arthritis to most rheumatologists do not include a formal quantitative joint count. Ann Rheum Dis. 2006;65(6):820–2.
122. Sokka T, Pincus T. Most patients receiving routine care for rheumatoid arthritis in 2001 did not meet inclusion criteria for most recent clinical trials or American College of Rheumatology criteria for remission. J Rheumatol. 2003;30(6):1138–46.
123. Gogus F, Yazici Y, Yazici H. Inclusion criteria as widely used for rheumatoid arthritis clinical trials: patient eligibility in a Turkish cohort. Clin Exp Rheumatol. 2005;23(5):681–4.
124. Pincus T, Bergman MJ. Quantitative recording of physician clinical estimates, beyond a global estimate and formal joint count, in usual care: applying the scientific method, using a simple one-page worksheet. Rheum Dis Clin North Am. 2009;35(4):813–7. x.
125. van der Heijde DM, Van't Hof M, van Riel PL, van de Putte LB. Development of a disease activity score based on judgment in clinical practice by rheumatologists. J Rheumatol. 1993;20(3):579–81.

126. Prevoo ML, van't Hof MA, Kuper HH, van Leeuwen MA, van de Putte LB, van Riel PL. Modified disease activity scores that include twenty-eight-joint counts. Development and validation in a prospective longitudinal study of patients with rheumatoid arthritis. Arthritis Rheum. 1995;38(1):44–8.
127. Aletaha D, Smolen J. The simplified disease activity index (SDAI) and the clinical disease activity index (CDAI): a review of their usefulness and validity in rheumatoid arthritis. Clin Exp Rheumatol. 2005;23(5 Suppl 39):S100–8.
128. Pincus T, Yazici Y, Bergman MJ. RAPID3, an index to assess and monitor patients with rheumatoid arthritis, without formal joint counts: similar results to DAS28 and CDAI in clinical trials and clinical care. Rheum Dis Clin North Am. 2009;35(4):773–8. viii.
129. Wolfe F, Michaud K, Pincus T. A composite disease activity scale for clinical practice, observational studies, and clinical trials: the patient activity scale (PAS/PAS-II). J Rheumatol. 2005;32(12):2410–5.
130. Fleischer Jr AB, Feldman SR, Rapp SR, Reboussin DM, Exum ML, Clark AR, et al. Disease severity measures in a population of psoriasis patients: the symptoms of psoriasis correlate with self-administered psoriasis area severity index scores. J Investig Dermatol. 1996;107(1):26–9.
131. Fransen J, Antoni C, Mease PJ, Uter W, Kavanaugh A, Kalden JR, et al. Performance of response criteria for assessing peripheral arthritis in patients with psoriatic arthritis: analysis of data from randomised controlled trials of two tumour necrosis factor inhibitors. Ann Rheum Dis. 2006;65(10):1373–8.
132. Hawker G, Gabriel S, Bombardier C, Goldsmith C, Caron D, Gladman D. A reliability study of SLEDAI: a disease activity index for systemic lupus erythematosus. J Rheumatol. 1993;20(4):657–60.
133. Hay EM, Bacon PA, Gordon C, Isenberg DA, Maddison P, Snaith ML, et al. The BILAG index: a reliable and valid instrument for measuring clinical disease activity in systemic lupus erythematosus. Q J Med. 1993;86(7):447–58.
134. Swaak AJ, van den Brink HG, Smeenk RJ, Manger K, Kalden JR, Tosi S, et al. Systemic lupus erythematosus. Disease outcome in patients with a disease duration of at least 10 years: second evaluation. Lupus. 2001;10(1):51–8.
135. Petri M, Hellmann D, Hochberg M. Validity and reliability of lupus activity measures in the routine clinic setting. J Rheumatol. 1992;19(1):53–9.
136. Mosca M, Bencivelli W, Vitali C, Carrai P, Neri R, Bombardieri S. The validity of the ECLAM index for the retrospective evaluation of disease activity in systemic lupus erythematosus. Lupus. 2000;9(6):445–50.
137. Bencivelli W, Vitali C, Isenberg DA, Smolen JS, Snaith ML, Sciuto M, et al. Disease activity in systemic lupus erythematosus: report of the Consensus Study Group of the European Workshop for Rheumatology Research. III. Development of a computerised clinical chart and its application to the comparison of different indices of disease activity. The European Consensus Study Group for Disease Activity in SLE. Clin Exp Rheumatol. 1992;10(5):549–54.
138. Gladman DD, Urowitz MB, Goldsmith CH, Fortin P, Ginzler E, Gordon C, et al. The reliability of the systemic lupus international collaborating clinics/American College of Rheumatology damage index in patients with systemic lupus erythematosus. Arthritis Rheum. 1997;40(5):809–13.
139. Karlson EW, Daltroy LH, Rivest C, Ramsey-Goldman R, Wright EA, Partridge AJ, et al. Validation of a systemic lupus activity questionnaire (SLAQ) for population studies. Lupus. 2003;12(4):280–6.
140. Garrett S, Jenkinson T, Kennedy LG, Whitelock H, Gaisford P, Calin A. A new approach to defining disease status in ankylosing spondylitis: the bath ankylosing spondylitis disease activity index. J Rheumatol. 1994;21(12):2286–91.

141. Calin A, Garrett S, Whitelock H, Kennedy LG, O'Hea J, Mallorie P, et al. A new approach to defining functional ability in ankylosing spondylitis: the development of the bath ankylosing spondylitis functional index. J Rheumatol. 1994;21(12):2281–5.
142. Jenkinson TR, Mallorie PA, Whitelock HC, Kennedy LG, Garrett SL, Calin A. Defining spinal mobility in ankylosing spondylitis (AS). The bath as metrology index. J Rheumatol. 1994;21(9):1694–8.
143. Lukas C, Landewe R, Sieper J, Dougados M, Davis J, Braun J, et al. Development of an ASAS-endorsed disease activity score (ASDAS) in patients with ankylosing spondylitis. Ann Rheum Dis. 2009;68(1):18–24.
144. Dougados M, Gueguen A, Nakache JP, Nguyen M, Mery C, Amor B. Evaluation of a functional index and an articular index in ankylosing spondylitis. J Rheumatol. 1988;15(2):302–7.
145. Luqmani RA, Bacon PA, Moots RJ, Janssen BA, Pall A, Emery P, et al. Birmingham vasculitis activity score (BVAS) in systemic necrotizing vasculitis. QJM. 1994;87(11):671–8.
146. Exley AR, Bacon PA, Luqmani RA, Kitas GD, Gordon C, Savage CO, et al. Development and initial validation of the vasculitis damage index for the standardized clinical assessment of damage in the systemic vasculitides. Arthritis Rheum. 1997;40(2):371–80.
147. Stone JH, Hoffman GS, Merkel PA, Min YI, Uhlfelder ML, Hellmann DB, et al. A disease-specific activity index for Wegener's granulomatosis: modification of the Birmingham vasculitis activity score. International network for the study of the systemic vasculitides (INSSYS). Arthritis Rheum. 2001;44(4):912–20.
148. Seo P, Min YI, Holbrook JT, Hoffman GS, Merkel PA, Spiera R, et al. Damage caused by Wegener's granulomatosis and its treatment: prospective data from the Wegener's Granulomatosis Etanercept Trial (WGET). Arthritis Rheum. 2005;52(7):2168–78.
149. Bellamy N, Buchanan WW, Goldsmith CH, Campbell J, Stitt LW. Validation study of WOMAC: a health status instrument for measuring clinically important patient relevant outcomes to antirheumatic drug therapy in patients with osteoarthritis of the hip or knee. J Rheumatol. 1988;15(12):1833–40.
150. Burckhardt CS, Clark SR, Bennett RM. The fibromyalgia impact questionnaire: development and validation. J Rheumatol. 1991;18(5):728–33.
151. van Riel PL. Provisional guidelines for measuring disease activity in clinical trials on rheumatoid arthritis. Br J Rheumatol. 1992;31(12):793–4.
152. Tugwell P, Boers M. Omeract conference on outcome measures in rheumatoid arthritis clinical trials: introduction. J Rheumatol. 1993;20(3):528–30.
153. Wells GA, Boers M, Shea B, Brooks PM, Simon LS, Strand CV, et al. Minimal disease activity for rheumatoid arthritis: a preliminary definition. J Rheumatol. 2005;32(10):2016–24.
154. Sharp JT. Scoring radiographic abnormalities in rheumatoid arthritis. J Rheumatol. 1989;16(5):568–9.
155. Sharp JT. Assessment of radiographic abnormalities in rheumatoid arthritis: what have we accomplished and where should we go from here? J Rheumatol. 1995;22(9):1787–91.
156. Sharp JT, Lidsky MD, Collins LC, Moreland J. Methods of scoring the progression of radiologic changes in rheumatoid arthritis. Correlation of radiologic, clinical and laboratory abnormalities. Arthritis Rheum. 1971;14(6):706–20.
157. van der Heijde D. How to read radiographs according to the Sharp/van der Heijde method. J Rheumatol. 2000;27(1):261–3.
158. Landewe R, van der Heijde D. Radiographic progression in rheumatoid arthritis. Clin Exp Rheumatol. 2005;23(5 Suppl 39):S63–8.
159. Larsen A. How to apply Larsen score in evaluating radiographs of rheumatoid arthritis in long-term studies. J Rheumatol. 1995;22(10):1974–5.
160. Larsen A, Dale K, Eek M. Radiographic evaluation of rheumatoid arthritis and related conditions by standard reference films. Acta Radiol. 1977;18(4):481–91.
161. Rau R, Wassenberg S, Herborn G, Stucki G, Gebler A. A new method of scoring radiographic change in rheumatoid arthritis. J Rheumatol. 1998;25(11):2094–107.

162. Clegg DO, Reda DJ, Weisman MH, Blackburn WD, Cush JJ, Cannon GW, et al. Comparison of sulfasalazine and placebo in the treatment of ankylosing spondylitis. A Department Of Veterans Affairs Cooperative Study. Arthritis Rheum. 1996;39(12):2004–12.
163. Calin A, Nakache JP, Gueguen A, Zeidler H, Mielants H, Dougados M. Defining disease activity in ankylosing spondylitis: is a combination of variables (bath ankylosing spondylitis disease activity index) an appropriate instrument? Rheumatology (Oxford). 1999;38(9):878–82.
164. Creemers MC, Franssen MJ, van't Hof MA, Gribnau FW, van de Putte LB, van Riel PL. Assessment of outcome in ankylosing spondylitis: an extended radiographic scoring system. Ann Rheum Dis. 2005;64(1):127–9.
165. Calin A, Mackay K, Santos H, Brophy S. A new dimension to outcome: application of the bath ankylosing spondylitis radiology index. J Rheumatol. 1999;26(4):988–92.
166. Whiting-O'Keefe QE, Stone JH, Hellmann DB. Validity of a vasculitis activity index for systemic necrotizing vasculitis. Arthritis Rheum. 1999;42(11):2365–71.
167. Smolen JS, Aletaha D, Bijlsma JW, Breedveld FC, Boumpas D, Burmester G, et al. Treating rheumatoid arthritis to target: recommendations of an international task force. Ann Rheum Dis. 2010;69(4):631–7.
168. Boutry N, Hachulla E, Flipo RM, Cortet B, Cotten A. MR imaging findings in hands in early rheumatoid arthritis: comparison with those in systemic lupus erythematosus and primary Sjögren syndrome. Radiology. 2005;236(2):593–600.

Chapter 4
PROMs for Rheumatoid Arthritis

Yasser El Miedany

Introduction

Rheumatoid arthritis (RA) has become a major health concern due to the finding that the aging of the population has led to a marked increase in the prevalence of the disease with its consequences [1]. In the meantime, the medical research has brought about major advances to the therapeutic tools for RA; resulting in significant change in the disease treatment paradigms. Earlier, more aggressive and timely treatment has made remission a realistic target. These advances led to transformation of the arthritic patients' management pathways, and the development of new models of integrated care in inflammatory arthritis (Fig. 4.1) [2]. Furthermore, these advances mandated a redefinition of health outcomes for RA patients' management, which has expanded to include: disease activity remission, structural remission, patient remission, medication compliance, as well as low incidence of comorbidities (Fig. 4.2) [3].

The interest in patient-reported outcomes in inflammatory arthritis started in the early 1990s. The World Health Organization/International League of Associations for Rheumatology (WHO–ILAR) core set of outcome measures to be reported in RA randomized trials was published in 1994 [4] and, since then, various organization authorities have made further recommendations regarding the reporting of RA-specific disease states. The American College of Rheumatology (ACR) core set of RA outcomes was published in 1993 and included 7 parameters namely: tender and swollen joints, physician global assessment, inflammatory markers, as well as patient global assessment, pain score, and functional disability [5]. Although fatigue

Y. El Miedany (✉)
Honorary Senior Clinical Lecturer, King's College London, London, UK

Professor of Rheumatology and Rehabilitation, Ain Shams University, Cairo, Egypt

Department of Rheumatology, Darent Valley Hospital, Gravesend, Kent, UK
e-mail: drelmiedany@rheumatology4u.com

Y. El Miedany (ed.), *Patient Reported Outcome Measures in Rheumatic Diseases*,
DOI 10.1007/978-3-319-32851-5_4

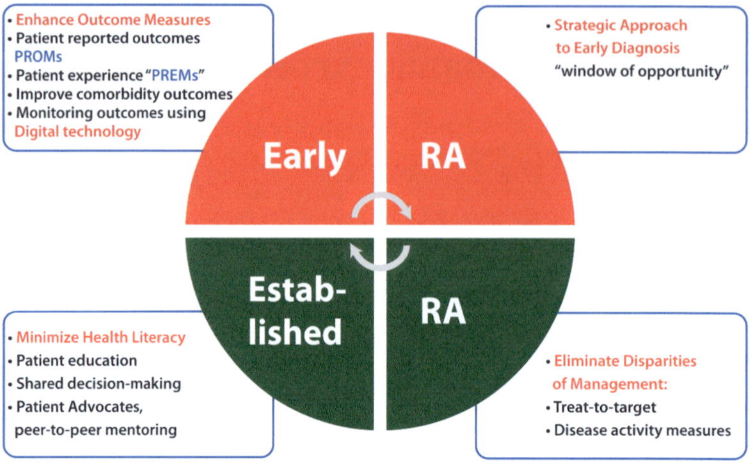

Fig. 4.1 Transformation of rheumatoid arthritis patients' management: new model of integrated care

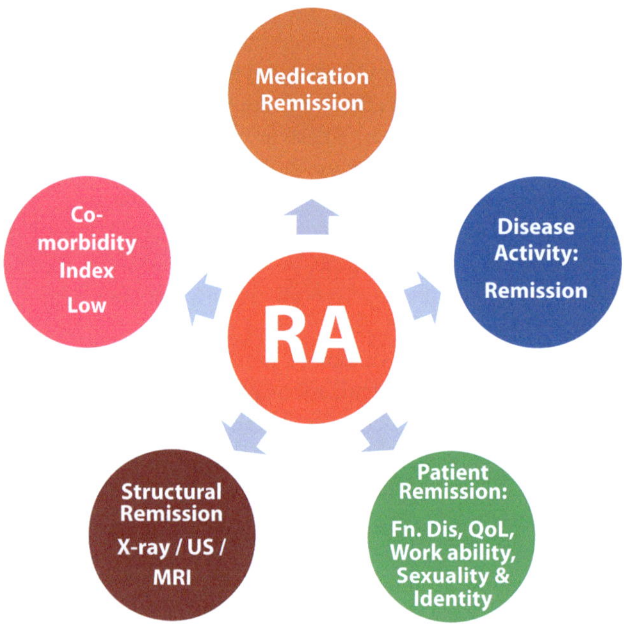

Fig. 4.2 Redefining health outcomes: management outcomes of rheumatoid arthritis

is not part of the ACR core set of RA outcomes, outcome measures in rheumatology (OMERACT), in 2006, endorsed the inclusion of fatigue in their core set [6]. Later on and in concordance with the OMERACT recommendation, both the European league against rheumatism (EULAR) and ACR recommended that fatigue should be reported within the domain of disease activity in every randomized clinical trial [7].

Gradually, patient-reported outcomes in RA gained momentum as research studies documented its value in standard clinical practice [8, 9]. The new global trend toward "Patient-Centered Care" has endorsed patient-reported outcomes measures (PROMs) use in routine healthcare. Effectiveness of care from the patient's own perspective, measured by a patient-reported outcome measure, has become actively involved in quality measurement and service improvement [10]. This chapter will highlight the value of PROMs for RA patients, its impact on both the short-term as well as long-term patients' management. It will also discuss patient-reported outcome tools available for RA patients and the differences amongst them and the possibility of using PROMs as biomarker for RA patients.

Patient-Reported Outcomes in Rheumatoid Arthritis

Classifying Disease Activity State

Patient-reported outcomes have been investigated in terms of their relations with the disease activity. Several studies showed their significant association with disease activity parameters [11–13]. However, as early arthritis and disease remission became the targets of management, the interest has shifted toward specific patient-reported symptoms such as pain, fatigue, duration of morning stiffness, quality of life, as well as functional ability. Patient-reported tender joints were also introduced into standard clinical practice as well as research trials and were found comparable to the physician-reported joint tenderness [14]. Assessing patient global is essential to calculate the disease activity score (DAS-28) [15]. Similarly, in the American College of Rheumatology core set of disease activity measures, three elements pertain to the patients' perspective; these elements are: pain, functional capacity, and patient global assessment [5]. The RAPID3 (routine assessment of patient index data 3) questionnaire incorporates three patient-reported outcomes from the RA core set (namely pain, function, and patient global assessment), and this tool has been shown to provide similar information to clinician-scored indices of disease activity, namely: CDAI (Clinical Disease Activity Index) = Tender Joint Count, Swollen Joint Count, physician global and patient global assessment; SDAI (Simplified Disease Activity Index) = Tender Joint Count, Swollen Joint Count, physician global, patient global assessment as well as CRP; DAS-28: Disease Activity Scale with 28 joint count = Tender Joint Count, Swollen Joint Count, CRP, patient global [16]. The development of multidimensional patient-reported outcome measures, which has been validated [6, 17, 18], facilitated the inclusion of such parameters in standard day-to-day practice and paved the way for a more active role for patient involvement in monitoring their disease activity. This could enhance treatment by providing early warning when targets are not met and indicating the need for a physician visit to re-evaluate treatment.

Prognostic Marker

The introduction of the early arthritis concept and the "window of opportunity" widened the scope to include disease parameters to help identify the patient subgroup suffering from persistent inflammatory arthritis. The EPISA study [19], carried out to predict persistent inflammatory arthritis disease course, identified duration of morning stiffness, deterioration of functional disability over 3 months, as well as anti-cyclic citrullinated peptide (CCP) antibodies as the three main poor prognostic manifestations in this subgroup of patients. This important role of functional disability was also highlighted by studies that linked increased mortality to greater functional disability in arthritis patients [20]. Recently, the American College of Rheumatology guidelines (2015) for management of inflammatory arthritis [21] identified functional disability, seropositivity for rheumatoid factor or anti-CCP, presence of bony erosions, as well as the presence of extra-articular manifestations as poor prognostic features in arthritic patients.

The discrepancy between the clinicians and the patient global assessment especially early in the disease course can be attributed to the fact that both clinicians and patients have different perspectives on outcomes. A recent study [22] was carried out aiming at assessment of the concurrence and non-concurrence of patient and physician global assessment in early rheumatoid arthritis patients both in disease activity and in remission. Retrospective analysis of 480 patients diagnosed according to the 2010 ACR/EULAR criteria [23] for early inflammatory arthritis revealed that global estimates of both patients and physicians vary according to disease activity status. In patients with moderate to highly active disease (DAS-28 > 3.2), the mean patient global assessment score was significantly higher than the physician global score, whereas in disease remission, there was no significant difference. Furthermore, results revealed that parameters such as sleep, fatigue, self-helplessness, and work ability had a significant impact on the patients with active disease and should be considered by the treating physician. Whilst the health assessment questionnaire (HAQ) assesses the patients' functional ability, quality of life assessment should be also added to the standard clinical assessment.

A Potential Disease-Modifying Role

Recording patient-reported outcomes has traditionally been looked at as a one-stop assessment. In relation to the patient's ever-changing condition characteristic for RA, recording PROMs at each patient's visit adds to its dynamic plasticity. This highlights the importance of keeping a record of these outcomes over longer periods of time for further analysis. A recent study [24] looked into sharing the patients' consecutive PROMs scores recorded with them. Electronic recording of the data obtained facilitated expressing these figures as easy-to-read charts. Results revealed that this new e-approach helped the patients to visualize the progress of their disease activity course and response to therapy. Monitoring real-time changes in disease activity provided patients with visual evidence of their responses to treatment at different time points. Following 1-year of management, statistically significant differences were seen in disease activity parameters and patients' willingness to remain on treatment favoring the visual feedback approach. In addition, the study depicted that viewing previous PROMs records (1) helped the patients understand the effect of treatment on disease activity, (2) helped in medication adherence, (3) improved trust in the treating physician, (4) alleviated concerns about the future, and (5) helped in coping with daily life and disease. These findings highlight that keeping a record of the patient outcome measures and sharing it with the patients not only is politically correct, in that the patients were involved in the treatment, but the statistically significant differences suggest that this adjunctive therapy based on PROMs recordings may actually also have disease-modifying potential.

Patient Education

Over the past years, there has been a significant change in patient education approaches. Traditionally, in standard clinical practice, patient education tended to focus on helping patients to understand their disease and to give information regarding the medication prescribed or interventions being used. This usually is carried out using pre-prepared information leaflets. On the other hand, in research studies, patient education targeted behavior changes and enhancement of a general sense of control as well as skill in coping with the disease and its sequelae [25–27]. The newly adopted patient-centered care approach emphasized the positive role of the patient in their treatment, or what is called "self-management." The recently published guidelines from the National Institute for Health and Clinical Excellence (NICE) [28] and EULAR [29] for inflammatory arthritis addressed the different aspects that need to be tackled by the appropriate patient education programs. This includes major risk factors, such as cardiovascular, falls, and osteoporosis/fracture risks, which may also account for increased mortality, poor quality of life, and work disability, as well as comorbidities. Therefore, patient educational programs should be tailored to the patient's needs. Recent studies [30, 31] showed that PROMs can be used as a link between the disease outcomes and patient education as it enables the treating physician and the patient to identify the main points that need tackling. The integration of the PROMs and patient education offered a new opportunity toward patient self-efficacy in disease management. A recently introduced patient education program, the "joint fitness program" adopted PROMs to identify the patient's educational needs [32].

Cost-Effectiveness

Cost-effectiveness is not a straightforward concept as it encompasses elements not directly measurable in currency, such as morbidity, mortality, and reduction in quality of life. Recently, the American College of Physicians recommended the establishment of an organization for the generation and review of cost-effectiveness analyses [33]. In England and Wales, the National Institute for Health and Clinical Excellence (NICE) was established to balance the financial costs and clinical benefits of health technologies and evaluate their cost-effectiveness [34]. The health status information collected from patients by way of PROMs questionnaires before and after an intervention provides an indication of the outcomes or quality of care delivered to the patients. The PROMs used to collect data from patients will comprise a condition-specific instrument, in addition to more general patient-specific information. There are intentions to link payments to PROMs data: "payments to hospitals will be conditional on the quality of care given to patients as well as the volume. A range of quality measures covering safety, clinical outcomes, patient experience, and patient's views about the success of their treatment (known as Patient-reported outcome measures or PROMs) will be used [35]." A recent study [36] revealed how PROMs can be cost-effective. In that study, arthritic patients could achieve better control of their disease by showing them a comparison between previous PROMs taken when their disease activity was at its peak and their current PROMs. This was achieved by helping them to be more adherent to their medications and less likely to stop due to intolerance. It also helped to give them the ability to cope with their activities of daily living, achieve fewer visits to their general practitioners (GPs), and become less concerned about their future. Medication compliance was significantly correlated with changes in all measured disease parameters as well as ability to work.

Patient-Reported Outcome Measures in the Assessment of Comorbidities

The relation of RA and comorbid conditions can be complex. This might be attributed to different types of comorbidities and their pathogenesis. In type-I comorbidity, there is no relation between RA and the comorbid condition that is detected. For example, trauma and certain cancers are unrelated to the presence of RA. Type-II comorbidity occurs when the comorbid condition leads to an increase in an RA outcome: for example, persons with depression and RA are more likely to become work disabled than persons without depression. Type-III comorbidity (RA consequences) occurs when an RA outcome leads to an increase in a comorbid condition, for example, gastrointestinal ulceration and herpes zoster. Type-IV comorbidity (RA illness) occurs when RA causes (at least in part) the comorbid conditions; e.g., myocardial infarction and lymphoma. Type-V comorbidity (RA treatment) occurs when RA treatment causes or contributes to comorbidity development; e.g., steroids and infection. Finally, type-VI comorbidity (common external factor) occurs when a common condition leads both to RA and the comorbidity; e.g., smoking, RA, and lung cancer [37]. The potential role of PROMs in the assessment of comorbidities in arthritic patients is an example of the PROMs' dynamic nature [38]. Recent PROMs questionnaires allow the treating clinician to assess for RA-associated comorbidities at each visit. In its early stages, inflammatory arthritis patients may not have significant comorbidities that warrant further management. However, as the disease progresses and becomes more active, the patient can be prone to 1 or more of these comorbidities. Screening for these symptoms is highly recommended on a regular basis for every patient. Furthermore, this approach would also facilitate on-the-spot assessment for cardiovascular risk, falls risk, osteoporosis as well as depression [39]. This dynamic impact of PROMs plays an important role on the long-term patients' care.

Patient-Reported Outcome Measures for Rheumatoid Arthritis

Quantitative measurement in many rheumatic diseases has progressed following two inspiring conferences held in 1982 [40, 41], which endorsed proposals for outcome measures assessment in rheumatoid arthritis [4, 15, 32, 42–45]; osteoarthritis [46]; fibromyalgia [47]; systemic lupus erythematosus [48–53]; ankylosing spondylitis [54, 55]; as well as vasculitis [56–58]. However, unfortunately, most rheumatology patient care continues to run largely without quantitative measures other than laboratory tests, which may not be available at the time of a patient visit and often give false-positive or false-negative results [59, 60].

According to Bowling [61], PROMs can be stratified in terms of their disease specificity (generic or disease-specific), measurement objectives (discrimination, evaluation, and prediction) and what they intend to measure (quality of life, health-related quality of life, or health status) [62, 63]. The multidimensional measurement scale involves more than one item of these outcome measures and therefore can be categorized broadly into two main categories: generic health status and condition-specific measures. Generic instruments comprise items intended to be relevant to the widest range of patients' conditions and the general population. On the other hand, condition-specific instruments are often more focused on a particular disease or health condition (e.g., rheumatoid arthritis or spondyloarthritis), a patient population (e.g., older adults), a specific problem or symptom (e.g., pain or fatigue), or a described function (e.g., activities of daily living) [64]. Disease-specific tools tend to be multidimensional [65] (Table 4.1) [12, 13, 18, 62, 63, 66–69].

For any given area of health, condition-specific instruments may have greater clinical appeal due to incorporation of content specific to the particular conditions, and the likelihood of increased responsiveness to interventions. In view of the fact that there is no single measure that can serve as a gold standard in all patients suf-

Table 4.1 Patient-reported outcome measures for rheumatoid arthritis

Type	Measure	Score	Generic	Specific tools
Unidimensional	Single construct	Items (questions) are added to yield overall score	• EurQoL [62] • Nottingham Health Profile [63]	• Pain questionnaire [12] • Bristol rheumatoid arthritis fatigue numerical rating scales (BRAF-NRS) [66] • Rheumatoid arthritis-specific work productivity survey (WPS-RA) [67]
Multidimensional	Health concepts of relevance to a wide range of patients	Specific score for each domain	• -SF-36 [13] • -MDHAQ [68]	• MDPROMs-RA [18] • Bristol rheumatoid arthritis fatigue multidimensional questionnaire (BRAF-MDQ) [66] • Rheumatic arthritis impact of disease (RAID) [69]

fering from inflammatory arthritic conditions, a mutual index of several measures has been recommended for assessment of disease activity and monitoring response to therapy. The most widely used indices in RA are the ACR core dataset, disease activity score (DAS-28), and clinical disease activity index (CDAI) [4, 42, 43, 45, 46]. Specific multidimensional PROMs have been developed to capture those elements of health outcome measures of relevance to a specific patient group. Therefore, it represents the best available tool offering a quantitative "gestalt" impression of the outcome measures for a specific condition. Multidimensional PROMs questionnaire are already available for rheumatoid arthritis (examples are shown in Table 4.1 [12, 13, 18, 62, 63, 66–69]). In all these conditions, PROMs has shown both a diagnostic value in helping to identify those who might be suffering from early inflammatory condition and a therapeutic impact as it helps to monitor response to therapy over time [65].

Patient-Reported Outcome Measures Evolving from Static to Dynamic

In acute diseases in hospital settings (the primary setting of most traditional medical practice, education, training, and research) quantitative data regarding blood pressure, temperature, and body weight come as a priority, whereas no data are collected concerning functional status or pain since success or failure of the treatment is obvious within a short period. However, in chronic diseases such as in the standard rheumatology outpatient setting (the primary locale of almost all contemporary rheumatologic care), such information is critical for the documentation of patient outcomes and results of care. An earlier report [70] highlighted that pain, function, and RAPID scores should be considered as vital signs in chronic diseases, analogous to pulse and temperature in acute disease and blood pressure and cholesterol in long-term health conditions. However, whilst more attention has been paid to the long-term value of PROMs (functional disability is the most significant predictor of mortality in RA), its short-term value in routine clinical care, role in enhancing the patient-centered care approach, as well as improving patients' experience, came to light recently. This was supported by the results of a recent report [71] that emphasized the expansion of PROMs from the static phase of capturing and measuring outcomes at a single point of time to a more dynamic role over a long period. Another study [24], which looked into sharing the patients' previous PROMs records with them either in a paper or electronic format (visual feedback), revealed that viewing previous PROMs records had a significant positive impact on their disease activity control as well as compliance to therapy. This was achieved by helping the patients to be more adherent to their medications and less likely to stop due to intolerance.

The Biomarker Concept in Rheumatoid Arthritis

Better understanding of the disease pathology and the implementation of recent radiographic tools (such as ultrasound [US] and magnetic resonance imaging [MRI]) lead to the concept that RA is a syndrome with different clinical stages. During the course of the disease (Table 4.2), there are four major time points when crucial decisions are required. First, the stage of early inflammatory arthritis, in particular before the diagnostic criteria are fulfilled where markers for prognosis are especially needed at this stage. Second, once the diagnosis is established, markers of disease activity and severity are needed. Third, screening tests for prediction of response to therapy and progression of the disease, and finally, later in the disease course, markers/predictors of comorbidities and mortality are required to establish rules to increase treatment success and reduce safety concerns. Therefore, the proposed biomarker(s) should be able to identify these new subsets at the different critical time points [72]. The proper timing at this stage creates the so-called "window of opportunity."

Table 4.2 The biomarker concept in RA: patient-reported outcome (PRO) parameters in relation to the 4 major time points in the disease process

Stage	Disease process	Relevant PRO parameter
First stage	Early inflammatory arthritis	Functional disability, morning stiffness, quality of life
Second stage	Established disease activity	Patient global assessment, pain score, patient self-reported joint tenderness
Third stage	Prediction of response	Functional disability, quality of life
Fourth stage	Predictor of co-morbidity	Co-morbidity screen, functional disability

Application of the Concept of Personalized Medicine in Rheumatoid Arthritis

The healthcare services worldwide are now both looking at the use of personalized medicine to provide better care. One of the first applications of personalized medicine was for breast cancer [31], where identification of molecular targets inside the tumor tissue is now mandatory for the use of targeted treatments. This practice has reached the regulatory level and drug trials are ongoing based on targeted biomarkers. Some of these aspects can be applied to RA. A tailored approach to treatment can be envisioned, based, for example, on combinations of biologics or sequential therapies guided by biomarkers. Maintaining a clinical balance between applying timely and effective treatment and avoiding ineffective, costly, and potentially aggressive treatment at the personal level is at present one of the main challenges in RA management. Unfortunately, the optimal tools for diagnosis, prognosis, treatment selection, and efficacy measurement are not yet at hand. The search for biomarkers identifying key targets for the assessment of major outcomes in rheumatoid arthritis became a hot issue over the past few years. The National Institutes of Health biomarkers definition working group [73] defines a biomarker as "a characteristic that is objectively measured and evaluated as an indicator of normal biological processes, pathogenic processes, or pharmacologic responses to a therapeutic intervention."

Patient-Reported Outcome Measures as a Biomarker in Rheumatoid Arthritis

In RA, which is a major leading cause of disability, proposed biomarkers should help the identification of the patients suffering from persistent inflammatory arthritis in its early stages. Biomarkers also should help to identify those who would require aggressive forms of therapy (whether through a combination of disease-modifying antirheumatic drugs [DMARDs] or early biologic therapy), and show variation with the disease activity with the possibility of adopting patient-centered care into standard clinical practice. Biomarkers should also be able to identify those patients prone to sustaining structural joint damage early in the disease course. The possibility of identifying the individual RA patient's future disease severity could guide the choice of the best treatment strategy and during the disease course could help in tailoring a treatment plan aiming at stopping the joint damage.

Change from baseline for patient-reported outcomes was assessed in four treat-to-target studies (Table 4.3) [74–77]. Recent studies [22, 78] assessed biomarkers and a patient-tailored approach in rheumatoid arthritis and whether PROMs are the missing biomarkers. Changes from baseline to week 76 of clinical variables, patient-reported outcome measures, and measures of radiographic progression were assessed in 481 subjects suffering from early inflammatory arthritis (disease duration <6 months) diagnosed according to the ACR/EULAR criteria 2010 and treated

Table 4.3 Change from baseline for patient-reported outcomes in 4 treat-to-target studies

Study	Target	Tender J. count	Pain score (VAS: 0–100)	Patient global assessment (VAS: 0–100)	Fatigue score (VAS: 0–100)	Morning stiffness (min)	HAQ (0–3)
TICORA [74]	DAS < 2.4	−12	−43	−52	NR	NR	−0.8
CAMERA [75]	ACR remission	−11	−36	−32	NR	−63	−0.4
ESPOIR-GUEPARD [76]	DAS-28 < 3.2	−10.1	−44.8	−46.6	−37.1	NR	−0.9
Schipper et al. [77]	DAS-29 < 2.6	−4	−30	−32	NR	NR	−0.5

Values are expressed as mean difference from baseline, *NR* not reported, *VAS* visual analogue scale, *TICORA* Tight Control for Rheumatoid Arthritis, *CAMERA* Computer-Assisted Management in Early Rheumatoid Arthritis to target. Results revealed that the crude functional disability score as well as the percentage changes at 3 and 6 months showed a significant increase in the group with persistent inflammatory synovitis compared to the self-limiting arthritis group. Using binary logistic regression analyses to assess the association between functional disability and disease activity flare up revealed that a flare was associated with poor baseline function and quality of life measures: functional disability (OR per 0.1 unit = 1.8 [1.06–1.54], $p = 0.004$) and quality of life (OR = 1.12 [1.01–1.23], $p = 0.024$). Patient global assessment and pain score were associated significantly with scores of DAS-28, ACR response, systemic manifestations, and work ability. Changes in the functional disability scores correlated significantly to changes in PD scores ($p < 0.01$). In multiple conditional logistic regression analysis, factors associated with the development of joint space narrowing were worsening of functional disability score by > 0.5/3, synovial thickening and synovial PD score ≥ 2 at both baseline and 6 months of treatment. The discriminative power had an AUC of 0.864 (95 % CI 0.765–0.937), with sensitivity 84 %, specificity 92 %, and likelihood ratio + 5.6. Another study [39] assessed the use of PROMs to assess for comorbidity. Results revealed that PROMs questionnaire were able to identify patients at high cardiovascular risk, high falls as well as infection risk. In view of these data, PROMs met the criteria of a valid marker for rheumatoid arthritis, being objectively measured, indicator of normal and pathologic joint affection, as well as a sensitive and specific marker for response to therapy and poor prognosis.

Embedding Patient-Reported Outcome Measures in the Decision-Making Process

The expansion in use of economic evaluation by health agencies has mirrored the growing recognition of the usefulness of health-related quality of life as an important indicator of outcome of disease treatment among clinicians and patients [33, 79, 80]. Patient-reported experience measures (PREMs) became an independent assessment tool to measure management outcomes [81]. A cornerstone of such analysis is the quality-adjusted life year (QALY), which is formed by the arithmetic product of quantity and quality of life. Such economic implication raised the issue of shared decision-making between the patient and the treating physician as the recommended approach in clinical practice. Shared decision-making is a process in which patients are encouraged to participate in selecting appropriate treatments or management options. The constituent elements of QALY are: health-related quality of life measures and survival. In the UK, the mechanics for collecting patient-based HRQOL assessments have been presaged in the National Health Service from 2009, requiring both pre- and post-surgery PROMs assessment of health status in selected procedures [82]. Embedding such data within national health information systems would facilitate an easier interpretation of QALY-based information. Furthermore, assimilating health-related quality of life into routine clinical rheumatology practice will assist not only the quality of care provided but also the longer-term development of other uses for those data. This represents another new evolving role for PROMs, which can facilitate incorporating information on HRQOL and quality of life in treatment decision-making of RA patients, improving the relevance of the QALY as a composite measure to those groups of users. Data derived from a PROMs questionnaire should provide the guide for the treating clinician in making decisions about different clinical inputs as well as for monitoring the outcomes and response to treatment. By implementing PROMs routinely in standard clinical practice, it can help to set up a management plan tailored to the patient's needs. In addition to its value in providing a baseline assessment of the health status, quality of life, and patient satisfaction or well-being, it helps to improve the patient physician communication, identifying new comorbidities that might have developed over the past few months prior to the clinic visit and the assessment of different procedure effectiveness.

Electronic Patient-Reported Outcome Measures in Rheumatoid Arthritis

Electronic health recording started to have its place in standard rheumatology practice. Direct provision of patient-reported outcomes via standardized electronic questionnaires was suggested as a tool to improve the efficiency, completeness, and accuracy of data collection. This overall approach is consistent with a broader movement in the healthcare delivery toward a patient-centered approach, quality of care provided, as well as the functioning of electronic health recording. For several years, a key barrier to the use of ePROMs data in clinical care settings was the difficulty of transforming the paper-based questionnaires into an instantly accessible application [83]. With the rapid expansion of Internet-connected gadgets and mobile devices, both at home and in the clinical setting, it became possible to develop online systems with a broad range of implementations in standard clinical practice. However, it has to be noted that an ePROMs system does not replace the patient–clinician clinical assessment and discussion, but it helps to focus the dialogue on symptoms that need consideration and allow the clinician to quickly determine whether the patient's symptoms are worsening or improving over time, therefore it has a time saving impact on clinic visits.

Earlier reports raised the concern that paper-based questionnaires might need to be altered to be presented in electronic formats. As this could change the way patients respond to the questions, PROMs methodologists have outlined the reasons and approaches for evaluating the equivalence of the questionnaire data across each mode of administration [84]. Earlier studies carried out in oncology clinical practice [85–87] revealed that these smart electronic systems supported multiple clinical activities, including assessment of symptoms and toxicities related to chemotherapy and radiation, postoperative surveillance, and symptom management during palliative care and hospice. A recent study [88] was carried out to assess the use of electronic patient-reported outcome measures in the standard clinical care setting of early arthritis patients. Results revealed that an ePROMs questionnaire could be administered through tablet computers, Web pages, and smart phones. In comparison to the paper format, there were insignificant differences between the paper and online formats in terms of disease activity measures assessed in this work. On the other hand, the electronic format helped to handle the complex skip patterns, provided accurate time and date of recording, achieved higher patient compliance versus paper with better data quality recorded, and facilitated the availability of an outbound calling option. The equality between the electronic and paper-based PROMs reported in this study is in agreement with the results of an earlier study, which showed that paper- and Web-based surveys provide data that are essentially equivalent [89].

As far as disease management and monitoring response to therapy, it was feasible, using ePROMs, to sum the patient's disease activity parameters, and based on the scores calculated, clinical relevant actions tailored to the patient's disease activity were taken that have reflected on the disease control and target achieved. In addition to its value in monitoring disease activity in standard clinical practice, ePROMs helped to optimize the patients' adherence to their treatment. This agrees with the outcome of earlier studies that reported that by using an iterative design process that focuses on patient outcome measures and disease activity parameters, the patients' perception of their therapy was augmented with sensor technology [18, 90]. In addition to the reported finding that implementing a PROMs system in standard clinical practice did improve patient–rheumatologist communication during clinic visits [91–93], results of this work showed that ePROMs was able to alert clinicians to acute needs for symptom management between visits. This comes in agreement with outcomes of earlier studies revealing values of electronic systems in the management of patients' chronic conditions in between their clinic visits [87, 94–98]. Furthermore, some systems have been designed to provide educational materials to patients, tailored to their reported symptoms and needs, right after they complete a survey [95, 97]. The electronic format enabled the treating rheumatologist(s) to have systematically collected symptom data that can support clinical decision-making. These features have been found to improve patient satisfaction with their care and have the potential to improve symptom management [99, 100]. On another front, the significant correlation between adherence to therapy and the information the patient gets about his medication, as well as the patient's contribution in the decision-making, highlight the importance of Shared Decision-Making in the management process.

Conclusion

The field of PROs in RA is of great interest, and is clearly relevant in these days of patient-centered care. Assessments based on patients' opinions (PROMs) have received increasing recognition as being critically important end points in both clinical trials and standard rheumatology practice for rheumatoid arthritis patients in the last decade. PROMs' role has expanded from merely assessing disease activity parameters at a certain time of management, to playing an active role in the diagnosis, assessment of disease activity, monitoring of comorbidities, adherence to therapy, and patient self-management. PROMs also evolved from the generic phase into a disease-specific era. Embedding PROMs in the decision-making process has facilitated filling the gap between the standard clinical practice and the growing role of health economics.

References

1. Arthritis Alliance of Canada. The impact of arthritis in Canada: today and over the next 30 years. 2011. http://www.arthritisnetwork.ca/downloads/20111022_Impact_of_arthritis.pdf. Accessed 20 Jul 2012.
2. El Miedany Y. Comorbidity index in rheumatoid arthritis. Time to think. Clin Rheumatol. 2015;34:1995–2000.
3. Palmer D, El Miedany Y. Shared decision making for patients living with inflammatory arthritis. Br J Nurs. 2016;25(1):2–6.
4. Boers M, Tugwell P, Felson DT, van Riel PL, Kirwan JR, Edmonds JP, et al. World Health Organization and International League of Associations for Rheumatology core endpoints for symptom modifying antirheumatic drugs in rheumatoid arthritis clinical trials. J Rheumatol. 1994;21 Suppl 41:86–9.
5. Felson DT, Anderson JJ, Boers M, Bombardier C, Chernoff M, Fried B, et al. The American College of Rheumatology preliminary core set of disease activity measures for rheumatoid arthritis clinical trials. The committee on outcome measures in rheumatoid arthritis clinical trials. Arthritis Rheum. 1993;36:729–40.
6. Gossec L, Dougados M, Rincheval N, Balanescu A, Boumpas DT, Canadelo S, et al. Elaboration of the preliminary rheumatoid arthritis impact of disease (RAID) score: a EULAR initiative. Ann Rheum Dis. 2009;68(11):1680–5.
7. Aletaha D, Landewe R, Karonitsch T, Bathon J, Boers M, Bombardier C, et al. Reporting disease activity in clinical trials of patients with rheumatoid arthritis: EULAR/ACR collaborative recommendations. Ann Rheum Dis. 2008;67:1360–4.
8. Pincus T, Wolfe F. Patient questionnaires for clinical research and improved standard patient care: is it better to have 80% of the information in 100% of patients or 100% of the information in 5% of patients? J Rheumatol. 2005;32:575–7.
9. El Miedany Y, El Gaafary M, Ahmed I, Youssef S, Nasr A. US guided treat-to-target approach in early RA: implications for uncoupling of disease activity and structural joint damage. Curr Rheumatol Rev. 2015;11:18–27.
10. Saag KG, Yazdany J, Alexander C, Caplan L, Coblyn J, Desai SP, American College of Rheumatology Quality Measurement White Paper Development Workgroup, et al. Defining quality of care in rheumatology: the American College of Rheumatology white paper on quality measurement. Arthritis Care Res (Hoboken). 2011;63(1):2–9.
11. Cadena J, Vinaccia S, Pérez A, Rico MI, Hinojosa R, Anaya JM. The impact of disease activity on the quality of life, mental health status and family dysfunction in Colombian patients with rheumatoid arthritis. J Clin Rheumatol. 2003;9(3):142–50.
12. Smedstad LM, Vaglum P, Kvien TK, Moum T. The relationship between self-reported pain and sociodemographic variables, anxiety and depressive symptoms in rheumatoid arthritis. J Rheumatol. 1995;22(3):514–20.
13. Birrell FN, Hassell AB, Jones PW, Dawes PT. How does the short form 36 health questionnaire (SF-36) in rheumatoid arthritis relate to RA outcome measures and SF-36 population values? A cross sectional study. Clin Rheumatol. 2000;19(3):195–9.

14. El Miedany Y, Palmer D, Jilani A, El Gaafary M. Outcome measures in rheumatoid arthritis in standard clinical practice: patient self report joint tenderness Vs physician performed joint evaluation. Rheumatology (Oxford). 2008;47(S2):ii141.
15. van der Heijde DM, Van't Hof M, van Riel PL, van de Putte LB. Development of a disease activity score based on judgment in clinical practice by rheumatologists. J Rheumatol. 1993;20:579–81.
16. Pincus T, Yazici Y, Bergman MJ. RAPID3, an index to assess and monitor patients with rheumatoid arthritis, without formal joint counts: similar results to DAS28 and CDAI in clinical trials and clinical care. Rheum Dis Clin North Am. 2009;35:773–8.
17. Pincus T. A multidimensional health assessment questionnaire (MDHAQ) for all patients with rheumatic diseases to complete at all visits in standard clinical care. Bull NYU Hosp Jt Dis. 2007;65(2):150–60.
18. El Miedany Y, El Gaafary M, Youssef S, Palmer D. Incorporating patient reported outcome measures in clinical practice: development and validation of a questionnaire for inflammatory arthritis. Clin Exp Rheumatol. 2010;28:734–44.
19. El Miedany Y, El Gaafary M, Youssef S, Mehanna AN. Development of a scoring system for assessment of outcome of early undifferentiated inflammatory synovitis. Jt Bone Spine. 2008;75(2):155–62.
20. Pincus T, Callahan LF, Sale WG, Brooks AL, Payne LE, Vaughn WK. Severe functional declines, work disability, and increased mortality in seventy-five rheumatoid arthritis patients studied over nine years. Arthritis Rheum. 1984;27(8):864–72.
21. Singh JA, Saag KG, Bridges Jr SL, Akl EA, Bannuru RR, Sullivan MC, et al. American College of Rheumatology guideline for the treatment of rheumatoid arthritis. Arthritis Care Res. 2016;68(1):1–26.
22. El Miedany Y, El Gaafary M, Youssef S, Palmer D. Physician versus patient global assessment in early rheumatoid arthritis: putting the cart before the horse. Ann Rheum Dis. 2014;73 Suppl 2:616–7.
23. Aletaha D, Neogi T, Silman AJ, Funovits J, Felson DT, Bingham 3rd CO, et al. Rheumatoid arthritis classification criteria an American College of Rheumatology/European league against rheumatism collaborative initiative. Arthritis Rheum. 2010;62(9):2569–81.
24. El Miedany Y, El Gaafary M, Palmer D. Assessment of the utility of visual feedback in the treatment of early rheumatoid arthritis patients: a pilot study. Rheumatol Int. 2012;32(10):3061–8.
25. Rimer B, Jones WL, Keintz MK, Catalono RB, Engstrom PF. Informed consent: a crucial step in cancer patient education. Health Educ Q. 1984;10(Suppl):30–42.
26. Heneghan K, Sachdeva A, McAninch J. Transformation to a system that supports full patient participation. Bull Am Coll Surg. 2009;91(6):12–20.
27. Hardware B, Lacey E, Shewan J. Towards the development of a tool to assess educational needs in patients with arthritis. Clin Eff Nurs. 2004;8:111–7.
28. National Institute for Health and Clinical Excellence. The management of rheumatoid arthritis in adults. Clinical guideline 79. 2012. http://tiny.cc/lbah0. Accessed 14 Nov 2012.
29. Smolen JS, Landewé R, Breedveld FC, Dougados M, Emery P, Gaujoux-Viala C, et al. EULAR recommendations for the management of rheumatoid arthritis with synthetic and biological disease-modifying antirheumatic drugs. Ann Rheum Dis. 2010;69(6):964–75.
30. Ndosi M, Adebajo A. Patient education in rheumatoid arthritis: is the needs-based approach the way forward? Clin Rheumatol. 2015;34(11):1827–9.
31. Palmer D, El Miedany Y. PROMs: a novel approach to arthritis self-management. Br J Nurs. 2012;21(10):601–5.
32. El Miedany Y, El Gaafary M, El Arousy N, Ahmed I, Youssef S, Palmer D. Arthritis education: the integration of patient reported outcome measures and patient self-management. Clin Exp Rheumatol. 2012;30(6):899–904.
33. American College of Physicians. Information on cost effectiveness: an essential product of a national comparative effectiveness program. Ann Intern Med. 2008;148:956–61.
34. Rawlins MD, Culyer AJ. National Institute for Clinical Excellence and its value judgments. Br Med J. 2004;329:224–7.

35. British Thoracic Society. Jargon buster. British Thoracic Society reports 2010; 2(1). http://www.impressresp.com/index.php?export=pdf&no_html=1&option=com_glossary&task=list&letter=P&Itemid=2. Accessed 13 Nov 2012.
36. El Miedany Y, El Gaafary M, Youssef S, Palmer D. Patient reported outcome measures: its impact on disease activity and adherence to therapy in inflammatory arthritis. Arthritis Rheum. 2011;63(S10):1753–8.
37. Michaud K, Wolfe F. Comorbidities in rheumatoid arthritis. Best Pract Res Clin Rheumatol. 2007;21(5):885–906.
38. El Miedany Y. PROMs in inflammatory arthritis: moving from static to dynamic. Clin Rheumatol. 2013;32(6):735–42.
39. El Miedany Y, El Gaafary M, Youssef S, Palmer D. Answering the difficult question: how to identify rheumatoid arthritis patients at higher risk of cardiovascular disease in the standard practice? Ann Rheum Dis. 2009;68 Suppl 3:78.
40. Tugwell P, Bombardier C. A methodologic framework for developing and selecting endpoints in clinical trials. J Rheumatol. 1982;9:758–62.
41. Bomardier C, Tugwell P. A methodological framework to develop and select indices for clinical trials: statistical and judgmental approaches. J Rheumatol. 1982;9:753–7.
42. Tugwell P, Boers M. OMERACT Committee. Proceedings of the OMERACT conferences on outcome measures in rheumatoid arthritis clinical trials, Maastrict, Netherlands. J Rheumatol. 1993;20:527–91.
43. van der Heijde DM, Van't Hof MA, van Riel PL, Theunisse LA, Lubberts EW, van Leeuwen MA, et al. Judging disease activity in clinical practice in rheumatoid arthritis: first step in the development of a disease activity score. Ann Rheum Dis. 1990;49:916–20.
44. Prevoo ML, Van't Hof MA, Kuper HH, van Leeuwen MA, van de Putte LB, van Riel PL. Modified disease activity scores that include twenty-eight-joint counts: development and validation in a prospective longitudinal study of patients with rheumatoid arthritis. Arthritis Rheum. 1995;38(1):44–8.
45. Aletaha D, Smolen J. The simplified disease activity index (SDAI) and the clinical disease activity index (CDAI): a review of their usefulness and validity in rheumatoid arthritis. Clin Exp Rheumatol. 2005;23:S100–8.
46. Bellamy N, Buchanan WW, Goldsmith CH, Campbell J, Stitt LW. Validation study of WOMAC: a health status instrument for measuring clinically important patient relevant outcomes to antirheumatic drug therapy in patients with osteoarthritis of the hip or knee. J Rheumatol. 1988;15(2):1833–40.
47. Burckhardt CS, Clark SR, Bennett RM. The fibromyalgia impact questionnaire: development and validation. J Rheumatol. 1991;18:728–33.
48. Hawker G, Gabriel S, Bombardier C, Goldsmith C, Caron D, Gladman D. A reliability study of SLEDAI: a disease activity index for systemic lupus erythematosus. J Rheumatol. 1993;20:657–60.
49. Hay EM, Bacon PA, Gordon C, Isenberg DA, Maddison P, Snaith ML, et al. The BILAG index: a reliable and valid instrument for measuring clinical disease activity in systemic lupus erythematosus. Q J Med. 1993;86(7):447–58.
50. Swaak AJ, van den Brink HG, Smeenk RJ, Manger K, Kalden JR, Tosi S, et al. Systemic lupus erythematosus: disease outcome in patients with a disease duration of at least 10 years: second evaluation. Lupus. 2001;10(1):51–8.
51. Petri M, Hellmann DB, Hochberg M. Validity and reliability of lupus activity measures in the routine clinic setting. J Rheumatol. 1992;19:53–9.
52. Mosca M, Bencivelli W, Vitali C, Carrai P, Neri R, Bombardieri S. The validity of the ECLAM index for the retrospective evaluation of disease activity in systemic lupus erythematosus. Lupus. 2000;9(6):445–50.
53. Bencivelli W, Vitali C, Isenberg DA, Smolen JS, Snaith ML, Sciuto M, et al. Disease activity in systemic lupus erythematosus: report of the consensus study group of the European workshop for rheumatology research. III. Development of a computerised clinical chart and its application to the comparison of different indices of disease activity. The European consensus study group for disease activity in SLE. Clin Exp Rheumatol. 1992;10(5):549–54.

54. Calin A, Garrett S, Whitelock H, Kennedy LG, O'Hea J, Mallorie P, et al. A new approach to defining functional ability in ankylosing spondylitis: the development of the bath ankylosing spondylitis functional index. J Rheumatol. 1994;21(12):2281–5.
55. Machado P, Landewé R, Lie E, Kvien TK, Braun J, Baker D, et al. Ankylosing spondylitis disease activity score (ASDAS): defining cut-off values for disease activity states and improvement scores. Ann Rheum Dis. 2011;70(1):47–53.
56. Luqmani RA, Bacon PA, Moots RJ, Janssen BA, Pall A, Emery P, et al. Birmingham vasculitis activity score (BVAS) in systemic necrotizing vasculitis. Q J Med. 1994;87(11):671–8.
57. Whiting O'Keefe QE, Stone JH, Hellmann DB. Validity of a vasculitis activity index for systemic necrotizing vasculitis. Arthritis Rheum. 1999;42:2365–71.
58. Stone JH, Hoffman GS, Merkel PA, Min YI, Uhlfelder ML, Hellmann DB, et al. A disease-specific activity index for Wegener's granulomatosis: modification of the Birmingham vasculitis activity score. Arthritis Rheum. 2001;44(4):912–20.
59. Pincus T, Yazici Y, Sokka T. Quantitative measures of rheumatic diseases for clinical research versus standard clinical care: differences, advantages and limitations. Best Pract Res Clin Rheumatol. 2007;21(4):601–28.
60. Wolfe F, Michaud K. The clinical and research significance of the erythrocyte sedimentation rate. J Rheumatol. 1994;21:1227–37.
61. Bowling A. Measuring disease: a review of disease-specific quality of life measurement scales, vol. 2. Buckingham: Open University Press; 2001. p. 25–6.
62. Brooks R. EuroQol: the current state of play. Health Policy. 1996;37(1):53–72.
63. Ebrahim S, Barer D, Nouri F. Use of the Nottingham Health Profile with patients after a stroke. J Epidemiol Community Health. 1986;40(2):166–9.
64. Meadows K. Patient-reported outcome measures: an overview. Br J Community Nurs. 2011;16(3):146–51.
65. Pincus T, Yazici Y, Bergman M. Development of a multi-dimensional health assessment questionnaire (MDHAQ) for the infrastructure of standard clinical care. Clin Exp Rheumatol. 2005;23 Suppl 39:S19–28.
66. Nicklin J, Cramp F, Kirwan J, Greenwood R, Urban M, Hewlett S. Measuring fatigue in rheumatoid arthritis: a cross-sectional study to evaluate the Bristol rheumatoid arthritis fatigue multi-dimensional questionnaire, visual analog scales, and numerical rating scales. Arthritis Care Res. 2010;32:1559–68.
67. Osterhaus JT. Discriminant validity, responsiveness and reliability of the rheumatoid arthritis-specific work productivity survey (WPS-RA). Arthritis Res Ther. 2009;11:R73.
68. Pincus T, Swearingen C, Wolfe F. Toward a multidimensional health assessment questionnaire (MDHAQ): assessment of advanced activities of daily living and psychological status in the patient-friendly health assessment questionnaire format. Arthritis Rheum. 1999;42:2220–30.
69. Gossec L, Paternotte S, Aanerud GJ, Balanescu A, Boumpas DT, Carmona L, et al. Finalisation and validation of the rheumatoid arthritis impact of disease score, a patient-derived composite measure of impact of rheumatoid arthritis: a EULAR initiative. Ann Rheum Dis. 2011;70(6):935–42.
70. Pincus T. Pain, function, and RAPID scores: vital signs in chronic diseases, analogous to pulse and temperature in acute diseases and blood pressure and cholesterol in long-term health. Bull NYU Hosp Joint Dis. 2008;66(2):155–65.
71. El Miedany Y, Palmer D, El Gaafary M. Further analysis of helplessness measurement in inflammatory arthritis/spondyloarthritis: the development of the modified rheumatology attitude index. Rheumatology (Oxford). 2010;49(S1):162.
72. Maksymowych WP, Fitzgerald O, Wells GA, Gladman DD, Landewé R, Ostergaard M, et al. Proposal for levels of evidence schema for validation of a soluble biomarker reflecting damage endpoints in rheumatoid arthritis, psoriatic arthritis, and ankylosing spondylitis, and recommendations for study design. J Rheumatol. 2009;36(8):1792–9.
73. Biomarkers Definition Working Group. Biomarkers and surrogate endpoints: preferred definitions and conceptual framework. Clin Pharmacol Ther. 2001;69(3):89–95.

74. Grigor C, Capell H, Stirling A, McMahon AD, Lock P, Vallance R, et al. Effect of a treatment strategy of tight control for rheumatoid arthritis (the TICORA study): a single-blind randomised controlled trial. Lancet. 2004;364(9430):263–9.
75. Verstappen SM, Jacobs JW, van der Veen MJ, Heurkens AH, Schenk Y, ter Borg EJ, Utrecht Rheumatoid Arthritis Cohort study group, et al. Intensive treatment with methotrexate in early rheumatoid arthritis: aiming for remission. Computer Assisted Management in Early Rheumatoid Arthritis (CAMERA, an open-label strategy trial). Ann Rheum Dis. 2007;66(11):1443–9.
76. Soubrier M, Lukas C, Sibilia J, Fautrel B, Roux F, Gossec L, et al. Disease activity score driven therapy versus routine care in patients with recent-onset active rheumatoid arthritis: data from the GUEPARD trial and ESPOIR cohort. Ann Rheum Dis. 2011;70(4):611–5.
77. Schipper LG, Vermeer M, Kuper HH, Hoekstra MO, Haagsma CJ, Den Broeder AA, et al. A tight control treatment strategy aiming for remission in early rheumatoid arthritis is more effective than usual care treatment in daily clinical practice: a study of two cohorts in the Dutch Rheumatoid Arthritis Monitoring registry. Ann Rheum Dis. 2012;71(6):845–50.
78. El Miedany Y, El Gaafary M, Sayed S, Palmer D. Biomarkers and patient tailored approach in rheumatoid arthritis. Can PROMs be the missing biomarker. Ann Rheum Dis. 2015;74:1002.
79. Aspinall SL, Good CB, Glassman PA, Valentino MA. The evolving use of cost-effectiveness analysis in formulary management within the Department of Veterans Affairs. Med Care. 2005;43:20–6.
80. Alishiri GH, Bayat N, Fathi Ashtiani A, Tavallaii SA, Assari S, Moharamzad Y. Logistic regression models for predicting physical and mental health-related quality of life in rheumatoid arthritis patients. Mod Rheumatol. 2008;18(6):601–8.
81. El Miedany Y, El Gaafary M, Youssef S, Ahmed I, Palmer D. The arthritic patients' perspective of measuring treatment efficacy: patient reported experience measures (PREMs) as a quality tool. Clin Exp Rheumatol. 2014;32(4):547–52.
82. Department of Health. Guidance on the routine collection of patient reported outcome measures (PROMs). Available from: http://www.dh.gov.uk/en/Publicationsandstatistics/Publications/Publications/PolicyAndGuidance/DH_091451. Accessed 19 Jun 2014.
83. Cramer JA, Roy A, Burrell A, Fairchild CJ, Fuldeore MJ, Ollendorf DA, Wong PK. Medication compliance and persistence: terminology and definitions. Value Health. 2008;11:44–7.
84. Luqmani R, Hennell S, Estrach C, Birrell F, Bosworth A, Davenport G, British Society for Rheumatology, British Health Professionals in Rheumatology Standards, Guidelines and Audit Working Group, et al. British Society for Rheumatology and British Health Professionals in Rheumatology guideline for the management of rheumatoid arthritis (the first two years). Rheumatology (Oxford). 2006;45(9):1167–9.
85. Zbrozek A, Hebert J, Gogates G, Thorell R, Dell C, Molsen E, et al. Validation of electronic systems to collect patient-reported outcome (PRO) data-recommendations for clinical trial teams: report of the ISPOR ePRO systems validation good research practices task force. Value Health. 2013;16(4):480–9.
86. Bennett A, Jensen R, Basch E. Electronic patient-reported outcome systems in oncology clinical practice. CA Cancer J Clin. 2012;62:336–47.
87. Maguire R, McCann L, Miller M, Kearney N. Nurse's perceptions and experiences of using of a mobile-phone-based advanced symptom management system (ASyMS) to monitor and manage chemotherapy related toxicity. Eur J Oncol Nurs. 2008;12:380–6.
88. El Miedany Y, El Gaafary M, Sayed S, Palmer D. Electronic patient reported outcome measures (e-PROMs) for early arthritis in standard clinical practice: a pilot study. Ann Rheum Dis. 2015;74 Suppl 2:65.
89. Coons SJ, Gwaltney CJ, Hays RD, Lundy JJ, Sloan JA, Revicki DA. et al; ISPOR ePRO task force. Recommendations on evidence needed to support measurement equivalence between electronic and paper based patient-reported outcome (PRO) measures: ISPOR ePRO good research practices task force report. Value Health. 2009;12(4):419–29.
90. Horevoorts N, Vissers P, Mols F, et al. Response rates for patient-reported outcomes using web-based versus paper questionnaires: comparison of two invitational methods in older colorectal cancer patients. J Med Internet Res. 2015;17(5), e111. doi:10.2196/jmir.3741.

91. Huffstutter J, Craig WD, Schimizzi G, Harshbarger J, Lisse J, Kasle S, et al. A multicenter, randomized, open study to evaluate the impact of an electronic data capture system on the care of patients with rheumatoid arthritis. Curr Med Res Opin. 2007;23(8):1967–79.
92. Detmar SB, Muller MJ, Schornagel JH, Wever LD, Aaronson NK. Health-related quality-of-life assessments and patient physician communication: a randomized controlled trial. JAMA. 2002;288:3027–34.
93. McCann L, Maguire R, Miller M, Kearney N. Patients' perceptions and experiences of using a mobile phone-based advanced symptom management system (ASyMS) to monitor and manage chemotherapy related toxicity. Eur J Cancer Care (Engl). 2009;18:156–64.
94. Velikova G, Booth L, Smith AB, Brown PM, Lynch P, Brown JM, et al. Measuring quality of life in routine oncology practice improves communication and patient well-being: a randomized controlled trial. J Clin Oncol. 2004;22:714–24.
95. El Miedany Y, Palmer D. Can standard rheumatology clinical practice be patient-based? Br J Nurs. 2008;17(10):673–5.
96. Dy SM, Roy J, Ott GE, McHale M, Kennedy C, Kutner JS, Tien A. Tell Us™: a Web-based tool for improving communication among patients, families, and providers in hospice and palliative care through systematic data specification, collection, and use. J Pain Symptom Manage. 2011;42(4):526–34.
97. Gibson F, Aldiss S, Taylor RM, Maguire R, Kearney N. Involving health professionals in the development of an advanced symptom management system for young people: the ASyMS-YG study. Eur J Oncol Nurs. 2009;13:187–92.
98. McCall K, Keen J, Farrer K, Maguire R, McCann L, Johnston B, et al. Perceptions of the use of a remote monitoring system in patients receiving palliative care at home. Int J Palliat Nurs. 2008;14(9):426–31.
99. Snyder CF, Jensen R, Courtin SO, Wu AW, Website for Outpatient QOL Assessment Research Network. Patient Viewpoint: a website for patient-reported outcomes assessment. Qual Life Res. 2009;18:793–800.
100. Palmer D, El Miedany Y. EROMIA in inflammatory arthritis: the next step in standard practice. Br J Nurs. 2010;19(1):42–6.

Chapter 5
PROMs for Spondyloarthritis

Uta Kiltz, Laure Gossec, Xenofon Baraliakos, and Jürgen Braun

Introduction

Patients with spondyloarthritis (SpA) constitute a heterogeneous group of rheumatic diseases with a partially common genetic background, represented by HLA-B27 and IL23 receptor polymorphisms, and rather specific clinical features such as inflammation and ankylosis of the axial skeleton but also peripheral manifestations (arthritis or enthesitis) [1]. In addition, SpA patients often suffer from extra-articular symptoms such as uveitis, psoriasis, or chronic inflammatory bowel disease (IBD) [2]. The clinical picture and the course of SpA is rather variable. Patients with SpA may have predominant axial (axSpA) or peripheral disease (pSpA), but mixed forms occur frequently. The disease course of patients with axSpA is often characterized by inflammatory changes in the spine, which may develop into areas of new bone formation. This pathognomonic process is often associated with pain, functional disability, restricted mobility, fatigue, and decreased quality of life. The classification of patients with axSpA includes the classical ankylosing spondylitis (AS) and non-radiographic axSpA—in case no structural changes are yet present. Furthermore, psoriatic arthritis (PsA), arthritis related to IBD, reactive arthritis (ReA), and juvenile SpA can be differentiated (Table 5.1), but clinical overlaps are not infrequent. Ankylosing spondylitis has always been considered as the prototype of the SpA

U. Kiltz (✉) • J. Braun
Rheumazentrum Ruhrgebiet, Herne, Germany
e-mail: Uta.kiltz@elisabethgruppe.de

L. Gossec
Department of Rheumatology, AP-HP, Pitié Salpêtrière Hospital, UPMC Univ Paris 06, Sorbonne Universitées, Paris, France

X. Baraliakos
Rheumazentrum Ruhrgebiet, Herne, Germany

Ruhr-University Bochum, Bochum, Germany

Y. El Miedany (ed.), *Patient Reported Outcome Measures in Rheumatic Diseases*,
DOI 10.1007/978-3-319-32851-5_5

Table 5.1 The different spondyloarthritis subtypes

Predominantly axial SpA	Predominantly peripheral SpA
Non-radiographic SpA	Psoriatic arthritis
Radiographic axial SpA (Ankylosing Spondylitis)	Reactive arthritis
	Arthritis associated with inflammatory bowel disease
	Undifferentiated pSpA

SpA spondyloarthritis

spectrum and, together with PsA, it is the best studied subtype so far. Patients with pSpA who fulfill the classification criteria for SpA but do not have psoriasis, IBD, or a preceding infection are classified as undifferentiated pSpA.

AxSpA can be classified according to the Assessment of Spondyloarthritis International Society (ASAS) classification criteria [3, 4]. Thus, patients with structural changes in conventional radiographs of the sacroiliac joints (classified as established AS) and patients who do not have such changes (classified as non-radiographic axSpA [nr-axSpA]) are covered by this concept, which is based on the idea of a disease continuum. Nevertheless patients do show a similar disease burden independent of a particular stage [5]. The disease spectrum of pSpA [4] is partly overlapping with the concept of PsA, which also can be well classified according to the Classification of Psoriatic Arthritis (CASPAR) criteria [6]. Patients with PsA have peripheral arthritis, skin psoriasis, dactylitis, and enthesitis as predominant features, but they also may have axial features and/or other extra-articular features of SpA [6]. PsA is usually associated with skin psoriasis (sometimes also with nail lesions), but those changes do not occur in all patients.

Patient reported outcomes (PROs) are at the core of assessing disease status and/or treatment response with patient assessments of global health, pain, stiffness, physical function, and decreased health-related quality of life (HRQoL). The majority of established questionnaires used for axSpA have been developed based on evaluation of patients with established AS. AS is the showcase of axSpA and has been known for decades, but some PROs have also been tested in the whole group of axSpA patients. For patients with PsA, some of the measures of the clinical domains have been successfully adapted from measures used in the assessment of rheumatoid arthritis or AS or even psoriasis. To capture all patient-perceived consequences of SpA across the disease spectrum, major efforts have been made to develop valid and reliable questionnaires assessing PROs such as pain, stiffness, fatigue, and QoL in patients with SpA.

Here we review the PROs used for patients with SpA, separately for axSpA and PsA. No validated instrument is currently available for patients with pSpA, but some work has been done to establish such an instrument [7].

In the present chapter, we discuss the most widely used and/or best-validated questionnaires including the psychometric information available for these questionnaires. Furthermore, we discuss the measures that are of relevance for clinical practice. The selection of questionnaires was limited to those related to musculoskeletal manifestations. Thus, questionnaires focusing on gastrointestinal, cutaneous, or eye manifestations are not reviewed in this chapter.

Axial Spondyloarthritis

Clinical Picture of Axial SpA

The most significant clinical symptoms of patients with axSpA are back pain and peripheral, usually asymmetric oligoarthritis of the lower limbs and enthesitis [1]. Because of the underlying inflammation, the back pain is often worse at night (nocturnal pain) and may lead to various degrees of morning stiffness (>30 min). Major concerns of patients with axSpA are spinal pain and stiffness either due to inflammation or ankylosis in the axial skeleton, which may also result in impaired spinal mobility and decreased physical function. These impairments often lead to limitations of activities and social participation [8]. Reduced work participation is of major importance for our patients, who classically start with the first symptoms of the disease in the second or third decade of life [9].

Assessment of Patients with axSpA

The clinical features to be assessed in patients with axSpA include symptoms, disease activity, physical function, and HRQoL. The ASAS group has defined a number of core sets of areas of disease that should be measured in different situations, including the ASAS cores set for clinical record keeping (Table 5.2) [10].

Five out of the eight domains are patient-reported outcomes and will be addressed in the following chapters. Although enthesitis is frequent, no validated PRO is available for this disabling aspect. Validated indices comprises physical examination of the entheses with documentation of pain and tenderness.

Table 5.2 ASAS core set for clinical record keeping

Domain	Instrument
Physical function	*BASFI or Dougados Functional Index*
Pain	*VAS/NRS past week in spine, at night, due to AS and VAS/NRS past week, in spine due to AS*
Spinal mobility	Chest expansion and modified Schober and occiput-to-wall distance and lateral spinal flexion
Patient global assessment	*VAS/NRS past week*
Morning stiffness	*Duration of morning stiffness in spine past week*
Fatigue	*VAS/NRS past week*
Peripheral joints and entheses	Number of swollen joints (44 joint count). Validated enthesis indexes
Acute phase reactants	ESR

Adapted from Ref. [10]
Domains in italics are PRO
AS ankylosing spondylitis, *BASFI* Bath AS Functional Index, *ESR* erythrocyte sedimentation rate, *NRS* numerical rating scale, *VAS* visual analogue scale

PRO in Axial SpA

Instruments currently available for the assessment of patients with axSpA focus predominantly on specific aspects of health—such as pain, disease activity, and physical function—and measure specific concepts such as physical function and HRQoL. All measures were designed for use in AS, but they can also be used in other SpA conditions according to the presence or absence of axial symptoms.

Single Measures for Assessing Symptoms (Pain, Stiffness, Fatigue)

In patients with axial involvement, the degree of both night pain and spinal pain during the day is measured by using either a visual analogue scale (VAS) or a numerical rating scale (NRS). In general, the use of an NRS is preferred by patients and doctors. Morning stiffness in the spine is usually assessed for aspects, duration, and severity. In addition to the Bath Ankylosing Spondylitis Disease Activity Index (BASDAI) result, a value over 4 on a pain scale from 0 to 10 is usually considered as reflecting "active" disease. Pain and stiffness have a considerable influence on HRQoL in AS patients. Overall, 83 % of patients report problems related to pain, and for 1/3 of them this aspect is considered very important [11]. Women are 2–3 times more likely to have high levels of pain than men. Patients with AS report significantly more back pain than patients with RA (44 vs. 25 mm on VAS pain), while pain in peripheral joints is comparable in the two groups [12].

Fatigue has been described as a major issue in AS, with up to 65 % of the patients reporting this symptom [13]. The scores on the fatigue question of the BASDAI have been shown to be significantly associated with scores on several dimensions of the 36-question Short Form Health Survey (SF-36) and with the AS-specific Quality of Life (ASQoL) instrument, suggesting that HRQoL is influenced by the degree of fatigue [14]. Fatigue is most often assessed by using item 1 of the disease-specific questionnaire for assessing disease activity in AS patients: the BASDAI (see next section). The degree of fatigue has also been assessed in controlled trials by using the functional assessment of chronic illness Therapy-Fatigue subscale (FACIT-fatigue) [15].

Disease Activity

BASDAI

BASDAI is a fully patient-reported measure. It is simple to use since it comprises only six questions (see Appendix 1) [16]:

- Fatigue
- Axial involvement
- Peripheral articular involvement

- Localized tenderness/enthesopathy
- Morning stiffness (2 questions)

The answers to these questions are scored on a 0–10 NRS, which is anchored by 0 (*none*) to 10 (*very severe*). The BASDAI sum score is calculated by the sum of questions 1–4 plus the mean of questions 5 and 6, then the total is divided by 5. The sum score ranges from 0 to 10; higher values indicate more active disease. A BASDAI score ≥ 4/10 is considered as the threshold above which a disease status can be considered as "active" [17]. However, this value has been proposed arbitrarily and its validity has not been formally established [18]. Nevertheless, a BASDAI value of 3.9/10 discriminated between patients with well-controlled and poorly controlled symptoms in AS [19].

A change of at least 50 % in the BASDAI is usually considered as reflecting a clinically relevant improvement [17]. The minimum clinically important difference (MCID) between measurements has been reported as a change in BASDAI of ≥1/10 units on NRS or ≥10 mm on VAS or a score difference of 22.5 % between two different examinations of the same patient, with a sensitivity of 0.65 and a specificity of 0.82 [20].

However, BASDAI scores do not seem to not correlate well with symptoms and clinical measurements of disease activity and/or MRI scores [21–23]. Furthermore, the degree of spinal inflammation seems to be largely similar in patients with AS and nr-axSpA, irrespective of the corresponding BASDAI level, which challenges the concept of the (initially arbitrarily) chosen cutoff of BASDAI ≥ 4 for definition of high disease activity [24].

The BASDAI is the most frequently used measure of disease activity in daily care and in clinical trials. In most countries a BASDAI ≥ 4 is mandatory before prescription of tumor-necrosis-factor inhibitors (TNFi). Because of the limitation of this threshold, expert opinion is mandatory in order to prescribe TNFi. There is some evidence that patients with AS may respond to TNF inhibitors despite not fulfilling the ASAS criteria for initiating TNFi therapy [25], but this, however, represents an off-label use.

Ankylosing Spondylitis Disease Activity Score

Since the BASDAI is a purely patient-based questionnaire without any objective parameters of disease activity, a new measure, the AS Disease Activity Score (ASDAS) recently has been proposed [26]. This composite index takes into account some questions of the BASDAI (Q2: total back pain, Q3: peripheral pain, and Q6: morning stiffness), patient's global assessment and C-reactive protein (CRP) or erythrocyte sedimentation rate (ESR) values. The statistical background of the ASDAS to ensure that each item of ASDAS adds extra information not yet captured by the other items, and, thus, is not redundant. Response to the items and value of serological markers are weighted and calculated to give the final ASDAS score. The score is most easily calculated using a calculator (online via www.asas-group.org). Scores range from 0 (no disease activity) to infinite (being determined by the level of CRP or ESR). The cutoffs between the disease activity states are: inactive disease ≤1.3, moderate 1.3–2.0, high 2.1–3.5, and very high ≥3.5. The ASDAS cutoff for clinically important improvement between examinations is ≥1.1 and the cutoff for a major improvement is ≥2.0. The ASDAS has been extensively validated. It has been shown to be reliable, discriminative, and sensitive [27–29].

Physical Function (BASFI, DFI, HAQ-S)

Limited spinal mobility and decrease in function is a major and also clinically a poor prognostic sign of axial SpA. Consequently, physical function is considered as a major outcome for patients with SpA. Patients with AS report significantly impaired health on all scales of the Short Form (SF-36) as compared to the general population or patients with other medical conditions. Patients with AS also have rather low scores in physical domains [30]. Studies have shown an association between spinal mobility measures and radiographic damage in patients with AS [31, 32]. However, physical function in patients with AS is influenced not only by structural damage but also by disease activity (inflammation) [32, 33]. It is important to realize that the term "function" is frequently limited to physical function in this context, ignoring the complexity of global functioning. However, the influence of other factors, such as psychological factors, has only rarely been studied in AS.

Bath Ankylosing Spondylitis Functional Index

The most frequently used tool to asses function in axial SpA is the BASFI (Bath Ankylosing Spondylitis Functional Index), which measures the functional status as a self-report. It contains ten questions on activities of daily living, which are scored with a rating scale from 0 (no functional impairments) to ten (maximal impairment) [34]. Domains addressed in the questionnaire are:

- Bending
- Reaching
- Getting up
- Putting on socks
- Climbing stairs
- Looking over the shoulder

The mean of the individual scores is calculated to give the overall index score. The sum score ranges from 0 to 10, with higher values indicating worse functioning. The MCID has been reported at 7 mm or change of 17.5 % with a sensitivity of 0.60 and a specificity of 0.85 [20]. The BASFI is reliable, sensitive to change, and feasible to use in patients with AS in clinical practice. However, since the median score of the BASFI has been reported as 2.0 with clustering at the lower end of the scale, the questionnaire may not be sufficiently sensitive to detect changes in functioning in patients without severe impairments.

Dougados Functional Index

It contains 20 questions on activities of daily living, addressing aspects of dressing, bathing, standing, climbing stairs, bending, changing position, doing housework, coughing, and breathing deeply [35]. The value of the 3-point Likert scale is added to give a total sum score between 0 and 40; higher values reflecting higher functional impairment. The Dougados Functional Index (DFI) has been used in studies of disease outcome and in clinical trials.

Health Assessment Questionnaire for the Spondyloarthropathies

See later section: Assessment in Patients with SpA (axSpA and PsA) with Generic Tools

Functioning and Quality of Life (ASQoL, ASAS HI)

The most prevalent symptoms in patients with AS are pain, stiffness, fatigue, and sleep problems [11]. On the other hand, other aspects, such as having energy for social activities or work participation, also have been mentioned as very important for patients with SpA [8, 36]. Instruments currently available for the assessment of patients with SpA focus predominantly on physical function, taking into account that the overall picture of impairments, limitations, and restrictions in activities or social participation of patients with established AS are not adequately assessed in general SpA questionnaires and none of the questionnaires measures the entire range of functional disability [37].

Ankylosing Spondylitis Quality of Life Questionnaire

The most frequently used HRQoL instrument in SpA trials so far is the ASQoL [38, 39]. The 18 items that are being addressed here include aspects such as pain, fatigue, dressing, emotional functions, and social community. The items can be summed up to give a total score ranging from 0 to 18—with a lower score reflecting a higher HRQoL.

ASAS Health Index

The ASAS Health Index (ASAS HI) overcomes these limitations by using the International Classification of Functioning, Disability and Health (ICF) as a conceptualized basis (see Appendix 2) [40]. The ASAS HI is an instrument for patients with established AS but also nr-axSpA that assesses functioning and health as operationalized by the ICF core set for AS [41]. It is a linear composite measure and contains 17 items (dichotomous response option: "I agree" and "I do not agree") that cover most of the ICF core set (see Appendix 2). The items are addressed aspects as pain, emotional functions, sleep, sexual functions, mobility, self-care, and participation in the community life. The items can be summed up to give a total score ranging from 0 to 17, with a lower score indicating a better and a higher score indicating an inferior health status. Preliminary validity has been confirmed in a field test in four English-speaking countries. The ASAS HI has been translated so far into 15 languages and the psychometric properties of the ASAS HI and its translations are tested in a large ongoing trial worldwide [42]. It is important to emphasize that the ASAS HI is a health index and not a HRQoL instrument. Health is thereby operationalized through the ICF concept of functioning. With the ASAS HI, the occurrence of problems is captured in different categories of functioning and are not depending on the subjective experience of the patients, which is a prerequisite of a HRQoL instrument.

Psoriatic Arthritis

Clinical Picture of PsA

Psoriatic arthritis (PsA) is a heterogeneous disease, which includes varying levels of peripheral joint involvement and skin manifestations. Musculoskeletal involvement is characterized by synovitis, enthesitis, dactylitis, and spondylitis. The manifestation can present as an asymmetric oligoarthritis, a polyarthritis as an axial manifestation [43]. Therefore, the key clinical features of PsA that should be assessed in order to determine disease severity and effect of treatment include peripheral arthritis, skin and nail psoriasis, axial disease, enthesitis, and dactylitis. The impact of PsA is wide-reaching, and both physical and mental aspects of quality of life can be modified by this disease. Thus, the measurement of the patient's status rests in part on the assessment of patient reported outcomes, i.e., questionnaires to assess different aspects of life.

Here, we will review different patient-reported questionnaires that are either specific to PsA, or generic, and which are used to assess people with PsA.

Assessment of Patients with PsA

The Core Set: Several years ago, the international group Outcome Measures in Rheumatology (OMERACT) and the Group for Research and Assessment of Psoriasis and Psoriatic Arthritis (GRAPPA) decided through consensus on a Core Set of variables to be collected in clinical trials of PsA [44]. These experts have proposed six core domains (*inner circle*) to be measured in clinical trials and observational studies of PsA: peripheral joint activity, skin activity, pain, patient global assessment (PGA), physical function, and HRQoL (Fig. 5.1) [44]. The "outer circle" corresponds to domains that are not necessary to assess in PsA trials or domains that are still under evaluation.

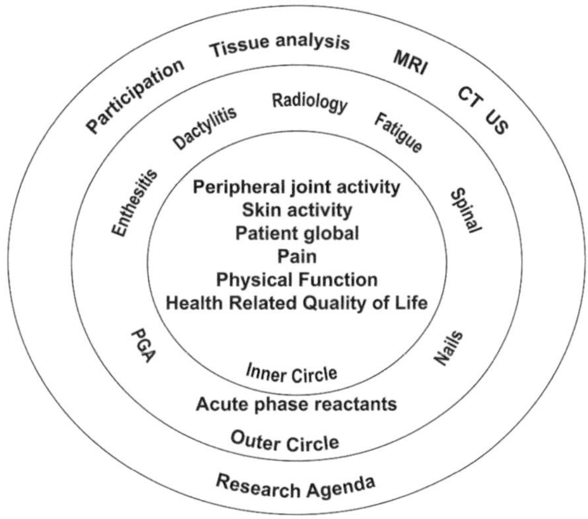

Fig. 5.1 The OMERACT Core Set of outcome measures for PsA [44]. All Rights Reserved

Table 5.3 Domains of health reported in 58 publications of PsA published 2006–2010

Patient-reported domain of health	Articles reporting the domain *N* (% of 58 articles)
Function/disability	28 (48.0)
Pain	27 (46.6)
Patient's global assessment	23 (39.6)
Quality of life	22 (37.9)
Skin	2 (3.4)
Fatigue	9 (15.5)
Composite scores	6 (10.3)
Morning stiffness	6 (10.3)
Utility/productivity	4 (6.9)
Other	2 (3.4)
Coping/self efficacy	1 (1.7)

Over the last years, and based in particular on input from patient research partners, the Core Set is being revisited in particular to identify "missing" domains that are important to patients [45]. One of the domains that is increasingly considered as important is fatigue, as will be discussed later in this chapter [46]. Other outcomes that were brought forward for consideration in the new Core Set are dactylitis, enthesitis, and work participation [47].

Which of These Outcome Measures Are Used?

A systematic literature review was performed regarding clinical outcomes in PsA analyzing 58 articles published on PsA in 2006–2010 [48]. Of these studies, around half reported functional disability, pain, and PGA; other domains of health were less frequently reported, including, for example, fatigue reported in only 15 % of the studies (Table 5.3).

Domains of Health Important for People Living with PsA

Qualitative methodology (such as focus groups or individual in-depth interviews) provides the opportunity to explore the perspective of those who experience the disease, i.e., the patient's perspective in detail. Such studies have yielded a wealth of information in RA. In PsA, however, there have been few published qualitative studies to date, although several are ongoing [45, 49, 50].

A systematic literature review reported on 11 studies assessing impact of PsA from the patient's perspective [45, 51]. Impact of PsA was shown to be wide-reaching. The most frequently reported dimensions of health were mainly related to the consequences and societal aspects of the disease (i.e., ability to work, social participation, and leisure) followed by physical aspects (i.e., functional capacity; pain; fatigue) and emotional aspects (such as coping mechanisms; emotional problems such as anger, anxiety, fear; and embarrassment and shame due to appearance).

Two questionnaires have been developed specifically for PsA and used qualitative methods in their elaboration. In the elaboration of the PsA Impact of Disease (PsAID) [52], 16 domains of health that were considered important by patients were identified (Table 5.4). Similarly, the development of the PsA Quality of Life (PsAQoL) questionnaire yielded domains of health that could be categorized into four main experiences: reaction to diagnosis, life changes, adaptation and acceptance, and concerns for the future (Table 5.4) [53]. These included as expected pain or skin disease, but also other domains, such as fatigue, coping, emotional, and social problems.

The domains of impact important for patients should be taken into consideration particularly in PsA where quality of life instruments should reflect both rheumatic and dermatological impact on patients [49].

PROMs Specifically Developed for PsA

There are very few questionnaires that have been developed specifically for PsA; we will review two of them here.

The PsAQoL Questionnaire

The Psoriatic Arthritis Quality of Life (PsAQoL) assesses quality of life defined as the extent to which needs are fulfilled and reflects impact from the perspective of the patient [53]. Its content was derived from unstructured, qualitative interviews conducted with patients with PsA, which generated a 51-item questionnaire. Face and content validity were assessed by field test interviews with another sample of PsA patients. Then a postal survey was conducted and the resulting analysis led to a

Table 5.4 Domains of health important for patients with PsA as reflected in two patient-derived questionnaires assessing impact of PsA

Domains of health	16 Domains identified in the PsAID development process [52]	20 Domains of health included in the PsAQoL [53]
Pain	X	
Skin problems	X	
Fatigue	X	X
Ability to work/leisure	X	
Functional capacity (capacity to perform daily physical activities, loss of independence)	X	X
Feeling of discomfort	X	
Mobility		X
Morning stiffness		X
Sleep disturbance	X	
Anxiety, fear, and uncertainty	X	
Anger, irritation		X
Coping	X	X
Embarrassment and/or shame due to appearance	X	
Social participation	X	X
Depression	X	X
Relationship with family	X	X
Concentration difficulties	X	
Rejection and discrimination due to appearance	X	
Sexual life	X	

PsA psoriatic arthritis, *PsAID* Psoriatic Arthritis Impact of Disease, *PsAQoL* Psoriatic Arthritis Quality of Life

35-item version of the questionnaire. Finally a test–retest postal survey was conducted to improve the scaling properties, reliability, internal consistency, and validity. Rasch analysis of data from this postal survey identified a 20-item version with good item fit and excellent psychometric properties (internal consistency 0.91, test–retest reliability 0.89, and good external construct validity). The final 20 items of the questionnaire consisted, as far as possible, of wording taken from the transcripts. They cover various domains of impact such as physical problems, fatigue, emotional, and social problems (Table 5.4).

Sensitivity and responsiveness to change have been further assessed in 28 PsA patients, demonstrating significant change at 3 and 6 months after change of disease modifying therapy ($p<0.01$ and $p<0.05$, respectively) [54]. Standardized response mean was large at 3 months (0.71) and small at 6 months (0.41). The PsAQoL has been translated and validated in Dutch and Swedish [55, 56]. In summary, the PsAQoL is a disease-specific instrument that is derived directly from qualitative interviews, has good psychometric properties, and is quick and easy to complete, making it suitable for use in both research and clinical settings. However, the PsAQoL has been little used to date [57–61]. Furthermore, it is subject to copyright.

The PsAID Questionnaire

The European League Against Rheumatism (EULAR) recently developed the PsAID (Psoriatic Arthritis Impact of Disease) questionnaire, a multidimensional patient-reported questionnaire to assess the impact of PsA from the patient's perspective [52]. The objective was to develop a questionnaire that can be used to calculate a score, reflecting the impact of PsA based on the patients' perspective. The questionnaire has been developed by a mixed group of rheumatologists/researchers, patient research partners, and health professionals, including an International Classification of Health and Functioning expert and a nurse practitioner/researcher. Compared to existing instruments, the PsAID score is unique because it has been developed with the active involvement of 11 patient research partners from 11 European countries. Therefore the instrument is fully based on the patient perspective of the illness [62].

First, the 11 patient research partners identified 16 domains (areas of health) important for patients with PsA; then 139 patients prioritized the 16 domains according to importance and the lowest priority 4 domains were excluded from the next steps. NRS questions were developed, one for each of the 12 domains of health. To combine the domains into a single score, relative weights were determined for each domain, based on relative importance as reported by 474 PsA patients from across Europe. At the same time, an international cross-sectional and longitudinal validation study was performed in 13 countries (474 patients) to validate the PsAID in terms of psychometric properties, regarding cross-sectional relation with other well-known outcome measures, and longitudinal validation for reliability and sensitivity to change in smaller samples ($N = 80$ and 71, respectively). The measures performed well; reliability was high (intra-class correlation coefficient, 0.95, 95 % confidence interval 0.92–0.96) and so was sensitivity to change (standardized response mean 0.90) [52].

There are two versions of the PsAID. For clinical practice the 12-item version is recommended. This version covers pain, skin problems, fatigue, work and/or leisure activities, functional capacity, discomfort, sleep disturbance, anxiety/fear and uncertainty, coping, embarrassment and/or shame, social participation, and depression (Table 5.4, Appendix 3).

For clinical research (clinical trials and longitudinal observational studies) the 9-item version (which is shorter and does not contain the last 3 items: embarrassment and/or shame, social participation, and depression) is recommended. The PsAID score provides information on each individual item as well as one overall score. The PsAID score gives a number between 0 and 10. A higher score on the PsAID indicates more impact of the disease. A score below 4 out of 10 is considered a patient-acceptable status. A change of 3 or more points is considered a relevant absolute change [63]. The PsAID questionnaires are available online free of charge with their available translations.

Dermatological Life Quality Index

The Dermatological Life Quality Index (DLQI) was not developed for PsA: It is a psoriasis questionnaire. The DLQI is a 10-item questionnaire assessing the effect of psoriasis on daily activities and level of disability over the previous 7 days [64]. The DLQI questions are grouped into six subcategories: symptoms and feelings, daily activities, leisure, work/school, personal relationships, and treatment. DLQI is a validated questionnaire with scores ranging from 0 to 30, with higher scores indicating more impairment. Although the DLQI is not *per se* a function tool, it has been used in some studies as a measure of dermatological-related functional limitations [65]. The MCID for the DLQI has not been established for PsA, but in psoriasis patients it has been estimated as a 5-point improvement [66].

Widely Used, Nonspecific PROs in PsA

We will review here some of the generic PROs most frequently used in the context of PsA, in particular in PsA clinical trials [48].

Single Questions Used in PsA

Single questions are usually in the format of VAS or NRS. Both of these are reported with a figure from 0 to 10, or 0 to 100, where 0 is usually perfect status, and 10 or 100 usually the worst status [67].

Patient Global Assessment

PGA is one of the most widely used PROs in PsA [48, 68] and is usually assessed by the following question: "Considering all the ways psoriatic arthritis has affected you during the last week, circle the number that best describes how you have been doing" [67].

PGA is an overall measure of the patient status, and is included in several composite measures of disease activity such as the Psoriatic Arthritis Disease Activity Score (PASDAS) or the definition of Minimal Disease Activity [69–71].

Recently GRAPPA has also suggested using other "patient global" questions specific to joints and skin. The joint and skin patient assessments, respectively, ask the following questions: "Considering all the ways your joints have affected you during the last week, circle the number that best describes how you have been doing" and "Considering all the ways psoriasis (skin disease) has affected you during the last week, circle the number that best describes how you have been doing" [52, 67, 68].

In an initial study, PGA appeared to be related to both of these patient assessments [68].

We recently showed in 223 PsA patients that intra-class correlation between PGA and joint or skin patient assessment were, respectively, 0.71 (95 % confidence interval, 0.64–0.77) and 0.52 (95 % confidence interval, 0.42–0.60) [72]. This indicates the joint global assessment proposed by GRAPPA may be redundant with PGA, whereas the skin global assessment may bring additional and different information. Furthermore, in multivariate analysis PGA was explained (R^2 of model 0.75) by coping (β[beta] = 0.287), pain (β[beta] = 0.240), work and/or leisure activities (β[beta] = 0.141), and anxiety (β[beta] = 0.109) [72]. Thus PGA in PsA is explained by physical aspects of impact, such as pain and activities, but also psychological aspects: coping and anxiety. In this study, skin impact was not an additional explanatory factor of PGA, perhaps because many of the patients had limited skin involvement [49].

Pain

Pain is a widely assessed outcome in PsA, often using a single question VAS or NRS though the wording may vary slightly. One validated formulation of the pain question is the following: "Circle the number that best describes the pain you felt due to your psoriatic arthritis during the last week" with anchors going from "none" to "extreme."

Pain is a major component of the impact of PsA and is reported by patients as the most important domain of health in this disease, as is also the case in RA [52, 73, 74].

The interpretation of improvement in pain in PsA rests on the Minimal Clinically Important Difference cutoff, which has been validated as an improvement from baseline of at least 10 points on a 0-100 scale [75].

Fatigue

Fatigue is a subjective experience that can be described as an overwhelming, sustained sense of exhaustion and decreased capacity for physical and mental work. Levels of fatigue in PsA are elevated: in a large cross-sectional cohort almost 50 % of PsA patients reported moderate fatigue and 29 % experienced severe fatigue [76]. The importance attributed to fatigue is also high: In a priority exercise of 474 patients with PsA from 13 countries, patients ranked fatigue as the second most important domain after pain and before skin problems [52].

There is no consensus regarding which instrument should be used to assess fatigue in PsA. In a systematic literature review on clinical outcomes in PsA, the most frequently used tools were VAS and NRS single questions [14, 48]. Fatigue assessed with NRS was shown to be an independent outcome measure and sensitive to change in patients with PsA [77]. Fatigue can also be assessed using more complex scales that were adapted and validated for patients with PsA, namely the modified Fatigue Severity Scale (mFSS) and the Functional Assessment of Chronic Illness Therapy—Fatigue (FACIT—Fatigue) [78]. The SF-36 vitality subscale has a high correlation ($r = -0.76$) with fatigue measures such as the FSS [79]. FACIT-Fatigue demonstrated good reliability and validity and has the advantage of covering a broader concept of fatigue. However, good correlations have been shown between the fatigue NRS and more complex scales, and the fatigue VAS is reported to perform as well as or better than longer scales [14, 80].

Assessment in Patients with SPA (axSpA and PsA) with Generic Questionnaires

Health Assessment Questionnaire

The Stanford Health Assessment Questionnaire Disability Index (HAQ-DI) is currently the most widely used measure of functioning and disability across rheumatic diseases, and in PsA studies as well [48, 81, 82]. Although the HAQ was originally developed for RA, it is validated in PsA. The HAQ contains 20 items that deal with difficulties experienced with 8 categories of daily living. The HAQ results in a total score between 0 (no disability) and 3 (severe disability) [73]. The HAQ has good psychometric properties. In different contexts, this measure is sensitive to change and is a good predictor of future disability and costs. Specifically in PsA, the HAQ has been shown to be reliable, valid, and sensitive to change in several PsA trials [65, 70, 71, 83, 84]. The interpretation of the HAQ is slightly different in PsA than in RA. Whereas in RA, the cutoff for a minimally important difference (MID) is 0.25, in PsA it is higher and has been suggested to be about 0.35 [84].

The Health Assessment Questionnaire for the Spondyloarthropathies (HAQ-S) (S = spondyloarthritis) is an adaptation based on the original HAQ [81], incorporating issues of physical functioning specific to patients with axial SpA. Items concerning dressing, arising, eating, walking, hygiene, reaching, gripping, and errands and chores have been taken unchanged from the original HAQ. In the HAQ-S, 5 specific items concerning neck function and static posture (driving a car, using a rear-vision mirror, carrying heavy groceries, sitting for long periods, and working at a desk) were added [85]. Ward et al. showed in a large US American cohort that the values of HAQ-S increased over a median of 5 years at an average rate of 0.0168 units per year [86].

Medical Outcomes Study Short Form-36

The Short Form-36 (SF-36) is a generic health profile that has been developed with the aim to compare various aspects of health status across a general and broad patient population [87]. Generic health profiles are questionnaires that provide assessment of more than one dimension of health status and the SF-36 is intended to measure "general health concepts not specific to any disease, or treatment group." The SF-36 has 36 items that are divided into eight subdomains: physical functioning (PF), role limitations due to physical problems (RP), bodily pain (BP), general health (GH), vitality (VT), social functioning (SF), role limitations due to emotional problems (RE), and mental problems (MH). The SF-36 has been used to capture health-related outcomes in a variety of rheumatic conditions, e.g., AS and PsA [88].

The SF-36 has been validated in PsA, and is often used in clinical trials to assess the domain of health-related quality of life in PsA populations [46, 48, 89]. A comparative study of quality of life in patients with PsA versus RA or psoriasis indicated significant alteration of quality of life in particular in RA and PsA, with great alterations in the mental components for patients with RA [90].

In clinical settings, large intra-individual variations in the SF-36 scale scores and its low ability to detect deterioration make it unsuitable for use with individual patients, although the scale appears to have satisfactory ability to detect treatment-related improvements in health at a group level. In research settings, the SF-36 can be used to compare disease groups with the general population [5].

Conclusion

Patient assessment in SpA is multidimensional, and the evaluation of disease status is challenging because of the large phenotypic heterogeneity of the disease. The principal clinical features in patients with SpA are pain, stiffness, and fatigue, which are clearly patient-reported complaints. Therefore, assessing these complaints with PROs is straightforward and will help to quantify the current disease state, to follow the disease progression, and to measure the effect of any intervention. The major decisions facing the clinician are what to measure and what is the best way to measure it? The ASAS core set for AS patients and the OMERACT outcome measures core set for PsA should be regarded as a guide to minimum recommended practice. Physical function, pain, patient global, and joint measures are recommended for clinical record keeping in both core sets.

PRO measures that are currently used and widely available can provide important perspectives not captured in composite clinical response criteria with the potential of better informing treatment decisions in clinical practice.

Acknowledgments We wish to thank Maarten de Wit (Netherlands) and Tania Gudu (Romania) for their help and participation in the psoriatic arthritis chapter.

Appendix 1: BASDAI

BASDAI

Please draw a mark on each line below to indicate your situation in the past 7 days?

1. How would you describe the overall level of fatigue/tiredness you have experienced?

None	Very severe
	0 — 1 — 2 — 3 — 4 — 5 — 6 — 7 — 8 — 9 — 10

2. How would you describe the overall level of AS neck, back, or hip pain you have had?

None	Very severe
	0 — 1 — 2 — 3 — 4 — 5 — 6 — 7 — 8 — 9 — 10

3. How would you describe the overall level of pain/swelling in joints other than the neck, back, or hips you have had?

None	Very severe
	0 — 1 — 2 — 3 — 4 — 5 — 6 — 7 — 8 — 9 — 10

4. How would you describe the overall level of discomfort you have had from any areas tender to touch or pressure?

None	Very severe
	0 — 1 — 2 — 3 — 4 — 5 — 6 — 7 — 8 — 9 — 10

5. How would you describe the overall level of morning stiffness you have had from the time you wake up?

None	Very severe
	0 — 1 — 2 — 3 — 4 — 5 — 6 — 7 — 8 — 9 — 10

6. How long does your morning stiffness last from the time you wake up?

In hours	Hours or more
	0 — ¼ — ½ — ¾ — 1 — 1¼ — 1½ — 1¾ — ≥2

Appendix 2: ASAS Health Index

ASAS
Assessment of SpondyloArthritis international Society

ASAS Health Index

Date: ______________________________

Name: ______________________________

Please answer all statements by placing one check mark per statement to indicate which response best applies to you **at this moment in time** taking into account your rheumatic disease (the term "rheumatic disease" contains all forms of spondyloarthritis including ankylosing spondylitis) .

1. Pain sometimes disrupts my normal activities.

   ☐ I agree

   ☐ I do not agree

2. I find it hard to stand for long.

   ☐ I agree

   ☐ I do not agree

3. I have problems running.

   ☐ I agree

   ☐ I do not agree

4. I have problems using toilet facilities.

   ☐ I agree

   ☐ I do not agree

5. I am often exhausted.

   ☐ I agree

   ☐ I do not agree

6. I am less motivated to do anything that requires physical effort.

   ☐ I agree

   ☐ I do not agree

7. I have lost interest in sex.

   ☐ I agree

   ☐ I do not agree

   ☐ Not applicable, I do not want to answer

8. I have difficulty operating the pedals in my car.

   ☐ I agree

   ☐ I do not agree

   ☐ Not applicable, I cannot / do not drive

Developed by Assessment of SpondyloArthritis International Society (ASAS)

ASAS Assessment of SpondyloArthritis international Society

ASAS Health Index

9. I am finding it hard to make contact with people.

   ☐ I agree

   ☐ I do not agree

10. I am not able to walk outdoors on flat ground.

   ☐ I agree

   ☐ I do not agree

11. I find it hard to concentrate.

   ☐ I agree

   ☐ I do not agree

12. I am restricted in traveling because of my mobility.

   ☐ I agree

   ☐ I do not agree

13. I often get frustrated.

   ☐ I agree

   ☐ I do not agree

14. I find it difficult to wash my hair.

   ☐ I agree

   ☐ I do not agree

15. I have experienced financial changes because of my rheumatic disease.

   ☐ I agree

   ☐ I do not agree

16. I sleep badly at night.

   ☐ I agree

   ☐ I do not agree

17. I cannot overcome my difficulties.

   ☐ I agree

   ☐ I do not agree

Thank you for answering this questionnaire.

Developed by Assessment of SpondyloArthritis International Society (ASAS)

Appendix 3: PSAID

The EULAR Psoriatic Arthritis Impact of Disease: PsAID12 for clinical practice

We want you to indicate how much your psoriatic arthritis impacts your health. Please tell us how you have been feeling this last week.

1. Pain

Circle the number that best describes the pain you felt due to your psoriatic arthritis during the last week:

None	0	1	2	3	4	5	6	7	8	9	10	Extreme	For office use only Result ×3 ☐

2. Fatigue

Circle the number that best describes the overall level of fatigue due to your psoriatic arthritis you have experienced during the last week:

No fatigue	0	1	2	3	4	5	6	7	8	9	10	Totally exhausted	Result ×2 ☐

3. Skin problems

Circle the number that best describes the skin problems including itching you felt due to your psoriatic arthritis during the last week:

None	0	1	2	3	4	5	6	7	8	9	10	Extreme	Result x2 ☐

4. Work and/or leisure activities

Circle the number that best describes the difficulties you had to participate fully in work and/or leisure activities due to your psoriatic arthritis during the last week:

None	0	1	2	3	4	5	6	7	8	9	10	Extreme	Result ×2 ☐

5. Functional capacity

Circle the number that best describes the difficulty you had in doing daily physical activities due to your psoriatic arthritis during the last week:

No difficulty	0	1	2	3	4	5	6	7	8	9	10	Extreme difficulty	Result ×2 ☐

6. Discomfort

Circle the number that best describes the feeling of discomfort and annoyance with everyday tasks due to your psoriatic arthritis during the last week:

None	0	1	2	3	4	5	6	7	8	9	10	Extreme	Result ×2 ☐

7. Sleep disturbance

Circle the number that best describes the sleep difficulties (i.e., resting at night) you felt due to your psoriatic arthritis during the last week:

No difficulty	0	1	2	3	4	5	6	7	8	9	10	Extreme difficulty	Result ×2 ☐

8. Coping

Considering your psoriatic arthritis overall, how well did you cope (manage, deal, make do) with your psoriatic arthritis during the last week?

Very well	0	1	2	3	4	5	6	7	8	9	10	Very poorly	For office use only Result ×1 ☐

9. Anxiety, fear, and uncertainty

Circle the number that best describes the level of anxiety, fear, and uncertainty (for example, about the future, treatments, fear of loneliness) due to your psoriatic arthritis you have experienced during the last week:

None	0	1	2	3	4	5	6	7	8	9	10	Extreme	Result ×1 ☐

10. Embarrassment and/or shame

Considering your psoriatic arthritis overall, circle the number that best describes the level of embarrassment and/or shame due to your appearance experienced during the last week:

None	0	1	2	3	4	5	6	7	8	9	10	Extreme	Result ×1 ☐

11. Social participation

Circle the number that best describes the difficulties you had to participate fully in social activities (including relationships with family and/or people very close to you) due to your psoriatic arthritis during the last week:

None	0	1	2	3	4	5	6	7	8	9	10	Extreme	Result ×1 ☐

12. Depression

Circle the number that best describes the level of depression due to your psoriatic arthritis you have experienced during the last week:

THANK YOU FOR ANSWERING THIS QUESTIONNAIRE

None	0	1	2	3	4	5	6	7	8	9	10	Extreme	Result ×1 ☐

References

1. Dougados M, Baeten D. Spondyloarthritis. Lancet. 2011;377(9783):2127–37.
2. Stolwijk C, van Tubergen A, Castillo-Ortiz JD, Boonen A. Prevalence of extra-articular manifestations in patients with ankylosing spondylitis: a systematic review and meta-analysis. Ann Rheum Dis. 2013;74:65–73.
3. Rudwaleit M, van der Heijde D, Landewe R, Listing J, Akkoc N, Brandt J, et al. The development of assessment of spondyloarthritis international society classification criteria for axial spondyloarthritis (part ii): validation and final selection. Ann Rheum Dis. 2009;68(6):777–83 [Multicenter Study Research Support, Non-U.S. Gov't Validation Studies].
4. Rudwaleit M, van der Heijde D, Landewe R, Akkoc N, Brandt J, Chou CT, et al. The assessment of spondyloarthritis international society classification criteria for peripheral spondyloarthritis and for spondyloarthritis in general. Ann Rheum Dis. 2011;70(1):25–31 [Research Support, Non-U.S. Gov't].
5. Kiltz U, Baraliakos X, Karakostas P, Igelmann M, Kalthoff L, Klink C, et al. Do patients with non-radiographic axial spondylarthritis differ from patients with ankylosing spondylitis? Arthritis Care Res. 2012;64(9):1415–22 [Comparative Study Research Support, Non-U.S. Gov't].
6. Taylor W, Gladman D, Helliwell P, Marchesoni A, Mease P, Mielants H, et al. Classification criteria for psoriatic arthritis: development of new criteria from a large international study. Arthritis Rheum. 2006;54(8):2665–73.
7. Turina MC, Ramiro S, Baeten DL, Mease P, Paramarta JE, Song IH, et al. A psychometric analysis of outcome measures in peripheral spondyloarthritis. Ann Rheum Dis. 2015.
8. Dagfinrud H, Kjeken I, Mowinckel P, Hagen KB, Kvien TK. Impact of functional impairment in ankylosing spondylitis: impairment, activity limitation, and participation restrictions. J Rheumatol. 2005;32(3):516–23 [Research Support, Non-U.S. Gov't].
9. Boonen A, Brinkhuizen T, Landewe R, van der Heijde D, Severens JL. Impact of ankylosing spondylitis on sick leave, presenteeism and unpaid productivity, and estimation of the societal cost. Ann Rheum Dis. 2010;69(6):1123–8.

10. van der Heijde D, van der Linden S, Dougados M, Bellamy N, Russell AS, Edmonds J. Ankylosing spondylitis: plenary discussion and results of voting on selection of domains and some specific instruments. J Rheumatol. 1999;26(4):1003–5 [Review].
11. Ward MM. Health-related quality of life in ankylosing spondylitis: a survey of 175 patients. Arthritis Care Res. 1999;12(4):247–55 [Research Support, Non-U.S. Gov't].
12. Verstappen SM, Jacobs JW, van der Heijde DM, van der Linden S, Verhoef CM, Bijlsma JW, et al. Utility and direct costs: ankylosing spondylitis compared with rheumatoid arthritis. Ann Rheum Dis. 2007;66(6):727–31.
13. Jones SD, Koh WH, Steiner A, Garrett SL, Calin A. Fatigue in ankylosing spondylitis: its prevalence and relationship to disease activity, sleep, and other factors. J Rheumatol. 1996;23(3):487–90 [Research Support, Non-U.S. Gov't].
14. van Tubergen A, Coenen J, Landewe R, Spoorenberg A, Chorus A, Boonen A, et al. Assessment of fatigue in patients with ankylosing spondylitis: a psychometric analysis. Arthritis Rheum. 2002;47(1):8–16.
15. Revicki DA, Rentz AM, Luo MP, Wong RL. Psychometric characteristics of the short form 36 health survey and functional assessment of chronic illness therapy-fatigue subscale for patients with ankylosing spondylitis. Health Qual Life Outcomes. 2011;9:36 [Research Support, Non--U.S. Gov't Validation Studies].
16. Garrett S, Jenkinson T, Kennedy LG, Whitelock H, Gaisford P, Calin A. A new approach to defining disease status in ankylosing spondylitis: the bath ankylosing spondylitis disease activity index. J Rheumatol. 1994;21(12):2286–91 [Comparative Study Research Support, Non-U.S. Gov't].
17. Braun J, Brandt J, Listing J, Zink A, Alten R, Golder W, et al. Treatment of active ankylosing spondylitis with infliximab: a randomised controlled multicentre trial. Lancet. 2002;359(9313):1187–93 [Clinical Trial Multicenter Study Randomized Controlled Trial Research Support, Non-U.S. Gov't].
18. Brandt J, Haibel H, Cornely D, Golder W, Gonzalez J, Reddig J, et al. Successful treatment of active ankylosing spondylitis with the anti-tumor necrosis factor alpha monoclonal antibody infliximab. Arthritis Rheum. 2000;43(6):1346–52.
19. Cohen JD, Cunin P, Farrenq V, Oniankitan O, Carton L, Chevalier X, et al. Estimation of the bath ankylosing spondylitis disease activity index cutoff for perceived symptom relief in patients with spondyloarthropathies. J Rheumatol. 2006;33(1):79–81.
20. Pavy S, Brophy S, Calin A. Establishment of the minimum clinically important difference for the bath ankylosing spondylitis indices: a prospective study. J Rheumatol. 2005;32(1):80–5 [Research Support, Non-U.S. Gov't].
21. Machado P, Landewe RB, Braun J, Baraliakos X, Hermann KG, Hsu B, et al. MRI inflammation and its relation with measures of clinical disease activity and different treatment responses in patients with ankylosing spondylitis treated with a tumour necrosis factor inhibitor. Ann Rheum Dis. 2012;71(12):2002–5 [Randomized Controlled Trial Research Support, Non-U.S. Gov't].
22. Sieper J, Baraliakos X, Listing J, Brandt J, Haibel H, Rudwaleit M, et al. Persistent reduction of spinal inflammation as assessed by magnetic resonance imaging in patients with ankylosing spondylitis after 2 yrs of treatment with the anti-tumour necrosis factor agent infliximab. Rheumatology. 2005;44(12):1525–30.
23. Maksymowych WP, Salonen D, Inman RD, Rahman P, Lambert RG. Low-dose infliximab (3 mg/kg) significantly reduces spinal inflammation on magnetic resonance imaging in patients with ankylosing spondylitis: a randomized placebo-controlled study. J Rheumatol. 2010;37(8):1728–34 [Randomized Controlled Trial Research Support, Non-U.S. Gov't].
24. Kiltz U, Baraliakos X, Karakostas P, Igelmann M, Kalthoff L, Klink C, et al. The degree of spinal inflammation is similar in patients with axial spondyloarthritis who report high or low levels of disease activity: a cohort study. Ann Rheum Dis. 2012;71(7):1207–11 [Comparative Study Research Support, Non-U.S. Gov't].
25. Fagerli KM, Lie E, van der Heijde D, Heiberg MS, Kaufmann C, Rodevand E, et al. Selecting patients with ankylosing spondylitis for TNF inhibitor therapy: comparison of ASDAS and BASDAI eligibility criteria. Rheumatology. 2012;51(8):1479–83.

26. Lukas C, Landewe R, Sieper J, Dougados M, Davis J, Braun J, et al. Development of an ASAS-endorsed disease activity score (ASDAS) in patients with ankylosing spondylitis. Ann Rheum Dis. 2009;68(1):18–24 [Validation Studies].
27. Aydin SZ, Can M, Atagunduz P, Direskeneli H. Active disease requiring TNF-alpha-antagonist therapy can be well discriminated with different ASDAS sets: a prospective, follow-up of disease activity assessment in ankylosing spondylitis. Clin Exp Rheumatol. 2010;28(5):752–5 [Validation Studies].
28. Nas K, Yildirim K, Cevik R, Karatay S, Erdal A, Baysal O, et al. Discrimination ability of ASDAS estimating disease activity status in patients with ankylosing spondylitis. Int J Rheum Dis. 2010;13(3):240–5 [Comparative Study Multicenter Study].
29. Pedersen SJ, Sorensen IJ, Hermann KG, Madsen OR, Tvede N, Hansen MS, et al. Responsiveness of the ankylosing spondylitis disease activity score (ASDAS) and clinical and MRI measures of disease activity in a 1-year follow-up study of patients with axial spondyloarthritis treated with tumour necrosis factor alpha inhibitors. Ann Rheum Dis. 2010;69(6):1065–71 [Multicenter Study Research Support, Non-U.S. Gov't Validation Studies].
30. Kiltz U, van der Heijde D. Health-related quality of life in patients with rheumatoid arthritis and in patients with ankylosing spondylitis. Clin Exp Rheumatol. 2009;27(4 Suppl 55):S108–11 [Review].
31. Wanders A, Landewe R, Dougados M, Mielants H, van der Linden S, van der Heijde D. Association between radiographic damage of the spine and spinal mobility for individual patients with ankylosing spondylitis: can assessment of spinal mobility be a proxy for radiographic evaluation? Ann Rheum Dis. 2005;64(7):988–94 [Evaluation Studies].
32. Machado P, Landewe R, Braun J, Hermann KG, Baker D, van der Heijde D. Both structural damage and inflammation of the spine contribute to impairment of spinal mobility in patients with ankylosing spondylitis. Ann Rheum Dis. 2010;69(8):1465–70.
33. Landewe R, Dougados M, Mielants H, van der Tempel H, van der Heijde D. Physical function in ankylosing spondylitis is independently determined by both disease activity and radiographic damage of the spine. Ann Rheum Dis. 2009;68(6):863–7.
34. Calin A, Garrett S, Whitelock H, Kennedy LG, O'Hea J, Mallorie P, et al. A new approach to defining functional ability in ankylosing spondylitis: the development of the bath ankylosing spondylitis functional index. J Rheumatol. 1994;21(12):2281–5 [Comparative Study Research Support, Non-U.S. Gov't].
35. Dougados M, Gueguen A, Nakache JP, Nguyen M, Mery C, Amor B. Evaluation of a functional index and an articular index in ankylosing spondylitis. J Rheumatol. 1988;15(2):302–7.
36. Boonen A, Chorus A, Miedema H, van der Heijde D, van der Tempel H, van der Linden S. Employment, work disability, and work days lost in patients with ankylosing spondylitis: a cross sectional study of Dutch patients. Ann Rheum Dis. 2001;60(4):353–8.
37. Sigl T, Cieza A, van der Heijde D, Stucki G. ICF based comparison of disease specific instruments measuring physical functional ability in ankylosing spondylitis. Ann Rheum Dis. 2005;64(11):1576–81 [Comparative Study].
38. Doward LC, Spoorenberg A, Cook SA, Whalley D, Helliwell PS, Kay LJ, et al. Development of the ASQoL: a quality of life instrument specific to ankylosing spondylitis. Ann Rheum Dis. 2003;62(1):20–6 [Research Support, Non-U.S. Gov't].
39. Doward LC, McKenna SP, Meads DM, Twiss J, Revicki D, Wong RL, et al. Translation and validation of non-English versions of the ankylosing spondylitis quality of life (ASQoL) questionnaire. Health Qual Life Outcomes. 2007;5:7 [Multicenter Study Research Support, Non-U.S. Gov't].
40. Kiltz U, van der Heijde D, Boonen A, Cieza A, Stucki G, Khan MA, et al. Development of a health index in patients with ankylosing spondylitis (ASAS hi): final result of a global initiative based on the ICF guided by ASAS. Ann Rheum Dis. 2015;74(5):830–5.
41. Boonen A, Braun J, van der Horst Bruinsma IE, Huang F, Maksymowych W, Kostanjsek N, et al. ASAS/who ICF core sets for ankylosing spondylitis (as): how to classify the impact of as on functioning and health. Ann Rheum Dis. 2010;69(1):102–7 [Consensus Development Conference].

42. Kiltz U, van der Heijde D, Boonen A, Bautista-Molano W, Burgos-Vagas R, Chiowchanwisawakit P, et al. Translation and cross-cultural adaptation of the ASAS health index and the environmental item set into 15 languages. Arthritis Rheum. 2014;66(10):557.
43. Mease PJ. Psoriatic arthritis: update on pathophysiology, assessment and management. Ann Rheum Dis. 2011;70 Suppl 1:i77–84.
44. Gladman DD, Mease PJ, Strand V, Healy P, Helliwell PS, Fitzgerald O, et al. Consensus on a core set of domains for psoriatic arthritis. J Rheumatol. 2007;34(5):1167–70.
45. Stamm TA, Nell V, Mathis M, Coenen M, Aletaha D, Cieza A, et al. Concepts important to patients with psoriatic arthritis are not adequately covered by standard measures of functioning. Arthritis Rheum. 2007;57(3):487–94.
46. Tillett W, Eder L, Goel N, De Wit M, Gladman DD, FitzGerald O, et al. Enhanced patient involvement and the need to revise the core set—report from the psoriatic arthritis working group at OMERACT 2014. J Rheumatol. 2015;42:2198–203.
47. Orbai AM, Mease P, De Wit M. The GRAPPA OMERACT psoriatic arthritis working group report from the grappa 2015 annual meeting. J Rheumatol. 2016;43:965–9.
48. Palominos PE, Gaujoux-Viala C, Fautrel B, Dougados M, Gossec L. Clinical outcomes in psoriatic arthritis: a systematic literature review. Arthritis Care Res. 2012;64(3):397–406.
49. Tillett W, Adebajo A, Brooke M, Campbell W, Coates LC, FitzGerald O, et al. Patient involvement in outcome measures for psoriatic arthritis. Curr Rheumatol Rep. 2014;16(5):418.
50. Moverley AR, Vinall-Collier KA, Helliwell PS. It's not just the joints, it's the whole thing: qualitative analysis of patients' experience of flare in psoriatic arthritis. Rheumatology. 2015;54(8):1448–53.
51. Gudu T, Kiltz U, Palimos PE, Gossec L. Impact of psoriatic arthritis: linking the domains of health which are important for patients with psoriatic arthritis to the international classification of functioning, disability and health. 2015.
52. Gossec L, de Wit M, Kiltz U, Braun J, Kalyoncu U, Scrivo R, et al. A patient-derived and patient-reported outcome measure for assessing psoriatic arthritis: elaboration and preliminary validation of the psoriatic arthritis impact of disease (PSAID) questionnaire, a 13-country EULAR initiative. Ann Rheum Dis. 2014;73(6):1012–9.
53. McKenna SP, Doward LC, Whalley D, Tennant A, Emery P, Veale DJ. Development of the PsAQoL: a quality of life instrument specific to psoriatic arthritis. Ann Rheum Dis. 2004;63(2):162–9.
54. Healy PJ, Helliwell PS. Psoriatic arthritis quality of life instrument: an assessment of sensitivity and response to change. J Rheumatol. 2008;35(7):1359–61.
55. Billing E, McKenna SP, Staun M, Lindqvist U. Adaptation of the psoriatic arthritis quality of life (PsAQoL) instrument for Sweden. Scand J Rheumatol. 2010;39(3):223–8.
56. Wink F, Arends S, McKenna SP, Houtman PM, Brouwer E, Spoorenberg A. Validity and reliability of the Dutch adaptation of the psoriatic arthritis quality of life (PsAQoL) questionnaire. PLoS One. 2013;8(2), e55912.
57. Marzo-Ortega H, McGonagle D, Rhodes LA, Tan AL, Conaghan PG, O'Connor P, et al. Efficacy of infliximab on MRI-determined bone oedema in psoriatic arthritis. Ann Rheum Dis. 2007;66(6):778–81.
58. Gladman D, Fleischmann R, Coteur G, Woltering F, Mease PJ. Effect of certolizumab pegol on multiple facets of psoriatic arthritis as reported by patients: 24-week patient-reported outcome results of a phase III, multicenter study. Arthritis Care Res. 2014;66(7):1085–92.
59. Tezel N, Yilmaz Tasdelen O, Bodur H, Gul U, Kulcu Cakmak S, Oguz ID, et al. Is the health-related quality of life and functional status of patients with psoriatic arthritis worse than that of patients with psoriasis alone? Int J Rheum Dis. 2015;18(1):63–9.
60. Osterhaus JT, Purcaru O. Discriminant validity, responsiveness and reliability of the arthritis-specific work productivity survey assessing workplace and household productivity within and outside the home in patients with axial spondyloarthritis, including nonradiographic axial spondyloarthritis and ankylosing spondylitis. Arthritis Res Ther. 2014;16(4):R164.
61. Gezer O, Batmaz I, Sariyildiz MA, Sula B, Ucmak D, Bozkurt M, et al. Sleep quality in patients with psoriatic arthritis. International journal of rheumatic diseases. Int J Rheum Dis. 2014.

62. De Wit M, Kvien T, Gossec L. Patient participation as an integral part of patient reported outcomes development guarantees the representativeness of the patient voice: a case-study from the field of rheumatology. RMD Open. 2015;1(1), e000129.
63. European League Against R. Tools and products. 2015. http://www.eular.org/tools_products_.cfm. Accessed 4 Sep. 2015.
64. Finlay AY, Khan GK. Dermatology life quality index (DLQI): a simple practical measure for routine clinical use. Clin Exp Dermatol. 1994;19(3):210–6.
65. Gladman DD, Mease PJ, Cifaldi MA, Perdok RJ, Sasso E, Medich J. Adalimumab improves joint-related and skin-related functional impairment in patients with psoriatic arthritis: patient-reported outcomes of the adalimumab effectiveness in psoriatic arthritis trial. Ann Rheum Dis. 2007;66(2):163–8.
66. Feldman SR, Kimball AB, Krueger GG, Woolley JM, Lalla D, Jahreis A. Etanercept improves the health-related quality of life of patients with psoriasis: results of a phase iii randomized clinical trial. J Am Acad Dermatol. 2005;53(5):887–9.
67. Katz PP. Introduction to special issue: patient outcomes in rheumatology, 2011. Arthritis Care Res. 2011;63 Suppl 11:S1–3.
68. Cauli A, Gladman DD, Mathieu A, Olivieri I, Porru G, Tak PP, et al. Patient global assessment in psoriatic arthritis: a multicenter GRAPPA and OMERACT study. J Rheumatol. 2011;38(5):898–903.
69. Helliwell PS, FitzGerald O, Fransen J, Gladman DD, Kreuger GG, Callis-Duffin K, et al. The development of candidate composite disease activity and responder indices for psoriatic arthritis (grace project). Ann Rheum Dis. 2013;72(6):986–91.
70. Coates LC, Fransen J, Helliwell PS. Defining minimal disease activity in psoriatic arthritis: a proposed objective target for treatment. Ann Rheum Dis. 2010;69(1):48–53.
71. Coates LC, Helliwell PS. Validation of minimal disease activity criteria for psoriatic arthritis using interventional trial data. Arthritis Care Res. 2010;62(7):965–9.
72. Tälli S, Etcheto A, Fautrel B, et al. Patient global assessment in psoriatic arthritis—what does it mean? An analysis of 223 patients from the psoriatic arthritis impact of disease (PsAID) study. Joint Bone Spine. 2016;83:335–40.
73. Arthritis R and Aging Medical Information System. http://aramis.Stanford.Edu/downloads/haq%20instructions%20%28aramis%29%206-30-09.Pdf. Stanford: Stanford University.
74. Gossec L, Paternotte S, Aanerud GJ, Balanescu A, Boumpas DT, Carmona L, et al. Finalisation and validation of the rheumatoid arthritis impact of disease score, a patient-derived composite measure of impact of rheumatoid arthritis: a EULAR initiative. Ann Rheum Dis. 2011;70(6):935–42.
75. Dworkin RH, Turk DC, Wyrwich KW, Beaton D, Cleeland CS, Farrar JT, et al. Interpreting the clinical importance of treatment outcomes in chronic pain clinical trials: impact recommendations. J Pain. 2008;9(2):105–21.
76. Husted JA, Tom BD, Schentag CT, Farewell VT, Gladman DD. Occurrence and correlates of fatigue in psoriatic arthritis. Ann Rheum Dis. 2009;68(10):1553–8.
77. Minnock P, Kirwan J, Veale D, Fitzgerald O, Bresnihan B. Fatigue is an independent outcome measure and is sensitive to change in patients with psoriatic arthritis. Clin Exp Rheumatol. 2010;28(3):401–4.
78. Chandran V, Bhella S, Schentag C, Gladman DD. Functional assessment of chronic illness therapy-fatigue scale is valid in patients with psoriatic arthritis. Ann Rheum Dis. 2007;66(7):936–9.
79. Husted JA, Tom BD, Farewell VT, Gladman DD. Longitudinal analysis of fatigue in psoriatic arthritis. J Rheumatol. 2010;37(9):1878–84.
80. Wolfe F. Fatigue assessments in rheumatoid arthritis: comparative performance of visual analog scales and longer fatigue questionnaires in 7760 patients. J Rheumatol. 2004;31(10):1896–902.
81. Fries JF, Spitz P, Kraines RG, Holman HR. Measurement of patient outcome in arthritis. Arthritis Rheum. 1980;23(2):137–45.

82. Bruce B, Fries JF. The health assessment questionnaire (HAQ). Clin Exp Rheumatol. 2005;23(5 Suppl 39):S14–8.
83. Blackmore MG, Gladman DD, Husted J, Long JA, Farewell VT. Measuring health status in psoriatic arthritis: the health assessment questionnaire and its modification. J Rheumatol. 1995;22(5):886–93.
84. Mease PJ, Woolley JM, Bitman B, Wang BC, Globe DR, Singh A. Minimally important difference of health assessment questionnaire in psoriatic arthritis: relating thresholds of improvement in functional ability to patient-rated importance and satisfaction. J Rheumatol. 2011;38(11):2461–5.
85. Daltroy LH, Larson MG, Roberts NW, Liang MH. A modification of the health assessment questionnaire for the spondyloarthropathies. J Rheumatol. 1990;17(7):946–50 [Research Support, Non-U.S. Gov't Research Support, U.S. Gov't, P.H.S.].
86. Ward MM. Predictors of the progression of functional disability in patients with ankylosing spondylitis. J Rheumatol. 2002;29(7):1420–5 [Comparative Study Research Support, Non-U.S. Gov't].
87. Ware Jr JE, Sherbourne CD. The MOS 36-item short-form health survey (SF-36). I. Conceptual framework and item selection. Med Care. 1992;30(6):473–83.
88. Heiberg, M. S., Nordvag, B. Y., Mikkelsen, K., Rodevand, E., Kaufmann, C., Mowinckel, P., Kvien, T. K. The comparative effectiveness of tumor necrosis factor-blocking agents in patients with rheumatoid arthritis and patients with ankylosing spondylitis: a six-month, longitudinal, observational, multicenter study. Arthritis Rheum 2005;52:2506–12.
89. Husted JA, Gladman D, Farewell VT, Long JA, Cook RJ. Validating the sf-36 health survey questionnaire in patients with psoriatic arthritis. J Rheumatol. 1997;24(3):511–7.
90. Strand V, Sharp V, Koenig AS. Comparison of health related quality of life in rheumatoid arthritis, psoriatic arthritis and psoriasis and effects of etanercept treatment. Ann Rheum Dis. 2012;71:1143–50.

Chapter 6
PROMs for Systemic Lupus Erythematosus

Brian Bekker Hansen and Lise Højbjerre

Introduction and Background

Systemic Lupus Erythematosus (SLE) is a heterogeneous, inflammatory, multisystem autoimmune disease. Symptoms include joint pain and swelling, skin rash, and fatigue [1]. These symptoms impact daily and leisure activities, work productivity, emotional well-being, relationships, physical functioning, and social functioning. The symptoms of SLE appear to occur in "flares." Subsequently, the impact of SLE can vary over time, depending on whether symptoms are present and/or more intense in severity. In addition to joint inflammation, SLE often impacts the heart, skin, lungs, blood vessels, liver, kidneys, and nervous system of patients [1]. The symptoms of SLE contribute to a substantially reduced health-related quality of life (HRQoL) [2]. A number of patient reported outcome measures (PROMs) have been used to assess the burden of SLE on patients, including measurements of fatigue, pain, emotional/psychological well-being, and work productivity. Furthermore, both SLE-specific and generic PROMs measuring HRQoL have been used.

Treatment of the more severe cases of SLE involves a balance between suppressing the signs and symptoms of the disease and minimizing the toxicities of the drugs used. With treatment, disease activity indices might improve but the patient might feel potentially worse due to the side effects of the medication. In the evaluation of patients with SLE, it is important to measure the patients' perspective because the disease is likely to have a significant impact on physical, social, and psychological aspects impacting the patients' HRQoL. Improvements in clinical outcome measures (e.g., lab tests, clinical evaluation) in patients with SLE may not always translate to improvements in how patients feel or function. PROMs can be used to measure all relevant and important SLE symptoms and patient-perceived abilities to function and perform daily activities.

B.B. Hansen (✉) • L. Højbjerre
Global Market Access, Novo Nordisk A/S, Søborg, Denmark
e-mail: bbkh@novonordisk.com; lhbj@novonordisk.com

Y. El Miedany (ed.), *Patient Reported Outcome Measures in Rheumatic Diseases*,
DOI 10.1007/978-3-319-32851-5_6

Conceptual Model for SLE

A conceptual model can be used to illustrate the humanistic and economic burden of key symptoms and their impact. Such models are valuable in terms of identifying key measurement concepts, which can be used to demonstrate treatment benefit, providing insight into how best to measure particular concepts, and providing a contextual basis for interpreting patient reported findings. The conceptual model (Fig. 6.1) published by Holloway et al. (2014) [3] is based on a structured literature review of qualitative and quantitative articles and can be used to assess whether available disease-specific PROMs target key symptoms and impacts of SLE. The resulting conceptual model shows the symptoms and impacts identified as key concepts related to SLE (Fig. 6.1) [3].

Fatigue and pain are two of the most important and frequent symptoms for patients with SLE [4–10]. Specifically, patients describe mental and physical symptoms of fatigue including impacts on social life [4], emotional well-being [4, 11], physical functioning [4, 12], sleep [9, 13–15], and the ability to complete daily tasks and leisure activities [16, 17]. Important cognitive symptoms include being "unable to think clearly" and memory loss [12]. Other SLE symptoms include skin rash [16, 17], weight gain [4, 16], and hair loss [5, 16]. Symptoms impact all areas of HRQoL, with detrimental consequences observed in the physical, emotional, and social functioning of

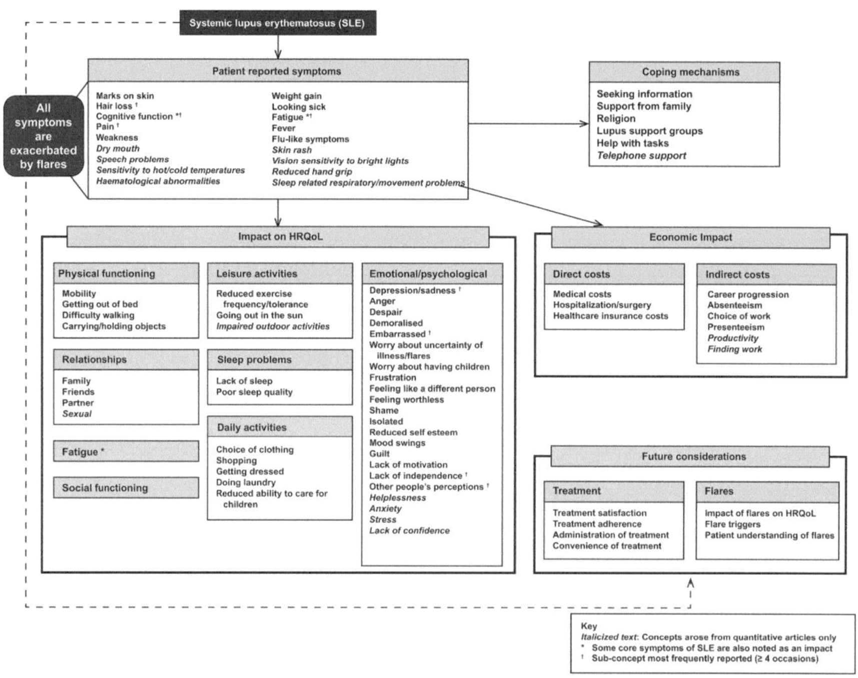

Fig. 6.1 Conceptual model [3]. Reprinted with permission from Holloway et al. [3]

SLE patients, as well as in their working life. In terms of the impact on emotional well-being, patients with SLE frequently feel sad, depressed, angry, and demoralized [4, 5, 8, 12, 18, 19]. In particular, patients feel embarrassed [4–6] or self-conscious, or they lack self-esteem, primarily because of the changes in their appearance (such as hair loss and skin manifestations) [6, 12]. Patients fear their disease worsening, and experience anxiety or stress related to the symptoms and the unpredictability of SLE [8, 16, 18, 19]. Many also experience feelings of frustration and a lack of: (1) confidence, (2) independence, (3) control over one's life, and (4) belonging [20]. SLE has a significant negative impact on patients' physical functioning, such as walking difficulty and other mobility problems [2, 12, 21, 22]. This affects various daily activities including opening jars and moving heavy objects [22], shopping [12], doing laundry [6], getting dressed [6], and caring for their children [4, 6]. Wider impacts on social functioning and working life are also reported [7, 20]. Specifically, patients have difficulty maintaining family and sexual relationships [4, 6, 18]. SLE also impacts negatively on patients' career progression [5], absence from work [12], difficulty concentrating at work or study [6, 10, 12], and their choice of work [6, 16].

The conceptual model presented suggests that patients use various coping mechanisms for the unpredictability of flares, including: (1) seeking and using information, (2) seeking emotional and practical help via the Internet, (3) receiving support from hospital meetings, (4) receiving support from family, (5) attending lupus support groups, and (6) religious practice [4, 6, 16]. The conceptual model also includes concepts such as treatment satisfaction, adherence, and the impact of flares in a "future considerations" box. There was a lack of evidence pertaining to these concepts in the currently available literature.

The conceptual model also demonstrates the economic burden of disease, in particular the high medical costs associated with SLE compared to other chronic diseases [23]. Substantial levels of inpatient care, medication/prescriptions, and visits to healthcare professionals (HCP), which are all increased by "flares," are the main drivers of direct costs in the treatment of SLE [24]. The conceptual model also shows that SLE is associated with high indirect costs due to lost productivity [25] resulting from unemployment and absenteeism [26], with "in-flare" patients with SLE having increased frequency and duration of time off work [27, 28].

Patient Reported Outcome Measures

Fatigue

Fatigue is one of the most important and frequent symptoms for patients with SLE. For many patients it is the most enduring complaint [15, 18]. Fatigue is described in various ways including tiredness, reduced energy, and mental fatigue, and it often impacts the HRQoL in patients with SLE [9, 20]. The lack of a clear definition of fatigue is evident in the literature and reflects the complex nature of the concept. Furthermore, there is a lack of consistent definition from patients and clinicians in terms of what fatigue really means to patients and how it differs from other related concepts such as "normal tiredness" and "energy." As a result, there is a notable variety and disparity in the content of the various PROMs developed to measure fatigue.

Several PROMs measuring fatigue exist. Some of the most frequently used are the Multidimensional Fatigue Inventory (MFI), Multidimensional Assessment of Fatigue (MAF), Fatigue Severity Scale (FSS), and the Functional Assessment of Chronic Illness Therapy—Fatigue scale (FACIT-Fatigue). For none of the listed fatigue PROMs the content and face validity have been established in patients with SLE using qualitative and cognitive debriefing methodologies in the development process. Of the fatigue measures, FACIT-Fatigue (Appendix 1) is currently one of the most frequently applied in recent clinical trials of belimumab [29, 30], and has been extensively validated within rheumatic diseases [31–33]. In a qualitative research study, patients with SLE perceived FACIT-Fatigue as a relevant and appropriate measure of fatigue in SLE [17].

FACIT-Fatigue is a one-dimensional 13-item PROM assessing self-reported fatigue and its impact upon functioning and daily activities. It asks patients to indicate how true each statement is on a 5-point Likert scale from 0 (*Not at all*) to 4 (*Very much*) with a 7-day recall period (see Table 6.1 and Appendix 1). The estimated completion time for the patient is 3–5 min, which limits the burden to both patient and medical staff at the clinic. The written instructions to the patient appear clear and no complex clinical terminology is included. In general the item-wording is written in a simple and understandable language for most patients.

FACIT-Fatigue has demonstrated the strong psychometric properties in terms of evidence of internal consistency, reliability, known-groups validity, concurrent validity, and ability to detect change in patients with SLE (Box 6.1) [31]. Further, test–retest reliability has been demonstrated in patients with psoriatic arthritis [32]. A minimal clinically important difference (MCID) has not been established in patients with SLE; however, in patients with rheumatoid arthritis the MCID has been estimated to be a 3–4 point change from a baseline in the score [33].

Table 6.1 Characteristics of functional assessment of chronic illness therapy—fatigue scale (FACIT-Fatigue)

Instrument characteristics	Description
Target population	Patients experiencing fatigue; no specific age range
Number of items	13
Completion time	3–5 min
Recall period	Past 7 days
Format and layout	The format and layout of the questionnaire appear simple and straightforward
Coverage	For example, fatigue, energy, tiredness, and impact on frustration and social activities
Response options	5-Point Likert scale: "Not at all", "A little bit", "Somewhat", "Quite a bit", and "Very much"
Mode of administration	Self-administered by the patient
Content validation	No patients with SLE were involved in qualitative research in the development phase

Box 6.1: Fatigue
Fatigue is one of the most frequent symptoms reported by patients with SLE.

The Functional Assessment for Chronic Illness Therapy — Fatigue scale (FACIT-Fatigue) is a well-established fatigue measure in SLE, and its psychometric properties in SLE has been established. It consists of 13 items written in a simple language without complex clinical terminology.

Pain

Pain is one of the most common complaints for patients with SLE and is described as "pain," "hurt," or "ache" and some patients speak specifically of "joint pain" [4–6]. Due to the subjective and variable nature of pain, it is best evaluated using patient-reported assessments.

In a review of previous studies involving SLE patients, it was reported that amongst a mean of 460 patients per study, 71–89 % of patients reported experiencing pain [7]. Many publications suggest there is an association of pain with fatigue [13–15, 34] and between pain and poor sleep quality [15]. PROMs specific to pain include the McGill Pain Questionnaire (MPQ) and the Brief Pain Inventory (BPI) (Table 6.2).

The MPQ exists as both a standard form (20 items) [35] and a short form (15 items) [36]. The standard form is more comprehensive. The MPQ is a multidimensional instrument designed to measure the physical and emotional components of pain. The MPQ was developed with minimal patient input ($n = 10$) and the patient group or inclusion/exclusion criteria was not specified. The instrument can be administered in any mode (e.g., self-administered or by a clinician), but the selected mode of administration should be consistent. The item and response wording is very clinical and patients with a low reading ability are likely to not understand the terminology. The recall period for assessment is "currently" or "presently." The MPQ focuses on pain, primarily assessing descriptors of pain. Some impacts of pain are assessed including pain-related fatigue and emotional impacts. However, in the literature review for the conceptual model, it was found that SLE patients tended to discuss SLE-related pain in terms of its location—for example, muscle pain, joint pain, or headaches—rather than how it feels (i.e., aches or discomfort), which could be problematic as the MPQ does not assess where pain occurs. The recall period of current/present pain may not be appropriate for SLE, given that symptoms may arise at any time and, unless the patient is experiencing symptoms during completion, such episodes could be missed. The Brief Pain Inventory (Appendix 2) is a PROM designed to assess the intensity of pain and the extent to which pain interferes with normal function [37]. The BPI is available as a standard form and a short form. The shorter version (BPI-SF) has become the standard for use in clinical and research applications [38] and is the focus for this review (Box 6.2). The BPI-SF focuses on pain and assesses various aspects of pain including the location, severity, and the impact of pain on patients' HRQoL. In line with the conceptual model (Fig. 6.1), the impact concepts assessed include daily activities, emotional/psycho-

Table 6.2 Characteristics of McGill Pain Questionnaire (MPQ) and Brief Pain Inventory (BPI-SF)

Instrument characteristics	Description (MPQ)	Description (BPI-SF)
Target population	Adults, all patients groups	Adults, all patients groups
Number of items	20	15
Completion time	10–15 min	5 min
Recall period	Asks patients to think about "present pain"	24 h
Format and layout	The format varies in different versions that are available online	The format of the questionnaire is clear and simple to follow
Coverage	Three sections:	1. Pain severity
	1. What does your pain feel like?	2. Extent to which pain interferes with daily life
	2. How does your pain change with time?	
	3. How strong is you pain?	
Response options	Likert scales from 2-point to 6-point scales	Twelve items ask patients to respond on a 0–10 scale. One item comprises a binary yes/no response and one item includes a diagram of a person that patients are asked to shade where they feel pain. The shading item is for informative purposes only and is not included in the scoring
Mode of administration	Self-administered or clinician administered (different version)	Self-administered by the patient
Content validation	The MPQ involved in-depth interviews with 10 patients, and health care professionals. No SLE patient input	No patients with SLE were involved in qualitative research in the development phase

logical impacts, physical functioning, relationships, and sleep problems. With a focus on pain, the BPI-SF has good concept coverage, assessing not only descriptors of pain, but also the location of pain and the impact on patients' HRQoL. Most items have an 11-point rating scale; for severity, 0 = no pain and 10 = pain as bad as you can imagine; and for interference, 0 = does not interfere and 10 = completely interferes. One item has a binary yes/no response and another asks patients to shade a diagram to show where they have pain. One item has a 0–100 % scale increasing in 10 % increments. The format of the questionnaire is clear and simple to follow, and thus does not appear to pose any problems for comprehension or accurate completion. BPI-SF has demonstrated strong psychometric properties in terms of internal consistency [39], test–retest reliability [37], construct [39–41] and discriminant [37, 42] validity and responsiveness [42], and a recent study confirmed the findings in an SLE population [43]. The BPI-SF appears to be the strongest measure of pain of the 2 reviewed.

Box 6.2: Pain

Pain is one of the most common complaints for patients with SLE in qualitative research and is associated with fatigue and poor sleep quality.

The **Brief Pain Inventory (BPI-SF)** can be recommended for use in patients with SLE to assess the intensity of pain and the extent to which pain interferes with normal function.

Further, qualitative research and validation of the psychometric properties of BPI are recommended to be explored in patients with SLE.

Emotional Well-Being and Depression

SLE has been shown to impact patient's emotional well-being. Changes in appearance due to the disease and side effects of treatment affect the patient's perception of their body image and sexuality, which in turn impacts their emotional well-being [8]. Patients with SLE frequently feel sad, depressed, angry, embarrassed, and have lack of self-esteem [4–6, 12]. Emotional well-being is a very broad term, and the focus of this discussion will be on anxiety and depression as it arose most frequently in the qualitative literature of patients with SLE.

Two frequently used PROMs assessing anxiety and depression are Beck's Depression Inventory (BDI) and the Hospital Anxiety and Depression Scale (HADS). Neither BDI nor HADS have been validated in patients with SLE. However, both instruments are suitable to use in clinical practice in patients with SLE who experience an impact on anxiety and depression. However, HADS could be considered over BDI, as the instructions are more detailed and straightforward and the item wording is clearer. Further, the response options in the HADS are worded simply and clearly defined, and thus should not pose any problems for patients with SLE.

HADS is a 14-item PROM assessing self-reported anxiety and depression (Box 6.3). Patients should indicate to which degree each of the 14 statements applies on a 4-point Likert-scale with a recall period of a week [44, 45] (Table 6.3). It consists of two domains (anxiety and depression) with seven items each. The estimated completion time is 2–5 min, which provides a limited burden to both patient and medical staff at clinic.

No evidence of validation of the psychometric properties of HADS has been published in patients with SLE [3]. The HADS has demonstrated strong psychometric properties in a general population and in patients with psychiatric disorders. Evidence of the ability to detect change in response to an intervention has been established in various diseases such as depression, neurotic disorder, and cancer [46].

Box 6.3: Anxiety and Depression

Anxiety and depression is frequently expressed by patients with SLE in qualitative research.

The **Hospital Anxiety and Depression Scale (HADS)** can be recommended for use in patients with SLE where the medical staff suspects that the patient's emotional well-being is impacted by anxiety or depression.

Further, qualitative research and validation of the psychometric properties of HADS are recommended to be explored in patients with SLE.

Table 6.3 Characteristics of Hospital Anxiety and Depression Scale (HADS) and Becks Depression Inventory (BDI)

Instrument characteristics	Description (HADS)	Description (BDI)
Target population	Adults	Adults
Number of items	14	21
Completion time	2–5 min	5–10 min
Recall period	Past week	Not specified
Format and layout	Acceptable format and layout; the items are fairly close together	The format is generally simple to follow
Coverage	Depression: 7 items, anxiety: 7 items	Depression total score
Response options	4-point Likert scale: (0–3 response). Response options differ depending on item	4-point Likert scale: (0–3 response). Response options differ depending on item
Mode of administration	Self-administered by the patient	Self-administered by the patient or interviewer administered
Content validation	No patients with SLE involved in qualitative research in the development phase. Developed based on clinician observations, however not specific for SLE	No patients with SLE involved in qualitative research in the development phase. Developed based on clinician observations, however not specific for SLE

Health-Related Quality of Life

HRQoL in patients with SLE is influenced by treatment, disease activity, and symptoms of fatigue, depression, pain, sleep disturbances, and cognitive dysfunction [47]. Due to the radical nature of the disease, HRQoL is an important outcome measure in patients with SLE. HRQoL can be accessed through generic or disease-specific PROMs.

Generic Assessment of HRQoL

The generic HRQoL measure selected for review is the 36-item Short Form Health Survey version 2 (SF-36v2) (Table 6.4). SF-36v2 has been validated in many different health conditions and is a widely used and accepted measure of HRQoL [40, 48]. This PROM covers many domains of importance to patients including physical function, social function, pain, vitality (fatigue and energy), and mental health, and distinguishes limitation on activities by physical and emotional factors. This is

Table 6.4 Characteristics of the short form (36 item) Health Survey version 2 (SF-36v2) and the Lupus quality of life (LupusQoL)

Instrument characteristics	Description (SF-36v2)	Description (LupusQoL)
Target population	Generic, for use in all disease populations. Adult and adolescents ≥ 14 years	SLE patients, adults
Number of items	36	34
Completion time	5–10 min	Less than 10 min
Recall period	Standard 4-week recall or Acute 1-week recall version	Last 4 weeks
Format and layout	The layout of the items is straightforward and the formatting of the instrument makes rating each item a relatively simple task	The format of the questionnaire does not appear to pose any problems for comprehension or accurate completion. However, the response options are displayed a little close, making the instrument appear slightly overcrowded
Coverage	Physical functioning, bodily pain, vitality, social functioning, mental health, general health perceptions, role limitations due to physical problems, role limitations due to emotional problems, plus an item to measure reported health transition (health compared to 1 year ago)	Physical health; pain; planning; intimate relationships; burden to others; emotional health; body image; fatigue
Response options	3 and 5-point Likert scales	5-point scale ranging from "never" to "all of the time"
Mode of administration	Self-administered by the patient as well as Interviewer/Telephone/ Computer administered	Self-administered by the patient
Content validation	No patients were included in the development of the measure [52] but the SF-36 has been widely used in general health populations since its development	Items generated with input from 30 SLE patients Pilot tested with 20 SLE patients to assess face and content validity [51]

crucial in a chronic disease such as SLE where the disease, as well as the therapies used, may cause physical and emotional effects; SF-36v2 makes it possible to assess these different aspects of health status and quality of life separately.

The SF-36v2 has 36-items; 26 are rated on a 5-point scale and 10 are rated on a 3-point scale. These items and response options are generally clear and easy to understand, and the instructions are simple and straightforward to follow. In terms of the recall period of the questionnaire, both a 4-week recall and an acute 1-week recall version exist. A recall period of the past 7 days may be more appropriate, given the fluctuating nature of the condition—patient's symptoms and limitations may vary significantly from day to day. SF-36v2 has demonstrated good psychometric properties in terms of internal consistency, reliability, and test–retest reliability, construct validity, and concurrent validity in the general population [48, 49]. More importantly, in an SLE population, the SF-36v2 has demonstrated evidence of internal consistency reliability, concurrent validity, and known groups validity [50]. Of note, the SF36v2 is able to detect change in many conditions [48, 51] and distribution and anchor-based estimates suggest Minimal Clinically Important Differences (MCIDs) of approximately 3–6 points in an SLE population [50]. SF-36v2 is able to discriminate between levels of disease severity, which is important for assessing change. Patients were not involved in the initial development, but the SF-36v2 has been widely used in general health populations since its development.

SLE-Specific Assessment of HRQoL

Several disease-specific instruments have been designed to assess HRQoL in SLE: Lupus Quality of Life (LupusQoL), L-QoL, SLE-QoL, and Lupus-PRO. The LupusQoL is the strongest of the disease-specific HRQoL measures in terms of development, conceptual coverage, and validation and will be the focus for this review. The LupusQoL (Appendix 3, Table 6.4) is a 34-item questionnaire designed to assess SLE patients' HRQoL (Box 6.4). Concept elicitation interviews were conducted with 30 SLE patients to gather information regarding concepts that are relevant to patients [52]. The LupusQoL comprises 8 domains: physical health, pain, planning, intimate relationships, burden to others, emotional health, body image, and fatigue [52]. It emphasizes areas such as sleep, body image, and sexual health, which are not specifically queried in SF-36v2. LupusQoL has demonstrated good internal consistency, test–retest reliability, and concurrent validity with the generic SF-36v2 [52].

The response options are clearly worded and appear to be easy for patients to understand. The item wording is clear and simple to understand, however the response options may be somewhat skewed toward the higher end of the severity spectrum and some options could be difficult to differentiate between. Patients are required to think over the past 4 weeks. This is a fairly long period and may elicit inaccurate responses, as some patients may forget the impact that their illness had over this time. LupusQoL has good psychometric properties in terms of reliability, construct validity, discriminant validity, and concurrent/convergent validity [52]. No evidence is available on ability to detect change.

Box 6.4: Health-Related Quality of Life

Health-Related Quality of Life (HRQoL) in patients with SLE is influenced by treatment, disease activity, and symptoms of fatigue, depression, pain, sleep disturbances, and cognitive dysfunction.

The **Short Form Health Survey (SF-36v2)** can be recommended to assess different aspects of general health status and quality of life.

The **LupusQoL** can be used to assess the impact that SLE has upon patients' HRQoL and it emphasizes areas such as sleep, body image, and sexual health, which are not specifically queried in SF-36v2.

Reflections and Considerations for the Future

To understand the value of therapies for SLE from the patient perspective, PROMs should be included in clinical practice in conjunction with well-established clinical assessments. The selection of suitable measures to assess SLE-related symptoms and impacts in clinical practice requires careful consideration [53, 54]. This chapter therefore presented a conceptual model of the key symptoms and impacts associated with SLE. The key patient-reported concepts identified within the model were fatigue, pain, cognition, daily activities, emotional well-being, physical/social functioning, and work productivity. The subjective nature of many SLE symptoms and impacts requires accurate and reliable measurement of these symptoms based on patient self-report. In light of this, it is important to also review and evaluate the content validity and psychometric properties of PROMs that may be appropriate for use in an SLE population.

The FACIT-Fatigue, LupusQoL, BPI, SF-36v2, and LupusQoL appear to be the strongest PROMs as measures of the key concepts identified in the conceptual model and all had evidence of the psychometric validity. In addition, the generic SF-36v2 is widely used in randomized clinical trials with patients with SLE and is recognized and accepted by clinical, patient, regulatory, reimbursement, and academic communities. FACIT-Fatigue has proven to be a valid measure of fatigue through a qualitative study [17] and the psychometric properties in an SLE population are well documented [31]. Of the PROMs reviewed, only the LupusQoL has documented evidence of qualitative input from patients with SLE in the development process.

In clinical standard practice it could be an advantageous if all of the key symptoms and impacts were covered in one single PROM. Some PROMs have recently been developed for this purpose such as the Multi-Dimensional Questionnaire for Patient Reported Outcome Measures-SLE (MDPROMs SLE) [55] and Lupus Impact Tracker (LIT) [56]. Further research and experience with the use of multidimensional measures in clinical practice are needed.

It is important to acknowledge that patients with SLE may experience many symptom-free days, followed by a severe flare. Flares are likely to impact patients'

HRQoL [2, 57]. Therefore, further research in developing PROMs that capture the impact of flares should be considered in the future. SLE often involves day-to-day symptom fluctuations due to these flares, thus the recall period of the measurement instrument is also an important consideration. PROs with shorter recall periods may underestimate symptom burden and may place undue demand on patients; however, longer recall period may not allow for reliable symptom and impact reporting.

The recommended PROMs in this chapter have been selected on the basis of identification of key SLE symptoms and impacts in the conceptual model. PROMs of other symptoms of SLE not reported in the conceptual model were thus deprioritized and therefore not included. Appropriate and validated PROMs for some key concepts identified in the model (e.g., skin manifestations of the disease, impact of flares, and treatment satisfaction) were not identified, or no PROMs have been used to measure these concepts in patients with SLE. This represents a gap in knowledge that may benefit from further research. PROMs are in this context considered complementary to more objective measures and should be incorporated into clinical practice.

Conclusion

SLE is a condition associated with high unmet need and considerable burden to patients, as demonstrated by the conceptual model presented in this chapter. This review highlights some of the existing PROMs of SLE signs and symptoms and HRQoL that demonstrate appropriate content validity and are psychometrically adequate for a population of patients with SLE, and as a result such measures may be suitable for use in clinical practice for patients with SLE.

Both generic and disease-specific PROMs were reviewed. Those PROMs included HRQoL, measures of fatigue, pain, and depression/anxiety. The Functional Assessment for Chronic Illness Therapy Fatigue scale (FACIT-fatigue) is the strongest fatigue measure in terms of psychometric properties and conceptual coverage. The Brief Pain Inventory (BPI-SF) is the strongest pain instrument in terms of content validity. However, qualitative research in patients with SLE is needed to ensure the applicability of the items and the appropriateness of the recall period. The Hospital Anxiety and Depression Scale (HADS) is the recommended PROM for measurement of anxiety and depression as the instructions and response options are straightforward and clearly defined. The LupusQoL is the strongest HRQoL measure in terms of the development, conceptual coverage, and validation. It might be favorable in standard clinical practice to consider including 1 cohesive PROM for the assessment of patient reported key symptoms and impacts in SLE. However, further research and validation studies as well as experience with the use of these "all-in-one" PROMs in clinical practice are needed.

Appendix 1: FACIT-Fatigue is presented with permission from the copyright holder. Potential users

Potential users should go to http://www.facit.org/FACITOrg and contact copyright holder for permission before using FACIT-Fatigue in studies and clinical practice.

FACIT Fatigue Scale (Version 4)

Below is a list of statements that other people with your illness have said are important. **Please circle or mark one number per line to indicate your response as it applies to the** ***past 7 days***.

		Not at all	A little bit	Some-what	Quite a bit	Very much
HI7	I feel fatigued	0	1	2	3	4
HI12	I feel weak all over	0	1	2	3	4
An1	I feel listless (*washed out*)	0	1	2	3	4
An2	I feel tired	0	1	2	3	4
An3	I have trouble *starting* things because I am tired	0	1	2	3	4
An4	I have trouble *finishing* things because I am tired	0	1	2	3	4
An5	I have energy	0	1	2	3	4
An7	I am able to do my usual activities	0	1	2	3	4
An8	I need to sleep during the day	0	1	2	3	4
An12	I am too tired to eat	0	1	2	3	4
An14	I need help doing my usual activities	0	1	2	3	4
An15	I am frustrated by being too tired to do the things I want to do	0	1	2	3	4
An16	I have to limit my social activity because I am tired	0	1	2	3	4

Appendix 2: Brief Pain Inventory—Short Form

BPI-SF is presented with permission from the copyright holder. Potential users should go to www.mdanderson.org/departments/prg and contact copyright holder for permission before using BPI-SF in studies and clinical practice.

STUDY ID #:__________ DO NOT WRITE ABOVE THIS LINE HOSPITAL #: __________

Brief Pain Inventory (Short Form)

Date: ____/____/____ Time: _______

Name: __________________ __________________ ______________

Last First Middle Initial

1. Throughout our lives, most of us have had pain from time to time (such as minor headaches, sprains, and toothaches). Have you had pain other than these every-day kinds of pain today?

   1. Yes 2. No

2. On the diagram, shade in the areas where you feel pain. Put an X on the area that hurts the most.

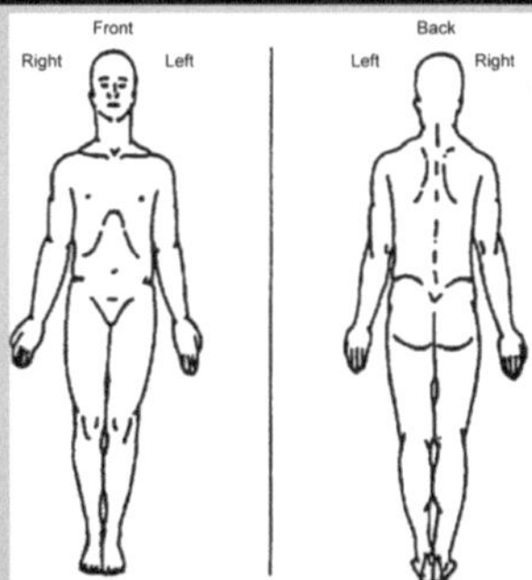

3. Please rate your pain by circling the one number that best describes your pain at its **worst** in the last 24 hours.

   0 1 2 3 4 5 6 7 8 9 10
   No Pain — Pain as bad as you can imagine

4. Please rate your pain by circling the one number that best describes your pain at its **least** in the last 24 hours.

   0 1 2 3 4 5 6 7 8 9 10
   No Pain — Pain as bad as you can imagine

5. Please rate your pain by circling the one number that best describes your pain on the **average.**

   0 1 2 3 4 5 6 7 8 9 10
   No Pain — Pain as bad as you can imagine

6. Please rate your pain by circling the one number that tells how much pain you have **right now.**

   0 1 2 3 4 5 6 7 8 9 10
   No Pain — Pain as bad as you can imagine

Page 1 of 2

STUDY ID #:__________ DO NOT WRITE ABOVE THIS LINE HOSPITAL #:__________

Date: ____/____/____ Time: ________

Name: __________________ __________________ ______________

Last First Middle Initial

7. What treatments or medications are you receiving for your pain?

____

____

8. In the last 24 hours, how much relief have pain treatments or medications provided? Please circle the one percentage that most shows how much **relief** you have received.

0%	10%	20%	30%	40%	50%	60%	70%	80%	90%	100%
No Relief										Complete Relief

9. Circle the one number that describes how, during the past 24 hours, pain has interfered with your:

A. General Activity

0	1	2	3	4	5	6	7	8	9	10
Does not Interfere										Completely Interferes

B. Mood

0	1	2	3	4	5	6	7	8	9	10
Does not Interfere										Completely Interferes

C. Walking Ability

0	1	2	3	4	5	6	7	8	9	10
Does not Interfere										Completely Interferes

D. Normal Work (includes both work outside the home and housework)

0	1	2	3	4	5	6	7	8	9	10
Does not Interfere										Completely Interferes

E. Relations with other people

0	1	2	3	4	5	6	7	8	9	10
Does not Interfere										Completely Interferes

F. Sleep

0	1	2	3	4	5	6	7	8	9	10
Does not Interfere										Completely Interferes

G. Enjoyment of life

0	1	2	3	4	5	6	7	8	9	10
Does not Interfere										Completely Interferes

Page 2 of 2

Appendix 3: LupusQoL

LupusQoL is presented with permission from the copyright holders. Anyone running a commercially funded study must obtain a license for the LupusQoL and pay the license fee. Use is free for noncommercially funded studies but copyright holders requires that researchers contact the licensors for permission before using to ensure that researchers use the professionally developed and validated translations only.

Potential users should go to www.lupusqol.com for more information on using LupusQoL in studies and clinical practice.

LupusQoL©

LupusQoL Questionnaire

The following questionnaire is designed to find out how SLE affects your life. Read each statement and then circle the response, which is closest to how you feel. Please try to answer all the questions as honestly as you can.

How often over the last 4 weeks

1. Because of my Lupus I need help to do heavy physical jobs such as digging the garden, painting and/or decorating, moving furniture

All of the time | most of the time | a good bit of the time | occasionally | never

2. Because of my Lupus I need help to do moderate physical jobs such as vacuuming, ironing, shopping, cleaning the bathroom

All of the time | most of the time | a good bit of the time | occasionally | never

3. Because of my Lupus I need help to do light physical jobs such as cooking/preparing meals, opening jars, dusting, combing my hair or attending to personal hygiene

All of the time | most of the time | a good bit of the time | occasionally | never

4. Because of my Lupus I am unable to perform everyday tasks such as my job, childcare, housework as well as I would like to

All of the time | most of the time | a good bit of the time | occasionally | never

5. Because of my Lupus I have difficulty climbing stairs

All of the time | most of the time | a good bit of the time | occasionally | never

6. Because of my Lupus I have lost some independence and am reliant on others

All of the time | most of the time | a good bit of the time | occasionally | never

7. I have to do things at a slower pace because of my Lupus

All of the time | most of the time | a good bit of the time | occasionally | never

8. Because of my Lupus my sleep pattern is disturbed

All of the time | most of the time | a good bit of the time | occasionally | never

How often over the last 4 weeks

9. I am prevented from performing activities the way I would like to because of pain due to Lupus

All of the time | most of the time | a good bit of the time | occasionally | never

LupusQoL©

10.Because of my Lupus, the pain I experience interferes with the quality of my sleep

All of the time most of the time a good bit of the time occasionally never

11. The pain due to my Lupus is so severe that it limits my mobility

All of the time most of the time a good bit of the time occasionally never

12. Because of my Lupus I avoid planning to attend events in the future

All of the time most of the time a good bit of the time occasionally never

13. Because of the unpredictability of my Lupus I am unable to organise my life efficiently

All of the time most of the time a good bit of the time occasionally never

14. My Lupus varies from day to day which makes it difficult for me to commit myself to social arrangements

All of the time most of the time a good bit of the time occasionally never

15. Because of the pain I experience due to Lupus I am less interested in a sexual relationship

All of the time most of the time a good bit of the time occasionally never not applicable

16. Because of my Lupus I am not interested in sex

All of the time most of the time a good bit of the time occasionally never not applicable

17. I am concerned that my Lupus is stressful for those who are close to me

All of the time most of the time a good bit of the time occasionally never

18.Because of my Lupus I am concerned that I cause worry to those who are close to me.

All of the time most of the time a good bit of the time occasionally never

19. Because of my Lupus I feel that I am a burden to my friends and/or family

All of the time most of the time a good bit of the time occasionally never

Over the past 4 weeks I have found my Lupus makes me feel

20. Resentful

All of the time most of the time a good bit of the time occasionally never

21. So fed up nothing can cheer me up

All of the time most of the time a good bit of the time occasionally never

LupusQoL©

22. Sad

All of the time | most of the time | a good bit of the time | occasionally | never

23. Anxious

All of the time | most of the time | a good bit of the time | occasionally | never

24. Worried

All of the time | most of the time | a good bit of the time | occasionally | never

25. Lacking in self-confidence

All of the time | most of the time | a good bit of the time | occasionally | never

How often over the past 4 weeks

26 My physical appearance due to Lupus interferes with my enjoyment of life

All of the time | most of the time | a good bit of the time | occasionally | never

27. Because of my Lupus, my appearance (e.g. rash, weight gain/loss) makes me avoid social situations

All of the time | most of the time | a good bit of the time | occasionally | never | not applicable

28. Lupus related skin rashes make me feel less attractive

All of the time | most of the time | a good bit of the time | occasionally | never | not applicable

How often over the past 4 weeks

29. The hair loss I have experienced because of my Lupus makes me feel less attractive

All of the time | most of the time | a good bit of the time | occasionally | never | not applicable

30. The weight gain I have experienced because of my Lupus treatment makes me feel less attractive

All of the time | most of the time | a good bit of the time | occasionally | never | not applicable

31. Because of my Lupus I cannot concentrate for long periods of time

All of the time | most of the time | a good bit of the time | occasionally | never

LupusQoL©

32. Because of my Lupus I feel worn out and sluggish

All of the time most of the time a good bit of the time occasionally never

33. Because of my Lupus I need to have early nights

All of the time most of the time a good bit of the time occasionally never

34. Because of my Lupus I am often exhausted in the morning

All of the time most of the time a good bit of the time occasionally never

Please feel free to make any additional comments.

____

____

Please check that you have answered each question

Thank you, for completing this questionnaire

Appendix 4: Multidimensional Questionnaire for Patient Reported Outcome Measures—SLE

Multi-Dimensional Questionnaire for Patient Reported Outcome Measures – SLE

This questionnaire includes information not available from blood tests, X-rays, or any source other than you. Please try to answer each question. There is **no right or wrong answer.** Please answer exactly as **YOU** think or feel.

1. We are interested in learning how your illness affects your ability to function in daily life. Please tick (√) the ONE best answer that describes your usual abilities OVER THE PAST WEEK:

Over the **LAST WEEK** were you able to	Without ANY Difficulty	With SOME Difficulty	With MUCH Difficulty	Unable TO DO	**Fn. Dis.**
1. Get on and off the toilet?	....	....	....	....	
2. Use your grip strength; eg, open previously opened jars Or lift a saucepan during cooking?	....	....	....	....	**QoL**
3. Dress yourself, including tying shoelaces & doing buttons?	....	....	....	....	
4. Stand up from a chair without arms?	....	....	....	....	
5. Wait in a line for 15 minutes?	....	....	....	....	
6. Reach and get down a 5-pound object (such as a bag of sugar) from just above your head?	....	....	....	....	
7. Walk outdoors on flat ground?	....	....	....	....	
8. Go up 2 or more flights of stairs?	....	....	....	....	
9. Do housework/DIY jobs around the house?	....	....	....	....	
10. Move heavy objects?	....	....	....	....	
					Not Applicable
1. Get a good night's sleep?	....	....	....	....	....
2. Deal with the usual stresses of daily life?	....	....	....	....	....
3. Cope with social/family activities?	....	....	....	....	....
4. Deal with feelings of anxiety or being nervous?	....	....	....	....	....
5. Deal with feelings of low self-esteem or feeling blue?	....	....	....	....	....
6. Get going in the morning?	....	....	....	....	....
7. Do your work as you used to do?	....	....	....	....	....
8. Deal with any worries about your future?	....	....	....	....	....
9. Continue doing things you used to do, despite tiredness?	....	....	....	....	....
10. Continue your relationship with your partner (husband/wife)?	....	....	....	....	....

2. How much PAIN or body ache have you had because of Lupus disease OVER THE PAST WEEK? Please put a circle around the number that best indicates your level of pain: Pain

NO PAIN 0 0.5 1 1.5 2 2.5 3 3.5 4 4.5 5 5.5 6 6.5 7 7.5 8 8.5 9 9.5 10 PAIN As Bad As It Could Be

3. Considering all the ways Lupus may be affecting you AT THIS TIME, Please put a circle around the number that best indicates how well you are doing: PGA

VERY WELL 0 0.5 1 1.5 2 2.5 3 3.5 4 4.5 5 5.5 6 6.5 7 7.5 8 8.5 9 9.5 10 VERY POORLY

4. How much of a problem has UNUSUAL FATIGUE or tiredness been for you OVER THE PAST WEEK? (Please put a circle around the number that best indicates your fatigue) Fatigue

FATIGUE No Problem 0 0.5 1 1.5 2 2.5 3 3.5 4 4.5 5 5.5 6 6.5 7 7.5 8 8.5 9 9.5 10 A MAJOR Problem

5. OVER THE LAST WEEK when you awakened in the morning, did you feel stiff? MS

YES: □ Please indicate the number of minutes ...., or hours .... until you are as limber as you will be for the day.

NO: □

El Miedany et al. EULAR 2014

6. Please place an (X) in the appropriate box to indicate in which of your joints you feel painful TODAY.

Alternatively you can put a figure 1, 2, or 3 to describe the severity of the pain you feel in any joint as follows:

1 = mild pain
2 = moderate pain
3 = severe pain

Tender Joint count	
Pt.	Phys.

Shoulder
Elbow
Wrist
Knuckles/ Fingers
Hip
Knee
Ankle
Top Foot
Toes

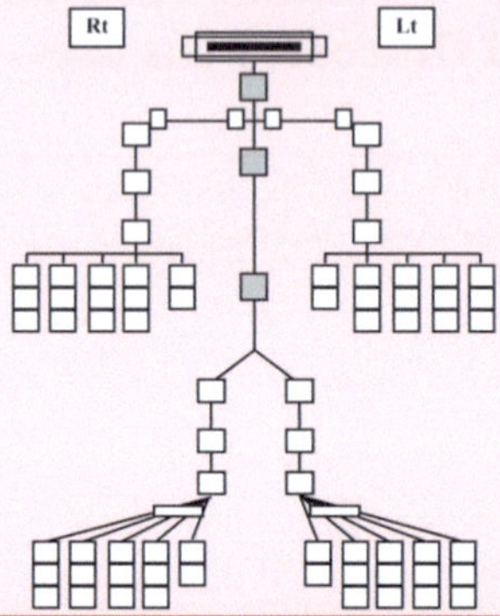

Neck
Shoulder Blade
Low Back

7. Please tick (√) if you have experienced any of the following OVER THE LAST 10 DAYS:

Fits/seizures	Tender finger nodules	Gynecological problem	Cardiovascular Risk Assessment
Hallucinations	Muscle pain	Short plans for having a baby	Age > 50 years old
Illogical thinking	Muscle weakness	Miscarriage	High blood pressure
Bizarre/disorganized behavior	New/recurrent skin rash	Sexual relationship problems	High cholesterol
Difficulty to focus	Patchy of diffuse loss of hair	Problems with passing water	Current smoker
Altered speech	Mouth ulcers	Dark/reddish urine/kidney problem	Ischemic heart disease
Insomnia	Wheezing/asthma	I worry about my appearance	Stroke
Daytime drowsiness	Cough/shortness of breath	Lost height	Irregular heart beats
Visual disturbance	Chest pain	Had a recent fracture	Diabetes mellitus
Double vision/squint	Feeling sickly/Nausea	Falls Risk Assessment	The section below is for official
Change in the look of your face	Dry eye	Loss of your balance	use. Please do not tick
Problems with hearing	Dry mouth	Problems with your sight	ESR: CRP:
Persistent headache	Fever	Weakness of your grip strength	WCC: Plt:
Migraine	Pulmonary embolism/DVT	> 1 fall in the last year	SLEDAI: BMI:
Finger ulcers/gangrene/dark spots	Diagnosed to have cancer	Change in gait/Slow walking speed	B/P: / Chol:

8. The statements below concern your personal beliefs. Please circle the number that best describes how you feel about the statement. 0 = Not at all; 10 = Strongly Agree

mRAI

1. My condition is controlling my life.	0 1 2 3 4 5 6 7 8 9 10
2. I would feel helpless if I could not rely on other people for help with my condition.	0 1 2 3 4 5 6 7 8 9 10
3. I am concerned that medicines cannot help me.	0 1 2 3 4 5 6 7 8 9 10
4. I've concerns regarding side effects of medications used to treat my condition.	0 1 2 3 4 5 6 7 8 9 10
5. I often do not take my medicines as directed.	0 1 2 3 4 5 6 7 8 9 10
6. No matter what I do, or how hard I try, I just cannot seem to get relief from my symptoms.	0 1 2 3 4 5 6 7 8 9 10
7. I am not coping effectively with my condition.	0 1 2 3 4 5 6 7 8 9 10
8. Sometimes I feel my condition is beyond both my and my doctor's control.	0 1 2 3 4 5 6 7 8 9 10
9. Sometimes my condition makes me feel like giving up.	0 1 2 3 4 5 6 7 8 9 10
10. Due to my condition, sometimes I feel I am a burden to those close to me.	0 1 2 3 4 5 6 7 8 9 10

Date: / /201_

□ I consent to my clinical data being used for research/audit.
Signature of the patient: ______________________

Patient:
D.O.B:

References

1. Manson JJ, Rahman A. Systemic lupus erythematosus. Orphanet J Rare Dis. 2006;1:6.
2. Jolly M, Pickard AS, Wilke C, Mikolaitis RA, Teh LS, McElhone K, Fogg L, Block J. Lupus-specific health outcome measure for US patients: the LupusQoL-US version. Ann Rheum Dis. 2010;69:29–33.

3. Holloway L, Humphrey L, Heron L, Pilling C, Kitchen H, Højbjerre L, Strandberg-Larsen M, Bekker Hansen B. Patient-reported outcome measures for systemic lupus erythematosus clinical trials: a review of content validity, face validity and psychometric performance. Health Qual Life Outcomes. 2014;12:116.
4. Beckerman NL. Living with lupus: a qualitative report. Soc Work Health Care. 2011;50:330–43.
5. McElhone K, Abbott J, Gray J, Williams A, Teh LS. Patient perspective of systemic lupus erythematosus in relation to health-related quality of life concepts: a qualitative study. Lupus. 2010;19:1640–7.
6. Robinson J, Aguilar D, Schoenwetter M, Dubois R, Russak S, Ramsey-Goldman R, Navarra S, Hsu B, Revicki D, Cella D, Rapaport MH, Renahan K, Ress R, Wallace D, Weisman M. Impact of systemic lupus erythematosus on health, family, and work: the patient perspective. Arthritis Care Res. 2010;62:266–73.
7. Schneider M, Schmeding A, Carnarius H, Ager M, McWade V. Systemic lupus erythematosus (SLE): understanding the burden. Value Health. 2010;13:A470.
8. Yee CS, McElhone K, Teh LS, Gordon C. Assessment of disease activity and quality of life in systemic lupus erythematosus—new aspects. Best Pract Res Clin Rheumatol. 2009;23:457–67.
9. Aberer E. Epidemiologic, socioeconomic and psychosocial aspects in lupus erythematosus. Lupus. 2010;19:1118–24.
10. Strand V, Galateanu C, Pushparajah DS, Nikai E, Sayers J, Wood R, van Vollenhoven RF. Limitations of current treatments for systemic lupus erythematosus: a patient and physician survey. Lupus. 2013;22:819–26.
11. Pettersson S, Lovgren M, Eriksson LE, Moberg C, Svenungsson E, Gunnarsson I, Henriksson EW. An exploration of patient-reported symptoms in systemic lupus erythematosus and the relationship to health-related quality of life. Scand J Rheumatol. 2012;41:383–90.
12. Gallop K, Nixon A, Swinburn P, Sterling KL, Naegeli AN, Silk ME. Development of a conceptual model of health-related quality of life for systemic lupus erythematosus (SLE) from the patients' perspective. Lupus. 2012;21:934–43.
13. Ad Hoc Committee on Systemic Lupus Erythematosus Response Criteria for Fatigue. Measurement of fatigue in systemic lupus erythematosus: a systematic review. Arthritis Care Res. 2007;57:1348–57.
14. Cleanthous S, Tyagi M, Isenberg DA, Newman SP. What do we know about self-reported fatigue in systemic lupus erythematosus? Lupus. 2012;21:465–76.
15. Ramsey-Goldman R, Rothrock N. Fatigue in systemic lupus erythematosus and rheumatoid arthritis. PM R. 2010;2:384–92.
16. Mattsson M, Moller B, Stamm T, Gard G, Bostrom C. Uncertainty and opportunities in patients with established systemic Lupus Erythematosus: a qualitative study. Musculoskeletal Care. 2012;10:1–12.
17. Kosinski M, Gajria K, Fernandes AW, Cella D. Qualitative validation of the FACIT-fatigue scale in systemic lupus erythematosus. Lupus. 2013;22:422–30.
18. Danoff-Burg S, Friedberg F. Unmet needs of patients with systemic lupus erythematosus. Behav Med. 2009;35:5–13.
19. Yazdany J, Yelin E. Health-related quality of life and employment among persons with systemic Lupus Erythematosus. Rheum Dis Clin North Am. 2010;36:15–32.
20. Doward LC, McKenna SP, Whalley D, Tennant A, Griffiths B, Emery P, Veale DJ. The development of the L-QoL: a quality-of-life instrument specific to systemic lupus erythematosus. Ann Rheum Dis. 2009;68:196–200.
21. Robinson M, Sheets CS, Currie LM. Systemic lupus erythematosus: a genetic review for advanced practice nurses. J Am Acad Nurse Pract. 2011;23:629–37.
22. Johnsson PM, Sandqvist G, Bengtsson A, Nived O. Hand function and performance of daily activities in systemic lupus erythematosus. Arthritis Rheum. 2008;59:1432–8.
23. Carls G, Li T, Panopalis P, Wang S, Mell AG, Gibson TB, Goetzel RZ. Direct and indirect costs to employers of patients with systemic lupus erythematosus with and without nephritis. J Occup Environ Med. 2009;51:66–79.

24. Zhu TY, Tam LS, Li EK. The socioeconomic burden of systemic lupus erythematosus: state-of-the-art and prospects. Expert Rev Pharmacoecon Outcomes Res. 2012;12:53–69.
25. Zhu TY, Tam LS, Li EK. Cost-of-illness studies in systemic lupus erythematosus: a systematic review. Arthritis Care Res (Hoboken). 2011;63:751–60.
26. Yelin E, Katz P. Introduction to special section: cost and social and psychological impact of rheumatic diseases. Arthritis Rheum. 2008;59:457.
27. Zhu TY, Tam LS, Lee VWY, Lee KKC, Li EK. The impact of flare on disease costs of patients with systemic lupus erythematosus. Arthritis Rheum. 2009;61:1159–67.
28. Aghdassi E, Zhang W, St. Pierre Y, Clarke AE, Morrison S, Peeva V, Landolt-Marticorena C, Su J, Reich H, Scholey J, Herzenberg A, Pope JE, Peschken C, Lunnet Canios I, Wither JE, Fortin PR. Healthcare cost and loss of productivity in a Canadian population of patients with and without lupus nephritis. J Rheumatol. 2011;38:658–66.
29. Strand V, Chu AD. Measuring outcomes in systemic lupus erythematosus clinical trials. Expert Rev Pharmacoecon Outcomes Res. 2011;11:455–68.
30. Furie R, Petri MA, Strand V, Gladman DD, Zhong ZJ, Freimuth WW. Clinical, laboratory and health-related quality of life correlates of Systemic Lupus Erythematosus Responder Index response: a post hoc analysis of the phase 3 belimumab trials. Lupus Sci Med. 2014;1, e000031.
31. Lai JS, Beaumont JL, Ogale S, Brunetta P, Cella D. Validation of the functional assessment of chronic illness therapy-fatigue scale in patients with moderately to severely active systemic lupus erythematosus, participating in a clinical trial. J Rheumatol. 2011;38:672–9.
32. Chandran V, Bhella S, Schentag C, Gladman DD. Functional assessment of chronic illness therapy-fatigue scale is valid in patients with psoriatic arthritis. Ann Rheum Dis. 2007;66:936–9.
33. Cella D, Yount S, Sorensen M, Chartash E, Sengupta N, Grober J. Validation of the Functional Assessment of Chronic Illness Therapy Fatigue Scale relative to other instrumentation in patients with rheumatoid arthritis. J Rheumatol. 2005;32:811–9.
34. Ozel F, Argon G. The effects of fatigue and pain on daily life activities in systemic lupus erythematosus. European J Internal Med. 2011;22:S70.
35. Melzack R. The McGill Pain Questionnaire: major properties and scoring methods. Pain. 1975;1(3):277–99.
36. Melzack R. The short-form McGill Pain Questionnaire. Pain. 1987;30(2):191–7.
37. Cleeland CS, Ryan KM. Pain assessment: global use of the Brief Pain Inventory. Ann Acad Med Singapore. 1994;23(2):129–38.
38. Cleeland CS. The brief pain inventory: user guide. 2009. 63 p. http://www.mdanderson.org/education-and-research/departments-programs-andlabs/departments-and-divisions/symptom-research/symptom-assessmenttools/BPI_UserGuide.pdf.
39. Cleeland CS, Gonin R, Hatfield AK, Edmonson JH, Blum RH, Stewart JA, Pandya KJ. Pain and its treatment in outpatients with metastatic cancer. N Engl J Med. 1994;330(9):592–6.
40. Food and Drug Administration. Guidance for industry: patient-reported outcome measures: use in medical product development to support labelling claims. Silver Spring, MD: Food and Drug Administration; 2009.
41. Atkinson TM, Rosenfeld BD, Sit L, Mendoza TR, Fruscione M, Lavene D, Shaw M, Li Y, Hay J, Cleeland CS, Scher HI, Breitbart WS, Basch E. Using confirmatory factor analysis to evaluate construct validity of the Brief Pain Inventory (BPI). J Pain Symptom Manage. 2011;41(3):558–65.
42. Daut RL, Cleeland CS, Flannery RC. Development of the Wisconsin Brief Pain Questionnaire to assess pain in cancer and other diseases. Pain. 1983;17(2):197–210.
43. Naegeli AN, Tomaszewski EL, Al Sawah S. Psychometric validation of the Brief Pain Inventory-Short Form in patients with systemic lupus erythematosus in the United States. Lupus. 2015;24:1377–83.
44. Zigmond AS, Snaith RP. The hospital anxiety and depression scale. Acta Psychiatr Scand. 1983;67:361–70.
45. Snaith RP. The hospital anxiety and depression scale. Health Qual Life Outcomes. 2002;1:29.

46. Herrmann C. International experiences with the Hospital Anxiety and Depression Scale-A review of validation data and clinical results. J Psychosom Res. 1997;42:17–41.
47. Garris CP, Oglesby AK. Assessment of health care resource utilization by level of flare severity in patients with systemic lupus erythematosus (SLE) in the managed care setting. J Manag Care Pharm. 2011;17:552.
48. QualityMetric Inc. User's manual for the SF-36v2 health survey. 3rd ed. **2011**. http://www.qualitymetric.com/WhatWeDo/ManualsUserGuides/UsersManualfortheSF36v2HealthSurvey/tabid/328/Default.aspx.
49. Brazier JE, Harper R, Jones NM, O'Cathain A, Thomas KJ, Usherwood T, Westlake L. Validating the SF-36 health survey questionnaire: new outcome measure for primary care. BMJ. 1992;305(6846):160–4.
50. Beaumont JLLJ, Cella D, Brunetta P, Ogale S. Validation of the SF-36 in patients with systemic lupus erythematosus (SLE). Arthritis Rheum. 2009;60:296.
51. Busija L, Pausenberger E, Haines TP, Haymes S, Buchbinder R, Osborne RH. Adult measures of general health and health-related quality of life: Medical Outcomes Study Short Form 36-Item (SF-36) and Short Form 12-Item (SF-12) Health Surveys, Nottingham Health Profile (NHP), Sickness Impact Profile (SIP), Medical Outcomes Study Short Form 6D (SF-6D), Health Utilities Index Mark 3 (HUI3), Quality of Well-Being Scale (QWB), and Assessment of Quality of Life (AQOL) [abstract]. Arthritis Care Res. 2011;63:S383–412.
52. McElhone K, Abbott J, Shelmerdine J, Bruce IN, Ahmad Y, Gordon C, Peers K, Isenberg D, Ferenkeh-Koroma A, Griffiths B, Akil M, Maddison P, Teh L-S. Development and validation of a disease-specific health-related quality of life measure, the LupusQoL, for adults with systemic lupus erythematosus. Arthritis Care Res. 2007;57:972–9.
53. Ware Jr JE, Sherbourne CD. The MOS 36-item short-form health survey (SF-36). I. Conceptual framework and item selection. Med Care. 1992;30(6):473–83.
54. Food and Drug Administration. Guidance for industry: systemic lupus erythematosus—developing medical products for treatment. 2010. http://www.fda.gov/downloads/Drugs/GuidanceComplianceRegulatoryInformation/Guidances/ucm072063.pdf.
55. European Medicines Agency. Guideline on clinical investigation of medicinal products for the treatment of systemic lupus erythematosus, cutaneous lupus and lupus nephritis (draft). 2013. http://www.ema.europa.eu/docs/en_GB/document_library/Scientific_guideline/2013/03/WC500139615.pdf.
56. El Miedany Y, El Gaafary M, El Yassaki A, Ahmed I, Youssef S, Hegazi MO, Palmer D. Incorporating patient reported outcome measures in clinical practice: development and validation of a PROMs questionnaire for SLE. Ann Rheum Dis. 2013;72 Suppl 3:484.
57. Jolly M, Garris CP, Mikolaitis RA, Jhingran PM, Dennis G, Wallace DJ, Clarke A, Dooley MA, Parke A, Strand V, Alárcon GS, Kosinski M. Development and validation of the Lupus Impact Tracker: a patient-completed tool for clinical practice to assess and monitor the impact of systemic lupus erythematosus. Arthritis Care Res (Hoboken). 2014;66(10):1542–50.
58. Ruperto N, Hanrahan LM, Alarcon GS, Belmont HM, Brey RL, Brunetta P, Buyon JP, Costner MI, Cronin ME, Dooley MA, Filocamo G, Fiorentino D, Fortin PR, Franks Jr AG, Gilkeson G, Ginzler E, Gordon C, Grossman J, Hahn B, Isenberg DA, Kalunian KC, Petri M, Sammaritano L, Sánchez-Guerrero J, Sontheimer RD, Strand V, Urowitz M, von Feldt JM, Werth VP, Merrill JT. International consensus for a definition of disease flare in lupus. Lupus. 2011;20:453–62.

Chapter 7
PROMs for Fibromyalgia

Loreto Carmona, Rafael J. Curbelo, and Concepción González Isabel

Introduction

Etymologically, the term "fibromyalgia" means pain in the muscle fibers, and was first used by Hench in 1976 [1]. In 1904, Gowers had named it "fibrositis" [2]; however, as peripheral inflammation has never been proven since, the suffix *–itis* was not established. The "Fibromyalgia syndrome" (FMS) was accepted by the World Health Organization (WHO) in 1992, with the code M79.7 of the International Classification of Diseases (ICD-10), as a nonarticular rheumatism [3]. Clinically, it is defined as "pain in the muscles, ligaments, and tendons," i.e., fibrous parts of the body.

According to the 1990 classification criteria of the American College of Rheumatology (ACR), FMS is characterized by the existence of widespread musculoskeletal pain, of unknown etiology, lasting for at least 3 months, with pain in no less than 11 out of 18 pressure points—also known as tender or trigger points [4]. However, in addition to increased sensitivity to pain, FMS may also cause stiffness, fatigue, cognitive impairment, paresthesia, bloating, hand swelling, and low-quality sleep, among other somatic symptoms, and in some patients other conditions exist concomitantly, such as irritable bowel syndrome, tension headaches with subsequent dominance, Raynaud's phenomenon, or temporomandibular joint pathology. That is the reason why in 2010 a new classification was proposed, including pain plus other symptoms [5]. These new criteria classify a patient with FMS if either high level of pain plus

L. Carmona, M.D., Ph.D. (✉) • R.J. Curbelo, M.Sc., Ph.D.
Instituto de Salud Musculoesquelética, Calle Conde de la Cimera, 6, Madrid 28040, Spain
e-mail: loreto.carmona@inmusc.eu; rafacurbelo@gmail.com

C.G. Isabel, Ph.D.
Instituto de Salud Osteoarticular, Conde de la Cimera 6, Madrid 28040, Spain
e-mail: cripb55@gmal.com

Y. El Miedany (ed.), *Patient Reported Outcome Measures in Rheumatic Diseases*,
DOI 10.1007/978-3-319-32851-5_7

moderate levels of other symptoms or moderate pain and high levels of other symptoms are present. Symptoms must be steadily present for at least 3 months and no disorder should explain the pain, hence, FMS remained an exclusion diagnosis. In 2011, the diagnostic criteria were revised to include 19 specific pain locations, and 6 self-administered symptoms questionnaires including sleep difficulty, fatigue, headache, depression, abdominal pain, and poor cognitive status [6].

The prevalence of FMS is remarkably high; it affects 2–5 % of the general population, mainly women—the men to women ratio being 1–9—and mostly people in their 40s, although cases among teenagers are increasing [7–11]. However, on using the 2010 classification, with a higher weight of somatic symptoms, the prevalence of FMS was reported to be even higher, particularly in men [10]. Not surprisingly, FMS is a costly condition, with an estimated cost of 10,000 Euros per patient per year [12, 13].

Some authors believe that FMS is a primary psychogenic disorder, as depression is commonly found in patients with FMS [14]. In their study, Hauser et al. [15] noted that psychological trauma caused by sexual abuse in childhood, as well as complex personalities, may both be risk factors for the development of FMS; furthermore, depression and posttraumatic stress disorder (PTSD) were depicted to have a negative impact on the outcome of FMS. In addition to psychosocial causes, genetic studies reported an association between FMS and some single nucleotide polymorphisms of genes encoding proteins involved in the neural synapse [16]. Other research work assessing genome-wide analysis and epigenetic modifications in FMS are currently under study [17].

In view of such a wide range of FMS symptoms, a multidisciplinary treatment approach has been recommended, including pharmacology, psychology, sport and physical medicine, nutrition, and alternative therapies such as acupuncture and balneotherapy.

Challenges in the Assessment of Fibromyalgia

Fibromyalgia is one of the most common forms of chronic pain disorders. Pain in FMS patients has been attributed to aberrant nociception due to altered central or peripheral control and a positive feedback mechanism that amplifies the sensation of pain [16]. Patients with FMS show signs of hyperalgesia and allodynia; often, simple things such as shopping or house chores cause an intense pain. Alterations in brain levels of substances such as growth hormone—which is secreted during the deeper stages of rapid eye movement (REM) sleep—are below normal limits. Serotonin, melatonin, substance P, and nerve growth factor may all be involved in sleep quality and clinical symptoms observed in FMS [18]. Plasma cytokines also may be associated with increased sensitivity to pain, fatigue, depression, and poor quality sleep [19]. However, all these "objective measures" are not specific to FMS and show high interindividual variability.

High Subjectivity

Given the fact that the symptoms of FMS are numerous and very subjective, and that there are no objective measures of disease evolution, such as biomarkers, the follow-up of FMS patients is complex. The following are the most typical symptoms present in FMS and a brief description of how they appear in the clinic.

Pain, as already noted, is a major symptom in FMS. It is typically widespread—whole body aches—and causes significant reduction in quality of life. It is often described as chronic and both "electrical" and "tingling," as it is often accompanied by paresthesia [20]. Notwithstanding, pain varies widely in intensity and quality from one patient to another.

Fatigue is another landmark in FMS. It can be physical (i.e., lack of energy, physical exhaustion), emotional (i.e., lack of motivation), or cognitive (inability to think or concentrate). Fatigue impacts on virtually any aspect of living, such as the ability to work, meet family needs, or engage in social activities [21]. Patients describe fatigue as "an inescapable or overwhelming feeling of deep physical tiredness," "weakness in the muscles," "an uncontrollable, unpredictable constant state of never being rested," "a ghastly sensation of being totally drained of every fiber of energy," "not proportional to effort exerted," "not relieved by rest," and as "an invisible foe that creeps upon (them) unannounced and without warning" [22].

Sleep. The FMS impact on sleep was defined in OMERACT (Outcome Measures in Rheumatology Clinical Trials) as difficulty falling asleep and staying asleep, and getting unrefreshing sleep [23]. More than 70 % of patients with FMS complain of poor sleep quality and associate this with feeling tired and difficulty in performing physical activity [24].

Cognitive impairment. Cognitive difficulties—specifically, longer reaction times, short-term memory deficits, and attention problems—are 2.5 times more prevalent in patients with FMS than with any other rheumatic condition. It has been estimated that 76.4–82.5 % of persons with FMS in a rheumatology practice may complain of cognitive difficulties [25, 26]. More than half of the persons with FMS report "mental confusion," now termed as "fibrofog," which in some cases may be more worrisome than pain [27]. Patients describe this state as "looking at life as through a haze" [27]. Patients with FMS have limited working and long-term memory, and this limitation is independent of, or on top of, anxiety or depression [28, 29]. Consequences of this limitation are a decline in attention and in executive function [25].

Gender Issues

FMS is believed to be a disease of women; however, the new classification has brought up a high prevalence in men as well [30]. Several studies have analyzed the differences of the syndrome between men and women. Apparently, men have lower health perception and more physical limitations, while women have greater life interference due to pain [31, 32]. In addition, women's pain threshold is significantly lower, and they suffer more diffuse pain, increased fatigue, and irritable bowel syndrome than men [22, 32, 33]. In addition, women with FMS feel fatigue more sharply than men with FMS [22, 33]. Prados et al. found that in FMS men, lower quality of sleep, with negative effects of somnolence, fatigue, decreased vigilance, etc. were the main predictors of pain [34]. Subsequent studies by this group showed that women tend to catastrophize and to consume more painkillers than men [35]. On the other hand, Racine et al. observed no gender differences in the extent (i.e., number of painful areas) and operation of pain (i.e., depressive symptoms, pain severity, and interference); however, they found differences in pain-related beliefs, as men were more likely to view pain as reflecting harm, and they were also more likely than women to use activity avoidance as a pain-coping strategy [36]. It was also reported that psychosocial distress impacts differently on men and women and thus produces different FMS pictures [11, 37].

Cultural Issues

In addition to the gender factor—in particular pain behavior that is usually more acceptable in women than in men—some of the symptoms in FMS, or their effect on daily life, may have a different expression in different cultures.

Illness perception, for instance, varies between Spanish and Dutch women with FMS, with the Spanish perceiving more symptoms and showing greater emotional representation than the Dutch; these latter presenting more positive beliefs about the controllability of the illness [38]. Fatigue has different impact and daily-living consequences in different countries and clearly affects work differently—depending mainly on availability of work adaptations or flexibility among countries—as well as care-seeking behavior [39–41].

Pain is perhaps the symptom with more clear cultural implications. Some cultures, for example, do not accept pain as desirable or acceptable [42, 43], and this may have an influence on reporting levels of pain; pain-coping strategies; activities of daily living that can be accomplished; or behaviors, such as victimizing or support seeking [43–46]. Very interestingly, linguistic reports and classifications of pain differ between cultures, with dozens of specific pain terms in some languages and a single inclusive term in others [47]. This must be taken into account when developing PROMs that include description of "pains."

Evidence on commonalities among cultures also exists. A comparative study between German and US patients with FMS showed that the reporting of childhood abuse was overlapping in the two countries, thus highlighting the importance of psychological distress in FMS [15].

Highly Correlated Symptoms

As previously noted, many of the symptoms experienced by FMS patients are intercorrelated. Restless sleep, for instance, is linked to daytime fatigue and musculoskeletal pain, and thus sleep, fatigue, and pain scores all will be affected [48]. Depression and anxiety are independently associated with the severity of pain symptoms in FMS [49]. In turn, depression is often associated with severe fatigue and poor quality sleep, whereas anxiety is more commonly linked to palpitations, dizziness, sweating, and paresthesia [24]. In addition, decreased cognitive function seems to be related to pain severity in various chronic pain populations [26].

Concomitant Diseases

Very importantly, FM may occur concomitantly with other articular diseases, such as lupus erythematosus, rheumatoid arthritis, and other systemic and chronic pain syndromes. The effect of FMS in all of them has been widely studied [50–57]. The opposite, however, that is the impact of other diseases on FMS has been less studied, but it can be anticipated that the measures of pain, daily functioning, and even fatigue will be clearly affected. Not only rheumatic diseases can appear concomitantly, but also other diseases, such as multiple sclerosis, that present with fatigue or other symptoms similar to those present in FMS may interfere with the disease outcome measures reported by the patient, e.g., through PROMs [58, 59]. The existence of concomitant diseases with similar symptoms may pose a double-sided management decision: to escalate the treatment of the non-FMS condition (i.e., biological therapy in inflammatory diseases) or to increase analgesia to treat FMS. A better approach would be to use cognitive-behavioral therapy to approach both conditions.

On the other hand, FMS is closely associated with other comorbid conditions. Reported co-prevalence for some of these diseases varies from 25 to 67 % for osteoarthritis, 10 to 42 % for hypertension, 12 to 40 % for osteoporosis, and 4 to 23 % for diabetes [60–62]. Not surprisingly, FMS is associated with other psychological disorders. Earlier reports revealed that FMS patients are at a higher risk of dying from suicide and accidents [63, 64]. In view of the fact that FMS patients are rarely admitted to hospital because of FM as the primary diagnosis, and that most, if not all, of these associated disease processes are treatable and often can be managed effectively on an outpatient basis, it is therefore important to take such symptoms seriously and explore FMS patients for the risk of having other associated ailments with views toward implementing effective prevention/management strategies.

Complex Constructs

Finally, FMS poses a challenge for measurement as it holds very complex constructs among its symptoms. Above all, cognitive impairment, recently added to the ACR diagnostic criteria [65], remains as the least assessed and treated FMS domain. This is the case both in general clinical practice and in research. This has been attributed, mainly, to the expertise and time required for neuropsychological tests for the different aspects of this domain, which includes attention, memory, processing speed, recognition, etc.

Available PROMs in FMS

PROMs are critical in FMS due to the challenges previously noted. Without the existence of these questionnaires it would be complicated to monitor evolution, progression, and treatment of FMS.

OMERACT established in 2004 the key domains for the measurement of FMS: pain, patient global assessment, fatigue, health-related quality of life, function (multidimensional), sleep, depression, and treatment side effects. Other important domains, not considered as essential, included physical function, tender point intensity, dyscognition, anxiety, and clinician global assessment [20]. In 2012 (OMERACT 9), the core-set finally included pain, fatigue, tenderness, overall patient, multidimensional function, and sleep disturbance [21, 23, 66] (see Fig. 7.1).

A wide variety of instruments have been used in FMS. Many of them were developed for generic use or have been borrowed from other clinical populations. The number of available PROMs specifically developed for FMS is surprisingly low for a syndrome that is so subjective. The existing instruments will be commented upon in detail and all are available at the EULAR Outcomes Measure Library [67]. They cover a wide range of domains and constructs as they are summarized in Table 7.1.

Fibromyalgia Impact Questionnaire

The Fibromyalgia Impact Questionnaire (FIQ) is a self-administered questionnaire with ten items that measure multiple domains of the FMS, such as the ability to perform large muscle tasks, work difficulty, pain, fatigue, morning tiredness, stiffness, anxiety, and depression [68, 69] (Appendix 1). It yields a score from 0 to 100, with higher scores indicating greater impact. It is widely used, probably due to its easiness of use and because it is free of charge. The FIQ has been validated in more than 46 languages, as it was the first PRO designed especially for FMS. As a limitation, it can underestimate the severity of the patient, as items that are not marked are deleted from the calculation; in addition, the FIQ has a gender bias, as it was

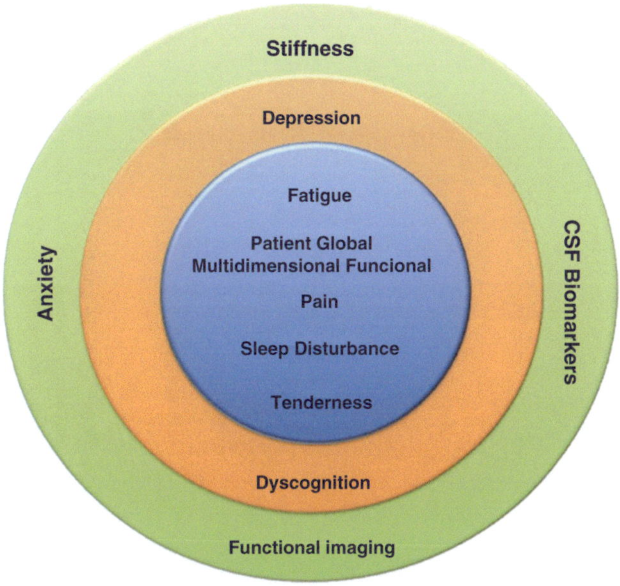

Fig. 7.1 Core-set measures established in OMERACT 9 for its use in clinical trials of FMS. Modified from Mease P, Arnold LM, Choy EH, Clauw DJ, Crofford LJ, Glass JM, et al. Fibromyalgia syndrome module at OMERACT 9: domain construct. J Rheumatol, 2009; 36(10):2318–29. [23]

developed originally for women. It has been used as the gold standard for several PRO validation studies, which has to be viewed with concern [68].

Revised Version of the Fibromyalgia Impact Questionnaire (FIQR)

The FIQR attempts to address the FIQ's original limitations, such as the complicated scoring and the gender bias, as well as tenderness. It is divided into three linked sets of domains: *Function,* which contains nine questions; *Overall impact*, with two questions related to the overall impact of FMS on functioning and overall symptom severity; and *Symptoms*, which contains ten questions, four of which are new and relate to memory, tenderness, balance, and environmental sensitivity (i.e., loud noises, bright lights, odors, and cold temperatures) [70]. Scoring has been simplified, and an online tool facilitates self-administration (http://fiqrinfo.ipage.com/). The FIQR takes approximately half as long to complete as the FIQ. Problems with translations into languages different from English and Spanish have been pointed out in the literature [71].

Table 7.1 Summary of domains evaluated in the PROMs specific for FMS

	FIQ	FIQ-R	FFS	FBI	ICAF	VASFIQ	FSQ	FHAQ	PROMs-FM
Pain	X	X	X		X	X	X		X
ADL	X	X	X		X	X	X	X	X
Global assessment	X	X	X		X				X
Fatigue	X	X	X		X	X	X		X
Anxiety or depression	X	X	X		X	X			X
Social function	X	X							X
Stiffness	X					X	X		X
Sleep			X		X	X	X		X
HRQoL					X				X
Cognitive aspects			X						
Coping					X				X
Other			Headache, autonomic disturbances, …	Urinary symptoms		Rigidity	Headache		Helplessness, symptoms

Abbreviations: *ADL* activities of daily living, *FIQ* fibromyalgia impact questionnaire, *FIQ-R* revised version of the FIQ, *ICAF* combined index of fibromyalgia, *FFS* fibrofatigue scale, *FBI* Fibromyalgia Bladder Index, *VASFIQ* FIQ in a visual analogue scale, *FHAQ* Fibromyalgia Health Assessment Questionnaire, *FSQ* Function and Symptom Questionnaire, *PROMs-FM* Multi-Dimensional Patient Reported Outcome Measures Questionnaire for Fibromyalgia, *HRQL* health related quality of life

Fibrofatigue Scale

A self-administered questionnaire, the Fibrofatigue Scale (FFS), was designed to measure the severity of symptoms in FMS as well as in chronic fatigue syndrome patients [72]. Consisting of 12 items, the scale evaluates pain, muscular tension, fatigue, concentration difficulties, failing memory, irritability, sadness, sleep disturbances, autonomic disturbances, irritable bowel, headache, and subjective experience of infection. Scale developers were specifically interested in creating a tool that could be used to monitor treatment outcomes. However, the scale requires a trained administrator, making it potentially unsuitable for large-scale studies or clinical practice [72].

Fibromyalgia Bladder Index

The Fibromyalgia Bladder Index (FBI) is a PRO specific for urinary symptoms in FMS with two subscales: bladder urgency/pain and frequency/nocturia. It has eight items, and the score ranges between 0 and 17. The main drawback is that it exists only in its English version [73].

Combined Index of Severity of Fibromyalgia

The Combined Index of Severity of Fibromyalgia (ICAF) is a self-administered questionnaire that evaluates FMS main symptoms through five domains: emotional (anxiety and depression), physical (pain, fatigue, sleep quality, and functional ability), active coping (positive coping strategies), passive coping, and global [74] (Appendix 2). It has 59 items and the score ranges from 0 to 89; its psychometric properties are very good; however, due to its length and complex scoring system, and to the fact that is only available in Spanish, the ICAF seldom has been used.

Visual Analogue Scale FIQ

The Visual Analogue Scale FIQ (VASFIQ) is a 7-item scale modified VAS of the FIQR that quantifies the severity of FMS. It enables rapid patient assessment and informed treatment decisions in busy clinics [75]. It is widely used in clinical practice and research, and has no floor or ceiling effect. However, its psychometric properties are far from excellent and it needs initial training. The VASFIQ should not be used isolatedly to make treatment decisions.

Fibromyalgia Health Assessment Questionnaire

The Fibromyalgia Health Assessment Questionnaire (FHAQ) is a subset of the original Health Assessment Questionnaire (HAQ) [76] that has been specially designed for FMS, adapting the original tool to measure more adequately the functional ability in FMS. It yields a score from 0 to 3 that reflects the patient's state of functional ability; the lower the score, the better the functional state.

Function and Symptom Questionnaire

The Function and Symptom Questionnaire (FSQ) is a 9-item questionnaire that covers current disability in daily activities, somatic symptoms, and sleep quality [77]. It is only available in English, and it is simple to use and very useful in clinical practice and research.

Multi-dimensional Questionnaire for Patient Reported Outcome Measures: Fibromyalgia (PROMs-FM)

A recent questionnaire, the Multi-dimensional Questionnaire, for PROMs-FM was developed specifically for fibromyalgia patients (Appendix 3). It has integrated the modified 2010 ACR criteria for FMS as well as the patient reported outcome measures in a multidimensional format. In addition to patient reported assessment of symptoms severity score and widespread pain index, it includes assessment for functional disability, quality of life, VAS (0–100) for sleep disturbance, waking feeling unrefreshed, global status, fatigue, body pain, and impact of mood changes, as well as assessment for FMS associated comorbidities such as falls, cardiovascular risks, sexual dysfunction, self-helplessness together with self-reported soft tissue painful areas [78]. Being short, rapid, and comprehensive, the questionnaire can be used for the diagnosis, monitoring of the disease progression, as well as response to therapy. It is only available in English in its original version.

Additional Considerations and Psychometric Properties of the Included PROMs

For the collection of PROMs in FMS, we performed a systematic review. Although we identified other questionnaires used for FMS patients, we decided to include PROMs that were specific for FMS only. Two indices that are widely used but that were not included in our review are worth mentioning: (1) the combined index of severity (the CODI index), which we excluded as it does not really fit the concept of

Table 7.2 Summary of the main psychometric properties of the available FMS questionnaires

	Aspect of validity tested	Internal consistency	Test–retest	Responsiveness
FIQ	Construct	+++	+++	+
FIQ-R	Construct	+++	++	NT
FFS	Face	+++	++	+
FBI	Face	++	++	NT
ICAF	Construct	+++	++	+++
VASFIQ	Construct	NT	NT	NT
FSQ	Face	NT	NT	+
FHAQ	NT	NT	NT	NT
PROMs-FM	Construct	+++	+++	++

Abbreviations: *FIQ* Fibromyalgia impact questionnaire, *FIQ-R* Revised version of the FIQ, *ICAF* Combined Index of Fibromyalgia, *FFS* Fibrofatigue Scale, *FBI* Fibromyalgia Bladder Index, *VASFIQ* FIQ in a visual analogue scale, *FSQ* Function and Symptom Questionnaire, *FHAQ* Fibromyalgia Health Assessment Questionnaire, *PROMs-FM* Multi-Dimensional Patient Reported Outcome Measures Questionnaire for Fibromyalgia, *NT* not tested, +++ high, ++ moderate, + poor

PROMs because it needs a physician's global assessment [79] and (2) the Central Sensitization Inventory (CSI) [80], because it is an index that combines various assessment tools, but it is not a PROMs in essence.

None of the aforementioned questionnaires developed for FMS had a full and proper validation process. This is partly due to the fact that many of the outcome measures currently used in FMS were developed and validated for use in other medical conditions, and were subsequently adopted for research and clinical practice. This aspect is not incorrect as it has facilitated basic exploration into the nature and impact of FMS. It also represents a methodological advance over previous non-standardized research. In addition, the validation of an instrument is a continuing process. Testing validity is not established based on just a single approach, but after a series of converging studies [81].

A summary of the psychometric properties of the PROMs will be discussed in the next section. Table 7.2 presents a summary of the psychometric properties of the main PROMs questionnaires developed for FMS patients.

Reliability

In general, internal consistency of the PROMs tools in FMS is good, with most of them showing Cronbach's α(alpha) > 0.8. The revised version of the FIQ shows the highest internal consistency with α(alpha) = 0.95, followed by the PROMs-FM (α[alpha] = 0.93) and FFS (α[alpha] = 0.92), although such high internal consistency may actually reflect overlapping of items or domains. The ICAF shows values from α(alpha) = 0.77–0.85, and an overall α(alpha) = 0.85, and the original FIQ an α(alpha) = 0.82 for all items. The FBI also has good consistency (Bladder Urgency and Pain α[alpha] = 0.76, Frequency and Nocturia α[alpha] = 0.76, and ICSI/ICPS α[alpha] = 0.81). Internal consistency was not available for VASFIQ, FSQ, or FHAQ.

Test–retest reliability was adequate in general, although evidence was not available for FHAQ or FSQ. Values for the intraclass correlation coefficient (ICC) for the FBI range from 0.73 to 0.84 whereas for PROMs-FM its range was 0.89–0.96. Reliability is expected to be measured by using ICC for continuous scales, ICC or weighted kappa for ordinal scales, and unweighted kappa for nominal scales. However, reliability was tested by means of correlation in the FIQ (Spearman correlation coefficient 0.85 [82]), the FIQ-R (Pearson's $r=0.83$ in its Turkish version [71]), and the ICAF.

Validity

The validity of the original version of the FIQ was not tested—or we were unable to find any published study—whereas the revised version showed strong correlation with the FIQ ($r=0.88$ $p<0.001$) and SF-36's physical function and pain subscales ($r=-0.80$ and $r=-0.60$, respectively; note that correlations are negative due to the fact that higher SF-36 scores relate to being healthier [70]). Total ICAF score shows a moderate correlation with the FIQ ($r=0.69$) and HAQ ($r=0.59$). While testing the construct validity of the FFS, Spearman correlation coefficient was computed between the FFS and the different symptoms of FMS, as measured by VAS scales. The correlations of the FFS items with pain score and the physical function subscale of the SF-36 ranged from 0.28 to 0.32 [83]. There was a positive correlation between the total FBI with the total King's Health Questionnaire—a questionnaire that measures bladder and bowel problems. Individual correlations between the FBI and the individual King's Health Questionnaire's domains ranged from 0.35 to 0.62 [73].

With regard to the global VASFIQ, its score correlates highly with FIQ scores at baseline ($r=0.94$). Change in global VASFIQ and FIQ scores correlates similarly to a Patients' Global Impression of Change scale ($r=0.58$). Individual VASFIQ scores correlate with corresponding full-length symptom questionnaire scores at baseline (VAS fatigue with MAF-GFI, $r=0.64$; VAS sleep with SPI, $r=0.50$; VAS depression with HADS-D, $r=0.43$; VAS anxiety with HADS-A, $r=0.47$). Content construct of the PROMs-FM scales for functional disability and quality of life revealed correlation with both SF-36 ($r=-0.86$) and EuroQoL-5D ($r=0.88$) scores [78]. The correlation between the FSQ and the clinical severity index was $r=0.53$, moderate.

Responsiveness

Regarding responsiveness, it was only tested in the FIQ, the FFS, and the ICAF. The approach to measure responsiveness in FIQ was rather weak in a clinical trial of acupuncture [84]. It showed an area under the curve of 0.77 to discriminate change, with no clear intervention or anticipated change. The FFS moved significantly (by Student's t test) in patients who improved the Clinical Global Impressions scale in a 24-week trial [85]. The FSS showed an area under the curve of 0.65 compared to the Clinical Severity Index [84]. The ICAF has also proven sensitivity to change

[74]. Changes in functional disability, quality of life, as well as self-helplessness scores in the PROMS-FM showed significant variation with disease activity status and response to therapy [78]; however, the study proving responsiveness is not fully available to assess potential biases.

Conclusion

FMS is a complex and highly subjective syndrome that poses many challenges to its measurement. The majority of PROMs available are not entirely adequate to measure the disease in full, but this is a problem common to most PROMs in rheumatology.

Appendix 1

The FIQ Directions and Questions

Directions: For questions 1–3, please circle the number that best describes how you did overall for the past week. If you don't normally do something that is asked, cross the question out.

Question 1.

Were you able to:	Always	Most	Occasionally	Never
1. Do shopping?	0	1	2	3
2. Do laundry with washer and dryer?	0	1	2	3
3. Prepare meals?	0	1	2	3
4. Wash dishes/cooking utensils by hand?	0	1	2	3
5. Vacuum a rug?	0	1	2	3
6. Make beds?	0	1	2	3
7. Walk several blocks?	0	1	2	3
8. Visit friends or relatives?	0	1	2	3
9. Do yard work?	0	1	2	3
10. Drive a car?	0	1	2	3
11. Climb stairs?	0	1	2	3

Question 2. *Of the 7 days in the past week, how many days did you feel good?*

0	1	2	3	4	5	6	7

Question 3. *How many days last week did you miss work, including housework, because of fibromyalgia?*

0	1	2	3	4	5	6	7

Directions: For the remaining items, mark the point on the line that best indicates how you felt overall of the past week.

Question 4. *When you worked, how much did pain or other symptoms of your fibromyalgia interfere with your ability to do your work, including housework?*

•— | — | — | — | — | — | — | — | — | — •

No problem with work	Great difficulty with work

Question 5. *How bad has your pain been?*

•— | — | — | — | — | — | — | — | — | — •

No pain	Very severe pain

Question 6. *How tired have you been?*

•— | — | — | — | — | — | — | — | — | — •

No tiredness	Very tired

Question 7. *How have you felt when you get up in the morning?*

•— | — | — | — | — | — | — | — | — | — •

Awoke well rested	Awoke very tired

Question 8. *How bad has your stiffness been?*

•— | — | — | — | — | — | — | — | — | — •

No stiffness	Very stiff

Question 9. *How nervous or anxious have you felt?*

•— | — | — | — | — | — | — | — | — | — •

Not anxious	Very anxious

Question 10. *How depressed or blue have you felt?*

•— | — | — | — | — | — | — | — | — | — •

Not depressed	Very depressed

Reprinted with permission of the developers Carol Burckhardt, Sharon Clark, and Robert Bennett at Oregon Health and Science University in Portland, Oregon

Appendix 2

http://www.msssi.gob.es/profesionales/prestacionesSanitarias/publicaciones/docs/fibromialgia.pdf

ICAF

INSTRUCTIONS

We would like to know how the symptoms of your disease were DURING THE LAST WEEK. Please circle only one response for each question.

PAIN SEVERITY

1. Please rate your pain by circling the one number that best describes your pain at its LEAST in the LAST WEEK.

0 1 2 3 4 5 6 7 8 9 10

No pain — Pain as bad as you can imagine

2. Please rate your pain by circling the one number that best describes your pain on the AVERAGE.

0 1 2 3 4 5 6 7 8 9 10

No pain — Pain as bad as you can imagine

SCORE 1
(Items 1+2)
Range 0-20

SLEEP QUALITY

3. Please circle the number that best describes HOW YOU SLEPT LAST WEEK.

0 1 2 3 4 5 6 7 8 9 10

Very well Very bad

SCORE 2
(Item 3)
Range 0-10

IMPACT

Please circle the number that best describes how you FELT OVERALL for the PAST WEEK

4. When you worked, how much did pain or other symptoms of your fibromyalgia INTERFERE with your ability to do YOUR WORK, INCLUDING HOUSEWORK?

0 1 2 3 4 5 6 7 8 9 10

No problem with work Great difficulty With work

5. How TIRED have you been?

0 1 2 3 4 5 6 7 8 9 10

No tiredness Very tired

6. How have you felt when you GOT UP IN THE MORNING?

0	1	2	3	4	5	6	7	8	9	10

Awoke well rested — Awoke very tired

SCORE 3
(Items 4+5+6)
Range 0-30

FATIGUE

Please circle the number that best describes how you usually FELT for PAST WEEK.

	Never	Sometimes	Regularly	Often	Always
7. I am bothered by fatigue	0	1	2	3	4
8. I get tired very quickly	0	1	2	3	4
9. I don't do much during the day	0	1	2	3	4
10. Physically, I feel exhausted	0	1	2	3	4
11. I have problems starting things	0	1	2	3	4

SCORE 4
(Items 7-11)
Range 0-20

PHYSICAL FUNCTION

Please check the one response that best describes YOUR USUAL ABILITIES over the PAST WEEK

Are you able to…	Without ANY difficulty	With SOME difficulty	With MUCH difficulty	UNABLE to do
12. Dress yourself, including tying shoelaces and doing buttons	0	1	2	3
13. Wash and dry your entire body?	0	1	2	3
14. Reach and get down a 5-pound object (such as a bag of sugar) from just above your head?	0	1	2	3
15. Get in and out of a car?	0	1	2	3
16. Do chores such as vacuuming or yardwork?	0	1	2	3

SCORE 5
(Items 12-16)
Range 0-15 ☐

ANXIETY AND DEPRESSION

Read each item and mark the reply that comes closest to how you have been FEELING in the PAST WEEK.

17. I feel tense or "wound up":

(3)☐ Most of the time

(2)☐ A lot of the time

(1)☐ From time to time, occasionally

(0)☐ Not at all

18. I still enjoy the things I used to enjoy:

(0)☐ Definitely as much

(1)☐ Not quite so much

(2) ☐ Only a little

(3) ☐ Hardly at all

19. I can laugh and see the funny side of things:

(0) ☐ As much as I always could

(1) ☐ Not quite so much now

(2) ☐ Definitely not so much now

(3) ☐ Not at all

20. Worrying thoughts go through my mind:

(3) ☐ A great deal of the time

(2) ☐ A lot of the time

(1) ☐ From time to time, but not too often

(0) ☐ Only occasionally

21. I look forward with enjoyment to things:

(0) ☐ As much as I ever did

(1) ☐ Rather less than I used to

(2) ☐ Definitely less than I used to

(3) ☐ Hardly at all

22. I get sudden feelings of panic:

(3) ☐ Very often indeed

(2) ☐ Quite often

(1) ☐ Not very often

(0) ☐ Not at all

SCORE 6
(Items 17-22)
Range 0-18

GENERAL HEALTH

We should like to know if you have had any medical complaints and how your health has been in general over the past week.

23. Felt constantly under strain?

(0) ☐ Not at all

(1) ☐ No more than usual

(2) ☐ Rather more than usual

(3) ☐ Much more than usual

24. Been getting edgy and bad-tempered?

(0) ☐ Not at all

(1) ☐ No more than usual

(2) ☐ Rather more than usual

(3) ☐ Much more than usual

25. Found everything getting on top of you?

(0) ☐ Not at all

(1) ☐ No more than usual

(2) ☐ Rather more than usual

(3) ☐ Much more than usual

26. Been feeling nervous and strung-up all the time?

(0) ☐ Not at all

(1) ☐ No more than usual

(2) ☐ Rather more than usual

(3) ☐ Much more than usual

27. Felt on the whole you were doing things well?

(0) ☐ Better than usual

(1) ☐ About the same

(2) ☐ Less well than usual

(3) ☐ Much less well

28. Been satisfied with the way you've carried out your task?

(0) ☐ More satisfied

(1) ☐ About same as usual

(2) ☐ Less satisfied than usual

(3) ☐ Much less satisfied

29. Been able to enjoy your normal day-to-day activities?

(0) ☐ More so than usual

(1) ☐ Same as usual

(2) ☐ Less so than usual

(3) ☐ Much less than usual

30. Felt that life isn't worth living?

(0) ☐ Not at all

(1) ☐ No more than usual

(2) ☐ Rather more than usual

(3) ☐ Much more than satisfied

31. Though of the possibility that you might make away with yourself?

(0) ☐ Definitely not

(1) ☐ I don't think so

(2) ☐ Has crossed my mind

(3) ☐ Definitely have

32. Found yourself wishing you were dead and away from it all?

(0) ☐ Not at all

(1) ☐ No more than usual

(2) ☐ Rather more than usual

(3) ☐ Much more than satisfied

33. Found that the idea of taking your own life kept coming into your mind?

(0) ☐ Definitely not

(1) ☐ I don't think so

(2) ☐ Has crossed my mind

(3) ☐ Definitely have

SCORE 7
(Items 23-33)
Range 0-33 ☐

COPING STRATEGIES

During the PAST WEEK, how many days did you use each of the following at least once in the day to cope with your pain? (Please indicate the number of days you used each strategy for pain, whether or not you were experiencing pain at the time.)

		Number of days							
		0	1	2	3	4	5	6	7
34	Imagined a calming or distracting image to help me relax								
35	Ignored the pain								
36	Asked someone to do something for me								
37	Focused on relaxing my muscles								
38	Held on to something when getting up or sitting down								
39	Told myself things will get better								
40	I got support from a family member								
41	Thought about all the good things I have								
42	Asked for help in carrying, lifting, or pushing something								
43	Told myself the pain will get better								
44	Avoided putting weight on feet or legs								
45	I didn't let the pain interfere with my activities								
46	Limited my walking because of pain								
47	Just didn't pay attention to the pain								
48	Talked to a friend or family member for support								
49	I just kept going								
50	Lay down on a bed								
51	Reminded myself about things that I have going for me such as intelligence, good looks, and good friends								

52	Got together with a family member								
53	Used deep, slow breathing to relax								
54	Went into a room by myself to rest								
55	Did not let the pain affect what I was doing								

<u>SCORE 8</u>
(Items in blank
34+35+37+39+41+43+45+47+49+51+53+55)
Range 0-84

<u>SCORE 9</u>
(Items in gray
36+38+40+42+44+46+48+50+52+54)
Range 0-70

SELF EFFICACY

We should like to know your opinion about YOUR ABILITY TO CONTROL FIBROMYALGIA SYMPTOMS.

Please circle the number that corresponds to how certain you are that you can do the following tasks regularly at the present time.

56. How certain are you that you can decrease your pain quite a bit?

0 1 2 3 4 5 6 7 8 9 10

Very uncertain Very certain

57. How certain are you that you can keep your fibromyalgia pain from interfering with your sleep?

0 1 2 3 4 5 6 7 8 9 10

Very uncertain Very certain

58. How certain are you that you can do something to help yourself feel better if you are feeling blue?

0 1 2 3 4 5 6 7 8 9 10

Very uncertain Very certain

59. As compared with other people with fibromyalgia like yours, how certain are you that you can manage pain during your daily activities?

0 1 2 3 4 5 6 7 8 9 10

Very uncertain Very certain

SCORE 10
(Items 56-59)
Range 0-40

ICAF SCORING SHEET

Physical		Active coping	
Direct score (1+2+3+4+5)		**Direct score** (8+10)	
Z score[1] (Direct - 61.7) / 13.43		Z score[1] (Direct - 63.99) / 24.04	
T score[2] (z * 10) + 50		T score[2] (z * 10) + 50	
Emotional		**Passive coping**	
Direct score (6+7)		**Direct score** (9)	
Z score[1] Direct - 23.84) / 13.43		Z score[1] (Direct – 37.06) / 14.38	
T score[2] (z * 10) + 50		T score[2] (z * 10) + 50	

For ICAF TOTAL calculation, **use direct scores** in the following formula:

Physical * 0.23		Emotional * 0.53		Passive coping * 0.1		Active coping * 0.14		**Direct score**
	+		+		-		=	

ICAF

Z score[1]
(Direct – 21.38) / 9.8

T score[2]
(z * 10) + 50

[1] Z scores are based in a previous study with 301 patients with fibromyalgia (Vallejo MA, Rivera J, Esteve-Vives J, Group ICAF: Development of a self-reporting tool to obtain a Combined Index of Severity of Fibromyalgia (ICAF). Health Qual Life Outcomes 2010; 8:2. http://www.hqlo.com/content/8/1/2)

[2] T scores have a media = 50, and a standard deviation = 10.

Reprinted with permission from *Fibromyalgia,* published by the Spanish Ministry of Health: http://www.msssi.gob.es/profesionales/prestacionesSanitarias/publicaciones/docs/fibromialgia.pdf

Appendix 3: Multi-dimensional Questionnaire for Patient Reported Outcome Measures: Fibromyalgia

Multi-Dimensional Questionnaire for Patient Reported Outcome Measures – Fibromyalgia

This questionnaire includes information not available from blood tests, X-rays, or any source other than you. Please try to answer each question. There is **no right or wrong answer.** Please answer exactly as **YOU** think or feel.

1. We are interested in learning how your illness affects your ability to function in daily life. Please tick (☒) the ONE best answer that describes your usual abilities OVER THE PAST WEEK:

Over the **LAST WEEK** were you able to	Without ANY Difficulty	With SOME Difficulty	With MUCH Difficulty	Unable TO DO	
1. Get on and off the toilet	....	....	....	....	
2. Dress yourself, including tying shoelaces & putting on socks	....	....	....	....	
3. Bend down to pick up object off the floor	....	....	....	....	
4. Sit for long periods of time; eg, working on flat-topped table or desk	....	....	....	....	
5. Lie down/sleep on your back	....	....	....	....	
6. Stand up from chair without arms	....	....	....	....	
7. Walk outdoors on flat ground including crossing the road	....	....	....	....	
8. Play with/look after children	....	....	....	....	
9. Go up 2 or more flights of stairs	....	....	....	....	
10. Do outside work (such as DIY/gardening/lifting)	....	....	....	....	
					Not Applicable
1. Get a good night's sleep?	....	....	....	....	....
2. Deal with the usual stresses of daily life?	....	....	....	....	....
3. Cope with social/family activities?	....	....	....	....	....
4. Deal with feelings of anxiety or being nervous?	....	....	....	....	....
5. Deal with feelings of low self-esteem or feeling blue?	....	....	....	....	....
6. Get going in the morning?	....	....	....	....	....
7. Do your work as you used to do?	....	....	....	....	....
8. Deal with any worries about your future?	....	....	....	....	....
9. Continue doing things you used to do, despite tiredness?	....	....	....	....	....
10. Continue your relationship with your partner (husband/wife)?	....	....	....	....	....

Fn. Disability [ ]

QoL [ ]

2. How much of a problem has SLEEP (ie, resting at night) been for you OVER THE PAST WEEK?

NO Prob. 0 5 10 15 20 25 30 35 40 45 50 55 60 65 70 75 80 90 95 100 SEVERE Prob.

3. How much of a problem has waking up UN-REFRESHED been for you OVER THE PAST WEEK?

NO Prob. 0 5 10 15 20 25 30 35 40 45 50 55 60 65 70 75 80 85 90 95 100 SEVERE Prob.

← Mild →← Mod →← Severe →

Sleep [ ] Unref. sleep [ ]

4. Considering all the ways your Symptoms may be affecting you AT THIS TIME Please put a circle around the number that best indicates how well you are doing:

VERY WELL 0 5 10 15 20 25 30 35 40 45 50 55 60 65 70 75 80 85 90 95 100 VERY POORLY

PGA [ ]

5. How much of a problem has UNUSUAL FATIGUE or tiredness been for you OVER THE PAST WEEK?

No Fatigue 0 5 10 15 20 25 30 35 40 45 50 55 60 65 70 75 80 85 90 95 100 Severe Fatigue

← Mild →← Mod. →← Severe →

6. How much of a problem has Trouble Thinking or remembering been for you OVER THE PAST WEEK?

NO Prob. 0 5 10 15 20 25 30 35 40 45 50 55 60 65 70 75 80 85 90 95 100 Severe Problem

← Mild →← Mod. →← Severe →

Fatigue [ ] Thinking [ ]

7. OVER THE PAST WEEK how would you rate the severity of your body PAIN?

No Pain 0 5 10 15 20 25 30 35 40 45 50 55 60 65 70 75 80 85 90 95 100 Severe Pain

Mild Mod.

8. OVER THE PAST WEEK how much of a problem has your mood (feeling down/anxious) affected you?

No Effect 0 1 2 2.5 3 4 5 6 7 7.5 8 9 10 Worst Effect

Mild Mod.

Pain [ ] Mood [ ]

Right	Left
Upper Limb	
Shoulder Girdle	Shoulder Girdle
Upper Arm	Upper Arm
Lower Arm	Lower Arm
Lower Limb	
Outer Hip Area	Outer Hip Area
Upper Leg	Upper Leg
Lower Leg	Lower Leg
Jaw	
Jaw (Rt.)	Jaw (Lt.)
Trunk	
Neck	Chest
Upper Back	Abdomen
Lower Back	*WPI score: /19*

Have you experienced any of these symptoms in the past months?	Yes	No
Pain or Cramps in the Lower Abdomen		
Depression		
Headache		

Please place (√) in front of the painful area(s) over your body that you feel painful TODAY

WPI score: (0-19)

Somatic Symp.:

Wolfe et al ACRS 2010

Please place (X) in the appropriate box to indicate in which of your JOINTS you feel painful TODAY

Tender Joints

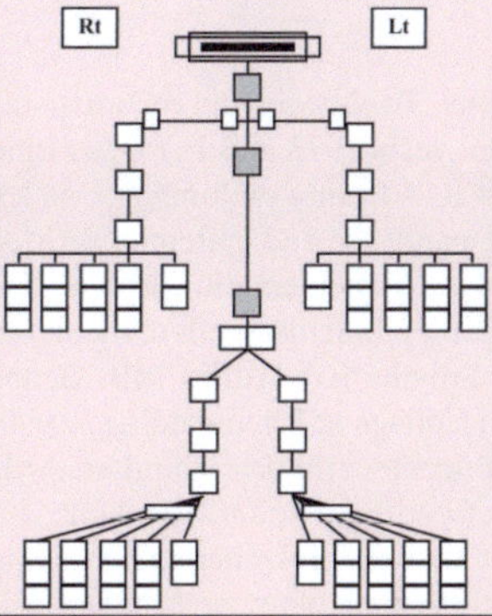

Neck
Shoulder
Shoulder Blade
Elbow
Wrist
Knuckles / Fingers
Low Back
Sacroiliac Joint
Hip
Knee
Ankle
Top Foot
Toes

Please tick (□) if you have experienced or diagnosed with any of the following OVER THE LAST 6 MONTHS:

Somatic Symptoms		Other Systemic Diseases	Cardiovascular Risk Assessment
Fever	Dry eye / Dry mouth	Loss of height/Vertebral fracture	Age > 50 years old
Hair loss	Mouth ulcers	Osteoporosis	High blood pressure
Muscle pain	Easy bruising	Recent fractures	High cholesterol
Muscle weakness	Irritable bowel syndrome	Vitamin D deficiency	Current smoker
Chest pain	Headache	Thyroid disease	Ischemic heart disease
Blurred vision	Wheezing in the chest	Parathyroid gland disease	Stroke
Hearing difficulties	Cough/Shortness of breath	Hepatitis C	Overweight/underweight
Itching	Heartburn	Diagnosed to have cancer	Diabetes mellitus
Loss of appetite	Dark or bloody stools	Absent from work due to body pains	**Falls Risk Assessment**
Pain/cramps in the abdomen	Feeling sickly/Nausea	Short plans for having a baby	> 1 fall in the last year
Rash	Constipation	Sexual relationship problems	Problems with your sight
Raynaud's phenomenon	Diarrhea	Problems with erection (for men)	Loss of your balance
Ringing in ears	Problems with urination	Psoriasis	Change in gait/Walking speed
Seizures	Bladder spasms	Coeliac disease	Weakness of your grip strength
Sun sensitivity	Numbness/tingling	Recent viral infection	For Official Use: Scores (0-3)
Taste changes/Loss of taste	Problems with thinking/memory	Registered disabled	Fatigue: Unrefresh.:
No Sympt.(0): □ Few Symp.(1): □	Mod. Symp.(2): □ Several Symp.(3): □	Recent viral infection	Cog. Symp.: WPI: /19

The statements below concern your personal beliefs. Please circle the number that best describes how you feel about the statement. 0 = Not at all; 10 = Strongly Agree

mRAI

1. My condition is controlling my life.	0 1 2 3 4 5 6 7 8 9 10
2. I would feel helpless if I could not rely on other people for help with my condition.	0 1 2 3 4 5 6 7 8 9 10
3. I am concerned that medicines cannot help me.	0 1 2 3 4 5 6 7 8 9 10
4. I've concerns regarding side effects of medications used to treat my condition.	0 1 2 3 4 5 6 7 8 9 10
5. I often do not take my medicines as directed.	0 1 2 3 4 5 6 7 8 9 10
6. No matter what I do, or how hard I try, I just cannot seem to get relief from my symptoms.	0 1 2 3 4 5 6 7 8 9 10
7. I am not coping effectively with my condition.	0 1 2 3 4 5 6 7 8 9 10
8. Sometimes I feel my condition is beyond both my and my doctor's control.	0 1 2 3 4 5 6 7 8 9 10
9. Sometimes my condition makes me feel like giving up.	0 1 2 3 4 5 6 7 8 9 10
10. Due to my condition, sometimes I feel I am a burden to those close to me.	0 1 2 3 4 5 6 7 8 9 10

References

1. Anonymous. Twenty-second rheumatism review. Review of the American and English literature for the years 1973 and 1974. Arthritis Rheum. [Review]. 1976;19(6 Suppl):973–1223.
2. Gowers WR. A lecture on lumbago: its lessons and analogues: delivered at the national hospital for the paralysed and epileptic. Br Med J. 1904;1(2246):117–21.
3. Anonymous. Implementation of the international statistical classification of diseases and related health problems, tenth revision (icd-10). Epidemiol Bull. 1997;18(1):1–4.
4. Wolfe F, Smythe HA, Yunus MB, Bennett RM, Bombardier C, Goldenberg DL, et al. The American College of Rheumatology 1990 criteria for the classification of fibromyalgia. Report of the multicenter criteria committee. Arthritis Rheum. [Comparative Study Research Support, Non-U.S. Gov't]. 1990;33(2):160–72.
5. Wolfe F, Clauw DJ, Fitzcharles MA, Goldenberg DL, Katz RS, Mease P, et al. The American College of Rheumatology preliminary diagnostic criteria for fibromyalgia and measurement of symptom severity. Arthritis Care Res. [Multicenter Study Research Support, Non-U.S. Gov't]. 2010;62(5):600–10.
6. Wolfe F, Clauw DJ, Fitzcharles MA, Goldenberg DL, Hauser W, Katz RS, et al. Fibromyalgia criteria and severity scales for clinical and epidemiological studies: a modification of the ACR preliminary diagnostic criteria for fibromyalgia. J Rheumatol. 2011;38(6):1113–22.
7. Katz JD, Mamyrova G, Guzhva O, Furmark L. Gender bias in diagnosing fibromyalgia. Gender Med. [Research Support, Non-U.S. Gov't]. 2010;7(1):19–27.
8. Yokota S, Kikuchi M, Miyamae T. Juvenile fibromyalgia: guidance for management. Pediatr Int. [Review]. 2013;55(4):403–9.
9. Mas AJ, Carmona L, Valverde M, Ribas B. Prevalence and impact of fibromyalgia on function and quality of life in individuals from the general population: results from a nationwide study in Spain. Clin Exp Rheumatol. [Research Support, Non-U.S. Gov't]. 2008;26(4):519–26.
10. Kashikar-Zuck S, Ting TV. Juvenile fibromyalgia: current status of research and future developments. Nat Rev Rheumatol. [Review]. 2014;10(2):89–96.
11. Lourenco S, Costa L, Rodrigues AM, Carnide F, Lucas R. Gender and psychosocial context as determinants of fibromyalgia symptoms (fibromyalgia research criteria) in young adults from the general population. Rheumatology (Oxford). 2015;54(10):1806–15.
12. Rivera J, Rejas-Gutierrez J, Vallejo MA, Esteve-Vives J, De Salas-Cansado M. Prospective study of the use of healthcare resources and economic costs in patients with fibromyalgia after treatment in routine medical practice. Clin Exp Rheumatol. [Multicenter Study Research Support, Non-U.S. Gov't]. 2012;30(6 Suppl 74):31–8.
13. Silverman S, Dukes EM, Johnston SS, Brandenburg NA, Sadosky A, Huse DM. The economic burden of fibromyalgia: comparative analysis with rheumatoid arthritis. Curr Med Res Opin. [Research Support, Non-U.S. Gov't]. 2009;25(4):829–40.
14. Thieme K, Turk DC, Flor H. Comorbid depression and anxiety in fibromyalgia syndrome: relationship to somatic and psychosocial variables. Psychosom Med. [Comparative Study Research Support, Non-U.S. Gov't]. 2004;66(6):837–44.
15. Hauser W, Hoffmann EM, Wolfe F, Worthing AB, Stahl N, Rothenberg R, et al. Self-reported childhood maltreatment, lifelong traumatic events and mental disorders in fibromyalgia syndrome: a comparison of US and German outpatients. Clin Exp Rheumatol. 2015;33(1 Suppl 88):S86–92.
16. Talotta R, Atzeni F, Bazzichi L, Giacomelli C, Di Franco M, Salaffi F, et al. Algo-dysfunctional syndromes: a critical digest of the recent literature. Clin Exp Rheumatol. [Review]. 2015;33(1 Suppl 88):S102–8.
17. Docampo E, Escaramis G, Gratacos M, Villatoro S, Puig A, Kogevinas M, et al. Genome-wide analysis of single nucleotide polymorphisms and copy number variants in fibromyalgia suggest a role for the central nervous system. Pain. [Multicenter Study Research Support, Non--U.S. Gov't]. 2014;155(6):1102–9.

18. Landis CA, Lentz MJ, Rothermel J, Riffle SC, Chapman D, Buchwald D, et al. Decreased nocturnal levels of prolactin and growth hormone in women with fibromyalgia. J Clin Endocrinol Metab. [Research Support, U.S. Gov't, P.H.S.]. 2001;86(4):1672–8.
19. Togo F, Natelson BH, Adler GK, Ottenweller JE, Goldenberg DL, Struzik ZR, et al. Plasma cytokine fluctuations over time in healthy controls and patients with fibromyalgia. Exp Biol Med (Maywood). [Research Support, N.I.H., Extramural Research Support, Non-U.S. Gov't]. 2009;234(2):232–40.
20. Mease PJ, Clauw DJ, Arnold LM, Goldenberg DL, Witter J, Williams DA, et al. Fibromyalgia syndrome. J Rheumatol. [Consensus Development Conference]. 2005;32(11):2270–7.
21. Vincent A, Benzo RP, Whipple MO, McAllister SJ, Erwin PJ, Saligan LN. Beyond pain in fibromyalgia: insights into the symptom of fatigue. Arthritis Res Ther. [Research Support, N.I.H., Extramural Review]. 2013;15(6):221.
22. Yunus MB, Inanici F, Aldag JC, Mangold RF. Fibromyalgia in men: comparison of clinical features with women. J Rheumatol. [Comparative Study]. 2000;27(2):485–90.
23. Mease P, Arnold LM, Choy EH, Clauw DJ, Crofford LJ, Glass JM, et al. Fibromyalgia syndrome module at omeract 9: domain construct. J Rheumat. [Consensus Development Conference Research Support, N.I.H., Extramural Research Support, Non-U.S. Gov't]. 2009;36(10):2318–29.
24. Coate L, S. Perrot, Choy E. Generalized pain syndromes Eular textbook on rheumatic diseases. UK: BMJ Group; 2012. p. 917–36.
25. Bertolucci PH, de Oliveira FF. Cognitive impairment in fibromyalgia. Curr Pain Headache Rep. [Review]. 2013;17(7):344.
26. Katz RS, Heard AR, Mills M, Leavitt F. The prevalence and clinical impact of reported cognitive difficulties (fibrofog) in patients with rheumatic disease with and without fibromyalgia. J Clin Rheumatol. 2004;10(2):53–8.
27. Kravitz HM, Katz RS. Fibrofog and fibromyalgia: a narrative review and implications for clinical practice. Rheumatol Int. 2015;35(7):1115–25.
28. Park DC, Glass JM, Minear M, Crofford LJ. Cognitive function in fibromyalgia patients. Arthritis Rheum. [Research Support, Non-U.S. Gov't Research Support, U.S. Gov't, P.H.S.]. 2001;44(9):2125–33.
29. Tesio V, Torta DM, Colonna F, Leombruni P, Ghiggia A, Fusaro E, et al. Are fibromyalgia patients cognitively impaired? Objective and subjective neuropsychological evidence. Arthritis Care Res. 2015;67(1):143–50.
30. Jones GT, Atzeni F, Beasley M, Fluss E, Sarzi-Puttini P, Macfarlane GJ. The prevalence of fibromyalgia in the general population: a comparison of the American College of Rheumatology 1990, 2010, and modified 2010 classification criteria. Arthritis Rheumatol. [Comparative Study Research Support, Non-U.S. Gov't]. 2015;67(2):568–75.
31. Hooten WM, Townsend CO, Decker PA. Gender differences among patients with fibromyalgia undergoing multidisciplinary pain rehabilitation. Pain Med. 2007;8(8):624–32.
32. Wolfe F, Ross K, Anderson J, Russell IJ. Aspects of fibromyalgia in the general population: Sex, pain threshold, and fibromyalgia symptoms. J Rheumatol. [Research Support, Non--U.S. Gov't Research Support, U.S. Gov't, P.H.S.]. 1995;22(1):151–6.
33. Yunus MB, Celiker R, Aldag JC. Fibromyalgia in men: comparison of psychological features with women. J Rheumatol. [Comparative Study]. 2004;31(12):2464–7.
34. Prados G, Miro E. [Fibromyalgia and sleep: a review]. Rev Neurol. [Research Support, Non--U.S. Gov't Review]. 2012;54(4):227–40.
35. Prados G, Miro E, Martinez MP, Sanchez AI, Lopez S, Saez G. Fibromyalgia: gender differences and sleep-disordered breathing. Clin Exp Rheumatol. [Comparative Study]. 2013;31(6 Suppl 79):S102–10.
36. Racine M, Castarlenas E, de la Vega R, Tome-Pires C, Sole E, Miro J, et al. Sex differences in psychological response to pain in patients with fibromyalgia syndrome. Clin J Pain. [Research Support, Non-U.S. Gov't]. 2015;31(5):425–32.

37. Miro E, Martinez MP, Sanchez AI, Prados G, Lupianez J. Men and women with fibromyalgia: relation between attentional function and clinical symptoms. Br J Health Psychol. 2015;20(3):632–47.
38. Ruiz-Montero PJ, Van Wilgen CP, Segura-Jimenez V, Carbonell-Baeza A, Delgado-Fernandez M. Illness perception and fibromyalgia impact on female patients from Spain and the Netherlands: do cultural differences exist? Rheumatol Int. 2015;13:1985–93.
39. Marques M, De Gucht V, Leal I, Maes S. A cross-cultural perspective on psychological determinants of chronic fatigue syndrome: a comparison between a Portuguese and a Dutch patient sample. Int J Behav Med. [Comparative Study Research Support, Non-U.S. Gov't]. 2013;20(2):229–38.
40. Karasz A, McKinley PS. Cultural differences in conceptual models of everyday fatigue: a vignette study. J Health Psychol. [Research Support, N.I.H., Extramural]. 2007;12(4):613–626.
41. Skapinakis P, Lewis G, Mavreas V. Cross-cultural differences in the epidemiology of unexplained fatigue syndromes in primary care. Br J Psychiatry. [Multicenter Study Research Support, Non-U.S. Gov't]. 2003;182:205–9.
42. Hobara M. Beliefs about appropriate pain behavior: cross-cultural and sex differences between Japanese and Euro-Americans. Eur J Pain. [Research Support, N.I.H., Extramural Research Support, Non-U.S. Gov't Research Support, U.S. Gov't, P.H.S.]. 2005;9(4):389–93.
43. Ferreira-Valente MA, Pais-Ribeiro JL, Jensen MP. Associations between psychosocial factors and pain intensity, physical functioning, and psychological functioning in patients with chronic pain: a cross-cultural comparison. Clin J Pain. [Comparative Study Research Support, Non--U.S. Gov't]. 2014;30(8):713–23.
44. Sanders SH, Brena SF, Spier CJ, Beltrutti D, McConnell H, Quintero O. Chronic low back pain patients around the world: cross-cultural similarities and differences. Clin J Pain. [Clinical Trial Comparative Study]. 1992;8(4):317–23.
45. Ferreira-Valente MA, Ribeiro JL, Jensen MP, Almeida R. Coping with chronic musculoskeletal pain in Portugal and in the United States: a cross-cultural study. Pain Med. [Research Support, N.I.H., Extramural Research Support, Non-U.S. Gov't Research Support, U.S. Gov't, Non-P.H.S.]. 2011;12(10):1470–80.
46. Koffman J, Morgan M, Edmonds P, Speck P, Higginson I. Cultural meanings of pain: a qualitative study of black Caribbean and white British patients with advanced cancer. Palliative Med. [Comparative Study Multicenter Study Research Support, Non-U.S. Gov't]. 2008;22(4):350–9.
47. Diller A. Cross-cultural pain semantics. Pain. [Comparative Study]. 1980;9(1):9–26.
48. Moldofsky H. The significance, assessment, and management of nonrestorative sleep in fibromyalgia syndrome. CNS Spectrums. [Review]. 2008;13(3 Suppl 5):22–26.
49. Kurtze N, Gundersen KT, Svebak S. The role of anxiety and depression in fatigue and patterns of pain among subgroups of fibromyalgia patients. Br J Med Psychol. [Research Support, Non--U.S. Gov't]. 1998;71 (Pt 2):185–194.
50. Wolfe F, Michaud K. Severe rheumatoid arthritis (ra), worse outcomes, comorbid illness, and sociodemographic disadvantage characterize ra patients with fibromyalgia. J Rheumatol. [Research Support, Non-U.S. Gov't]. 2004;31(4):695–700.
51. Ranzolin A, Brenol JC, Bredemeier M, Guarienti J, Rizzatti M, Feldman D, et al. Association of concomitant fibromyalgia with worse disease activity score in 28 joints, health assessment questionnaire, and short form 36 scores in patients with rheumatoid arthritis. Arthritis Rheum. [Research Support, Non-U.S. Gov't]. 2009;61(6):794–800.
52. Naranjo A, Ojeda S, Francisco F, Erausquin C, Rua-Figueroa I, Rodriguez-Lozano C. Fibromyalgia in patients with rheumatoid arthritis is associated with higher scores of disability. Ann Rheum Dis. [Letter]. 2002;61(7):660–1.
53. Dhir V, Lawrence A, Aggarwal A, Misra R. Fibromyalgia is common and adversely affects pain and fatigue perception in north Indian patients with rheumatoid arthritis. J Rheumatol. 2009;36(11):2443–8.
54. Almodovar R, Carmona L, Zarco P, Collantes E, Gonzalez C, Mulero J, et al. Fibromyalgia in patients with ankylosing spondylitis: prevalence and utility of the measures of activity, function and radiological damage. Clin Exp Rheumatol. 2010;28(6 Suppl 63):S33–9.

55. Aloush V, Ablin JN, Reitblat T, Caspi D, Elkayam O. Fibromyalgia in women with ankylosing spondylitis. Rheumatol Int. 2007;27(9):865–8.
56. Staud R. Are patients with systemic lupus erythematosus at increased risk for fibromyalgia? Curr Rheumat Rep. [Review]. 2006;8(6):430–35.
57. Bennett R. The concurrence of lupus and fibromyalgia: implications for diagnosis and management. Lupus. [Review]. 1997;6(6):494–9.
58. Pompa A, Clemenzi A, Troisi E, Pace L, Casillo P, Catani S, et al. Chronic pain in multiple sclerosis patients: utility of sensory quantitative testing in patients with fibromyalgia comorbidity. Eur Neurol. 2015;73(5–6):257–63.
59. Clemenzi A, Pompa A, Casillo P, Pace L, Troisi E, Catani S, et al. Chronic pain in multiple sclerosis: is there also fibromyalgia? An observational study. Med Sci Monitor. [Observational Study Research Support, Non-U.S. Gov't]. 2014;20:758–66.
60. Bennett RM, Jones J, Turk DC, Russell IJ, Matallana L. An internet survey of 2,596 people with fibromyalgia. BMC Musculoskelet Disord. 2007;8:27.
61. Wright M. Widespread body pain and mortality. Diagnosing fibromyalgia stops doctors from thinking. Br Med J. [Comment Letter]. 2002;324(7332):300.
62. Chamizo-Carmona E. [Is there an association between fibromyalgia and an increase in comorbidity: neoplastic and cardiovascular diseases, infections and mortality?]. Article in Spanish. Reumatol Clin. 2005;1(4):200–10.
63. Wolfe F, Hassett AL, Walitt B, Michaud K. Mortality in fibromyalgia: a study of 8,186 patients over thirty-five years. Arthritis Care Res. [Comparative Study]. 2011;63(1):94–101.
64. Dreyer L, Kendall S, Danneskiold-Samsoe B, Bartels EM, Bliddal H. Mortality in a cohort of Danish patients with fibromyalgia: increased frequency of suicide. Arthritis Rheum. [Research Support, Non-U.S. Gov't]. 2010;62(10):3101–8.
65. Bennett RM, Friend R, Marcus D, Bernstein C, Han BK, Yachoui R, et al. Criteria for the diagnosis of fibromyalgia: validation of the modified 2010 preliminary American College of Rheumatology criteria and the development of alternative criteria. Arthritis Care Res. 2014;66(9):1364–73.
66. Choy EH, Arnold LM, Clauw DJ, Crofford LJ, Glass JM, Simon LS, et al. Content and criterion validity of the preliminary core dataset for clinical trials in fibromyalgia syndrome. J Rheumatol. [Research Support, N.I.H., Extramural Research Support, Non-U.S. Gov't]. 2009;36(10):2330–4.
67. Castrejon I, Gossec L, Carmona L. The EULAR outcome measures library: an evolutional database of validated patient-reported instruments. Ann Rheum Dis. [Letter]. 2015; 74(2):475–6.
68. Bennett R. The fibromyalgia impact questionnaire (FIQ): a review of its development, current version, operating characteristics and uses. Clin Exp Rheumatol. 2005;23(5 Suppl 39):S154–62.
69. Burckhardt CS, Clark SR, Bennett RM. The fibromyalgia impact questionnaire: development and validation. J Rheumatol. 1991;18(5):728–33.
70. Bennett RM, Friend R, Jones KD, Ward R, Han BK, Ross RL. The revised fibromyalgia impact questionnaire (FIQR): validation and psychometric properties. Arthritis Res Ther. [Research Support, Non-U.S. Gov't Validation Studies]. 2009;11(4):R120.
71. Ediz L, Hiz O, Toprak M, Tekeoglu I, Ercan S. The validity and reliability of the Turkish version of the revised fibromyalgia impact questionnaire. Clin Rheumatol. [Validation Studies]. 2011;30(3):339–46.
72. Zachrisson O, Regland B, Jahreskog M, Kron M, Gottfries CG. A rating scale for fibromyalgia and chronic fatigue syndrome (the fibrofatigue scale). J Psychosom Res. [Clinical Trial Controlled Clinical Trial]. 2002;52(6):501–9.
73. Brand K, Littlejohn G, Kristjanson L, Wisniewski S, Hassard T. The fibromyalgia bladder index. Clin Rheumatol. 2007;26(12):2097–103.
74. Vallejo MA, Rivera J, Esteve-Vives J, Rejas J. A confirmatory study of the combined index of severity of fibromyalgia (ICAF*): factorial structure, reliability and sensitivity to change. Health Qual Life outcomes. [Research Support, Non-U.S. Gov't Validation Studies]. 2011;9:39.

75. Boomershine CS, Emir B, Wang Y, Zlateva G. Simplifying fibromyalgia assessment: The VASFIQ brief symptom scale. Ther Adv Musculoskelet Dis. 2011;3(5):215–26.
76. Fries JF. The hierarchy of quality-of-life assessment, the health assessment questionnaire (HAQ), and issues mandating development of a toxicity index. Control Clin Trials. [Research Support, U.S. Gov't, P.H.S.]. 1991;12(4 Suppl):106S–117S.
77. Wolfe F, Hawley DJ, Goldenberg DL, Russell IJ, Buskila D, Neumann L. The assessment of functional impairment in fibromyalgia (FM): Rasch analyses of 5 functional scales and the development of the FM health assessment questionnaire. J Rheumatol. [Evaluation Studies]. 2000;27(8):1989–99.
78. El Miedany Y, El Gaafary M, Youssef S, El Aroussy N, Ahmed I, Palmer D. Towards a multidimensional patient reported outcome measures assessment: Development and validation of a questionnaire for patients with fibromyalgia. EULAR: Ann Rheum Dis. 2013;72 Suppl 3:719.
79. Cuesta-Vargas A, Luciano JV, Penarrubia-Maria MT, Garcia-Campayo J, Fernandez-Vergel R, Arroyo-Morales M, et al. Clinical dimensions of fibromyalgia symptoms and development of a combined index of severity: the CODI index. Qual Life Res. [Research Support, Non-U.S. Gov't]. 2013;22(1):153–60.
80. Mayer TG, Neblett R, Cohen H, Howard KJ, Choi YH, Williams MJ, et al. The development and psychometric validation of the central sensitization inventory. Pain Pract. 2012;12(4): 276–85.
81. Mokkink LB, Terwee CB, Patrick DL, Alonso J, Stratford PW, Knol DL, et al. The COSMIN study reached international consensus on taxonomy, terminology, and definitions of measurement properties for health-related patient-reported outcomes. J Clin Epidemiol. 2010;63(7):737–45.
82. Rivera J, Gonzalez T. The fibromyalgia impact questionnaire: a validated spanish version to assess the health status in women with fibromyalgia. Clin Exp Rheumatol. [Clinical Trial Randomized Controlled Trial Validation Studies]. 2004;22(5):554–60.
83. Ablin JN, Odes L, Neumann L, Buskila D. The Hebrew version of the fibrofatigue scale: validation of a questionnaire for assessment of fibromyalgia and chronic fatigue syndrome. Rheumatol Int. [Validation Studies]. 2010;30(9):1173–6.
84. Finckh A, Morabia A, Deluze C, Vischer T. Validation of questionnaire-based response criteria of treatment efficacy in the fibromyalgia syndrome. Arthritis Care Res. 1998;11(2):116–23.
85. Sarzi-Puttini P, Atzeni F, Turiel M, Furlan R, Vulpio L, Carrabba M, et al. The Italian version of the fibrofatigue scale, a reliable tool for the evaluation of fibromyalgia symptoms. J Psychosom Res. [Validation Studies]. 2004;56(2):213–6.

Chapter 8
PROMs for Juvenile Idiopathic Arthritis

Alessandro Consolaro, Stefano Lanni, Angelo Ravelli, and Nicolino Ruperto

Introduction

Juvenile idiopathic arthritis (JIA) is the most common chronic rheumatic disease in children, with an incidence in Europe of about 16 to 150 per 100,000 per year, and is an important cause of short-term and long-term disability [1]. The International League of Associations for Rheumatology has defined JIA as arthritis with no apparent cause lasting more than 6 weeks with disease onset prior to age 16 [2]. Seven different subtypes of JIA are recognized, differing in genetic susceptibility, distribution, and severity of arthritis (Table 8.1). The prognosis of JIA is widely variable, depending on the subtype of the disease. In general, at least 50 % of children experience some form of the disease into adulthood and about one-third of patients diagnosed with JIA develops persisting functional and psychological disability, with many having limitations in daily activities impacting on health-related quality of life (HRQOL) [3, 4]. Although the recent advances and the newer therapeutic options, namely the biologic agents, have greatly improved the long-term outcome of this group of diseases, few chronic conditions may challenge the child and his family as much as severe JIA, a disease that, by its very nature, has a major impact on the everyday quality of life. The child has to face problems related to joint stiffness, pain, limitation of motion, alterations of his/her body image secondary to joint deformities, and growth problems that can lead to the impossibility of performing everyday activities in the same way as his peers. Moreover, these

A. Consolaro, M.D., Ph.D. • A. Ravelli, M.D.
Università degli studi di Genova, Genoa, Italy

Pediatria 2, Reumatologia, Istituto Giannina Gaslini, Genoa, Italy
e-mail: alessandroconsolaro@gaslini.org; angeloravelli@gaslini.org

S. Lanni, M.D. • N. Ruperto, M.D., M.P.H. (✉)
Pediatria 2, Reumatologia, Istituto Giannina Gaslini, Genoa, Italy
e-mail: stefanolanni@gaslini.org; nicolaruperto@gaslini.org

Y. El Miedany (ed.), *Patient Reported Outcome Measures in Rheumatic Diseases*,
DOI 10.1007/978-3-319-32851-5_8

Table 8.1 Frequency and sex distribution of categories of juvenile idiopathic arthritis according to the International League of Associations for Rheumatology (ILAR)

	Frequency (%)	Sex ratio
Systemic arthritis	4–17	F=M
Oligoarthritis	27–56	F≫M
Rheumatoid-factor-positive polyarthritis	2–7	F≫M
Rheumatoid-factor-negative polyarthritis	11–28	F≫M
Enthesitis-related arthritis	3–11	M≫F
Psoriatic arthritis	2–11	F>M
Undifferentiated arthritis	11–21	–

Modified from [1]

problems may heavily interfere with the development of independence and self-esteem, especially in adolescence.

A combined meeting held in 1997 by the World Health Organization (WHO) and the International League of Associations for Rheumatology (ILAR) [5] reached a consensus on the definitions of quality of life that is the perception of individuals of their own position in life in the context of culture and value systems in which they live and in relation to their goals, expectations, standard and concerns. HRQOL pertains to the physical, emotional, and social aspects of quality of life influenced by an individual's disease and/or its treatment; disability is the limitation in an individual's ability to act in a usual, customary, and personally desired way caused by one or more health conditions affecting physical or mental function.

As a consequence, in recent years, there has been a growing interest in the assessment of parent- and child-reported outcomes (PCROs) in pediatric rheumatic diseases. Incorporation of these measures in the routine clinical evaluation is considered important as they reflect the parent's and child's perception of the disease course and effectiveness of therapeutic interventions. Because parents and children (when mature enough to understand the clinical and therapeutic issues related to their disease) are asked with increasing frequency to actively participate in shared decision-making, integration of their perspective in clinical assessment may facilitate concordance with physician's choices and improve adherence to treatment [6–9]. In addition, the use of PCROs may help the physician to identify with greater accuracy the salient issues for each patient and to focus the attention on the relevant matters. Thus, information obtained from the parent or the child may contribute to the success of patient care. It is now agreed that the inclusion of PCROs in clinical practice may lead to improve the quality of care [10].

A number of tools for the assessment of PCROs in children with JIA are available, including visual analog scales (VAS) for rating of a child's overall well-being and intensity of pain, and questionnaires for the evaluation of functional ability and HRQOL [11–14]. The importance of the concepts of disability and HRQOL is directly reflected by the high number of references available in PubMed in the adult and pediatric rheumatology literature for the evaluation of the short- and long-term outcomes, in observation studies, and in clinical trials. More recently both concepts have been instrumental also for clinical trials since they have been included in the

Table 8.2 Measures contained in the Juvenile Idiopathic Arthritis (JIA) American College of Rheumatology (ACR) core set for the evaluation of response to therapy

The JIA ACR core set of response variables
1. Physician global assessment of disease activity
2. Parent/patient assessment of overall well-being
3. Functional ability (CHAQ)
4. Number of joints with active arthritis
5. Number of joints with limited range of motion
6. Index of inflammation (ESR or CRP)

CHAQ Childhood Health Assessment Questionnaire, *ESR* erythrocyte sedimentation rate, *CRP* C-reactive protein

six JIA core set of response variables for the evaluation of response to therapy [15–19] (Table 8.2), as well as in juvenile systemic lupus erythematosus (JSLE), and in juvenile dermatomyositis (JDM) [20–28].

This chapter describes the most recent and widely used PCROs for the management of children with JIA.

Parent/Patient Global Assessment

Parent or patient global assessment (PGA) is included in the JIA ACR core outcome variables for the evaluation of response to therapy [16] and is therefore considered a fundamental tool in the assessment of children with this disease. The parent of the JIA patient, or the child if aged appropriately, makes a global assessment of the child's overall well-being on a 10 cm VAS or on a 21-circle VAS (0 = very good, 10 = very poor) [29]. The 21-numbered circle VAS has at least 3 advantages over the traditional 10 cm horizontal line format: (1) the assessor can score the VAS without a ruler, implying a simpler and quicker calculation; (2) it eliminates the need to reproduce an exact 10 cm line in printing or photocopying questionnaires, averting the problem of minor distortion frequently seen with these procedures; (3) it is better understood by patients [30].

Of note, several studies show that the concordance between parent/patient and physician assessments of JIA disease activity is quite poor, closing 40 % [7, 31, 32]. It was observed that in patients meeting current definition of inactive disease in JIA, only 65 % of parents gave a score of zero in the PGA [7]. Parents' rating tended to be higher if their child has shorter disease duration, is taking second-line drug therapy, has increased reported pain, or has functional impairment. Alternatively, physicians consistently rate disease activity more highly than parents in the presence of any active joints [7, 31]. In a different chronic rheumatic condition such as JDM, Rider et al. found that physician and parent global ratings of disease activity were not collinear, and that the non-redundancy may be the result of each evaluating different aspects of the disease [33].

Pain

Pain is the major symptom of children with JIA [34]. Several studies have shown that pain is more prevalent in JIA than previously recognized and that a sizeable percentage of patients continues to report pain long after disease onset [35]. High levels of pain limit physical activities, disrupt school attendance, and contribute to psychosocial distress. These issues make reduction of pain a key goal of treatment [36].

The physician global rating of overall disease activity, the parent global rating of the child's overall well-being, and the parent rating of the intensity of child's pain on VAS are important quantitative measures used to assess the disease status in children with JIA. The 10 cm horizontal line VAS is traditionally used to make these assessments. However, as for the PGA, it has been suggested that the 21-numbered circle VAS may increase the precision of patient assessment [29].

Only a few studies of medications in JIA have reported their efficacy in controlling pain [37, 38]. This paucity of data might be partly due to the lack of inclusion of pain in the traditional outcome end points used in therapeutic studies in JIA, including the JIA ACR response criteria, the criteria for inactive disease and clinical remission or minimal disease activity, and the Juvenile Arthritis Disease Activity Score (JADAS) [11]. The impact of pain is presumed to be incorporated, at least in part, in the parent's or child's global rating of overall well-being. Furthermore, pain is known to be affected by many non-disease-related factors, which makes it an imperfect measure of disease activity. However, pain perception in children with chronic arthritis is multifactorial, and results from the integration of biological processes, psychological aspects, and sociocultural contexts [34]. Assessment of pain should, therefore, address its impact on a broad range of factors, including physical, social, and school activities; family and peer interactions; cognitive functioning; emotional distress; mood; behavior; and pain-coping strategies [35]. These issues make it clear that a reliable appraisal of pain in children with JIA requires the use of well-validated and developmentally based pediatric pain-assessment tools that can capture the multifaceted character of the pain experience.

Functional Ability

Functional ability/disability status or physical functioning are broad summary statements with respect to the effect of a disease on the patient's ability to carry out usual tasks, such as the activities of daily living [14]. The assessment of physical function is a fundamental component of the clinical evaluation of children with JIA.

Together with PGA, physical functioning assessment is also included among the ACR core outcome variables for JIA [16] (Table 8.2).

Childhood Health Assessment Questionnaire

The Childhood Health Assessment Questionnaire (CHAQ) [5] is the principal rheumatic "disease-specific" instrument to be used for studies involving patients with JIA and other pediatric rheumatic conditions (JDM, JSLE, etc.) [24, 39–44]. It measures functional ability in eight activities of daily living: dressing and grooming, arising, eating, walking, hygiene, reach, grip, and activities. In the CHAQ, several questions were added to the HAQ so that there is at least 1 question in each functional area that is relevant to children of all ages under 18. Each of the items within a single domain has 4 possible categories of answers: "without any difficulty" (score 0), "with some difficulty" (score 1), "with much difficulty" (score 2), and "unable to do" (score 3). The category "not applicable" was added for the items that may not apply due to the age of the child. Parents were instructed to take note only of impairment due to the disease in the preceding week. The items with the highest score in a domain determine the score for that domain, while the use of any aids or devices or help from another person is assigned a minimum score of 2 for that domain. These 8 domains are then averaged into a summary score called the disability index (DI), which may range from 0 to 3 with higher scores meaning higher disability. The CHAQ also provides an assessment of discomfort using a 10 cm VAS for the evaluation of pain and a 10 cm VAS for the evaluation of overall well-being.

Since its initial publication, the CHAQ has been translated into many languages and is used worldwide for assessing children with chronic musculoskeletal diseases [39]. A large number of studies have assessed the test–retest reliability, construct validity, minimal clinically important differences, and quality of the parent-proxy report of the CHAQ [39, 45, 46]. However, CHAQ has been demonstrated to suffer from a ceiling effect, with a tendency for scores to cluster at the normal end of the scale, particularly in patients with fewer joints involved [46, 47]. Another problem with the use of CHAQ is its length and complexity, including the requirement of a calculator to compute the scores. Mainly for these reasons, although the CHAQ has been found to have excellent measurement properties, it has remained essentially a research tool and is not routinely administered in most pediatric rheumatology centers. It also has been reported that the removal of aids/devices and help from the CHAQ does not alter the interpretation of disability at a group level, making the simplified CHAQ a more feasible and valid alternative for the evaluation of disability in JIA patients [43].

For the interpretation of the CHAQ scores, Dempster et al. [48] reported that the median CHAQ scores corresponding to mild, mild-to-moderate, and moderate disability were 0.13, 0.63, and 1.75, respectively. The minimal clinically important improvement was a reduction in score of 0.13.

Lam et al. [49] devised three modified versions of CHAQ that measure functional strengths as well as weaknesses (i.e., by using new response scales as well as by adding more challenging questions) to investigate whether they reduced the limitations of CHAQ, namely the ceiling effect and poor sensitivity for children with relatively good function. The new versions of CHAQ were found to suffer less from a ceiling effect and to be more normally distributed. Furthermore, they proved more sensitive at differentiating JIA patients from controls.

Juvenile Arthritis Functionality Scale

In 2007, Filocamo and coworkers developed a shorter and simpler questionnaire for the assessment of physical function in standard clinical care of children with JIA: the Juvenile Arthritis Functionality Scale (JAFS) [50]. The JAFS is a 15-item questionnaire in which functional activities are grouped in 3 functional areas, each composed of 5 items: (1) lower limbs, (2) hand-wrist, and (3) upper segment. The ability of the child to perform each task is scored as follows: 0 = without any difficulty, 1 = with difficulty, and 2 = unable to do. Questionnaire completers are asked to note only those difficulties that are caused by arthritis. An "unable to perform" column is included to designate the functions that cannot be performed because of developmental immaturity. The total score ranges from 0 to 30. A separate score for each area (range 0–10) can be calculated. Recently, a modified version of the JAFS has been devised, in which each item is scored on a 0–3 scale (0 = without any difficulty, 1 = with some difficulty, 2 = with much difficulty, and 3 = unable to do). The total score of the modified JAFS ranges from 0 to 45. The JAFS is proposed for use as both proxy report and patient self-report, with the suggested age range of 8–18 years for use as self-report. It has been argued that owing to the wide variability in the number and distribution of affected joints in children with JIA, functional questionnaires may contain some items that are irrelevant and uninformative for a particular patient [51]. Assessment of functional tasks that are unlikely to be affected in an individual child (e.g., "lift up a glass to mouth" in a child with arthritis only in the lower extremity joints or "walk on flat ground" in a child with arthritis only in the wrist and hand joints) may "dilute" the global score, leading to a potential underestimation of functional impairment. Thus, it would be desirable to ask only specific questions that are relevant for the patient's distribution of joint disease and to drop other questions. In this respect, the JAFS may be advantageous over the other physical function questionnaires as it explores functional activities grouped by the topography of involved joints or joint groups. Such structure enables a precise evaluation of the influence of impairment in individual joints on specific functions. Preliminary evidence was found that the JAFS captures with greater accuracy the functional impact of arthritis in specific body areas than does a standard questionnaire (the C-HAQ) in children with JIA [51]. The JAFS is currently being translated into several languages in the context of a multinational study set to evaluate the epidemiology treatment, and outcome of JIA worldwide [52].

Other Measures of Physical Function

Other validated tools for the assessment of functional ability in JIA patients include the Juvenile Arthritis Functional Assessment Scale (JAFAS), Juvenile Arthritis Functional Assessment Report (JAFAR), and the Juvenile Arthritis Self-Report Index (JASI). Developed in 1989, the JAFAS is an observer-based scale, which requires a trained observer and standardized equipment, and is based on timing on 10 physical tasks [53]. The JAFAR assesses the ability of children older than 7 years to perform physical tasks in 23 items; 2 versions are available, 1 for children (JAFAR-C) and 1 for parents (JAFAR-P) [54]. Finally, the JASI is a 100-item instrument that explores physical function in five domains. It is a very comprehensive, valid, and reliable tool, although it requires a long time to be completed [55]. The JASI is unique in that item generation took place through interviews with children, parents, teachers, and clinicians, although only the clinicians conducted item reduction.

To overcome the potential bias in answering that may be provided by subjective assessment of physical function, which can be influenced by level of understanding and emotional background of questionnaire completer, Iglesias and coworkers [56] designed an observational functional ability scale: the CAPFUN (capacidad funcional = functional ability). It consists of 20 items that assess 10 activities in the upper limbs or cervical spine and 10 in the lower limbs. Each item is scored as 0 when it is impossible to perform, as 1 when it is performed incompletely or with difficulty, and as 2 when it is well performed. The mean value of upper and lower limb scores is added and their mean value, which ranges from 0 to 2, is defined as the CAPFUN score. This tool, which has the advantage of providing an objective assessment of physical function, revealed good internal reliability and construct validity.

Health-Related Quality of Life

HRQOL is a multidimensional concept that incorporates measures of physical symptoms, functional status, and disease impact on psychological and social functioning [4, 39–41, 57–60]. JIA is a disease that influences all aspects of a child's life at a physical, social, and intellectual level [1, 61]. In chronic conditions such as JIA where mortality is not a major factor, HRQOL often serves as a primary measure of patient outcome. However, HRQOL should be defined, characterized, and measured in an appropriate way for it to be clinically useful.

In recent years, a number of HRQOL measures have been developed for use in children and are usually divided into 2 types: (1) disease-specific measures [14, 62–65], which are centered on a particular disease such as JIA and (2) generic, which measure quality of life independent of the underlying disease [66, 67].

On average, patients with JIA have a poorer HRQOL as compared with healthy peers in both physical and psychosocial domains, with physical health being more affected. In a recent multinational survey, the areas of HRQOL most affected by JIA (<2 SDs of the mean of healthy children) were global health, physical functioning, role social limitation (physical), and bodily pain/discomfort [41]. The results of this and other studies demonstrate that children with JIA have a greater impairment in physical well-being than in psychosocial health, and that physical disability and pain are important determinants of HRQOL [12, 41, 68].

When patients with JIA were divided according to ILAR category, it was found that those with persistent oligoarthritis had, on average, a better HRQOL than those with the other subtypes in all domains; the HRQOL of patients with systemic arthritis, polyarthritis, and extended oligoarthritis was similar in these three subtypes [41].

The Child Health Questionnaire

The Child Health Questionnaire (CHQ) is a generic health instrument designed to capture the physical and psychosocial well-being of children 5 years of age and older [66]. Parents are instructed to take into consideration the 4-week period preceding their compilation of the questionnaire. The CHQ measures by means of 50 items (questions) the following health concepts: global health (GGH); physical functioning (PF); role/social, emotional/behavioral limitations (REB); role/social physical limitations (RP); bodily pain discomfort (BP); behavior (BE); global behavior (GBE); mental health (MH); self-esteem (SE); general health perception (GH); change in health (CH); emotional impact on the parent (PE); impact on the parent's personal time (PT); limitations in family activities (FA); and family cohesion (FC). The 50 items are re-coded to ensure that all questions are positively scored, so that a higher score indicates better health, and recalibrated to ensure that the responses taken together represent a continuum. The scores for each health concept are then transformed according to the following formula: actual score (sum of the item responses divided by the number of completed items) minus the lowest possible score divided by the possible score range; the transformed scores are therefore on a scale ranging from 0 to 100, with a higher score indicating better functioning and well-being. The score for each health concept can be evaluated only if half or more of the items within a scale have been answered, or half plus one in the case of scales with an odd number of items. By means of two subsequent steps, two final grouping scores are then obtained by the procedures described below, namely the physical summary score (PhS) and the psychosocial summary score (PsS). As instructed by the developer of the CHQ, only 10 out of 15 possible health concepts are currently used to calculate the PhS and PsS summary scores: PF, RP, BP, GH, REB, PT, PE, SE, MH, BE. The use of the five remaining scales (GGH, GBE, CH, FA, FC) in calculating the PhS and PsS summary scores is still being evaluated and tested by the author of the CHQ. The first step is to calculate the standardized z-score for each of the ten health concepts using the following formula: the transformed score minus the estimated mean for that health concept in the reference population divided by the estimated standard deviation for the reference population. For the purposes of this project the means and standard deviation estimates were derived from the entire sample (that is all countries were combined and children with JIA and healthy children were also combined). The second step is to compute the aggregate summary scale scores (referred to as PhS RAW and PsS RAW) by multiplying the standardized z-score by its factor score coefficients (obtained by factor analysis; see later) and then summing the product of the 10 scales used. Finally, in the third step each aggregate score is transformed to the norm-based PhS and PsS scores that have a mean of 50, and a standard deviation of 10. This is done by multiplying each aggregate summary scale score by 10 and adding the resulting product to 50. CHQ scores were calculated using the proprietary algorithms and SAS programming code created specifically for the CHQ by its author.

The Juvenile Arthritis Quality of Life Questionnaire

The Juvenile Arthritis Quality of Life Questionnaire (JAQQ) was specifically developed for JIA patients [65]. It consists of 74 items grouped into 4 dimensions: gross motor function, fine motor function, psychosocial function, and general symptoms. A 100 mm VAS measure of pain is also included. Only the five most problematic items in each dimension are completed and scored by each patient. A substantially different instrument is, therefore, completed by each child. Indeed, this may complicate direct comparison of results among patients for research purposes. The JAQQ has been found to have moderate construct validity and responsiveness.

The Pediatric Rheumatology Quality of Life Scale

A shorter and simpler questionnaire for the assessment of HRQOL in routine care of patients with rheumatic diseases, the Pediatric Rheumatology Quality of Life Scale (PRQL) [69], was recently developed. As with the JAFS, the PRQL is currently being translated into several languages in the context of a multinational study set to evaluate the epidemiology treatment, and outcome of JIA worldwide [52]. The PRQL is a 10-item questionnaire that explores HRQOL in two domains: physical health (PhH) and psychosocial health (PsH). It is short, simple, and quick, taking <5 min to complete and score. It is proposed for use as both proxy report and patient self-report, with the suggested age range of 7–18 years for use as self-report. Validation of the parent proxy report and child self-report versions of the instrument was accomplished by evaluating 472 JIA patients and about 800 healthy children. As expected, both proxy- and self-reported HRQOL were found to be more impaired in JIA patients than in healthy children, with PhH being most involved. Surprisingly, however, the level of psychosocial well-being of JIA patients was comparable to (for parents' proxy reports) or even better than (for children's self-reports) that of healthy children. The poorer PsH seen in healthy children concerned predominantly the adolescent age group. This observation was attributed to the fact that most JIA patients currently seen in tertiary care pediatric rheumatology centers have well-controlled disease with little or no disease activity or disability. Children with chronic arthritis suffer in the active phase of their disease a considerable burden of symptoms, namely pain and stiffness, which affects many aspects of their lives. For these children, disease improvement represents a key priority. It is, therefore, conceivable that resolution of symptoms leads to a marked improvement in their mental and social health.

Compliance to Therapy

The first drug-specific and disease-specific questionnaire for the measurement of treatment tolerance in JIA was developed by Bulatovic and coworkers in 2011 [70]. They designed and validated a new questionnaire for methotrexate-related gastrointestinal and behavioral symptoms. Methotrexate is the first-choice disease-modifying antirheumatic drug for the treatment of JIA. Gastrointestinal adverse effects, which include nausea, abdominal pain, vomiting, or diarrhea, are quite common during methotrexate treatment. The Methotrexate Intolerance Severity Score (MISS) consists of 12 questions, assessing abdominal pain, nausea, and vomiting after or before (anticipatory) methotrexate intake and when thinking of methotrexate (associative). Furthermore, it assesses behavioral complaints associated with methotrexate intake, such as crying, restlessness, irritability, and refusal to take the drug. The score ranges between 0 and 36, and subjects with a score of ≥6, including at least 1 anticipatory, associative or behavioral symptom, were defined as methotrexate intolerant.

Multidimensional Tools and Composite Scores

The heterogeneous and multidimensional nature of JIA implies that numerous disease domains should be evaluated simultaneously to appraise the full extent of the illness [71]. In this respect, there are several PCROs not addressed by conventional instruments, such as evaluation of morning stiffness and overall level of disease activity, rating of disease status and course, proxy- or self-assessment of joint involvement and extra-articular symptoms, description of side effects of medications, assessment of therapeutic compliance, and satisfaction with the outcome of the illness, which may provide valuable insights into the influence of the disease and its treatment on a child's health.

A multidimensional questionnaire for the assessment of children with JIA in standard clinical care that incorporates most parent/child-reported outcomes has been recently validated. This tool has been named the Juvenile Arthritis Multidimensional Assessment Report (JAMAR) [72]. The JAMAR includes the following 15 measures/items: (1) assessment of physical function through the JAFS [50]; (2) rating of the intensity of a child's pain on a 21-numbered circle VAS [29]; (3) assessment of HRQOL, through the PRQL [69]; (4) rating of a child's overall well-being on a 21-numbered circle VAS [29]; (5) assessment of the presence of pain or swelling in the following joints or joint groups: cervical spine, lumbosacral spine, shoulders, elbows, wrists, small hand joints, hips, knees, ankles, and small foot joints; (6) assessment of morning stiffness; (7) assessment of extra-articular symptoms (fever and rash); (8) rating of the level of disease activity on a 21-numbered circle VAS [29]; (9) rating of disease status at the time of thc visit as remission, continued activity, or relapse; (10) rating of disease course from previous visit as much improved, slightly improved, stable, slightly worsened, or much worsened; (11) checklist of the medications the child is taking; (12) checklist of side effects of medications; (13) report of difficulties with medication administration; (14) report of disease-related school problems; and (15) a question about satisfaction with the outcome of the illness [73]. The JAMAR is conceived for use as both proxy-report and patient self-report, with the suggested age range of 7–18 years for use as self-report. The questionnaire format has been found to be very user-friendly, easy to understand, and readily responded to by parents and children. It is quick, taking less than 15 min to complete and can be scanned by a health professional for a clinical overview in a few seconds. Scoring of its components can be accomplished in less than 5 min.

The JAMAR has been selected for the assessment of PCROs in a multinational study aimed to investigate the EPidemiology, Treatment and Outcome of Childhood Arthritis throughout the world (EPOCA study) [52]. For the purposes of this study, the JAMAR has been or is currently being translated and cross-culturally adapted and validated in 45 national languages. One of the main objectives of the EPOCA study is to promote regular use of quantitative clinical measures and incorporation of PCROs in routine pediatric rheumatology practice.

Recently, composite disease activity scores for JIA entirely based on parent- or child-reported outcome measures included in the JAMAR were developed. These tools were named the Juvenile Arthritis Parent Assessment Index (JAPAI) and the Juvenile Arthritis Child Assessment Index (JACAI), respectively [74]. The JAPAI and JACAI are composed of the following items: (1) parent/child rating of overall well-being on a 0–10 cm VAS (0=best; 10=worst); (2) parent/child rating of pain intensity on a 0–10 cm VAS (0=no pain; 10=very severe pain); (3) assessment of physical function; and (4) assessment of HRQOL. Scores of physical function and HRQOL tools included in the composite scores are converted to a 0–10 score by means of specific formulae. Two different versions of the JAPAI and JACAI were devised: both the JAPAI-4 and JACAI-4 include all four items, whereas the JAPAI-3 and JACAI-3 include only the first three items (HRQOL assessment is excluded). After score adjustment, the JAPAI and JACAI scores are obtained as the simple linear sum of the scores of their components, which yields a global score of 0–40 for the 4-item versions and of 0–30 for the 3-item versions. The instruments were found to be feasible and to possess both face and content validity; they demonstrated good construct validity in both cross-sectional and longitudinal samples by yielding strong correlations with the JADAS [19] and fair correlations with JIA outcome measures not included in the indices. Furthermore, they exhibited good construct validity, discriminant validity, responsiveness to clinical change, and reliability in a large patient population.

Summary and Conclusions

In spite of their popularity and widespread use, most of the instruments used to assess PCROs have remained essentially research tools and are not routinely administered in most pediatric rheumatology centers. One of the reasons that may explain why these evaluations are uncommonly performed in daily clinical care is the length and complexity of some questionnaires, particularly those used for the assessment of physical function and HRQOL. Therefore, there is the concern that their regular administration may interfere with office routine and time management, with consequent increased costs and time.

Research in the field should therefore aim to simplify the assessment in order to facilitate the widespread use in routine clinical practice while maintaining the scientific integrity of the tools.

References

1. Ravelli A, Martini A. Juvenile idiopathic arthritis. Lancet. 2007;369:767–78.
2. Petty RE, Southwood TR, Manners P, Baum J, Glass DN, Goldenberg J, et al. International League of Associations for Rheumatology classification of juvenile idiopathic arthritis: second revision, Edmonton, 2001. J Rheumatol. 2004;31:390–2.
3. Foster HE, Marshall N, Myers A, Dunkley P, Griffiths ID. Outcome in adults with juvenile idiopathic arthritis—a quality of life study. Arthritis Rheum. 2003;48:767–75.
4. Ruperto N, Ravelli A, Levinson JE, Shear ES, Murray K, Tague BL, et al. Longterm health outcomes and quality of life in American and Italian inception cohorts of patients with juvenile rheumatoid arthritis. II. Early predictors of outcome. J Rheumatol. 1997;24:952–8.
5. Strand CV, Russell AS. WHO/ILAR taskforce on quality of life. J Rheumatol. 1997;24:1630–3.
6. Garcia-Munitis P, Bandeira M, Pistorio A, Magni-Manzoni S, Ruperto N, Schivo A, et al. Level of agreement between children, parents, and physicians in rating pain intensity in juvenile idiopathic arthritis. Arthritis Rheum. 2006;55:177–83.
7. Consolaro A, Vitale R, Pistorio A, Lattanzi B, Ruperto N, Malattia C, et al. Physicians' and parents' ratings of inactive disease are frequently discordant in juvenile idiopathic arthritis. J Rheumatol. 2007;34:1773–6.
8. Barton JL, Imboden J, Graf J, Glidden D, Yelin EH, Schillinger D. Patient-physician discordance in assessments of global disease severity in rheumatoid arthritis. Arthritis Care Res (Hoboken). 2010;62:857–64.
9. Luca N, Feldman BM. Pediatric rheumatology: improving the assessment of children with JIA. Nat Rev Rheumatol. 2011;7:442–4.

10. Berard R, Laxer RM. Improving the quality of care in children with juvenile idiopathic arthritis: a step in the right direction. J Rheumatol. 2011;38:789–90.
11. Brunner HI, Ravelli A. Developing outcome measures for paediatric rheumatic diseases. Best Pract Res Clin Rheumatol. 2009;23:609–24.
12. Brunner HI, Giannini EH. Health-related quality of life in children with rheumatic diseases. Curr Opin Rheumatol. 2003;15:602–12.
13. Filocamo G, Consolaro A, Solari N, Palmisani E, Dalprà S, et al. Recent advances in quantitative assessment of juvenile idiopathic arthritis. Ann Paediatr Rheum. 2012;1:84–96.
14. Duffy CM. Measurement of health status, functional status, and quality of life in children with juvenile idiopathic arthritis: clinical science for the pediatrician. Pediatr Clin North Am. 2005;52:359–72. v.
15. Chira P, Sandborg C. Adolescent rheumatology transitional care: steps to bringing health policy into practice. Rheumatology (Oxford). 2004;43:687–9.
16. Giannini EH, Ruperto N, Ravelli A, Lovell DJ, Felson DT, Martini A. Preliminary definition of improvement in juvenile arthritis. Arthritis Rheum. 1997;40:1202–9.
17. Wallace CA, Giannini EH, Huang B, Itert L, Ruperto N. American College of Rheumatology provisional criteria for defining clinical inactive disease in select categories of juvenile idiopathic arthritis. Arthritis Care Res (Hoboken). 2011;63:929–36.
18. Magni-Manzoni S, Ruperto N, Pistorio A, Sala E, Solari N, Palmisani E, et al. Development and validation of a preliminary definition of minimal disease activity in patients with juvenile idiopathic arthritis. Arthritis Rheum. 2008;59:1120–7.
19. Consolaro A, Ruperto N, Bazso A, Pistorio A, Magni-Manzoni S, Filocamo G, et al. Development and validation of a composite disease activity score for juvenile idiopathic arthritis. Arthritis Rheum. 2009;61:658–66.
20. Ruperto N, Ravelli A, Murray KJ, Lovell DJ, Andersson-Gare B, Feldman BM, et al. Preliminary core sets of measures for disease activity and damage assessment in juvenile systemic lupus erythematosus and juvenile dermatomyositis. Rheumatology (Oxford). 2003;42:1452–9.
21. Ruperto N, Ravelli A, Cuttica R, Espada G, Ozen S, Porras O, et al. The pediatric rheumatology international trials organization criteria for the evaluation of response to therapy in juvenile systemic lupus erythematosus: prospective validation of the disease activity core set. Arthritis Rheum. 2005;52:2854–64.
22. Ruperto N, Ravelli A, Oliveira S, Alessio M, Mihaylova D, Pasic S, et al. The Pediatric Rheumatology International Trials Organization/American College of Rheumatology provisional criteria for the evaluation of response to therapy in juvenile systemic lupus erythematosus. Prospective validation of the definition of improvement. Arthritis Rheum. 2006;55:355–63.
23. Ruperto N, Ravelli A, Pistorio A, Ferriani V, Calvo I, Ganser G, et al. The provisional Pediatric Rheumatology International Trial Organization/American College of Rheumatology/European League Against Rheumatism disease activity core set for the evaluation of response to therapy in juvenile dermatomyositis: a prospective validation study. Arthritis Rheum. 2008;59:4–13.
24. Apaz MT, Saad-Magalhaes C, Pistorio A, Ravelli A, de Oliveira SJ, Marcantoni MB, et al. Health-related quality of life of patients with juvenile dermatomyositis: results from the pediatric rheumatology international trials organisation multinational quality of life cohort study. Arthritis Rheum. 2009;61:509–17.
25. Hasija R, Pistorio A, Ravelli A, Demirkaya E, Khubchandani R, Guseinova D, et al. Approaches for the treatment of new onset and flared juvenile dermatomyositis: an international multicenter PRINTO study. Arthritis Rheum. 2011;63:3142–52.
26. Lazarevic D, Pistorio A, Palmisani E, Miettunen P, Ravelli A, Pilkington C, et al. The PRINTO criteria for clinically inactive disease in juvenile dermatomyositis. Ann Rheum Dis. 2013;72:686–93.
27. Ruperto N, Pistorio A, Ravelli A, Rider LG, Pilkington C, Oliveira S, et al. The pediatric rheumatology international trials organization provisional criteria for the evaluation of response to therapy in juvenile dermatomyositis. Arthritis Care Res. 2010;62:1533–41.

28. Miller FW, Rider LG, Chung YL, Cooper R, Danko K, Farewell V, et al. Proposed preliminary core set measures for disease outcome assessment in adult and juvenile idiopathic inflammatory myopathies. Rheumatology (Oxford). 2001;40:1262–73.
29. Filocamo G, Davi S, Pistorio A, Bertamino M, Ruperto N, Lattanzi B, et al. Evaluation of 21-numbered circle and 10-centimeter horizontal line visual analog scales for physician and parent subjective ratings in juvenile idiopathic arthritis. J Rheumatol. 2010;37:1534–41.
30. Pincus T, Bergman M, Sokka T, Roth J, Swearingen C, Yazici Y. Visual analog scales in formats other than a 10 centimeter horizontal line to assess pain and other clinical data. J Rheumatol. 2008;35:1550–8.
31. Sztajnbok F, Coronel-Martinez DL, Diaz-Maldonado A, Novarini C, Pistorio A, Viola S, et al. Discordance between physician's and parent's global assessments in juvenile idiopathic arthritis. Rheumatology (Oxford). 2007;46:141–5.
32. Miller ML, Ruprecht J, Wang D, Zhou Y, Lales G, McKenna S, et al. Physician assessment of disease activity in JIA subtypes. Analysis of data extracted from electronic medical records. Pediatr Rheumatol Online J. 2011;9:9.
33. Rider LG, Feldman BM, Perez MD, Rennebohm RM, Lindsley CB, Zemel LS, et al. Development of validated disease activity and damage indices for the juvenile idiopathic inflammatory myopathies: I. Physician, parent, and patient global assessments. Juvenile dermatomyositis disease activity collaborative study group. Arthritis Rheum. 1997;40:1976–83.
34. Kimura Y, Walco GA. Treatment of chronic pain in pediatric rheumatic disease. Nat Clin Pract Rheumatol. 2007;3:210–8.
35. Anthony KK, Schanberg LE. Pain in children with arthritis: a review of the current literature. Arthritis Rheum. 2003;49:272–9.
36. Consolaro A, Ravelli A. Paediatric rheumatology: juvenile idiopathic arthritis—are biologic agents effective for pain? Nat Rev Rheumatol. 2013;9:447–8.
37. Prince FH, Geerdink LM, Borsboom GJ, Twilt M, van Rossum MA, Hoppenreijs EP, et al. Major improvements in health-related quality of life during the use of etanercept in patients with previously refractory juvenile idiopathic arthritis. Ann Rheum Dis. 2010;69:138–42.
38. Ruperto N, Lovell DJ, Li T, Sztajnbok F, Goldenstein-Schainberg C, Scheinberg M, et al. Abatacept improves health-related quality of life, pain, sleep quality, and daily participation in subjects with juvenile idiopathic arthritis. Arthritis Care Res (Hoboken). 2010;62:1542–51.
39. Ruperto N, Ravelli A, Pistorio A, Malattia C, Cavuto S, Gado-West L, et al. Cross-cultural adaptation and psychometric evaluation of the childhood health assessment questionnaire (CHAQ) and the child health questionnaire (CHQ) in 32 countries. Review of the general methodology. Clin Exp Rheumatol. 2001;19:S1–9.
40. Gutierrez-Suarez R, Pistorio A, Cespedes CA, Norambuena X, Flato B, Rumba I, et al. Health-related quality of life of patients with juvenile idiopathic arthritis coming from 3 different geographic areas. The PRINTO multinational quality of life cohort study. Rheumatology. 2007;46:314–20.
41. Oliveira S, Ravelli A, Pistorio A, Castell E, Malattia C, Prieur AM, et al. Proxy-reported health-related quality of life of patients with juvenile idiopathic arthritis: the pediatric rheumatology international trials organization multinational quality of life cohort study. Arthritis Rheum. 2007;57:35–43.
42. Meiorin S, Pistorio A, Ravelli A, Iusan SM, Filocamo G, Trail L, et al. Validation of the childhood health assessment questionnaire in active juvenile systemic lupus erythematosus. Arthritis Rheum. 2008;59:1112–9.
43. Saad-Magalhaes C, Pistorio A, Ravelli A, Filocamo G, Viola S, Brik R, et al. Does removal of AIDS/devices and help make a difference in the childhood health assessment questionnaire disability index? Ann Rheum Dis. 2010;69:82–7.
44. Vilca I, Munitis PG, Pistorio A, Ravelli A, Buoncompagni A, Bica B, et al. Predictors of poor response to methotrexate in polyarticular-course juvenile idiopathic arthritis: analysis of the PRINTO methotrexate trial. Ann Rheum Dis. 2010;69:1479–83.
45. Huber AM, Hicks JE, Lachenbruch PA, Perez MD, Zemel LS, Rennebohm RM, et al. Validation of the childhood health assessment questionnaire in the juvenile idiopathic myopathies.

Juvenile dermatomyositis disease activity collaborative study group. J Rheumatol. 2001;28:1106–11.
46. Brunner HI, Klein-Gitelman MS, Miller MJ, Barron A, Baldwin N, Trombley M, et al. Minimal clinically important differences of the childhood health assessment questionnaire. J Rheumatol. 2005;32:150–61.
47. Ruperto N, Ravelli A, Migliavacca D, Viola S, Pistorio A, Duarte C, et al. Responsiveness of clinical measures in children with oligoarticular juvenile chronic arthritis. J Rheumatol. 1999;26:1827–30.
48. Dempster H, Porepa M, Young N, Feldman BM. The clinical meaning of functional outcome scores in children with juvenile arthritis. Arthritis Rheum. 2001;44:1768–74.
49. Lam C, Young N, Marwaha J, McLimont M, Feldman BM. Revised versions of the childhood health assessment questionnaire (CHAQ) are more sensitive and suffer less from a ceiling effect. Arthritis Rheum. 2004;51:881–9.
50. Filocamo G, Sztajnbok F, Cespedes-Cruz A, Magni-Manzoni S, Pistorio A, Viola S, et al. Development and validation of a new short and simple measure of physical function for juvenile idiopathic arthritis. Arthritis Rheum. 2007;57:913–20.
51. Meiorin S, Filocamo G, Pistorio A, Magni-Manzoni S, Sztajnbok F, Cespedes-Cruz A, et al. Impact of involvement of individual joint groups on subdimensions of functional ability scales in juvenile idiopathic arthritis. Clin Exp Rheumatol. 2009;27:527–33.
52. Consolaro A, Ruperto N, Filocamo G, Lanni S, Bracciolini G, Garrone M, et al. Seeking insights into the epidemiology, treatment and outcome of childhood arthritis through a multinational collaborative effort: introduction of the EPOCA study. Pediatr Rheumatol Online J. 2012;10:39.
53. Lovell DJ, Howe S, Shear E, Hartner S, McGirr G, Schulte M, et al. Development of a disability measurement tool for juvenile rheumatoid arthritis. The juvenile arthritis functional assessment scale. Arthritis Rheum. 1989;32:1390–5.
54. Howe S, Levinson J, Shear E, Hartner S, McGirr G, Schulte M, et al. Development of a disability measurement tool for juvenile rheumatoid arthritis. The juvenile arthritis functional assessment report for children and their parents. Arthritis Rheum. 1991;34:873–80.
55. Wright FV, Kimber JL, Law M, Goldsmith CH, Crombie V, Dent P. The juvenile arthritis functional status index (JASI): a validation study. J Rheumatol. 1996;23:1066–79.
56. Iglesias MJ, Cuttica RJ, Herrera CM, Micelotta M, Pringe A, Brusco MI. Design and validation of a new scale to assess the functional ability in children with juvenile idiopathic arthritis (JIA). Clin Exp Rheumatol. 2006;24:713–8.
57. Gong GW, Barrera M, Beyene J, Bhat S, Carcao M, Lord S, et al. The gap study (GapS) interview—developing a process to determine the meaning and determinants of quality of life in children with arthritis and rheumatic disease. Clin Exp Rheumatol. 2007;25:486–93.
58. Adunuri NR, Feldman BM. Critical appraisal of studies measuring quality of life in juvenile idiopathic arthritis. Arthritis Care Res (Hoboken). 2015;67:880–4.
59. DJ, Ruperto N, Mouy R, Paz E, Rubio-Pérez N, Silva CA, et al. Long-term safety, efficacy, and quality of life in patients with juvenile idiopathic arthritis treated with intravenous abatacept for up to seven years. Arthritis Rheumatol. 2015;67:275–970.
60. Cespedes-Cruz A, Gutierrez-Suarez R, Pistorio A, Ravelli A, Loy A, Murray KJ, et al. Methotrexate improves the health-related quality of life of children with juvenile idiopathic arthritis. Ann Rheum Dis. 2008;67:309–14.
61. Manners PJ, Diepeveen DA. Prevalence of juvenile chronic arthritis in a population of 12-year-old children in urban Australia. Pediatrics. 1996;98:84–90.
62. Tucker LB. Whose life is it anyway? Understanding quality of life in children with rheumatic diseases. J Rheumatol. 2000;27:8–11.
63. Burgos-Vargas R. Assessment of quality of life in children with rheumatic disease. J Rheumatol. 1999;26:1432–5.
64. Coulton CJ, Zborowsky E, Lipton J, Newman AJ. Assessment of the reliability and validity of the arthritis impact measurement scales for children with juvenile arthritis. Arthritis Rheum. 1987;30:819–24.

65. Duffy CM, Arsenault L, Duffy KN, Paquin JD, Strawczynski H. The juvenile arthritis quality of life questionnaire—development of a new responsive index for juvenile rheumatoid arthritis and juvenile spondyloarthritides. J Rheumatol. 1997;24:738–46.
66. Landgraf JM, Abetz L, Ware JE. The CHQ user's manual. 1st ed. Boston: The Health Institute, New England Medical Center; 1996.
67. Varni JW, Seid M, Knight TS, Burwinkle T, Brown J, Szer IS. The PedsQL(TM) in pediatric rheumatology—reliability, validity, and responsiveness of the pediatric quality of life inventory(TM) generic core scales and rheumatology module. Arthritis Rheum. 2002;46:714–25.
68. Arkela-Kautiainen M, Haapasaari J, Kautiainen H, Vilkkumaa I, Malkia E, Leirisalo-Repo M. Favourable social functioning and health related quality of life of patients with JIA in early adulthood. Ann Rheum Dis. 2005;64:875–80.
69. Filocamo G, Schiappapietra B, Bertamino M, Pistorio A, Ruperto N, Magni-Manzoni S, et al. A new short and simple health-related quality of life measurement for paediatric rheumatic diseases: initial validation in juvenile idiopathic arthritis. Rheumatology (Oxford). 2010;49:1272–80.
70. Bulatovic M, Heijstek MW, Verkaaik M, Van Dijkhuizen EH, Armbrust W, Hoppenreijs EP, et al. High prevalence of methotrexate intolerance in juvenile idiopathic arthritis: development and validation of a methotrexate intolerance severity score. Arthritis Rheum. 2011;63:2007–13.
71. Filocamo G, Consolaro A, Ferrari C, Ravelli A. Introducing new tools for assessment of parent- and child-reported outcomes in paediatric rheumatology practice: a work in progress. Clin Exp Rheumatol. 2013;31:964–8.
72. Filocamo G, Consolaro A, Schiappapietra B, Dalpra S, Lattanzi B, Magni-Manzoni S, et al. A new approach to clinical care of juvenile idiopathic arthritis: the juvenile arthritis multidimensional assessment report. J Rheumatol. 2011;38:938–53.
73. Filocamo G, Consolaro A, Schiappapietra B, Ruperto N, Pistorio A, Solari N, et al. Parent and child acceptable symptom state in juvenile idiopathic arthritis. J Rheumatol. 2012;39:856–63.
74. Consolaro A, Ruperto N, Pistorio A, Lattanzi B, Solari N, Galasso R, et al. Development and initial validation of composite parent- and child-centered disease assessment indices for juvenile idiopathic arthritis. Arthritis Care Res (Hoboken). 2011;63:1262–70.

Chapter 9
PROMs for Gouty Arthritis

Jasvinder Singh and Nipam Shah

Gout: The Disease and Its Manifestations

Gout is a debilitating, inflammatory arthritis. Gout is characterized by hyperuricemia and the related monosodium urate (MSU) crystal deposition within the joints and other tissues. MSU crystal deposition is associated with inflammatory arthritis, which leads to severe joint and bursa pain, subcutaneous deposits of urate (tophi), formation of urate calculi in kidneys and chronic systemic inflammation [1]. Gout can be acute or chronic in nature and is associated with substantial morbidity and impact on patient's health-related quality of life (HRQOL). The detection of needlelike MSU crystals in the joint or synovial fluid or aspirated material from a tophus showing strong negative birefringence by polarized microscopy is the diagnostic of gout [2].

Acute gout—also referred to as gout attacks, gouty arthritis, or gout flares—can involve synovial structures such as joints and tendons as well as bursa. Acute gout is induced by inflammatory cell reaction to joints/bursa associated with MSU crystal deposition. The clinical manifestations include acute inflammation joints/bursa associated with moderate to severe pain and activity limitation. The acute attacks involve peripheral joints and structures more commonly than the centrally located structures. A majority of the acute gout attacks involve a single joint. The involvement of metatarsophalangeal joint, especially the first metatarsophalangeal (MTP), also referred to as podagra, is a hallmark of gout.

Persistent clinical manifestations, also referred to as chronic gouty arthritis, occur due to chronic inflammation related to the continued deposition of MSU crystals and are the natural evolution of untreated hyperuricemia in patients with gout. Chronic gout is characterized by symmetric inflammatory polyarthritis associated

J. Singh (✉) • N. Shah
Department of Medicine, University of Alabama at Birmingham,
510 20th Street South, FOT 805B, Birmingham, AL 35294, USA
e-mail: Jasvinder.md@gmail.com

Y. El Miedany (ed.), *Patient Reported Outcome Measures in Rheumatic Diseases*,
DOI 10.1007/978-3-319-32851-5_9

with joint limitation, joint swelling, and deformity. Up to 50 % of patients with chronic gouty arthropathy have structural damage on radiographs [1]. Palpable tophi occur in various locations such as olecranon bursa, ear, and various joints. Urate nephropathy is a complication resulting from urate stones seen in 20 % of patients with gout [2].

Systemic manifestations including low-grade fever may also be seen, especially with a polyarticular gout flare. Chronic systemic inflammation, occurring with chronic uncontrolled gout, may also put patients at risk for increased cardiovascular morbidity and mortality, a topic of recent interest [3–5]. Regardless of whether gout is a risk factor for cardiovascular disease or is commonly associated with it due to a common underlying mechanism/risk factors [6], its increased prevalence in patients with gout is a cause for additional concern in patients with gout.

Due to multiple manifestations of gout, and its significant impact on HRQOL, studies of assessment of patient reported outcomes (PROs) in gout are key to our understanding its true impact on patient lives and associated morbidity [7, 8].

Patient Reported Outcomes: Definitions, Initiatives, and the Difference Between Outcomes and Outcome Measures

The term PRO was first coined in 2000 in order to avoid the confusion surrounding the term "quality of life" in the regulatory process as a part of clinical trials [9]. Historically, the use of PRO measures has been far less common in clinical practice than in clinical trials, where PROs are often selected as trial outcome measures [10].

The U.S. Food and Drug Administration (FDA) defined PRO as "a measurement of any aspect of a patient's health status that comes directly from the patient (i.e., without the interpretation of the patient's responses by a physician or anyone else)" [11, 12]. An FDA PRO consensus group defined PRO as a broad term that includes direct subjective assessment by the patient of elements of their health including: symptoms, function, well-being, perceptions about treatment, satisfaction with care received, and satisfaction with professional communication [13].

Patient Reported Outcomes Measures Information System (PROMIS), a leading research initiative by the National Institutes of Health (NIH), defined PRO as denoting health data that is provided by the patient through a system of reporting. A patient reported outcome is basically a patient's feedback on their feelings or what they are able to do as they are dealing with chronic diseases or conditions. PROs can also be measured when patients are undergoing treatment or are participating in a clinical trial [14]. Others have defined PRO as an umbrella term that can be applied to an array of different outcomes, including symptoms, functioning, perceived health status, and HRQOL [15].

Several recent efforts have highlighted the importance of measuring PROs as study outcomes. PROMIS is a system of highly reliable, precise measures of patient reported health status for physical, mental, and social well-being. PROMIS provides a "universal language" for evaluating health conditions, which are relevant to both the clinicians and researchers. Use of these standardized tools to measure health concepts helps in making comparisons across various populations, clinical practices, and research studies [16].

Patient Reported Outcomes vs. Patient Reported Outcome Measures

PROs are directly reported by patients without involvement of the clinician and these outcomes are measured in absolute terms. Patient reported outcome measures (PROMs) are the tools used to measure the PROs. These tools are validated questionnaires, which evaluate the patient's experience of symptoms, quality of care, and health-related behaviors. Thus, PROMs are the measurement of PROs. For example, pain severity is a PRO and pain Visual Analog Scale (VAS), a tool used to measure pain severity, is a PROM [17].

The Significance and Need for Patient Reported Outcomes in Gout

Why Are Patient Reported Outcomes Important in Gout?

There are several key reasons why PROs are important in chronic conditions such as gout. First, PROs help in detecting physical and/or psychological problems overlooked in day-to-day clinical assessments [18]. In absence of PROs, detection of these problems would likely require detailed communication between the physician and the patient. Time constraints of clinical encounters make this challenging. In many cases, even with availability of time during a clinic visit, these aspects of patient suffering and impact may go unreported and undetected. Thus, PROs facilitate this communication [18] and as standardized measures, help in detecting the progression of disease and also provide impact of prescribed treatment [18].

Second, physicians and patients may have different priorities regarding disease outcomes, as goals of treatment. This is particularly important in condition such as gout that has significant impact on pain and function, and mobility and affects middle-aged and sometimes young patients. For example, patients want physicians to ask about their feelings and the impact of gout on work productivity or social life more than about their physical examination or laboratory finding, which physicians might be more interested in [19]. Establishing a common understanding may be important for meeting patients' needs and for improving their satisfaction with health care and adherence to treatment. PRO measurement also may be used to monitor outcomes as a strategy for quality improvement or to reward presumed superior care in clinical practice [18].

Third, as a chronic disease, gout has a widespread impact. It not only affects a patient's life and his/her work, but also the family, the society, and the health care system [20–23]. Systematic reviews have demonstrated that gout has significant impact on the activities of daily living and HRQOL [24, 25]. Patients with gout suffer from severe pain, dependency, work disability, dietary restrictions, and social isolation [18]. This impact may differ by race/ethnicity and gender [23]. For example, compared to Caucasians with gout, African-Americans are more likely to report dietary restrictions due to gout, associated emotional burden, severe pain during gout flares, the need for canes/crutches during flares, and gout bringing their day to a halt [23]. Whether some of these differences may be partially attributable to lower adherence to urate-lowering therapy (ULT) in African-Americans is unclear [26].

Gout increases the dependency on family members for daily activities of life during the gout flares, but also due to the disability associated with chronic gout [23, 27]. Gout is associated with significantly higher number of days absent from work compared to those without gout in United States [28]. Also, the overall productivity at work is affected by gout. Employees with gout processed 3.5 % fewer units of work per hour compared to employees without gout [29]. Gout also leads to significant burden on the health care system. This burden is attributed to increase in the number of hospitalizations and cost of care. As per a U.S. Bone and Joint Decade report, gout and other crystal arthropathies accounted for 1.5 % of the 1.17 million nonfederal, short stay hospitalizations in 2007 [30]. Gout led to 2.3 million ambulatory care visits annually from 2001 to 2005 in the USA [31]. Using data from the Medical Expenditure Panel Survey (MEPS) a nationally representative survey of the US civilian, non-institutionalized population, the estimated all-cause annual cost of gout in the USA was $31.8 billion or $11,663 per person, using 2011 inflation adjusted dollars. Another study estimated that the estimated cost attributable to gout was 24 % of all-cause gout expenditures ($7.7 billion) [31]. Thus, in addition to associated personal and family suffering, gout is associated with significant societal and health care burden.

Lastly, PROs have been shown to have higher sensitivity to effects of treatment compared to physician reported measures in clinical trials [32]. PROs differ from physician reported outcomes in terms of disease/symptom presence, symptom frequency, and symptom severity, and therefore may lead to discordant reports [33]. For example, fatigue and symptom severity reporting were moderately discordant between physicians and patients [34, 35]. For conditions that are associated with pain, disability, and HRQOL deficits, such as gout, the best assessments for these outcomes are likely PROMs, rather than physician reported measures.

Recent Advances in PROs and PROMs in Gout

The Outcomes Measure in Rheumatology (OMERACT) Perspective

The Outcomes Measure in Rheumatology (OMERACT) gout special interest group (SIG) at the OMERACT-seven workshop identified five core domains for acute gout and nine core domains for chronic gout along with the instruments (core set for acute and chronic gout; Figs. 9.1 and 9.2). Pain, inflammation (joint swelling, joint tenderness), function, patient global, and safety were the five core outcome domains identified for acute gout (Fig. 9.1). Pain assessed by visual analog scale (VAS) or 4-point Likert scale, joint swelling or tenderness scored from 4-point Likert point scale, and patient global assessment on 5-point Likert scale were validated PROMs

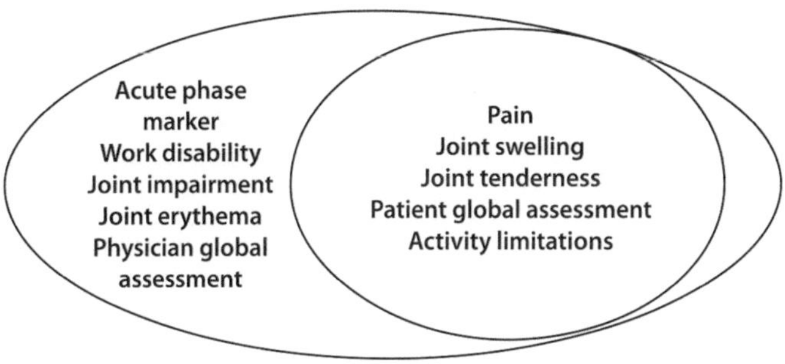

Fig. 9.1 Acute gout studies. Proposed outcome domains in studies of acute gout (domains in the inner oval are mandatory; in the outer oval, discretionary). Reprinted with permission from Schumacher HR, Taylor W, Edwards L, Grainger R, Schlesinger N, Dalbeth N, et al. Outcome domains for studies of acute and chronic gout. J Rheumatol 2009;36(10);2342–2345.

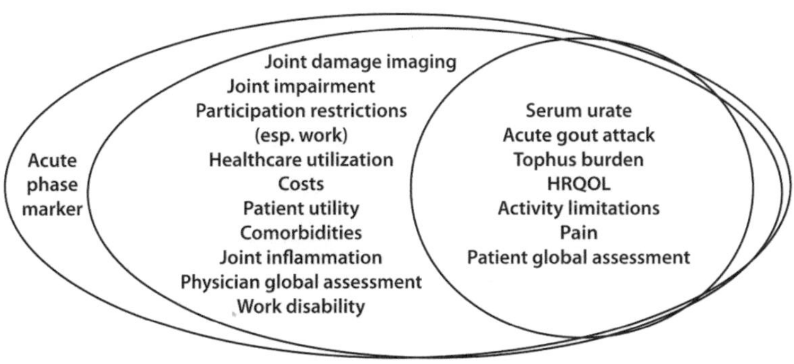

Fig. 9.2 Chronic gout studies. Proposed outcome domains in studies of chronic gout (domains in the inner circle are mandatory; in the next oval, discretionary; and in the outer oval, for research). Reprinted with permission from Schumacher HR, Taylor W, Edwards L, Grainger R, Schlesinger N, Dalbeth N, et al. Outcome domains for studies of acute and chronic gout. J Rheumatol 2009;36(10);2342–2345.

for the respective PROs at OMERACT-11 [36]. Function assessment by Health Assessment Questionnaire-Disability Index (HAQ-DI) was not endorsed as a valid measure, citing the need for more robust data [37]. Also, measures of non-core domains such as work disability, joint erythema, acute phase markers, and physician global still need validation [37].

The core set domains for chronic gout are serum urate, gout flare recurrence, tophus regression, joint damage imaging, health related quality of life, function, patient global assessment, participation, safety, and tolerability [38] (Fig. 9.2). VAS for pain and patient global, Short Form-36 (SF-36) for pain, and HAQ-DI for activity limitation were endorsed PROMs for these PROs [8]. Gout assessment questionnaire (GAQ) v2.0 for chronic gout needs future research and validation according to the discussions at OMERACT-10 [8].

Some concerns by patients with gout have emerged in the recent qualitative work, which had not emerged in previous qualitative work done at OMERACT. Therefore, these were not taken into account while developing the current gout core set domains endorsed by OMERACT. In particular, important areas identified to consider as potential domains or subdomains for the future are: difficulty wearing shoes, having to undertake a restrictive diet, and interference with sleep and sexual activity were ranked highly by patients and not included in OMERACT domains [39].

Each PROM for PRO endorsed for acute and chronic gout has been tested for validity, discriminative ability, and is feasible in randomized controlled trials (RCTs) in gout. The validation data for each of these measures is presented in Table 9.1 [8]. All the measures shown in Table 9.1 have been endorsed during the OMERACT gout workshops except GAQ v2.0, which was shown to have poor internal consistency and low validity [8, 40]. The scale of measurement, mean/median scores, and effect sizes for these PROMs are presented in Table 9.2 [7, 20, 21, 36, 41–45].

In the sections that follow, we describe the validity data for the PROMs for gout endorsed for measurement of each PRO, such as pain, function, HRQOL, mobility, and satisfaction.

PROMs for Pain

Pain is considered the fifth vital sign [46] and one of the commonest symptoms in the general population [47]. Due to its critical importance, it is measured at every patient encounter in the USA, alongside pulse rate, blood pressure, respiratory rate, and temperature. Pain is a subjective phenomenon and the current gold standard is the patient-report. Pain experience is unique to each person and is influenced by the patient's comorbidity and emotional and psychosocial experiences. Gout with its characteristic acute flares and chronic, inflammatory arthritis presentation has pain as a cardinal feature. The following sections summarize the data on pain outcome measures in patients with chronic and acute gout. The effects of various treatment regimens on VAS pain scores for acute and chronic gout are summarized in Table 9.3 [48–52] and Table 9.4 [9, 53], respectively.

Table 9.1 Validation data presented for patient reported outcomes in chronic gout

	Truth				Discrimination		
Instruments	Face validity	Content validity	Convergent/divergent	Internal inconsistency	Between treatments	Sensitivity to change	Feasibility
VAS pain	✓	✓	✓	✓	✓	✓	✓
SF-36 pain	✓	✓	✓	✓	✓	✓	✓
Patient global	✓	✓	✓	✓	✓	✓	✓
HAQ-DI	✓	✓	✓	✓	✓	✓	✓
GAQ v2.0	✓	✓	?[a]	?[b]	Not assessed	✓	?[c]

Reprinted with permission from Singh JA, Taylor WJ, Simon LS, Khanna PP, Stamp LK, McQueen FM, et al. Patient-reported outcomes in chronic gout: A report from omeract 10. The Journal of rheumatology. 2011 Jul;38(7):1452–1457. [8]

✓ Measure has been validated; ? uncertain

VAS Visual Analog Scale, *SF-36* Short Form-36, *HAQ-DI* Health Assessment Questionnaire-Disability Index, *GAQ v2.0* Gout Assessment questionnaire, version 2.0

[a]Correlations with SF-36 physical and mental component summary scores were low, raising issues regarding convergent validity

[b]Low for Unmet Gout Need subscale, but high for Gout Concern Overall and other subscales of the Gout Impact Section (GIS) of GAQ v2.0

[c]Feasibility has not been tested in research or clinical use settings

Table 9.2 Instruments for patient reported outcome measurements in gout

Instrument	Scale	Mean score	Effect size
VAS [7]	0–100		0.34
NRS [36]	0–10		1.62
HAQ [20]	0–3	0.59	0.62
GAQ [41]	0–100		
SF-36 [42]	0–100	40.37 (PCS)	0.91 to 1.09 (across all SF-36 domains)
		52.16 (MCS)	
SF-36 PF-10 [43]	0–100	61.96	
EQ-5D [21]	1–3	0.74	
SF-6D [21, 44]	0.29–1.00	0.67	
Mobility scale [45]	0–80	75.5 (median)	

VAS Visual Analog Scale, *NRS* Numeric Rating Scale, *HAQ-DI* Health Assessment Questionnaire-Disability Index, *GAQ v2.0* Gout Assessment questionnaire, version 2.0, *SF-36* Short Form-36, *SF-36 PF-10* Short Form-36 Physical Functioning Subscale, *EQ-5D* EuroQol-5 dimensions, *SF-6D* Short Form-6 Dimensions

Table 9.3 Visual analog scale scores for acute gout

Drugs/drug comparisons	Outcome	VAS score change/absolute in group 1	VAS score change/absolute in group 2	Mean change in VAS scores
Oral prednisolone plus IM Normal Saline (Grp 1) vs. oral indomethacin plus IM diclofenac (Grp 2) [48]	Pain at rest at 2 h	−9.5 mm per hour	−6.4 mm per hour	MD: 3.2 mm per hour[a]
				95 % CI: −0.78 to 7.14
$N=90$				$p=0.12$
	Pain with activity at 2 h	−19.2 mm per hour	−20.3 mm per hour	MD: 1.1 mm per hour[a]
				95 % CI: −5.34 to 3.24
				$p=0.63$
	Pain at rest after 2 weeks	−0.7 mm per day	−0.3 mm per day	MD: 0.5 mm per day[a]
				95 % CI: 0.03 to 0.89
				$p=0.04$
	Pain with activity after 2 weeks	−2.9 mm per day	−1.7 mm per day	MD: 1.2 mm per day[a]
				95 % CI: 0.44 to 2.00
				$p=0.026$
Oral prednisolone and colchicine vs. oral prednisolone and colchicine with topical ice [49]	Pain after 1 week	44.2 mm	77.5 mm	$p=0.021$[b]

(continued)

Table 9.3 (continued)

Drugs/drug comparisons	Outcome	VAS score change/absolute in group 1	VAS score change/absolute in group 2	Mean change in VAS scores
Subcutaneous canakinumab vs. intramuscular triamcinolone acetonide [50]	Pain at 72 h	35.7 mm	25.0 mm	Mean difference: 10.7 mm[c]
$N=443$				95 % CI: −15.4 to −6.0; $p<0.0001$
Drugs/drug comparisons	*Outcome*	*VAS score pretreatment*	*VAS score posttreatment*	*Mean change in VAS scores*
Intra-articular triamcinolone acetonide pre vs. post	Pain at 48 h	NR		Mean reduction from 88 (pre) to 0 (post)
$N=19$				
Subcutaneous anakinra pre vs. post [51]	Pain reduction at day 4	Pre: 73.5 mm	Post: 25.0 mm	Mean reduction: 48.5 mm[d]
		IQR: 70.0 to 80.0	IQR: 20.0 to 32.5	
$N=40$				$p<0.0001$
Intramuscular ketorolac pre vs. post [52]	Pain reduction at 90 min	Pre: 64.3 mm	Post: 10.1 mm	Mean reduction: 54.2 mm[e]
$N=9$				$p<0.01$

VAS visual analog scale, *MD* mean difference, *NR* not reported, *NSAIDs* nonsteroidal anti inflammatory drugs, *NNTB* number needed to treat to benefit

[a]The difference in mean pain score was at no time more than 13 mm, which was unlikely to be clinically relevant according to the authors

[b]4 of 16 patients required a second I-injection (I=intervention), 9 of 14 a second C injection (C=control). 3 patients required a third C-injection

[c]Absolute improvement: 11 % lower with canakinumab (15 to 6 % lower). Relative % change: 14 % more improvement with canakinumab (8 to 21 % more improvement) 2 NNTB 7 (95 % CI 5 to 12)

[d]Retrospective study

[e]No side effects were reported

Validation Data for VAS Pain in Acute Gout

Several studies have investigated whether VAS pain is a valid measure in acute gout by examining the effect of various therapies on VAS pain. Studies compared various treatments to each other or examined pre-to-post treatment change in VAS pain with a single intervention. These studies (summarized in the section that follows) have demonstrated the discriminative ability of pain measures in gout for different treatments and for different states with the same treatment.

Effect of treatments of acute gout on VAS pain (Table 9.3): A randomized study (RCT) compared oral prednisolone with oral diclofenac plus indomethacin in 90 patients with acute gout. Mean age was 65 years. After 2 weeks, the mean difference

Table 9.4 Visual analog scale scores in studies of chronic gout

Study/drug comparison	Outcome	VAS scores, placebo group/phase	VAS scores, intervention group/phase
Pegloticase biweekly vs. placebo [9]	Pain at 25 weeks	MCID for pain[a] achieved: 27 %	MCID for pain[a] achieved: 55 %
N=212			
Rilonacept vs. placebo cross-over study [53]	Pain reduction at 8 weeks	Median reduction: 50 mm	Median reduction: 13 mm[b]
N=10			

VAS Visual Analog Scale, *MCID* Minimal Clinically Important Difference
[a]MCID pain was defined as ≥10 points on a 100 mm VAS
[b]One withdrawal due to serious injection site erythema and induration

in pain reduction between the two groups was 0.5 mm per day for pain at rest and 1.2 mm for pain with activity, statistically significant during the follow phase (rest: $p=0.04$; activity: $p=0.026$) [48]. Thus, VAS pain has discriminant ability to distinguish between two effective therapies for acute gout.

A prospective study evaluated 19 patients with acute gout randomized into two groups, oral prednisolone with colchicine and oral prednisolone with colchicine and topical ice. Mean VAS pain (0–100 mm) reduction with oral prednisolone and colchicine treatment was 48.6 mm after 1 week (pretreatment: 96.0 mm; posttreatment: 47.4 mm); topical ice led to an *additional* reduction of 29 mm in pain VAS compared to control group (pretreatment: 85.5 mm; posttreatment: 8.0 mm). At 1 week, the VAS pain was significantly lower in the ice treatment group compared with the control ($p=0.021$) [49].

Two RCTs compared subcutaneous canakinumab 150 mg with intramuscular triamcinolone acetonide 40 mg in patients with acute gouty arthritis ($n=443$). Mean patient age was 53 years. The mean difference in VAS pain between canakinumab and triamcinolone acetonide groups posttreatment was 10.7 mm at 72 h (35.7 mm vs. 25.0 mm), with statistically significantly greater reduction in VAS pain with canakinumab than triamcinolone acetonide ($p<0.0001$). The mean difference was statistically significantly lower for canakinumab compared to triamcinolone acetonide at 24 h (mean difference: −10.2 (42.6 mm vs. 52.8 mm; $p=0.001$) [50].

Pre- and posttreatment studies of Pain VAS in acute gout (Table 9.3): 19 patients with acute gout received a single dose of intra-articular triamcinolone acetonide, which resulted in reduction in pain VAS from 88 mm (range: 82–93) at baseline to 0 mm (range: 0–21) at 48 h [54]. In a multicenter retrospective study of 40 patients who received subcutaneous anakinra for gouty arthritis, VAS pain score statistically significantly decreased from 73.5 mm (range: 70–80) at baseline to 25.0 mm (range: 20–32.5) at 4 days ($p<0.0001$) [51]. Nine patients with acute gouty arthritis were treated with intramuscular ketorolac injection. VAS pain decreased by 54.2 mm from 64.3 to 10.1 mm at 90 min, a statistically significant ($p<0.01$) [52].

Validation Data for VAS Pain in Chronic Gout

Construct Validity: VAS pain has statistically significant moderate correlation with tender joints, SF-36 Physical Component Score (PCS) and HAQ-DI scores (correlation coefficients, 0.42–0.56); and statistically significant low correlation with swollen joints and SF-36 Mental Component Summary (MCS) (correlation coefficient, 0.30–0.36) [7]. Moderate correlations were observed with SF-36 bodily pain subscale [7].

Reliability: Inter-rater or intra-rater assessments were not available for VAS pain in gout [7]. Intraclass correlation coefficient was 0.97 indicating high reliability of VAS pain for acute pain measurement in non-gout conditions and pain ratings are reproducible 90 % of the times [55].

Clinically meaningful change thresholds: The effect size (ES) and standardized response mean (SRM) for VAS pain in chronic gout were 0.34 and 0.30, respectively [7]. Minimal clinically important difference (MCID), moderate improvement, and really important difference (RID) thresholds for VAS pain scores were 22, 30, and 50 units, respectively, on a 0–100 mm scale [7].

Responsiveness to Change for VAS pain in chronic gout (Table 9.4): Chronic refractory gout patients were treated with pegloticase biweekly, pegloticase monthly vs. placebo ($N=212$; mean age, 55 years). At 25 weeks, the proportion of patients with pain improvement greater than or equal to MCID of ≥10 points on a 100 mm VAS was 55 % in pegloticase biweekly vs. 27 % in placebo, a statistically significantly result ($p=0.01$) [9]. A non-randomized crossover 8-week study compared rilonacept to placebo ($N=10$; mean age, 61 years) in patients with chronic active gouty arthritis. Median VAS pain scores decreased statistically significantly from baseline to 8 weeks, from 5.0 at baseline to 2.8 in placebo phase to 1.3 in rilonacept phase ($p<0.049$) [53].

Validation Data for Numeric Rating Scale Pain

Similar, but less robust data are available for Numeric Rating Scale (NRS) pain (0–10) as a PROM for gout. NRS pain had low correlation with activity limitations (correlation coefficient: 0.39). The effect size with NRS scale was 1.62 [36]. In a randomized trial of 152 patients with acute gout, the mean change in NRS pain from baseline to posttreatment was 4.3 with indomethacin and 1.8 with rilonacept (mean difference, 2.5), i.e., 25 % less improvement in pain with rilonacept [56].

In summary, VAS pain is a valid PROM in acute and chronic gout. NRS pain has similar properties, and more validation data are needed. These PROMs can differentiate between therapies as was evident in various treatment comparisons that showed statistically significant differences in PROMs in acute gout. A few examples include the following: (1) oral prednisolone was as effective as nonsteroidal anti-inflammatory drugs (NSAIDs) in the treatment of acute gout for reducing pain severity; (2) topical ice in combination with oral prednisolone and colchicine is a better modality than prednisolone and colchicine for the treatment of acute gout, since it is associated with greater VAS pain; (3) subcutaneous anakinra and intramuscular ketorolac were associated with statistically significant reductions in VAS pain scores in patients with acute gout; (4) rilonacept was associated with statistically significant reductions in VAS pain in patients with chronic gout compared to placebo whereas pain scores did not significantly differ by allopurinol use in chronic gouty arthritis patients; and (5) biweekly pegloticase was associated with greater VAS pain reduction in chronic gout patients compared to monthly pegloticase.

PROMs for Functional Limitation

Health Assessment Questionnaire-Disability Index (HAQ-DI)

HAQ-DI is a commonly used functional assessment in rheumatic conditions. Each item on HAQ-DI is scored from 0 to 3, with 0 being "no difficulty" to 3 being "unable to do [57]."

Validation Data for HAQ-DI in Chronic Gout

Construct Validity: HAQ-DI score was associated with disease characteristics such as tender joints, swollen joints, joints with limited mobility, and presence of tophi [20]. In a multicenter cohort study, data were collected at baseline and 6 months later for patients with gout. HAQ had high negative correlation (–0.69) with SF-36 physical functioning and bodily pain subscales, but low negative correlation with SF-36 mental health subscale (–0.23) [20]. The mean (±SD) HAQ-DI score was 0.59 ± 0.77 and the mean difference between HAQ-DI at baseline and at 6 months was 0.31 ± 0.58, the effect size being 0.62 [20]. The HAQ-DI improvements in patients with chronic gout on various treatment regimens are described in the following paragraph.

In another study, patients with chronic refractory gout were allocated to one of the three intervention groups: pegloticase biweekly, pegloticase monthly, and placebo. At 25 weeks, the proportion of patients with HAQ-DI greater than or equal to a minimum clinically important difference of ≥ 10 points on 100 mm-VAS was 45 %, 48 %, and 16 %, respectively [9], a difference that was statistically significant between pegloticase biweekly and placebo ($p < 0.003$) and pegloticase monthly and placebo ($p < 0.001$).

PROMs for Health Related Quality of Life (HRQOL)

Table 9.5 shows reliability, validity, and responsiveness to change for SF-36, PROMIS PF-10, and HAQ-DI as well as GAQ. A recent systematic review also summarized this evidence [58].

Generic HRQOL

SF-36 Scores

SF-36 consists of 36 items evaluating eight subscales with scores ranging from 0 to 100, with 100 being better health. The minimally clinically important difference (MCID) for the SF-36 scales was defined as improvement of >5 points on subscales and >2.5 points on summary scale scores [10].

Validation Data for SF-36 in Chronic Gout

Discrimination thresholds: An observational cohort study assessed whether long-term therapy with urate-lowering therapy (ULT) and colchicine lead to an improvement in HRQOL. The MCIDs were observed at first and second year. It was observed that at one year the effect sizes for SF-36 domains were large for PCS and pain, 0.91 and 1.09, respectively, whereas the effect sizes were smaller for physical function, general health, mental health, vitality social functioning, and emotional scales (0.20–0.49) [42]. For bodily pain scale, 69 % of patients achieved MCID, and for MCS 38 % patients achieved MCID [42].

At 12 weeks, 66 % of patients with acute gout in the canakinumab group had a greater than 10 point reduction in SF-36 bodily pain (range, 0–100; lower = less pain) compared to 57 % patients in the triamcinolone acetonide group [59]. Significant improvements were reported in a higher number of SF-36 domains (6 of 8) in the biweekly pegloticase compared to monthly pegloticase (3 of 8). Table 9.6 shows the changes from baseline to week 25 in all three groups: pegloticase biweekly, pegloticase monthly, and placebo [9].

SF-36 Physical Functioning (PF) Subscale Score

SF-36 PF-10 is a subscale of SF-36. The items on PF-10 are scored from 1 to 3 and the scores obtained on each item are summed and transformed to range from 0 to 100. The mean (SD) PF-10 score was 61.94 (29.33). PF-10 had a strong negative correlation with HAQ-DI and HAQ-II, –0.75 and –0.79, respectively, and positive correlations with other SF-36 domains ranging from 0.30 to 0.68 [43].

Table 9.5 Measurement values of instruments used to measure HRQOL

	Reliability		Validity				Scale development		Responsiveness
Measurement instrument	Internal consistency (Cronbach's a)	Test-retest (ICC)	Content	Construct (Pearson or Spearman's *r*)	Concurrent (Pearson or Spearman's *r*)	Hypothesis a priori	Confirmatory factor analysis	Rasch analysis	MCID, SDC, ES, Guyatt's RR or >20 % change in scores
GAQ 1.0	0.782–0.97	NR	Patients and rheumatologists	PCS (r=0.0220.34), MCS (r=0.01 to 0.23), MOS (r=0.0320.46)	NR	Yes	Yes	No	GRR 0.030 (1 month) to 1.142 (6 months) MCID 1.88212.33 (not significant in well-being for pain freq.)
HAQ-DI	0.81–0.97	0.68–0.84	Floor 20.5 %, Ceiling 34 %	Freq. of flares (r=0.41), physician global (r=0.4220.77), swollen joints (r=0.4020.62), painful joints (r=0.4620.650), joints with limited mobility (r=0.36), VAS pain (r=0.56), tophi (r=0.42), excellent/very good health=0.16, good=0.33, fair/poor=1.25	SF-36 (r=–0.41 to –0.67), PCS (r=–0.71), MCS (r=–0.56), DASH (r=0.81), Sollerman (r=–0.79), ACR functional class (r=0.79), HAQ II (r=0.87), PF 10 (r=–0.75)	Yes (55.5 % true)	Yes	Yes	Mean ES=0.62 (moderate), SDC=0.59 and GRR=1.91

SF-36	0.75–0.97	0.40–0.90	Ceiling	PCS: tophi (r=0.277), swollen joints (r=–0.334), painful joints (r=–0.544), flares last year (r=–0.369); MCS: painful joints (r=–0.436), freq. of flares (r=–0.321)	NR	NR	NR	NR	Colchicine: ES for PCS=0.3 (small), ES for MCS=0.16 (negligible)
			RP=18.4 %, SF=32.7 %, RE=58.6 %						Colchicine+ULT: ES for PCS=0.99 (large)
									ES for MCS=0.08 (negligible), MCID (all subjects) 70 % for PCS and 38 % in MCS
PF 10	0.94	NR	NR	Excellent/very good health=71.91, good=74.27, fair/poor=39.33	HAQ-DI (r=–0.75), SF-36 [0.30 (MH)-0.68 (RP)]	Yes	NR	NR	NR

Modified with permission from Chandratre P, Roddy E, Clarson L, Richardson J, Hider SL, Mallen CD. Health-related quality of life in gout: A systematic review. Rheumatology. 2013 Nov;52(11):2031–2040. By permission of Oxford University Press [58]

HAQ-DI Health Assessment Questionnaire-Disability Index; *GAQ* Gout Assessment Questionnaire, *SF-36* Short Form-36, *PF-10* Physical Functioning Subscale, *MCS* Mental Component Score, *PCS* Physical Component Score, *MCID* Minimal Clinically Important Difference, *NR* Not reported, *ES* Effect size

Table 9.6 Mean (±SD) change in SF-36 domain scores from baseline to week 25

Domain	PF	RP	BP	GH	VT	SF	RE	MH
Pegloticase biweekly, $n=61^{\dagger\dagger}$	11.8*†	15.4*†	24.3*†	7.7*	9.9*	13.5*†	8.2	10.1
	(24.1)	(27.8)	(25.5)	(17.5)	(20.1)	(28.9)	(30.6)	(19.2)
Pegloticase monthly, $n=63^{\dagger\dagger}$	9.5*	10.5*	17.9*	4.7	4.3	8.9	4.6	1.4
	(20.3)	(28.6)	(24.2)	(17.2)	(20.1)	(26.5)	(30.3)	(16.8)
Placebo, $n=38^{\dagger\dagger}$	0.25	1.15	−1.13	0.26	0.33	2.63	4.61	4.3
	(18.97)	(20.90)	(20.77)	(14.97)	(15.24)	(23.99)	(22.40)	(18.1)

Reprinted with permission from Strand V, Khanna D, Singh JA, Forsythe A, Edwards NL. Improved health-related quality of life and physical function in patients with refractory chronic gout following treatment with pegloticase: Evidence from phase iii randomized controlled trials. The Journal of Rheumatology. 2012 Jul;39(7):1450–1457. [9]

Shaded area shows changes in domain scores that are greater than or equal to minimum clinically important differences

SF-36 Short Form-36, *BP* bodily pain, *GH* general health, *MH* mental health, *PF* physical functioning, *RE* role emotional, *RP* role physical, *SF* social functioning, *VT* vitality

*p values < 0.05 based on independent-groups t tests of means for treatment groups compared to placebo

†Approached or met age/sex-matched normative values

††Number of subjects at Week 25; only patients with complete data through Week 25 are included in this analysis

Gout-Specific HRQOL Measure by Gout Assessment Questionnaire (GAQ)

GAQ been tested for validity, reliability, and representativeness in the patient with gout.

Validation Data for GAQ in Chronic Gout

Construct validity: SF-36 pain subscale had high correlation with well-being, productivity, gout concern, and gout pain and severity on GAQ (correlation coefficient ranging from 0.17 to 0.45). There was also high correlation between GAQ and SF-36 physical and social functioning domains. The mean change in GAQ scores for pain and severity were assessed in three groups based on serum uric acid levels. The three groups were clinically improved (<6 mg/dL), clinically stable (≥6.0 to <7.8 mg/dL), and clinically worse (≥7.8 mg/dL). The mean changes were similar at 1, 6, and 12 months in all groups. MCID was calculated using the patient-reported pain frequency and pain severity items from the GAQ as anchors. These items were used to assess the amount of change in the other scales associated with a minimum 1-point change in the pain scale (of a 5-point scale), using linear regression. The GAQ items for pain frequency and severity were well-being, productivity, and gout concern [41]. The minimal clinically important difference was statistically significantly >0 for all GAQ items for pain frequency and severity except well-being for pain frequency [41].

PROMs for Mobility

Mobility Scale

The Sollerman hand function test measures hand mobility. The scale has a score of 0–4 for each task performed with the total score out of 80 (higher score = full hand function). Other mobility measures are fingertip to palm (FTP) distance and grip strength. The serum urate concentrations correlated with the Sollerman score (correlation coefficient: –0.59) as well as arthritis severity measures such as pain visual analog scale, tender joint, and radiographic damage (correlation coefficient ranging from –0.71 to –0.67) [45].

PROMs for Satisfaction

Patient Satisfaction

Patient satisfaction is an important PRO. Patients with more comorbidities (cases) were more likely to have poor satisfaction with their health compared to those who did not (controls) (mean satisfaction with health; cases mean: 13.16; control mean: 14.45) [60], providing some evidence for construct validity.

PROMs for Global Disease Severity

Patient Global Disease Severity Score

The scores range from very well (score of 0) to very poor (score of 100). In patients with gout, patient global VAS scores had low correlations with domains such as tender and swollen joints, moderate correlations with SF-36 and HAQ scores, and no correlation with plasma urate levels, disease duration, recent gout flares, or comorbidities [7].

PROMs for Health Utility

Data on health utilities is limited due to their inclusion in only a few studies. Studies show a lower score in patients with gout compared to the general population, indicating their construct validity.

EQ-5D™

EQ-5D tests domains of mobility, self-care, daily activities, pain, and anxiety/depression. Each domain score ranges from 1 to 3, with 1 being no problems to 3 being severe problems. Patients with gout had a mean (interquartile range; IQR) EQ-5D of 0.74 (IQR: 0.69–0.84). The proportion of gout patients with moderate to severe problems on all the EQ-5D domains was higher than the general population. The individual domain proportions in gout patients with moderate/severe were 66 % for mobility, 24 % for self-care, 49 % for daily activity, 76 % for pain, and 18 % for anxiety/depression [21].

SF-6D

SF-6D is derived from SF-36 domains such as physical function, role limitations, social function, pain, mental health, and vitality. The SF-6D scores range from 0.29 to 1.00, with 1.00 corresponding to perfect health [44]. The mean value for SF-6D was 0.67 (0.59–0.81) in patients with gout [21]. This score is lower than the nationally representative sample of the US non-institutionalized civilian population, where the score was 0.80.

Applicability of PROMs in Research and Clinical Practice

PROMs have a wide range of applicability. PROMs are a valuable tool for evaluating patient-perceived benefits to key stakeholders. PROMs provide a meaningful way of assessing the disease condition and are likely to be just as applicable to clinicians as gout researchers. PROMs are particularly useful in gout wherein a key goal of clinical management is amelioration of symptoms and improvement of patients' quality of life.

PROMs in Research

PROMs provide important information about treatment effects and can help distinguish efficacy of various treatments. Depending on the differences in the mechanism of action, treatments can impact the PROMs differently. Regulatory authorities have mandated provision of patient-reported data in product development guidelines for use of PROMs for inclusion of PROMs in label of the approval of new drugs [61].

PROMs in Practice

PROMs can be used to screen for health problems in clinical practice, which can go undetected if patient participation is not involved. PROMs can be used to monitor progress of chronic disease phase and its impact over time helps the clinician to judge if the treatment is effective and modify the treatment when necessary. PROM data can also be used to compare the quality of care in the clinical practice as well, as clinicians can compare the outcomes to the benchmarks [62]. It remains to be seen whether regular use of PROM assessment in daily practice may improve patient–physician communication and may lead to better treatment adherence, by allowing choice of common goals during a clinic visit.

Summary and Conclusions

PROMs for gout have been tested for validity, reliability, and responsiveness to change in RCTs and observational studies and have been endorsed by OMERACT. VAS or SF-36 pain can be used as a measure of pain in patients with gout. HRQOL/function in patients with gout can be effectively measured by instruments such as HAQ-DI and/or SF-36. These PROMs are a useful source of information in addition to the physician-reported measures.

PROMs provide the patient's perspective regarding the disease and can provide important clues to managing a chronic disease, such as gout. PROMs are now recognized as important tools in understanding the impact of gout on patient lives and could assist in more patient-centered care for the management of patients with gout. However, at present PROMs are not widely integrated into clinical practice.

Therefore, assessment of PROMs and regular monitoring should be an integral part of modern day clinical practice of clinicians caring for patients with gout. Given the disparities observed between PROMs and physician-reported measures and the association of PROMs with higher patient satisfaction, we suggest that physicians should use PROMs to evaluate benefits/harms of therapies in gout and their acceptability to patients, and compliment this information with physician-assessed measures, such as serum uric acid and radiographic changes.

Future Directions and Identification of Gaps

As a chronic condition, gout requires frequent outpatient clinic visits, until allopurinol or other medications become effective. A change in PROMs over time may be due to effect of interventions or natural course of disease or measurement error. Further research is required to establish the ideal time point/s to administer the PROMs in primary care [63]. The relationship between PROMs and the quality of delivered care is also of interest for future studies [63].

PROMs have been extensively studied in clinical trials. However, there is scarcity of real world data on instruments used for PROMs. The real world data will identify any feasibility issues related to PROM administration, data capture and broad scale implementation [64]. Observational studies or national registries are required to capture PROM data to study feasibility and other relevant issues on PROM administration in clinical care.

PROM instruments can sometimes be too lengthy and difficult to administer in routine clinical care. Shorter versions for such instruments need to be developed and tested in clinical trials for routine use. Other measures such as GAQ are still in their infancy and more clinical trials are required before they can be adopted into clinical practice.

References

1. Perez-Ruiz F, Castillo E, Chinchilla SP, Herrero-Beites AM. Clinical manifestations and diagnosis of gout. Rheum Dis Clin North Am. 2014;40(2):193–206.
2. Grassi W, De Angelis R. Clinical features of gout. Reumatismo. 2011;63(4):238–45.
3. Krishnan E. Gout and coronary artery disease: epidemiologic clues. Curr Rheumatol Rep. 2008;10(3):249–55.
4. Krishnan E. Gout and the risk for incident heart failure and systolic dysfunction. BMJ Open. 2012;2(1), e000282.
5. Krishnan E, Baker JF, Furst DE, Schumacher HR. Gout and the risk of acute myocardial infarction. Arthritis Rheum. 2006;54(8):2688–96.
6. Singh JA. When gout goes to the heart: does gout equal a cardiovascular disease risk factor? Ann Rheum Dis. 2015;74(4):631–4.
7. Singh JA, Yang S, Strand V, Simon L, Forsythe A, Hamburger S, et al. Validation of pain and patient global scales in chronic gout: data from two randomised controlled trials. Ann Rheum Dis. 2011;70(7):1277–81.
8. Singh JA, Taylor WJ, Simon LS, Khanna PP, Stamp LK, McQueen FM, et al. Patient-reported outcomes in chronic gout: a report from OMERACT 10. J Rheumatol. 2011;38(7):1452–7.
9. Strand V, Khanna D, Singh JA, Forsythe A, Edwards NL. Improved health-related quality of life and physical function in patients with refractory chronic gout following treatment with pegloticase: evidence from phase iii randomized controlled trials. J Rheumatol. 2012;39(7):1450–7.
10. Strand V, Singh JA. Improved health-related quality of life with effective disease-modifying antirheumatic drugs: evidence from randomized controlled trials. Am J Manag Care. 2008;14(4):234–54.
11. Valderas JM, Alonso J. Patient reported outcome measures: a model-based classification system for research and clinical practice. Qual Life Res Int J Qual Life Asp Treat Care Rehab. 2008;17(9):1125–35.
12. Acquadro C, Berzon R, Dubois D, Leidy NK, Marquis P, Revicki D, et al. Incorporating the patient's perspective into drug development and communication: an ad hoc task force report of the patient-reported outcomes (pro) harmonization group meeting at the food and drug administration, February 16, 2001. Value Health. 2003;6(5):522–31.
13. Rothman ML, Beltran P, Cappelleri JC, Lipscomb J, Teschendorf B, Mayo FDAP-ROCMG. Patient-reported outcomes: conceptual issues. Value Health. 2007;10 Suppl 2:S66–75.
14. Patient Reported Outcome Measures Information System (PROMIS). Patient reported outcomes (PROs). 2015. http://www.nihpromis.org/patients/PROs.

15. McKenna SP. Measuring patient-reported outcomes: moving beyond misplaced common sense to hard science. BMC Med. 2011;9:86.
16. Bevans M, Ross A, Cella D. Patient-reported outcomes measurement information system (PROMIS): efficient, standardized tools to measure self-reported health and quality of life. Nurs Outlook. 2014;62(5):339–45.
17. Weldring T, Smith SM. Patient-reported outcomes (pros) and patient-reported outcome measures (proms). Health Serv Insights. 2013;6:61–8.
18. Valderas JM, Kotzeva A, Espallargues M, Guyatt G, Ferrans CE, Halyard MY, et al. The impact of measuring patient-reported outcomes in clinical practice: a systematic review of the literature. Qual Life Res. 2008;17(2):179–93.
19. Greenhalgh J, Meadows K. The effectiveness of the use of patient-based measures of health in routine practice in improving the process and outcomes of patient care: a literature review. J Eval Clin Pract. 1999;5(4):401–16.
20. Alvarez-Hernandez E, Pelaez-Ballestas I, Vazquez-Mellado J, Teran-Estrada L, Bernard-Medina AG, Espinoza J, et al. Validation of the health assessment questionnaire disability index in patients with gout. Arthritis Rheum. 2008;59(5):665–9.
21. Spaetgens B, Tran-Duy A, Wijnands JM, van der Linden S, Boonen A. Health and utilities in patients with gout under the care of a rheumatologist. Arthritis Care Res (Hoboken). 2015;67(8):1128–36.
22. ten Klooster PM, Vonkeman HE, Voshaar MA, Bode C, van de Laar MA. Experiences of gout-related disability from the patients' perspective: a mixed methods study. Clin Rheumatol. 2014;33(8):1145–54.
23. Singh JA. The impact of gout on patient's lives: a study of African-American and Caucasian men and women with gout. Arthritis Res Ther. 2014;16(3):R132.
24. Kim SY, Choi HK. Gout and quality of life. J Rheumatol. 2009;36(5):865–8.
25. Singh JA. Quality of life and quality of care for patients with gout. Curr Rheumatol Rep. 2009;11(2):154–60.
26. Solomon DH, Avorn J, Levin R, Brookhart MA. Uric acid lowering therapy: prescribing patterns in a large cohort of older adults. Ann Rheum Dis. 2008;67(5):609–13.
27. Lindsay K, Gow P, Vanderpyl J, Logo P, Dalbeth N. The experience and impact of living with gout: a study of men with chronic gout using a qualitative grounded theory approach. J Clin Rheumatol. 2011;17(1):1–6.
28. Edwards NL, Sundy JS, Forsythe A, Blume S, Pan F, Becker MA. Work productivity loss due to flares in patients with chronic gout refractory to conventional therapy. J Med Econ. 2011;14(1):10–5.
29. Kleinman NL, Brook RA, Patel PA, Melkonian AK, Brizee TJ, Smeeding JE, et al. The impact of gout on work absence and productivity. Value Health. 2007;10(4):231–7.
30. Anonymous. United states bone and joint decade: the burden of musculoskeletal diseases in the united states. Chapter 4. Arthritis and related conditions. Rosemont: American Academy of Orthopaedic Surgeons; 2008.
31. Center for Disease Control and Prevention (CDC). Gout 2015. http://www.cdc.gov/arthritis/basics/gout.htm.
32. Cohen SB, Strand V, Aguilar D, Ofman JJ. Patient- versus physician-reported outcomes in rheumatoid arthritis patients treated with recombinant interleukin-1 receptor antagonist (anakinra) therapy. Rheumatology. 2004;43(6):704–11.
33. Lubaczewski S, Shepherd J, Fayyad R, Guico-Pabia CJ. Real-world disparities between patient- and clinician-reported outcomes: results from a disease-specific program in depression and anxiety. Prof Case Manag. 2014;19(2):63–74.
34. Quinten C, Maringwa J, Gotay CC, Martinelli F, Coens C, Reeve BB, et al. Patient self-reports of symptoms and clinician ratings as predictors of overall cancer survival. J Natl Cancer Inst. 2011;103(24):1851–8.
35. Chalmers RL, Begley CG, Edrington T, Caffery B, Nelson D, Snyder C, et al. The agreement between self-assessment and clinician assessment of dry eye severity. Cornea. 2005;24(7):804–10.

36. Taylor WJ, Redden D, Dalbeth N, Schumacher HR, Edwards NL, Simon LS, et al. Application of the OMERACT filter to measures of core outcome domains in recent clinical studies of acute gout. J Rheumatol. 2014;41(3):574–80.
37. Singh JA, Taylor WJ, Dalbeth N, Simon LS, Sundy J, Grainger R, et al. OMERACT endorsement of measures of outcome for studies of acute gout. J Rheumatol. 2014;41(3):569–73.
38. Schumacher Jr HR, Edwards LN, Perez-Ruiz F, Becker M, Chen LX, Furst DE, et al. Outcome measures for acute and chronic gout. J Rheumatol. 2005;32(12):2452–5.
39. Diaz-Torne C, Pou MA, Castellvi I, Corominas H, Taylor WJ. Concerns of patients with gout are incompletely captured by OMERACT-endorsed domains of measurement for chronic gout studies. J Clin Rheumatol. 2014;20(3):138–40.
40. Taylor WJ. Gout measures: gout assessment questionnaire (gaq, gaq2.0), and physical measurement of tophi. Arthritis Care Res (Hoboken). 2011;63 Suppl 11:S59–63.
41. Colwell HH, Hunt BJ, Pasta DJ, Palo WA, Mathias SD, Joseph-Ridge N. Gout assessment questionnaire: initial results of reliability, validity and responsiveness. Int J Clin Pract. 2006;60(10):1210–7.
42. Khanna PP, Perez-Ruiz F, Maranian P, Khanna D. Long-term therapy for chronic gout results in clinically important improvements in the health-related quality of life: short form-36 is responsive to change in chronic gout. Rheumatology. 2011;50(4):740–5.
43. Ten Klooster PM, Oude Voshaar MA, Taal E, van de Laar MA. Comparison of measures of functional disability in patients with gout. Rheumatology. 2011;50(4):709–13.
44. Khanna D, Ahmed M, Yontz D, Ginsburg SS, Park GS, Leonard A, et al. The disutility of chronic gout. Qual Life Res. 2008;17(5):815–22.
45. Dalbeth N, Collis J, Gregory K, Clark B, Robinson E, McQueen FM. Tophaceous joint disease strongly predicts hand function in patients with gout. Rheumatology. 2007;46(12):1804–7.
46. Lanser P, Gesell S. Pain management: the fifth vital sign. Healthc Benchmarks. 2001;8(6):68–70. 62.
47. Breivik H, Collett B, Ventafridda V, Cohen R, Gallacher D. Survey of chronic pain in Europe: prevalence, impact on daily life, and treatment. Eur J Pain. 2006;10(4):287–333.
48. Man CY, Cheung IT, Cameron PA, Rainer TH. Comparison of oral prednisolone/paracetamol and oral indomethacin/paracetamol combination therapy in the treatment of acute goutlike arthritis: a double-blind, randomized, controlled trial. Ann Emerg Med. 2007;49(5):670–7.
49. Schlesinger N, Detry MA, Holland BK, Baker DG, Beutler AM, Rull M, et al. Local ice therapy during bouts of acute gouty arthritis. J Rheumatol. 2002;29(2):331–4.
50. Schlesinger N, Alten RE, Bardin T, Schumacher HR, Bloch M, Gimona A, et al. Canakinumab for acute gouty arthritis in patients with limited treatment options: results from two randomised, multicentre, active-controlled, double-blind trials and their initial extensions. Ann Rheum Dis. 2012;71(11):1839–48.
51. Ottaviani S, Molto A, Ea HK, Neveu S, Gill G, Brunier L, et al. Efficacy of anakinra in gouty arthritis: a retrospective study of 40 cases. Arthritis Res Ther. 2013;15(5):R123.
52. Shrestha M, Chiu MJ, Martin RL, Cush JJ, Wainscott MS. Treatment of acute gouty arthritis with intramuscular ketorolac tromethamine. Am J Emerg Med. 1994;12(4):454–5.
53. Terkeltaub R, Sundy JS, Schumacher HR, Murphy F, Bookbinder S, Biedermann S, et al. The interleukin 1 inhibitor rilonacept in treatment of chronic gouty arthritis: results of a placebo-controlled, monosequence crossover, non-randomised, single-blind pilot study. Ann Rheum Dis. 2009;68(10):1613–7.
54. Wechalekar MD, Vinik O, Schlesinger N, Buchbinder R. Intra-articular glucocorticoids for acute gout. Cochrane Database Syst Rev. 2013;4, CD009920.
55. Bijur PE, Silver W, Gallagher EJ. Reliability of the visual analog scale for measurement of acute pain. Acad Emerg Med Off J Soc Acad Emerg Med. 2001;8(12):1153–7.
56. Sivera F, Wechalekar MD, Andres M, Buchbinder R, Carmona L. Interleukin-1 inhibitors for acute gout. Cochrane Database Syst Rev. 2014;9, CD009993.
57. Taylor WJ, Colvine K, Gregory K, Collis J, McQueen FM, Dalbeth N. The health assessment questionnaire disability index is a valid measure of physical function in gout. Clin Exp Rheumatol. 2008;26(4):620–6.

58. Chandratre P, Roddy E, Clarson L, Richardson J, Hider SL, Mallen CD. Health-related quality of life in gout: a systematic review. Rheumatology. 2013;52(11):2031–40.
59. Hirsch JD, Gnanasakthy A, Lale R, Choi K, Sarkin AJ. Efficacy of canakinumab vs. Triamcinolone acetonide according to multiple gouty arthritis-related health outcomes measures. Int J Clin Pract. 2014;68(12):1503–7.
60. Roddy E, Zhang W, Doherty M. Is gout associated with reduced quality of life? A case-control study. Rheumatology. 2007;46(9):1441–4.
61. Baldwin M, Spong A, Doward L, Gnanasakthy A. Patient-reported outcomes, patient-reported information: from randomized controlled trials to the social web and beyond. Patient. 2011;4(1):11–7.
62. Snyder CF, Aaronson NK, Choucair AK, Elliott TE, Greenhalgh J, Halyard MY, et al. Implementing patient-reported outcomes assessment in clinical practice: a review of the options and considerations. Qual Life Res. 2012;21(8):1305–14.
63. Weenink JW, Braspenning J, Wensing M. Patient reported outcome measures (proms) in primary care: An observational pilot study of seven generic instruments. BMC Fam Pract. 2014;15:88.
64. National Quality forum. Pro's in performance measurement. 2013. http://www.google.com/url?sa=t&rct=j&q=&esrc=s&frm=1&source=web&cd=2&cad=rja&uact=8&ved=0CDUQFjAB&url=http%3A%2F%2Fwww.qualityforum.org%2FPublications%2F2012%2F12%2FPatient-Reported_Outcomes_Final_Report.aspx&ei=ZHYZVar6OZLRggTtl4PICQ&usg=AFQjCNHO3drQc9orjbBdR8O9P_TqJl9r0A&bvm=bv.89381419,d.eXY.

Chapter 10
PROMs for Osteoarthritis

Natalie J. Collins and Ewa M. Roos

Introduction

Of all rheumatic diseases, osteoarthritis (OA) is the most common [1]. The knee, hip, and hand joints are most commonly involved, with reported prevalence in various populations ranging from 20 to 30 % of adults [2]. Considering that age, obesity, and joint injury are among the biggest risk factors for OA [2], and that these are increasing in the population, it is not surprising that the proportion of people with symptomatic OA is expected to rise substantially in the coming years. The socio-economic burden of OA is well documented, in terms of healthcare expenditure and lost productivity. Alongside this, the individual burden of OA is profound, with OA being the eleventh leading cause of years lived with disability globally [3]. Although OA has typically been considered a disease of ageing, recent studies highlight the presence of OA in increasingly younger populations, such as those with anterior cruciate ligament (ACL) reconstructions [4], middle-aged adults with anterior knee pain [5], and young adults who have undergone hip arthroscopy [6].

N.J. Collins, PhD, MSports Physio, BPhty(Hons) (✉)
School of Health and Rehabilitation Sciences, The University of Queensland, St. Lucia, QLD, Australia
e-mail: n.collins1@uq.edu.au

E.M. Roos, Ph.D.
Department of Sports and Clinical Biomechanics, University of Southern Denmark, Odense, Denmark
e-mail: eroos@health.sdu.dk

Y. El Miedany (ed.), *Patient Reported Outcome Measures in Rheumatic Diseases*,
DOI 10.1007/978-3-319-32851-5_10

Why Are Patient-Reported Outcome Measures Important for Patients with Osteoarthritis?

Because of the progressive, degenerative nature of OA, patient-reported outcome measures (PROMs) play an important role in monitoring the course of the disease over time and the effectiveness of treatment. This is particularly the case for younger adults with OA, as the goal of management is to minimize symptoms, maximize function, and prolong the time until joint replacement surgery is required. Therefore, clinicians should use PROMs that can capture the natural course of the disease, from early or mild OA to severe end-stage joint disease, and to joint replacement and beyond. This will help to identify whether nonsurgical interventions are effective in managing symptoms, and may provide guidance when deciding whether a patient with OA is suitable for total joint replacement [7].

PROMs are also useful for OA patients to:

- Direct the focus of clinical appointments, goal setting, and management plans toward aspects that are of most concern to the patient
- Empower the patient to monitor their own health profile over time, by providing benchmarks for their ideal health state, their peers, and normative cohorts
- Provide a method of standardizing health status reporting, to allow pooling of data from international cohorts (e.g., joint replacement registries) and detection of clinical patterns that may impact on prognosis and treatment response

In parallel with our increased awareness that OA starts earlier than previously thought, and underpinned by the last 20 years of intensive research, treatment for OA has developed from joint replacement surgery for late stage disease to treatment guidelines recommending education, exercise, and weight loss as first-line treatment, followed by pharmacological treatments and, finally, surgical treatments. PROMs for use in OA should be able to pick up changes in symptoms, function, and quality of life relating to contemporary OA treatment.

Selecting PROMs for Use with Patients with Osteoarthritis

When selecting PROMs for clinical use, it is important to consider attributes that make a "good" PROM for patients with OA [8]:

1. Is it easy to use in the clinical setting?
2. Does it evaluate dimensions that are relevant for my OA patient? (*content validity*)
3. Does it measure what it is intended to measure? (*construct validity*)
4. Can I trust that the PROM is detecting true change in my patient, and is free from error? (*reliability*)
5. Is the PROM sensitive enough to detect real change in my patient's condition? (*responsiveness, floor/ceiling effects*)

Patient-Reported Outcome Measures for Patients with Osteoarthritis

Health professionals can use guidelines provided by OMERACT ("Outcome Measures in Rheumatology") to select PROMs that are most appropriate for patients with OA. Originally developed to guide selection of PROMs for clinical trials, the OMERACT Core Domain Set highlights elements that are important for patients with the condition of interest. For knee, hip, and hand OA, the most important core domains appropriate to PROMs are pain, physical function, and patient global assessment, while health-related quality of life (HRQOL) is strongly recommended [9].

There are a number of generic PROMs that are appropriate to measure the core domains in patients with OA. Visual analogue scales (VAS) and numeric rating scales (NRS) are commonly used to evaluate pain severity. In the absence of an established measure of global assessment, it is recommended that a single question be asked, using a VAS or Likert scale [10–12]. For example, clinicians could ask, "Considering all the ways your [knee] OA affects you, how have you been during the past [time frame]?" [11] It should be kept in mind, though, that the use of a single-item PROM can influence the reliability of the instrument. In measuring HRQOL, we encourage the reader to also consider generic quality of life (QOL) PROMs that can be used for multiple conditions, such as the EQ-5D (www.euroqol.org), Short Form-12 (SF-12) [13], Short Form-36 (SF-36) [14], and the Assessment of Quality of Life (AQoL) instrument [15]. However, it should be considered that little information is available regarding their measurement properties in patients with OA.

This chapter focuses on PROMs for knee, hip, and hand OA, as these are most commonly seen in the clinic. Examples of PROMs for other joints are listed at the end of the chapter. We have selected PROMs based on their fit with the OMERACT Core Domain Set. Where possible, we have focused on measures that were developed specifically for OA in the target joint to ensure that the content is relevant for patients. Because measurement properties are condition-specific and context-specific, where possible we present measurement properties that are specific to the joint and context (e.g., natural course or type of treatment) under study. The reader is encouraged to consider that not all measurement properties have been evaluated for all PROMs, and that the absence of evidence for particular measurement properties means that conclusions regarding these cannot be made at this time. For clarification regarding whether such evidence exists, we direct the reader to Table 10.1.

Patient-Reported Outcome Measures for Knee and Hip Osteoarthritis

Because the hip and knee undergo high loads during weight-bearing tasks such as gait, knee, and hip OA have a substantial impact on functional mobility. This limits an individual's ability to perform daily activities, occupational tasks, and exercise.

Table 10.1 Quick-reference guide for satisfying the requirements of a "good" PROM for use in individual patients with OA (as opposed to groups where some requirements are lower)

PROM	Subscale	Content validity	Internal consistency	Test-retest reliability^	Construct validity	Floor effects (≥15% score lowest score)#	Ceiling effects (≥15% score highest score)#	Missing items
Knee OA								
WOMAC	Pain	✓	✓/×	✓/×	✓	✓	19-41% (post-TKR)	1-3%
	Stiffness	✓	✓/×	×	✓	15-19%	19% (pre-TKR); 16-67% (post-TKR)	
	Function	✓	✓/×	✓/×	✓	✓	45% (post-TKR)	
KOOS	Pain	✓		✓/×	✓	✓	15-22% (post-TKR)	0-5%
	Symptoms	✓	✓	✓/×	✓	✓	✓	
	ADL	✓	✓	✓/×	✓	✓	✓	
	Sport/rec	✓	✓	×	✓	16-73%	16-20% (post-HTO; post-TKR)	
	QoL	✓	✓	×	✓	15% (post-HTO)	17% (post-TKR)	
KOOS-PS		✓	✓	×	✓	✓	✓	0%
Oxford Knee Score		✓	✓	✓	✓	✓	27% (post-TKR)	0-5%
ICOAP (knee version)	Constant	✓	✓	✓/×	✓	33% (knee OA)	✓	0%
	Intermittent	✓	✓	×	✓	✓	✓	
	Total	✓	✓/×	✓/×	✓	✓	✓	
Hip OA								
WOMAC	Pain	✓	✓	✓/×	✓	✓	34-38% post-THR	?
	Stiffness	✓	✓	×	✓	✓	28-31% post-THR	?
	Function	✓	×	✓	✓	✓	✓	11%^
HOOS	Pain	✓	✓	✓/×	✓	✓	19-47% (post-THR)	0.08-3.6%
	Symptoms	✓	✓	✓/×	✓	✓	29.1% (post-THR)	
	ADL	✓	×	✓/×	✓	✓	✓	
	Sport/rec	✓	✓	✓/×	✓	17.8% (pre-THR)	✓	
	QoL	✓	✓	✓/×	✓	✓	✓	
HOOS-PS		✓	?	✓	✓	✓	✓	0%

(continued)

Table 10.1 (continued)

Oxford Hip Score		✓	?	✓	✓	✓	19.9% (1-11 years post-THR)	0%
ICOAP (hip version)	Constant	✓	✓	✓	✓	?	?	?
	Intermittent	✓	✓	✓	✓	?	?	
	Total	✓	✓	✓	✓	?	?	
Hip/knee OA								
OAKHQOL	Physical activities	✓	×	✓/×	✓	✓	✓	4.4-8.6%
	Pain	✓	✓	×	✓	✓	✓	
	Mental health	✓	✓	✓/×	✓	✓	✓	
	Social activities	✓	✓/×		✓	✓	✓	
	Social support	✓	✓/×	✓/×	✓	✓	✓	
Mini-OAKHQOL	Physical activities	✓	✓	×	✓	✓	?	?
	Pain	✓	✓	×	✓	✓	?	
	Mental	✓	✓	×	✓	✓	?	
	health	✓	✓	×	✓	✓		
	Social activities	✓	×	×	✓	✓	?	
	Social support	✓	✓	×	✓	✓	?	
Hand OA								
AUSCAN	Pain	✓	✓/×	×	✓	?	?	2%
	Stiffness	✓	n/a	×	✓	?	?	1-2.5%
	Function	✓	✓/×	✓/×	✓	?	?	0-3%
FIHOA		×	?	✓	✓	?	?	3-6%
Cochin Scale		×	?	✓	✓	?	?	?

Green represents adequate properties, *yellow* represents mixed findings, and *red* represents inadequate properties. Please note that properties are specific for the context in which they have been determined. Acceptable test–retest reliability (column 5) refers to values for use in individuals (ICC ≥0.9). Mixed or inadequate findings for test–retest reliability (column 5) were found for most instruments. Clinicians can use minimal detectable change (MDC) or smallest detectable difference (SDD) values to determine whether an individual patient's scores represent a real change. Where available, these are provided in the text for each PROM. Several instruments have high floor/ceiling effects (column 7 and 8) seen prior to and following total joint replacement (TJR). Considering that TJR is appropriate for advanced stages of OA, it is as expected that >15 % would report worst possible pain/function, and, considering the good clinical treatment effect from TJR, it is to be expected that >15 % report no pain/no functional limitations postoperatively. While clinicians should be aware of the floor and ceiling effects >15 % from TJR common in many measures of pain and function, it should not preclude evaluation of pain and function by PROMs in TJR

ADL, activities of daily living; *OA*, osteoarthritis; *VAS*, visual analogue scale; *QoL*, quality of life; *HTO*, high tibial osteotomy; *TKR*, total knee replacement; *THR*, total hip replacement; ?, no data available; n/a, not applicable

#For floor and ceiling effects, a white box with red highlighting indicates that data is only available for total joint replacement, and that inadequate properties are specific to total joint replacement. Data is not available for nonsurgical OA populations

Harris Hip Score and modified Harris Hip Score are not reported as their measurement properties in OA have not been established vNonsurgical interventions, such as education, exercise therapy, diet, and pharmacological interventions, have small-to-moderate effects and are recommended as the first-line treatment for knee and hip OA. Those with end-stage knee or hip OA typically undergo total joint replacement surgery.

The similarities in symptoms and functional impairments between knee and hip OA are reflected in the high degree of overlap between PROMs for the two conditions. Some PROMs were developed with the intention to be used in either knee or hip OA patients. Thus, we will consider PROMs for knee and hip OA together in this chapter. These will be discussed under two headings: disease-specific PROMs, which are intended for use in patients with OA, and intervention-specific PROMs, which are intended for use in patients who are undergoing specific interventions for OA. We have selected the most commonly used PROMs for knee and hip OA, with a particular focus on those that have established measurement properties. Table 10.2 summarizes the characteristics of recommended PROMs for knee and hip OA, whereas Table 10.1 provides a quick-reference guide regarding the evidence for whether the PROMs satisfy the requirements of a "good" PROM for knee and hip OA. All PROMs described in this section were developed with input from patients with knee and/or hip OA, ensuring their content validity.

Patient-Reported Outcome Measures Specific for Hip and/or Knee Osteoarthritis

Western Ontario and McMaster Universities Osteoarthritis Index (WOMAC)

The WOMAC was developed for patients with knee or hip OA [16]. It comprises 24 items assessing pain, stiffness, and function in activities of daily living (ADL). Patients respond to each item based on the previous 48 hours, which reduces recall bias. WOMAC is available in a variety of formats (Likert scale and VAS) and has been validated in paper, electronic (e.g., computer and smartphone), and telephone versions [17–20]. This enhances its clinical use, especially for patients with communication difficulties. It takes less than 12 min for patients to complete, and 5 min for clinicians to calculate the three subscale scores (manual/computer). For missing items, the mean value of all answered items within the subscale should be entered [21]. Subscale scores should not be calculated if two or more pain items, both stiffness items, or four or more physical function items are missing [22, 23]. Higher scores represent worse outcome.

There are considerations regarding the content of WOMAC. There is a high degree of overlap between the pain and ADL subscales [24]. This is likely due to the nature of the pain questions, which ask about the severity of pain during particular functional activities for which the corresponding difficulty is the focus of the ADL subscale (e.g., pain during walking). This suggests that the pain subscale should be considered more of a measure of pain during ADL, as it does not consider how OA pain impacts on other areas of life (e.g., sleep and mood) [24, 25]. There may also be issues of content validity for more active patients with OA, especially younger adults with post-traumatic OA, as there are no items in either the pain or function subscales that relate to more vigorous activities (e.g., running).

All three WOMAC subscales demonstrate adequate reliability for use in groups of patients with hip OA (intraclass correlation coefficient [ICC] ≥ 0.8). The function subscale is sufficiently reliable for groups of patients with knee OA, but there is conflicting evidence for the pain and stiffness subscales. Clinicians wishing to use WOMAC in individual patients also need to consider the evidence regarding test–retest reliability. While the function subscale consistently demonstrates adequate reliability for use in individual patients with hip OA (ICC ≥ 0.9), there is conflicting evidence for knee OA. For the pain subscale in both hip and knee OA, some studies show adequate reliability, and others inadequate reliability. The stiffness subscale consistently demonstrates inadequate reliability for individual patients with knee or hip OA. This may be because this subscale only contains two items. Therefore, clinicians should be aware of the likelihood that changes in WOMAC scores observed in individual patients may represent error in the instrument, rather than true change in the patient's condition.

Clinicians can use values for measurement error (minimal detectable change [MDC]) to determine the minimum score that represents a true change in an individual patient's condition. In 95 % of cases (MDC_{95}), individual patients with hip OA will have experienced a real change if their function subscale score has changed by at least 9.1 points (when scored using the Likert version, score range 0–68) [26]. Values for the pain and stiffness subscales are unknown for patients with hip OA. For individual patients with knee OA, the change in pain subscale score should exceed 18.8, stiffness 27.1, and function 13.3 to be considered a real change in condition, when evaluated using the 11-point numerical rating scale version (scores converted to 0–100) [27].

All three subscales of the WOMAC are able to detect improvements with exercise and physical therapy, pharmacological interventions, and total joint replacement [28]. The pain and function subscales have no floor and ceiling effects in patients with hip and knee OA, meaning that these subscales can monitor deterioration and improvement in a patient's condition over time. Ceiling effects have only been noted after total joint replacement. In contrast, the stiffness subscale has demonstrated both floor and ceiling effects in patients with knee OA [24] and may not be an ideal tool to evaluate change over time.

A major limitation of WOMAC is that it is protected by copyright and trademark, and therefore requires permission for use. Although licensing and costs are determined on each individual request, clinicians should be aware that there may be fees associated with the use of WOMAC with patients. This restricts the accessibility of WOMAC to all patients with hip/knee OA, despite the multitude of language versions available.

Table 10.2 Characteristics of recommended PROMs for hip and knee OA

PROM	Dimensions evaluated (*indicates OMERACT core domain*)	Intended population	How to administer	Patient burden	Scoring	How to obtain	Available language translations
Specific for hip/knee OA							
WOMAC	*Pain* Stiffness *Physical function* (ADL)	Hip and knee OA	Patient-completed or interviewer-administered	• 24 items – Pain (5) – Stiffness (2) – Function (17) • Recall previous 48 h • 5–12 min to complete	• 5 min to score • Manual or computer calculation (sum of all items in each subscale) • 3 individual subscales • Likert version: – Pain 0–20 – Stiffness 0–8 – Function 0–68 • VAS version: – Pain 0–500 – Stiffness 0–200 – Function 0–1700 • Higher scores indicate worse pain, stiffness or function	http://www.womac.org (licensing and fee information, permission to use)	Available in >80 languages

KOOS	*Pain* Symptoms *Function in ADL* *Function in sport/ recreation* *Knee-related QoL*	Post-traumatic knee OA and preceding conditions	Patient-completed	• 42 items – Pain (9) – Symptoms (7) – ADL (17) – Sport/rec (5) – QoL (4) • Recall previous week • 10 min to complete	2–3 min to score using scoring spreadsheet; 10–15 min using manual scoring sheet (www.koos.nu) • 5 individual subscales • 0–100 • Higher scores indicate better pain, symptoms, function, QoL	Freely available (www.koos.nu)	Arabic (Egypt, Saudi Arabia), Bengali, Czech, Chinese, Croatian, Danish, Dutch, Estonian, English, Filipino, French, German (Germany, Austria), Greek, Hindi, Icelandic, Italian, Japanese, Kannada, Korean, Latvian, Lithuanian, Malayalam, Malay, Marathi, Persian, Portuguese (Portugal, Brazil), Polish, Russian, Singapore English, Slovakian, Slovenian, Spanish (Spain, Peru, USA), Swedish, Tamil, Telugu, Thai, Turkish, Ukrainian, Urdu, Vietnamese, Zulu
KOOS-PS	*Physical function* (ADL, sport/ recreation)	Knee OA	Patient-completed	• 7 items • Recall previous week • 2 min to complete	• <5 min to score using table [68] • Single score • 0–100 • Higher score indicates better function	Freely available (www.koos.nu)	Chinese, Dutch, English, French, German, Hindi, Italian, Korean, Norwegian, Portuguese Singapore English, Spanish, Swedish, Turkish

(continued)

Table 10.2 (continued)

PROM	Dimensions evaluated (*indicates OMERACT core domain*)	Intended population	How to administer	Patient burden	Scoring	How to obtain	Available language translations
OAKHQOL	*QoL* (physical activity, pain, mental health, social support, social activities, additional items regarding relationships, sexuality, employment)	Hip and knee OA	Patient-completed	• 43 items (version 2.3) – Physical activities (16) – Mental health (13) – Pain (4) – Social support (4) – Social functioning (3) – 3 additional items • Recall previous 4 weeks • 12–20 min to complete	• Score using manual calculation (mean item score for each subscale) • 5 individual subscales + 3 supplementary items • Normalized to 0–100 • Higher scores indicate better QoL	Freely available; French version in development publication [37]	Arabic (Morocco), Chinese, French, Persian, Spanish
Mini-OAKHQOL	*QoL* (physical activity, pain, mental health, social support, social activities, additional items regarding relationships, sexuality, employment)	Hip and knee OA	Patient-completed	• 20 items – Physical activities (7) – Mental health (3) – Pain (3) – Social support (2) – Social functioning (2) – 3 additional items • Recall previous 4 weeks • <10 min to complete	• Score using manual calculation (mean item score for each subscale) • 5 individual subscales + 3 supplementary items • Normalized to 0–100 • Higher scores indicate better QoL	Freely available [38] (email corresponding author francis.guillemin@univ-lorraine.fr)	French

HOOS	*Pain* Symptoms *Function in ADL*	Adults with hip disability with or without OA	Patient-completed	• 40 items – Pain (10) – Symptoms (5)	2–3 min to score using scoring spreadsheet; 10–15 min using manual scoring sheet (www.koos.nu) • 5 individual subscales • 0–100	Freely available (www.koos.nu)	Chinese, Danish, Dutch, English, Farsi (Persian), French, German, Greek, Italian, Japanese, Korean, Lithuanian, Norwegian, Polish, Portuguese (Portugal, Brazil), Spanish, Swedish, Turkish, Vietnamese
	Function in sport/ recreation *Hip-related QoL*			– ADL (17) – Sport/rec (4) – QoL (4) • Recall previous week • 10–15 min to complete	• Higher scores indicate better pain, symptoms, function, and QoL		
	Physical function (ADL, sport/ recreation)	Hip OA	Patient-completed	• 5 items • Recall previous week • 2 min to complete	• <5 min to score using table [68] • Single score • 0–100 • Higher score indicates better function	Freely available (www.koos.nu)	Danish, Dutch, English, French, German, Italian, Norwegian, Polish, Swedish, Turkish
ICOAP	*Pain* (intermittent, constant)	Hip and knee OA (separate versions)	Interviewer-administered (in person; telephone); can be patient-completed	• 11 items – Intermittent (5) – Constant (6) • Recall previous week • <10 min to complete	• Easy to score using manual calculation • 2 individual subscales • Normalized to 0–100 • Higher scores indicate a worse pain experience	Freely available (www.oarsi.org)	Czech, Dutch, English, French, German, Greek, Italian, Norwegian, Portuguese, Romanian, Russian, Spanish (Castilian; North and Central America), Swedish

(continued)

Table 10.2 (continued)

PROM	Dimensions evaluated (*indicates OMERACT core domain*)	Intended population	How to administer	Patient burden	Scoring	How to obtain	Available language translations
Specific for total joint replacement							
Oxford Knee Score	*Pain* *Physical function* (ADL)	Patients post-TKR	Patient-completed	• 12 items • Recall previous 4 weeks • 5–10 min to complete	• <5 min to score using manual calculation • Single score • 0–48 (revised scoring) • Higher scores indicate better outcomes	Documents and permission to use from http://isis-innovation.com/health-outcomes/patient-reported-outcome-measures; fees apply for some uses (e.g., commercial use, industry-funded research)	Chinese (Hong Kong, Malaysia, Singapore), Dutch (Netherlands, Belgium), English, French, German (Germany, Austria, Swiss), Gujarati, Hindi, Japanese, Korean, Malay (Malaysia, Singapore), Polish, Punjabi, Spanish, Swedish, Thai
Oxford Hip Score	*Pain* *Physical function* (ADL)	Patients post-THR	Patient-completed	• 12 items • Recall previous 4 weeks • 2–15 min to complete	• <5 min to score using manual calculation • Single score • 0–48 (revised scoring) • Higher scores indicate better outcomes	Documents and permission to use from: http://isis-innovation.com/health-outcomes/patient-reported-outcome-measures; fees apply for some uses (e.g., commercial use and industry-funded research)	Chinese, Danish, Dutch, English, Finnish, French, German, Hindi, Italian, Japanese, Korean, Malayalam, Tamil, Korean, Russian, Spanish, Turkish

ADL activities of daily living, *OA* osteoarthritis, *VAS* visual analogue scale, *QoL* quality of life, *TKR* total knee replacement, *THR* total hip replacement

Knee Injury and Osteoarthritis Outcome Score (KOOS) and Hip Disability and Osteoarthritis Outcome Score (HOOS)

The KOOS (Appendix 1) and HOOS were developed as extensions of the WOMAC 3.0 and intended for use in adults of all ages, from young adults with joint injury that may lead to OA, to elderly patients with OA. Dimensions of function in sport/recreation activities and knee/hip-related QOL were added to the WOMAC domains of pain and function in ADL. In addition, the pain subscale was extended to incorporate pain frequency (KOOS/HOOS), and pain when bending (KOOS/HOOS), extending (KOOS/HOOS), twisting on knee (KOOS), and when walking on hard surfaces and uneven surface (HOOS). The stiffness subscale was expanded to incorporate other joint-specific symptoms, for example, range of motion (KOOS/HOOS), grinding/clicking (KOOS/HOOS), catching (KOOS), and swelling (KOOS). Both the KOOS and HOOS contain the original WOMAC 3.0 version in its entirety.

The KOOS contains 42 items, while the HOOS contains 40 items. Patients respond to each item based on their knee/hip condition over the previous week, on 5-point Likert scales. Both are intended to be patient-completed, and paper and electronic versions have been validated [29]. Completion time for patients is typically 10–15 min. Scoring can be performed in 2–3 min using a scoring spreadsheet (freely available at www.koos.nu). Higher scores represent better outcome. The KOOS and HOOS are intended to be scored as five individual subscales, and the use of one aggregate score is discouraged [30]. Clinicians should be aware that only 50 % of items are required to formulate a subscale score. This means that items that are not relevant for particular patients can be left out as required (e.g., patients who do not have a bathtub can leave out ADL item 13, which relates to problems getting in and out of the bath). If more than 50 % of items are missing, a subscale score should not be calculated.

The HOOS and KOOS are freely available (www.koos.nu), and have no fees associated with their use. The Website also provides multiple language versions of each PROM. This enhances their accessibility for clinical use. Although associated with longer completion times, the HOOS and KOOS provide information of five dimensions deemed important to patients, compared to other PROMs that evaluate fewer dimensions or give one aggregated score for a more general outcome such as "knee function" (where items including pain, other symptoms and difficulty with ADL function may be included). The latter case may make clinical interpretation more difficult. Users should balance patient burden alongside information provided.

In contrast to WOMAC, the HOOS and KOOS have content validity for younger adults who are more physically active. This is represented in the sport/recreation function subscale. Importantly, the use of both functional scales (ADL and sport/recreation) in younger patients with hip/knee problems allows clinicians to track their function over time, from immediately post-injury to the onset and progression of OA development. For example, the KOOS can be used to monitor patients who have sustained ACL or meniscal injuries. However, clinicians should keep in mind that the sport/recreation subscale may not be appropriate for older patients with more severe hip or knee osteoarthritis who are unable or unwilling to participate in more vigorous physical activity.

Because the KOOS/HOOS pain and function in ADL subscales are comprised largely of the corresponding WOMAC subscales, clinicians should be aware that overlap between the two subscales is still a consideration. Although the KOOS and HOOS have an additional item relating to frequency of knee/hip pain, the pain subscale is still predominantly related to pain during ADL.

For all KOOS and HOOS subscales in knee and hip OA, respectively, there is conflicting evidence regarding test–retest reliability. Although all subscales are sufficiently reliable for use in groups, findings are mixed for use in individual patients. Clinicians can account for this when interpreting an individual patient's KOOS scores by ensuring that changes exceed the MDC. For an individual patient with knee OA, the change in pain score should exceed 26.4, symptoms 21.2, ADL 23.8, sport/recreation 49.1, and QOL 24.9, to be considered a real change in condition [31]. For an individual patient with hip OA, clinicians can use values for the smallest detectable difference (SDD) to decide whether changes in subscale scores represent real change in condition. This is 15.1 for pain, 10.5 for symptoms, 9.6 for ADL, 15.5 for sport/recreation, and 16.2 for QOL [32]. Clinicians should note that differences in methods used to calculate the MDC and SDD mean that these values should not be compared.

The HOOS is responsive to improvements with pharmacological interventions and total hip replacement in patients with hip OA, whereas the KOOS can detect improvements with physical therapy and total knee replacement in patients with knee OA. The responsiveness of the HOOS following physical therapy has not been evaluated in a psychometric study. A large number of clinical trial reports, however, find significant improvements from a multitude of treatments when evaluated by the KOOS or HOOS. Floor effects associated with the sport/recreation subscales of the HOOS and KOOS in patients with more severe OA mean that this subscale may not be able to detect deterioration. However, it is also likely that this subscale is not relevant for this whole patient population. Ceiling effects have not been detected in patients with OA, but are possible after total joint replacement (Table 10.1).

KOOS Physical Function Short Form (KOOS-PS) and HOOS Physical Function Short Form (HOOS-PS)

An Osteoarthritis Research Society International (OARSI)/OMERACT initiative, the KOOS-PS and HOOS-PS were developed as measures of physical function for people with knee and hip OA, respectively. Statistical analysis (Rasch analysis) was used to select items from the ADL and sport/recreation subscales of the KOOS and HOOS in order to provide a shorter, single measure of physical function. This was aimed at reducing item redundancy detected in the WOMAC and HOOS function subscales. Clinicians should be aware that the KOOS-PS and HOOS-PS do not evaluate pain, symptoms, or hip/knee-related quality of life.

The KOOS-PS contains seven items, whereas the HOOS-PS contains five items, relating to function over the previous week. They are intended to be patient-completed, taking approximately 2 min. Scoring can be performed in less than 5 min, with higher scores representing better function. All items must have a response in order to calculate a total score (i.e., no missing items). The KOOS-PS and HOOS-PS are available free of charge in a number of language versions (www.koos.nu).

The KOOS-PS and HOOS-PS provide short, quick measures of physical function, which reduces the likelihood of missing items. They do not have any floor or ceiling effects, meaning that they can detect deterioration or improvement in a patient's condition. The KOOS-PS is responsive to physical therapy, pharmacological interventions, and total knee replacement, whereas the HOOS-PS is responsive to changes following pharmacological interventions and total hip replacement in patients with hip OA. Responsiveness to other interventions is unknown.

Similar to the longer formats, a limitation of the physical function short forms is their reliability for use in individual patients. Although both are sufficiently reliable for use in groups of patients, the HOOS-PS has conflicting findings regarding test–retest reliability in patients with hip OA, whereas the KOOS-PS does not demonstrate adequate reliability for use in individual patients. Changes in an individual patient's KOOS-PS score of greater than 18.6 points represents a real change [31], but this has not been determined for HOOS-PS.

Measure of Intermittent and Constant Osteoarthritis Pain (ICOAP)

An OARSI/OMERACT initiative, the ICOAP was designed to comprehensively capture the pain experience of patients across the spectrum of knee or hip OA [33]. Patient focus groups identified two distinct types of OA pain: (1) constant aching pain and (2) less frequent, more intense pain that is often unpredictable [25]. The ICOAP evaluates the impact of intermittent and constant pain, with respect to intensity, frequency, and effect on mood, sleep, and QOL. Unlike WOMAC and KOOS, the ICOAP evaluates pain independent of physical function. It is intended to be used in conjunction with a measure of physical function such as KOOS-PS or HOOS-PS.

The ICOAP was designed for administration by a clinician (in person or by telephone), although it can be used in a patient-completed format. Patients respond to each of the 11 items with respect to their pain over the previous week. There are separate versions for knee and hip OA. It is easy for clinicians to score manually, by summing the items for each subscale. If the patient marks outside the box, the closest box is used, but if two boxes are marked, the item is considered missing. If one or two items are missing, these are replaced with the mean score of all other items. The patient's response is considered invalid if three or more items are missing. Scores are normalized to a score from 0 to 100, with higher scores indicating a worse pain experience. Although the original publication suggested that a total score could be calculated, subsequent statistical (Rasch) analysis indicated that, for people with knee OA, the subscales should not be combined, and two individual subscale scores should be calculated [34].

Developed as an OARSI/OMERACT initiative, the ICOAP has widespread accessibility, being freely available on the OARSI website (www.oarsi.org). It has been translated into at least 15 languages.

A limitation of the ICOAP is its reliability. The reliability of ICOAP is adequate for use in groups of patients with hip OA, but not sufficient to use in individual patients. For patients with knee OA, the constant pain subscale does not have adequate reliability for use in individual patients, while there are conflicting findings for the intermittent pain subscale. Accordingly, the minimal amount of change that clinicians can consider to represent real change in the condition of a patient with knee OA is high (MDC_{90}: constant pain 35.8, intermittent pain 39.3, total 29 out of 100 [35]). This limits the ability of the ICOAP to detect smaller, real changes after treatment with exercise, physical therapy, or pharmacology. The constant pain subscale also has large floor effects, reducing its ability to detect deterioration in a patient's condition. While known measurement properties favor the use of the ICOAP in patients with hip OA rather than knee OA, further evaluation of its measurement properties is required in both knee and hip OA cohorts.

Osteoarthritis of Knee Hip Quality of Life (OAKHQOL)

The OAKHQOL was developed specifically to evaluate QoL in patients with knee or hip OA [36]. It consists of 43 items across five subscales (physical activities, mental health, pain, social support, and social functioning) that are scored individually, as well as three supplementary items (professional activity, relationship with partner, and sexual activity) [37]. A short version of the OAKHQOL was recently developed to enhance the utility of the instrument. The Mini-OAKHQOL has 20 items that fit within the same domains and includes the same three supplementary items [38] (Table 10.2).

Patients complete the OAKHQOL and Mini-OAKHQOL independently, recalling the previous 4 weeks when responding to each item. Completion time is 12–20 min for the full version, and less than 10 min for the short version. Clinicians score the OAKHQOL and Mini-OAKHQOL manually, by calculating a mean item score for each subscale, and report the score for each of the three supplementary items individually. If 50 % or more of the items for an individual subscale are missing, the subscale score is not calculated. Scores are normalized to 0–100, with higher scores representing better QOL. The OAKQHOL and Mini-OAKHQOL are free to use in clinical settings. The items are presented in the development papers (French [37], English [38]), although instructions for participants are not available in English. Clinicians can email to receive the full version of the Mini-OAKHQOL (Table 10.2). At this time, the OAKHQOL and Mini-OAKHQOL have not been widely translated to other language versions.

Clinicians can be confident that the OAKQHOL and Mini-OAKHQOL subscales measure the QOL dimensions that they intend to measure, and that all items within the physical activities, pain, and mental health subscales measure the same constructs (Table 10.1).

The number of missing items associated with the full version of the OAKHQOL can be high, especially for the supplementary items (>50 %). Clinicians may choose to use the Mini-OAKHOL instead to minimize missing information. Although the supplementary questions are likely to be relevant for some patients with knee or hip

OA, asking patients about their relationship with their partner or their sexual activity may be irrelevant to others, or viewed as intrusive [37]. Clinicians should particularly consider the cultural implications of these items [39]. Because these items are not involved in the calculation of subscale scores, they can be omitted when not relevant for particular patients.

As with other PROMs discussed in this chapter, current information suggests that the OAKHQOL and Mini-OAKHQOL may not be sufficiently reliable for use in individual patients. For the full version of the OAKHQOL, the physical activities and mental health subscales show conflicting findings, whereas the pain subscale shows reliability values consistently below the cut-off deemed adequate for use in individuals. For the Mini-OAKHQOL, none of these three subscales are adequate for use in individual patients, although they can be used reliably in groups of patients. Clinicians should be aware that the reliability of the social functioning and social support subscales is consistently low for both the full and short versions of OAKHQOL, for use in individual patients and groups of patients. This may be due to the small number of items in the social subscales. This means that clinicians need to look for large changes in scores for individual patients to be confident that a real change in condition has occurred. Unfortunately, there is no data available at this time regarding the magnitude of these changes. This should be seen as an important limitation of the OAKHQOL.

The full version of the OAKHQOL demonstrates no floor effects, and only the social support subscale demonstrates ceiling effects. This means that the OAKHQOL is able to detect deterioration and, generally, improvement in a patient's condition over time. However, the subscales of the OAKHQOL differ in their ability to detect improvements following total joint replacement. While the physical activities and pain subscales, and to a lesser extent the mental health subscale, show reasonably large effects following total hip or knee replacement, the social functioning and social support subscales demonstrate small to minimal effects. Clinicians should consider that this might reflect the intention of joint replacement surgery (i.e., to improve pain and function), rather than a limitation of the measure itself. The responsiveness of the OAKHQOL to nonsurgical treatments has not been evaluated. At present, there is no information regarding these properties for the Mini-OAKHQOL.

While the OAKHQOL covers a wide variety of domains that are important to patients with knee and/or hip OA [40], clinicians should be aware of the limitations of both the full and short versions of the OAKHQOL in terms of their measurement properties. Further studies may help to clarify this in the future.

Patient-Reported Outcome Measures Specific for Total Joint Replacement

Oxford Knee Score (OKS) and Oxford Hip Score (OHS)

The Oxford Knee and Hip Scores (Appendix 2) were developed specifically to assess the outcome of total knee or total hip replacement, respectively. Both PROMs consist of 12 items covering symptoms and function, with a recall period covering the previous 4 weeks. Patient completion time has been reported to be 5–10 min for the OKS and 2–15 min for the OHS. The OKS and OHS were intended for patient completion. Although one study has shown that paper and telephone methods of completion are equivalent at the group level, this is not the case for use at the individual level [41]. Hence, clinicians should use one method consistently to monitor an individual patient and avoid using two methods interchangeably. Calculation of a single score takes clinicians less than 5 min to complete manually. Using the revised scoring system [42], scores range from 0 to 48, with higher scores indicating better outcomes.

Generally, low rates of missing data are reported (Table 10.1). The revised scoring guidelines suggest that if only one or two items of the 12 are unanswered, the mean of all other responses can be entered [42]. A total score should not be calculated if more than two items are unanswered. If a patient selects two answers to one item, clinicians should select the response indicating a worse health state.

The OKS and OHS are available in a number of different language versions. Clinicians should visit the Website listed in Table 10.2 to obtain a copyright license for use. No fees apply for the use of the OKS or OHS in public or private clinical settings, although support materials (e.g., comprehensive user manual) may need to be purchased. Patient-completed versions are available in computer, smartphone, and tablet platforms.

Both the OKS and OHS were intended to be single scores, and evaluation of measurement properties has been conducted on single scores. However, subsequent analysis of all 12 items of the OHS revealed two distinct factors: pain and functional impairment [43]. Thus, clinicians may choose to calculate an overall score, or report as two individual scores (OHS-pain and OHS-functional impairment), but should consider that the measurement properties of the two subscales are not yet established. It is not clear whether the OKS can be reported as two subscales, and so this should be avoided at this time.

Nearly all studies evaluating the reliability of the OKS and OHS demonstrate adequate reliability for use in individual patients. For the OKS, changes in individual patient scores greater than 6.1 points (scored using the old scale 12–60) can be considered to represent real changes in the patient's condition. Values for the OHS are unknown. The OHS is able to detect deterioration in symptoms prior to total hip replacement [44], as well as improvement with hyaluronic acid injection and total hip replacement. The OKS can detect improvement following total knee replacement. Responsiveness of the OKS and OHS to other interventions has not been evaluated.

Harris Hip Score (HHS) and Modified Harris Hip Score (mHHS)

The HHS was developed as a clinician-administered tool to evaluate patients undergoing total hip replacement, and is commonly used in the literature and clinical practice. While it contains eight items that can be answered by the patient (relating to pain and function), there are also two items regarding the presence of deformity and hip range of motion that are performed by the clinician. Thus, the HHS cannot be a solely patient-reported measure. Patients undergoing total hip replacement were not involved in the development of the HHS, meaning that content validity cannot be assumed. The HHS is also associated with high ceiling effects in patients undergoing total hip replacement [45].

The mHHS evolved from the HHS to remove the items assessed by the clinician. Thus, in comparison to the HHS, the mHHS can be patient-reported. However, the measurement properties of the mHHS have not been evaluated in patients with OA or those who have undergone total hip replacement. Rather, studies have evaluated its measurement properties in patients who have undergone hip arthroscopy, whereof a proportion have chondropathy [46]. On this basis, it is difficult to recommend the use of the HHS or mHHS in patients with hip OA at this time.

Patient-Reported Outcome Measures for Hand Osteoarthritis

Hand OA is a heterogeneous and often polyarticular condition consisting of several phenotypes, including interphalangeal OA, thumb base OA, and erosive OA [12]. The high burden of disease and reduced QOL in people with hand OA is attributable to its impact on dexterity and ability to perform daily and occupational tasks that involve the upper limb [47]. There is a paucity of evidence for effective management of hand OA, with pharmacological interventions providing only symptomatic relief, and limited surgical options [48].

As for knee and hip OA, the OMERACT core domains for hand OA are pain, physical function, and patient global assessment [49]. Although health-related QOL is also specified as a core domain for hand OA, at this time there is no reliable, valid, or disease-specific instrument available. This domain can be left out of patient evaluation, or alternatively, clinicians may choose to use a generic QOL measure, as mentioned earlier. The other core domains specified for hand OA are joint activity and hand strength [49]. As these cannot be evaluated using PROMs, they will not be considered further in this chapter.

Because the disability associated with hand OA is distinctly different to knee and hip OA, the content of PROMs appropriate for use in patients with hand OA should also differ. Although general PROMs for rheumatic diseases, such as the Health Assessment Questionnaire (HAQ) and Arthritis Impact Measurement Scales (AIMS-2), are widely used to assess patients with hand OA, it is unlikely that their content will be sufficient to capture the extent to which patients can use their hands [50]. Similarly, PROMs intended for use in various hand conditions, such as the Michigan Hand Outcomes Questionnaire, may not adequately capture symptoms associated with OA. Thus, we recommend the use of disease-specific PROMs for patients with hand OA. However, clinicians should keep in mind that the PROMs discussed were developed more than 10 years ago. As such, their content may not adequately reflect common daily tasks performed today, such as using a smartphone or computer keyboard or mouse. This should be a priority of future PROM development for this patient population.

An important consideration for patients with hand OA is the length of the PROM, and method of administration. It may not be appropriate, or indeed possible, for a patient with hand OA to fill in a paper questionnaire for 20 min. Where possible, it is recommended that shorter PROMs are utilized to reduce the functional burden on the patient. If clinicians wish to use a longer PROM, they should consider using an electronic version (e.g., tablet/touchscreen) to facilitate easier completion.

In selecting PROMs for use in patients with hand OA, clinicians should be aware that the literature is not as advanced as for knee and hip OA measures. We present information on two hand OA-specific PROMs, a PROM intended for hand OA or rheumatoid arthritis, and one PROM developed for rheumatoid arthritis that has been validated for patients with hand OA (Table 10.3). In contrast to knee and hip OA measures, their measurement properties for use in hand OA is less well established, as summarized in Table 10.1.

Patient-Reported Outcome Measures Specific for Hand Osteoarthritis

Australian Canadian Osteoarthritis Hand Index (AUSCAN)

The AUSCAN was developed for patients with hand OA, by the same group who developed WOMAC. AUSCAN resembles WOMAC in style and format. It comprises 15 items evaluating the same domains as WOMAC: pain, stiffness, and function in ADL. Clinicians can choose to use the Likert or VAS version, and administer as a patient-completed questionnaire or via interview. Patients recall the previous 48 hours when responding to items, and typically take 3–7 min to complete. Scoring takes approximately 5 min, via manual or computer calculation (sum of all items in each subscale). It is unclear how to handle missing items, although assumed that guidelines are provided in the user manual that can be purchased with the license for use. Higher scores represent worse outcome. Although the developers suggested that an overall score can be calculated by summing the three subscale scores [51], subsequent analysis found that the pain, stiffness, and function subscales represent three separate constructs, and recommended that they should not be combined in a total score [52]. Clinicians can use population-based normative data as a comparison for individual patient scores [53].

There is evidence that the AUSCAN subscales measure what they intend to measure. Because patients with hand OA were involved in development, the AUSCAN can be considered to have content that is relevant for patients with hand OA (content validity). However, as with WOMAC, there is a high correlation between the pain and function subscales [54], likely due to the pain items asking about pain during particular functional activities. Clinicians should therefore consider that the pain subscale is more a measure of pain during ADL and may wish to use an additional measure of the impact of pain on other areas of life (e.g., pain VAS). It is also possible that some of the items in the pain and function subscales are redundant.

Table 10.3 Characteristics of recommended PROMs for hand OA

PROM	Dimensions evaluated (*indicates OMERACT core domain*)	Intended population	How to administer	Patient burden	Scoring	How to obtain	Available language translations
Specific for hand OA							
AUSCAN	*Pain* Stiffness *Physical function* (ADL)	Hand OA	Patient-completed or interviewer-administered	• 15 items – Pain (5) – Stiffness (1) – Function (9) • Recall previous 48 h • 3–7 min to complete	• 5 min to score • Manual or computer calculation (sum of all items in each subscale) • 3 individual subscales • Likert version: – Pain 0–20 – Stiffness 0–4 – Function 0–36 • VAS version: – Pain 0–500 – Stiffness 0–100 – Function 0–900 • Higher scores indicate worse pain, stiffness, or function	http://www.auscan.org (licensing and fee information, permission to use)	Dutch, English, French, German, Italian, Korean, Norwegian, Spanish

Table 10.3 (continued)

PROM	Dimensions evaluated (*indicates OMERACT core domain*)	Intended population	How to administer	Patient burden	Scoring	How to obtain	Available language translations
FIHOA	*Function*	Hand OA	Interviewer-administered; can be patient-completed	• 10 items • No recall period specified • 2–3 min to complete	• 3 min to score • Manual calculation (sum of all items) • Single score • 0–30 • Higher scores indicate worse function	Available in original [69] and subsequent [70] publications; no fees	Dutch, English, French, Italian
Specific for hand arthritis							
Cochin Hand Function Scale	*Function*	Developed for hand RA; validated in hand OA	Interviewer-administered; can be patient-completed	• 18 items • No recall period specified • 3–5 min to complete (when interviewer-administered)	• 3–5 min to score • Manual calculation (sum of all items) • Single score • 0–90 • Higher scores indicate worse function	Available in original publication [57]; no fees	English, French, Italian

ADL activities of daily living, *OA* osteoarthritis, *RA* rheumatoid arthritis, *VAS* visual analogue scale

All three subscales of the AUSCAN are able to detect improvements with anti-inflammatory drug intervention up to 8 weeks, with larger effects seen in the pain and function subscales. No studies have investigated the responsiveness of the AUSCAN to other interventions, or whether there are floor or ceiling effects associated with the AUSCAN subscales.

Clinicians should be aware that there are limitations with test–retest reliability. The pain and stiffness subscales do not show adequate reliability for use in individual patients, whereas the function subscale shows mixed results. Clinicians should keep this in mind when interpreting change scores for an individual patient, as observed changes may represent error in the measure rather than real change. The stiffness subscale is also not sufficiently reliable for use in groups, whereas there are mixed findings for the pain and function subscales. At this time, there are no guidelines as to the minimum value that clinicians can use to represent a real change in the patient's condition. Additional questions can be used alongside AUSCAN to ascertain whether scores represent real change (e.g., VAS for global change).

The AUSCAN is available in multiple language versions. However, as for WOMAC, the AUSCAN is copyright-protected and may be associated with a fee for clinical use. This limits its accessibility to all patients with hand OA. Clinicians should enquire via the Website provided in Table 10.3 regarding permission to use AUSCAN and associated costs.

Functional Index for Hand Osteoarthritis (FIHOA)

The FIHOA was developed in 1995 to evaluate hand function in patients with hand OA. Although intended to be clinician-administered, it can be completed by the patient. The FIHOA is freely available in four language versions and is quick to use in clinical settings. It consists of ten items scored on 4-point Likert scales and can be completed in 2–3 min. Clinicians can calculate a single score in approximately 3 min by manually summing all items, to give a score from 0 to 30. Higher scores indicate worse function. There are no instructions on how to handle missing items.

Because patients were not involved in the development of the FIHOA, content validity cannot be assumed. Item 7 is split based on more traditional gender roles. Men respond to "are you able to use a screwdriver?" while women answer "are you able to sew?" Clinicians should consider that it is likely that these roles will not fit all patients, especially younger patients. It may be more appropriate to have patients choose the task most relevant for them. However, clinicians should be aware that the measurement properties of the FIHOA have been established with this item in its original format, and therefore these cannot be assumed to carry over to a modified version. There may also be cultural considerations with item 10 ("would you accept a handshake without reluctance?").

The FIHOA consistently demonstrates adequate reliability for use in individual patients and groups of patients with hand OA. Clinicians can consider that an individual patient's change score that exceeds 5.55 points represents a real change (SDD) [55]. Studies also support its construct validity, meaning that the FIHOA measures what it is intended to measure. Although the FIHOA is able to detect changes with pharmacological interventions of up to 8 weeks duration, it tends to be less responsive than the function subscale of the AUSCAN. The responsiveness of the FIHOA to other interventions, as well as floor and ceiling effects, have not been evaluated.

Patient-Reported Outcome Measures Specific for Hand Arthritis

Cochin Hand Function Scale

The Cochin Hand Function Scale was intended to measure hand function in people with rheumatoid arthritis and has since been validated for patients with hand OA [56]. It is also known by other names, including the Duruoz Hand Index and the Hand Function Disability Scale. While it was designed to be administered by an interviewer, it can be self-completed by the patient. The Cochin Scale contains 18 items relating to hand function, including kitchen, dressing, hygiene, office, and other tasks, and does not specify a recall period. When interviewer-administered, it takes approximately 3–5 min to complete. Scoring is performed manually by summing items and takes less than 5 min. Subscale scores can be calculated, along with a single score (0–90), with higher scores indicating worse hand function. The Cochin Scale is free to use, with French and English versions available in the original publication [57]. An Italian translation has been used in studies on scleroderma.

Clinicians should consider whether the items contained within the Cochin Scale are relevant for their patient with hand OA. Because the Cochin Scale was developed with input from patients with rheumatoid arthritis, content validity for patients with hand OA cannot be assumed. Furthermore, included items may need updating to reflect more modern daily upper limb tasks, such as computer and smartphone use.

The Cochin Scale has evidence of adequate reliability for use in individual patients and groups of patients with hand OA. It is able to detect deterioration in hand function over 6 months and can discriminate between patients with hand OA who improve or deteriorate [56]. However, there is no evidence regarding measurement error, floor or ceiling effects, missing items, or responsiveness to treatment. This limits the ability to recommend the Cochin Scale for use in patients with hand OA at this time.

Score for Assessment and Quantification of Chronic Rheumatic Affections of the Hands (SACRAH)

The SACRAH is a measure of pain, stiffness, and function that was developed as a patient-completed PROM for patients with hand OA or rheumatoid arthritis. The original version consists of 23 items, each scored on a VAS [58], and takes 3–5 min for patients to complete. Manual calculation of an average score for each subscale is performed (0–100), with higher scores indicating worse pain, stiffness, or function.

Because there appeared to be some item redundancy in the SACRAH, a modified version was developed by removing redundant items, leaving 12 items that take approximately 1–3 min to complete [59, 60]. This was followed by a short-form SACRAH, which consists of five items recalling the previous 48 hours and takes patients less than 1 min to complete [61]. Both reduced versions are scored in the same way as the full SACRAH. English and German versions are available.

The three versions of the SACRAH have the potential to be useful for clinical evaluation of patients with hand OA. SACRAH covers the same three domains as AUSCAN with some overlap in items and does not have fees associated with its use. Therefore, the SACRAH could represent an ideal alternative to the AUSCAN, especially considering the three different formats. However, it is difficult to access a complete version of the SACRAH. Although all included items are listed in the development papers, clinicians may have issues locating full versions that include instructions for patients, such as the recall period.

Importantly, there is minimal information available regarding the measurement properties of the full, modified, and short-form SACRAH in people with hand OA. Clinicians should be aware that the short-form SACRAH pain and stiffness subscales only contain one item each. While this minimizes completion time, it is also likely to substantially influence the reliability of these subscales for use in individual patients. Therefore, until further evidence regarding the measurement properties of SACRAH is available, we do not recommend any of the three versions for use in patients with hand OA at this time.

Patient-Reported Outcome Measures for Osteoarthritis in Other Joints

As for the knee, hip, and hand, there are some PROMs that have been developed specifically to evaluate patients with OA in other joints. However, their measurement properties are less well established.

We encourage the reader to consider generic PROMs that can be used to evaluate pain and function in patients with OA. Visual analogue scales or numeric rating scales are widely used in clinical practice and provide a simple method of capturing a patient's pain severity. They have established measurement properties across various health conditions, including musculoskeletal pain [33]. The Patient-Specific Functional Scale is a quick and easy measure of function for clinical use [62]. Importantly, content validity is ensured as the patients nominate their own problematic activities, which are tracked over time.

Other region-specific PROMs that may be considered for use in patients with OA are listed below. However, it is important to determine whether their measurement properties have been established for patients with OA, and use this information when deciding their suitability for clinical use.

- Neck Pain and Disability Scale [63]
- Neck OutcOme Score (NOOS) (www.koos.nu) [64]
- Disabilities of the Arm, Shoulder and Hand Questionnaire (DASH) [65]
- Ankle Osteoarthritis Scale [66]
- Foot and Ankle Outcome Score (FAOS) (www.koos.nu) [67]

Conclusion

This chapter has provided a detailed summary of a selected group of PROMs for knee, hip, and hand OA. Clinicians should carefully consider the known characteristics of each PROM, in the context of the patient's characteristics, when selecting the ideal PROM for specific patients. While further research is needed to establish the measurement properties of PROMs for OA, and develop additional PROMs to address gaps in available tools, clinicians can use the information provided to guide selection of appropriate tools for clinical management of patients with OA.

Appendix 1: Example of knee PROM—Knee injury and Osteoarthritis Outcome Score (KOOS)

KOOS KNEE SURVEY

Today's date: ____/_____/_____ Date of birth: ____/_____/_____

Name: ____

INSTRUCTIONS: This survey asks for your view about your knee. This information will help us keep track of how you feel about your knee and how well you are able to perform your usual activities.
Answer every question by ticking the appropriate box, only <u>one</u> box for each question. If you are unsure about how to answer a question, please give the best answer you can.

Symptoms
These questions should be answered thinking of your knee symptoms during the **last week**.

S1. Do you have swelling in your knee?

Never	Rarely	Sometimes	Often	Always
☐	☐	☐	☐	☐

S2. Do you feel grinding, hear clicking or any other type of noise when your knee moves?

Never	Rarely	Sometimes	Often	Always
☐	☐	☐	☐	☐

S3. Does your knee catch or hang up when moving?

Never	Rarely	Sometimes	Often	Always
☐	☐	☐	☐	☐

S4. Can you straighten your knee fully?

Always	Often	Sometimes	Rarely	Never
☐	☐	☐	☐	☐

S5. Can you bend your knee fully?

Always	Often	Sometimes	Rarely	Never
☐	☐	☐	☐	☐

Stiffness
The following questions concern the amount of joint stiffness you have experienced during the **last week** in your knee. Stiffness is a sensation of restriction or slowness in the ease with which you move your knee joint.

S6. How severe is your knee joint stiffness after first wakening in the morning?

None	Mild	Moderate	Severe	Extreme
☐	☐	☐	☐	☐

S7. How severe is your knee stiffness after sitting, lying or resting **later in the day**?

None	Mild	Moderate	Severe	Extreme
☐	☐	☐	☐	☐

Appendix 2: Example of knee PROM—Oxford Knee Score

Pain

P1. How often do you experience knee pain?

Never	Monthly	Weekly	Daily	Always
☐	☐	☐	☐	☐

What amount of knee pain have you experienced the **last week** during the following activities?

P2. Twisting/pivoting on your knee

None	Mild	Moderate	Severe	Extreme
☐	☐	☐	☐	☐

P3. Straightening knee fully

None	Mild	Moderate	Severe	Extreme
☐	☐	☐	☐	☐

P4. Bending knee fully

None	Mild	Moderate	Severe	Extreme
☐	☐	☐	☐	☐

P5. Walking on flat surface

None	Mild	Moderate	Severe	Extreme
☐	☐	☐	☐	☐

P6. Going up or down stairs

None	Mild	Moderate	Severe	Extreme
☐	☐	☐	☐	☐

P7. At night while in bed

None	Mild	Moderate	Severe	Extreme
☐	☐	☐	☐	☐

P8. Sitting or lying

None	Mild	Moderate	Severe	Extreme
☐	☐	☐	☐	☐

P9. Standing upright

None	Mild	Moderate	Severe	Extreme
☐	☐	☐	☐	☐

Function, daily living

The following questions concern your physical function. By this we mean your ability to move around and to look after yourself. For each of the following activities please indicate the degree of difficulty you have experienced in the **last week** due to your knee.

A1. Descending stairs

None	Mild	Moderate	Severe	Extreme
☐	☐	☐	☐	☐

A2. Ascending stairs

None	Mild	Moderate	Severe	Extreme
☐	☐	☐	☐	☐

For each of the following activities please indicate the degree of difficulty you have experienced in the **last week** due to your knee.

A3. Rising from sitting

None	Mild	Moderate	Severe	Extreme
☐	☐	☐	☐	☐

A4. Standing

None	Mild	Moderate	Severe	Extreme
☐	☐	☐	☐	☐

A5. Bending to floor/pick up an object

None	Mild	Moderate	Severe	Extreme
☐	☐	☐	☐	☐

A6. Walking on flat surface

None	Mild	Moderate	Severe	Extreme
☐	☐	☐	☐	☐

A7. Getting in/out of car

None	Mild	Moderate	Severe	Extreme
☐	☐	☐	☐	☐

A8. Going shopping

None	Mild	Moderate	Severe	Extreme
☐	☐	☐	☐	☐

A9. Putting on socks/stockings

None	Mild	Moderate	Severe	Extreme
☐	☐	☐	☐	☐

A10. Rising from bed

None	Mild	Moderate	Severe	Extreme
☐	☐	☐	☐	☐

A11. Taking off socks/stockings

None	Mild	Moderate	Severe	Extreme
☐	☐	☐	☐	☐

A12. Lying in bed (turning over, maintaining knee position)

None	Mild	Moderate	Severe	Extreme
☐	☐	☐	☐	☐

A13. Getting in/out of bath

None	Mild	Moderate	Severe	Extreme
☐	☐	☐	☐	☐

A14. Sitting

None	Mild	Moderate	Severe	Extreme
☐	☐	☐	☐	☐

A15. Getting on/off toilet

None	Mild	Moderate	Severe	Extreme
☐	☐	☐	☐	☐

For each of the following activities please indicate the degree of difficulty you have experienced in the **last week** due to your knee.

A16. Heavy domestic duties (moving heavy boxes, scrubbing floors, etc)

None	Mild	Moderate	Severe	Extreme
☐	☐	☐	☐	☐

A17. Light domestic duties (cooking, dusting, etc)

None	Mild	Moderate	Severe	Extreme
☐	☐	☐	☐	☐

Function, sports and recreational activities

The following questions concern your physical function when being active on a higher level. The questions should be answered thinking of what degree of difficulty you have experienced during the **last week** due to your knee.

SP1. Squatting

None	Mild	Moderate	Severe	Extreme
☐	☐	☐	☐	☐

SP2. Running

None	Mild	Moderate	Severe	Extreme
☐	☐	☐	☐	☐

SP3. Jumping

None	Mild	Moderate	Severe	Extreme
☐	☐	☐	☐	☐

SP4. Twisting/pivoting on your injured knee

None	Mild	Moderate	Severe	Extreme
☐	☐	☐	☐	☐

SP5. Kneeling

None	Mild	Moderate	Severe	Extreme
☐	☐	☐	☐	☐

Quality of Life

Q1. How often are you aware of your knee problem?

Never	Monthly	Weekly	Daily	Constantly
☐	☐	☐	☐	☐

Q2. Have you modified your life style to avoid potentially damaging activities to your knee?

Not at all	Mildly	Moderately	Severely	Totally
☐	☐	☐	☐	☐

Q3. How much are you troubled with lack of confidence in your knee?

Not at all	Mildly	Moderately	Severely	Extremely
☐	☐	☐	☐	☐

Q4. In general, how much difficulty do you have with your knee?

None	Mild	Moderate	Severe	Extreme
☐	☐	☐	☐	☐

Thank you very much for completing all the questions in this questionnaire.

Problems with your knee

Check (✓) one box for every question.

1. During the past 4 weeks...

How would you describe the pain you usually have from your knee?

None	Very mild	Mild	Moderate	Severe
☐	☐	☐	☐	☐

2. During the past 4 weeks...

Have you had any trouble with washing and drying yourself (all over) because of your knee?

No trouble at all	Very little trouble	Moderate trouble	Extreme difficulty	Impossible to do
☐	☐	☐	☐	☐

3. During the past 4 weeks...

Have you had any trouble getting in and out of a car or using public transportation because of your knee? (whichever you would tend to use)

No trouble at all	Very little trouble	Moderate trouble	Extreme difficulty	Impossible to do
☐	☐	☐	☐	☐

4. During the past 4 weeks...

For how long have you been able to walk before pain from your knee becomes **severe**? (with or without a cane)

No pain/more than 30 minutes	16 to 30 minutes	5 to 15 minutes	Around the house only	Not at all/severe pain when walking
☐	☐	☐	☐	☐

5. During the past 4 weeks...

After a meal (sitting at a table), how painful has it been for you to stand up from a chair because of your knee?

Not at all painful	Slightly painful	Moderately painful	Very painful	Unbearable
☐	☐	☐	☐	☐

6. During the past 4 weeks...

Have you been limping when walking because of your knee?

Rarely/ never	Sometimes, or just at first	Often, not just at first	Most of the time	All of the time
☐	☐	☐	☐	☐

7. During the past 4 weeks...

Could you kneel down and get up again afterwards?

Yes, easily	With little difficulty	With moderate difficulty	With extreme difficulty	No, impossible
☐	☐	☐	☐	☐

8. During the past 4 weeks...

Have you been troubled by pain from your knee in bed at night?

No nights	Only 1 or 2 nights	Some nights	Most nights	Every night
☐	☐	☐	☐	☐

9. During the past 4 weeks...

How much has pain from your knee interfered with your usual work (including housework)?

Not at all	A little bit	Moderately	Greatly	Totally
☐	☐	☐	☐	☐

10. During the past 4 weeks...

Have you felt that your knee might suddenly "give out" or let you down?

Rarely/ never	Sometimes, or just at first	Often, not just at first	Most of the time	All of the time
☐	☐	☐	☐	☐

11. During the past 4 weeks...

Could you do the grocery shopping <u>on your own</u>?

Yes, easily	With little difficulty	With moderate difficulty	With extreme difficulty	No, impossible
☐	☐	☐	☐	☐

12. During the past 4 weeks...

Could you walk down one flight of stairs?

Yes, easily	With little difficulty	With moderate difficulty	With extreme difficulty	No, impossible
☐	☐	☐	☐	☐

Finally, please check that you have answered each question.

Thank you very much.

References

1. Lawrence RC, Felson DT, Helmick CG, Arnold LM, Choi H, Deyo RA, et al. Estimates of the prevalence of arthritis and other rheumatic conditions in the United States. Part II. Arthritis Rheum. 2008;58(1):26–35.
2. Neogi T, Zhang Y. Epidemiology of osteoarthritis. Rheum Dis Clin North Am. 2013;39(1):1–19.
3. Vos T, Flaxman AD, Naghavi M, Lozano R, Michaud C, Ezzati M, et al. Years lived with disability (ylds) for 1160 sequelae of 289 diseases and injuries 1990–2010: a systematic analysis for the global burden of disease study 2010. Lancet. 2012;380(9859):2163–96.
4. Culvenor AG, Collins NJ, Guermazi A, Cook JL, Vicenzino B, Khan KM, et al. Early knee osteoarthritis is evident one year following anterior cruciate ligament reconstruction: a magnetic resonance imaging evaluation. Arthritis Rheum. 2015;67(4):946–55.
5. Hinman RS, Lentzos J, Vicenzino B, Crossley KM. Is patellofemoral osteoarthritis common in middle-aged people with chronic patellofemoral pain? Arthritis Care Res. 2014;66(8):1252–7.
6. Kemp JL, Makdissi M, Schache AG, Pritchard MG, Pollard TC, Crossley KM. Hip chondropathy at arthroscopy: prevalence and relationship to labral pathology, femoroacetabular impingement and patient-reported outcomes. Br J Sports Med. 2014;48(11):1102–7.
7. Gossec L, Paternotte S, Bingham 3rd CO, Clegg DO, Coste P, Conaghan PG, et al. Oarsi/omeract initiative to define states of severity and indication for joint replacement in hip and knee osteoarthritis. An omeract 10 special interest group. J Rheumatol. 2011;38(8):1765–9.
8. Collins NJ, Roos EM. Patient-reported outcomes for total hip and knee arthroplasty: commonly used instruments and attributes of a "good" measure. Clin Geriatr Med. 2012;28(3):367–94.
9. Bellamy N, Kirwan J, Boers M, Brooks P, Strand V, Tugwell P, et al. Recommendations for a core set of outcome measures for future phase III clinical trials in knee, hip, and hand osteoarthritis. Consensus development at omeract III. J Rheumatol. 1997;24(4):799–802.
10. Lane NE, Hochberg MC, Nevitt MC, Simon LS, Nelson AE, Doherty M, et al. Oarsi clinical trials recommendations: design and conduct of clinical trials for hip osteoarthritis. Osteoarthritis Cartilage. 2015;23(5):761–71.

11. McAlindon TE, Driban JB, Henrotin Y, Hunter DJ, Jiang GL, Skou ST, et al. Oarsi clinical trials recommendations: design, conduct, and reporting of clinical trials for knee osteoarthritis. Osteoarthritis Cartilage. 2015;23(5):747–60.
12. Kloppenburg M, Maheu E, Kraus VB, Cicuttini F, Doherty M, Dreiser RL, et al. Oarsi clinical trials recommendations: design and conduct of clinical trials for hand osteoarthritis. Osteoarthritis Cartilage. 2015;23(5):772–86.
13. Ware Jr J, Kosinski M, Keller SD. A 12-item short-form health survey: construction of scales and preliminary tests of reliability and validity. Med Care. 1996;34(3):220–33.
14. Ware Jr JE, Sherbourne CD. The mos 36-item short-form health survey (sf-36). I. Conceptual framework and item selection. Med Care. 1992;30(6):473–83.
15. Hawthorne G, Richardson J, Osborne R. The assessment of quality of life (aqol) instrument: a psychometric measure of health-related quality of life. Quality Life Res. 1999;8(3):209–24.
16. Bellamy N, Buchanan WW, Goldsmith CH, Campbell J, Stitt LW. Validation study of WOMAC: a health status instrument for measuring clinically important patient relevant outcomes to antirheumatic drug therapy in patients with osteoarthritis of the hip or knee. J Rheumatol. 1988;15(12):1833–40.
17. Bellamy N, Campbell J, Stevens J, Pilch L, Stewart C, Mahmood Z. Validation study of a computerized version of the western Ontario and McMaster universities va3.0 osteoarthritis index. J Rheumatol. 1997;24:2413–5.
18. Bellamy N, Wilson C, Hendrikz J, Whitehouse SL, Patel B, Dennison S, et al. Osteoarthritis index delivered by mobile phone (m-WOMAC) is valid, reliable, and responsive. J Clin Epidemiol. 2011;64(2):182–90.
19. Bellamy N, Campbell J, Hill J. A comparative study of telephone vs on-site completion of the womac 3.0 osteoarthritis index. J Rheumatol. 2002;29:783–6.
20. Theiler R, Spielberger J, Bischoff HA, Bellamy N, Huber J, Kroesen S. Clinical evaluation of the womac 3.0 oa index in numeric rating scale format using a computerized touch screen version. Osteoarthritis Cartilage. 2002;10(6):479–81.
21. Dowsey MM, Choong PF. The utility of outcome measures in total knee replacement surgery. Int J Rheum. 2013;2013:506518.
22. Bellamy N. Womac osteoarthritis index user guide. London: Victoria Hospital; 1995.
23. Ghomrawi HM, Mandl LA, Rutledge J, Alexiades MM, Mazumdar M. Is there a role for expectation maximization imputation in addressing missing data in research using womac questionnaire? Comparison to the standard mean approach and a tutorial. BMC Musculoskelet Disord. 2011;12:109.
24. Gandek B. Measurement properties of the western Ontario and McMaster universities osteoarthritis index: a systematic review. Arthritis Care Res. 2015;67(2):216–29.
25. Hawker GA, Stewart L, French MR, Cibere J, Jordan JM, March L, et al. Understanding the pain experience in hip and knee osteoarthritis—an oarsi/omeract initiative. Osteoarthritis Cartilage. 2008;16(4):415–22.
26. Pua YH, Cowan SM, Wrigley TV, Bennell KL. The lower extremity functional scale could be an alternative to the western ontario and mcmaster universities osteoarthritis index physical function scale. J Clin Epidemiol. 2009;62(10):1103–11.
27. Impellizzeri FM, Mannion AF, Leunig M, Bizzini M, Naal FD. Comparison of the reliability, responsiveness, and construct validity of 4 different questionnaires for evaluating outcomes after total knee arthroplasty. J Arthroplasty. 2011;26(6):861–9.
28. McConnell S, Kolopack P, Davis A. The western ontario and mcmaster universities osteoarthritis index (womac): a review of its utility and measurement properties. Arthritis Rheum. 2001;45(5):453–61.
29. Gudbergsen H, Bartels EM, Krusager P, Waehrens EE, Christensen R, Danneskiold-Samsoe B, et al. Test-retest of computerized health status questionnaires frequently used in the monitoring of knee osteoarthritis: a randomized crossover trial. BMC Musculoskelet Disord. 2011;12:190.
30. Roos EM, Lohmander LS. The knee injury and osteoarthritis outcome score (KOOS): from joint injury to osteoarthritis. Health Qual Life Outcomes. 2003;1:64.

31. Collins NJ, Prinsen CA, Christensen R, Bartels EM, Terwee CB, Roos EM. Knee Injury and Osteoarthritis Outcome Score (KOOS): systematic review and meta-analysis of measurement properties. Osteoarthritis Cartilage. 2016 Mar 21. pii: S1063-4584(16)01071-2. doi:10.1016/j.joca.2016.03.010. [Epub ahead of print].
32. Ornetti P, Parratte S, Gossec L, Tavernier C, Argenson JN, Roos EM, et al. Cross-cultural adaptation and validation of the French version of the hip disability and osteoarthritis outcome score (HOOS) in hip osteoarthritis patients. Osteoarthritis Cartilage. 2010;18(4):522–9.
33. Hawker GA, Mian S, Kendzerska T, French M. Measures of adult pain: Visual Analog Scale for Pain (VAS Pain), Numeric Rating Scale for Pain (NRS Pain), McGill Pain Questionnaire (MPQ), Short-Form McGill Pain Questionnaire (SF-MPQ), Chronic Pain Grade Scale (CPGS), Short Form-36 Bodily Pain Scale (SF-36 BPS), and Measure of Intermittent and Constant Osteoarthritis Pain (ICOAP). Arthritis Care Res. 2011;63 Suppl 11:S240–52.
34. Moreton BJ, Wheeler M, Walsh DA, Lincoln NB. Rasch analysis of the intermittent and constant osteoarthritis pain (ICOAP) scale. Osteoarthritis Cartilage. 2012;20(10):1109–15.
35. Robbins SM, Rastogi R, Howard J, Rosedale R. Comparison of measurement properties of the p4 pain scale and disease specific pain measures in patients with knee osteoarthritis. Osteoarthritis Cartilage. 2014;22(6):805–12.
36. Rat AC, Coste J, Pouchot J, Baumann M, Spitz E, Retel-Rude N, et al. Oakhqol: a new instrument to measure quality of life in knee and hip osteoarthritis. J Clin Epidemiol. 2005;58(1):47–55.
37. Rat AC, Pouchot J, Coste J, Baumann C, Spitz E, Retel-Rude N, et al. Development and testing of a specific quality-of-life questionnaire for knee and hip osteoarthritis: OAKHQOL (osteoarthritis of knee hip quality of life). Joint Bone Spine. 2006;73(6):697–704.
38. Guillemin F, Rat AC, Goetz C, Spitz E, Pouchot J, Coste J. The Mini-OAKHQOL for knee and hip osteoarthritis quality of life was obtained following recent shortening guidelines. J Clin Epidemiol. 2015;69:70–8.
39. Serhier Z, Harzy T, ELfakir S, Diouny S, El Rhazi K, Bennani Othmani M, et al. Cross-cultural adaptation and validation of the knee and hip health-related quality of life (OAKHQoL) in a Moroccan Arabic-speaking population. Rheumatology international. 2012;32(4):1015–23.
40. Rat AC, Guillemin F, Pouchot J. Mapping the osteoarthritis knee and hip quality of life (OAKHQOL) instrument to the international classification of functioning, disability and health and comparison to five health status instruments used in osteoarthritis. Rheumatology (Oxford). 2008;47(11):1719–25.
41. Abdel Messih M, Naylor JM, Descallar J, Manickam A, Mittal R, Harris IA. Mail versus telephone administration of the oxford knee and hip scores. J Arthroplasty. 2014;29(3):491–4.
42. Murray D, Fitzpatrick R, Rogers K, Pandit H, Beard D, Carr A, et al. The use of the oxford hip and knee scores. J Bone Joint Surg Br. 2007;89(8):1010–4.
43. Norquist JM, Fitzpatrick R, Dawson J, Jenkinson C. Comparing alternative RASCH-based methods vs raw scores in measuring change in health. Med Care. 2004;42(1 Suppl):I25–36.
44. Ostendorf M, Buskens E, van Stel H, Schrijvers A, Marting L, Dhert W, et al. Waiting for total hip arthroplasty: avoidable loss in quality time and preventable deterioration. J Arthroplasty. 2004;19(3):302–9.
45. Wamper KE, Sierevelt IN, Poolman RW, Bhandari M, Haverkamp D. The harris hip score: do ceiling effects limit its usefulness in orthopedics? Acta Orthop. 2010;81(6):703–7.
46. Kemp JL, Collins NJ, Roos EM, Crossley KM. Psychometric properties of patient-reported outcome measures for hip arthroscopic surgery. Am J Sports Med. 2013;41(9):2065–73.
47. Bukhave EB, Huniche L. Activity problems in everyday life—patients' perspectives of hand osteoarthritis: "try imagining what it would be like having no hands". Disabil Rehabil. 2014;36(19):1636–43.
48. Kloppenburg M, Kwok WY. Hand osteoarthritis—a heterogeneous disorder. Nat Rev Rheumatol. 2012;8(1):22–31.

49. Kloppenburg M, Boyesen P, Visser AW, Haugen IK, Boers M, Boonen A, et al. Report from the omeract hand osteoarthritis working group: set of core domains and preliminary set of instruments for use in clinical trials and observational studies. J Rheumatol. 2015;1.
50. O'Connor D, Kortman B, Smith A, Ahern M, Smith M, Krishnan J. Correlation between objective and subjective measures of hand function in patients with rheumatoid arthritis. J Hand Ther. 1999;12(4):323–9.
51. Bellamy N, Campbell J, Haraoui B, Buchbinder R, Hobby K, Roth JH, et al. Dimensionality and clinical importance of pain and disability in hand osteoarthritis: development of the Australian/Canadian (AUSCAN) osteoarthritis hand index. Osteoarthritis Cartilage. 2002;10(11):855–62.
52. Haugen IK, Moe RH, Slatkowsky-Christensen B, Kvien TK, van der Heijde D, Garratt A. The AUSCAN subscales, AIMS-2 hand/finger subscale, and FIOHA were not unidimensionalscales. J Clin Epidemiol. 2011;64(9):1039–46.
53. Bellamy N, Wilson C, Hendrikz J. Population-based normative values for the western ontario and mcmaster (Womac) osteoarthritis index and the Australian/Canadian (AUSCAN) hand osteoarthritis index functional subscales. Inflammopharmacology. 2010;18(1):1–8.
54. Moon KW, Lee SS, Kim JH, Song R, Lee EY, Song YW, et al. Cross-cultural adaptation, validation, and responsiveness of the Korean version of the auscan osteoarthritis index. Rheumatol Int. 2012;32(11):3551–7.
55. Moe RH, Garratt A, Slatkowsky-Christensen B, Maheu E, Mowinckel P, Kvien TK, et al. Concurrent evaluation of data quality, reliability and validity of the Australian Canadian osteoarthritis hand index and the functional index for hand osteoarthritis. Rheumatology (Oxford). 2010;49(12):2327–36.
56. Poiraudeau S, Chevalier X, Conrozier T, Flippo RM, Liote F, Noel E, et al. Reliability, validity, and sensitivity to change of the cochin hand functional disability scale in hand osteoarthritis. Osteoarthritis Cartilage. 2001;9(6):570–7.
57. Duruoz MT, Poiraudeau S, Fermanian J, Menkes CJ, Amor B, Dougados M, et al. Development and validation of a rheumatoid hand functional disability scale that assesses functional handicap. J Rheumatol. 1996;23(7):1167–72.
58. Leeb BF, Sautner J, Andel I, Rintelen B. SACRAH: a score for assessment and quantification of chronic rheumatic affections of the hands. Rheumatology (Oxford). 2003;42(10):1173–8.
59. Sautner J, Andel I, Rintelen B, Leeb BF. Development of the M-SACRAH, a modified, shortened version of SACRAH (score for the assessment and quantification of chronic rheumatoid affections of the hands). Rheumatology (Oxford). 2004;43(11):1409–13.
60. Sautner J, Andel I, Rintelen B, Leeb BF. A comparison of the modified score for the assessment of chronic rheumatoid affections of the hands and the australian/canadian osteoarthritis hand index in hand osteoarthritis patients. Int J Rheum. 2009;2009:249096.
61. Rintelen B, Haindl PM, Mai HT, Sautner J, Maktari A, Leeb BF. A tool for the assessment of hand involvement in rheumatic disorders in daily routine—the SF-SACRAH (short form score for the assessment and quantification of chronic rheumatic affections of the hands). Osteoarthritis Cartilage. 2009;17(1):59–63.
62. Chatman AB, Hyams SP, Neel JM, Binkley JM, Stratford PW, Schomberg A, et al. The patient-specific functional scale: measurement properties in patients with knee dysfunction. Phys Ther. 1997;77(8):820–9.
63. Wheeler AH, Goolkasian P, Baird AC, Darden 2nd BV. Development of the neck pain and disability scale. Item analysis, face, and criterion-related validity. Spine. 1999;24(13):1290–4.
64. Juul T, Sogaard K, Roos EM, Davis AM. Development of a patient-reported outcome: the neck outcome score (NOOS)—content and construct validity. J Rehabil Med. 2015;47(9):844–53.
65. McPhail SM, Bagraith KS, Schippers M, Wells PJ, Hatton A. Use of condition-specific patient-reported outcome measures in clinical trials among patients with wrist osteoarthritis: a systematic review. Adv Orthop. 2012;2012:273421.
66. Domsic RT, Saltzman CL. Ankle osteoarthritis scale. Foot Ankle Int. 1998;19(7):466–71.

67. Golightly YM, Devellis RF, Nelson AE, Hannan MT, Lohmander LS, Renner JB, et al. Psychometric properties of the foot and ankle outcome score in a community-based study of adults with and without osteoarthritis. Arthritis Care Res. 2014;66(3):395–403.
68. Davis AM, Perruccio AV, Canizares M, Tennant A, Hawker GA, Conaghan PG, et al. The development of a short measure of physical function for hip OA HOOS-Physical FunctionShortform (HOOS-PS): an OARSI/OMERACT initiative. Osteoarthritis Cartilage. 2008;16(5):551–9.
69. Dreiser RL, Maheu E, Guillou GB, Caspard H, Grouin JM. Validation of an algofunctional index for osteoarthritis of the hand. Rev Rhum Engl Ed. 1995;62(6 Suppl 1):43S–53.
70. Wittoek R, Cruyssen BV, Maheu E, Verbruggen G. Cross-cultural adaptation of the Dutch version of the functional index for hand osteoarthritis (FIHOA) and a study on its construct validity. Osteoarthritis Cartilage. 2009;17(5):607–12.

Chapter 11
PROMs for Systemic Sclerosis (Scleroderma)

Russell E. Pellar, Theresa M. Tingey, and Janet E. Pope

Introduction

Systemic sclerosis, otherwise known as scleroderma or SSc, is a rare multisystem connective tissue disease of unknown cause with fibrosis of the skin and internal organs, vascular disruption and damage, and the production of autoantibodies. These characteristic features lead to the development of many heterogeneous clinical features depending on the extent of disease and organs involved [1]. SSc is chronic in its course and is associated with significant morbidity and mortality and is one of the most severe connective tissue diseases [2–4].

Perhaps the most well recognized and universal physical manifestation of SSc is the progressive skin thickening and fibrosis [1]. This distinctive element of SSc classically involves the hands, but may also affect the arms, trunk, face, legs, and essentially any skin and carries the potential to cause substantial disfigurement and disability [5–7]. Due to the fibrosis, inflammation, pain, and joint contractures of SSc, patients often struggle with essential and basic tasks such as holding objects, reaching, eating, bathing, grooming, dressing, climbing stairs, and/or walking at all [8]. Because SSc is chronic and progressive, impaired function tends to worsen with time [9].

Although the clinical course is quite variable, SSc is typically classified as either limited cutaneous SSc (lcSSc) or diffuse cutaneous SSc (dcSSc), depending on the extent of skin involvement. In lcSSc, skin fibrosis not only is found distal to the

R.E. Pellar, B.E.Sc. (✉) • T.M. Tingey, B.Arts.Sc.
Schulich School of Medicine and Dentistry, University of Western Ontario, London, ON, Canada
e-mail: janet.pope@sjhc.london.on.ca

J.E. Pope, M.D., M.P.H., F.R.C.P.C.
Division of Rheumatology, Schulich School of Medicine and Dentistry, University of Western Ontario, London, ON, Canada

Division of Rheumatology, Department of Medicine, St. Joseph's Health Care London, London, ON, Canada

Y. El Miedany (ed.), *Patient Reported Outcome Measures in Rheumatic Diseases*,
DOI 10.1007/978-3-319-32851-5_11

elbows and knees, but may also affect the face and neck. In dcSSc, skin fibrosis is found both distally and proximally and represents the more severe form of SSc, with a more progressive course and earlier internal organ manifestations [10–13].

People with SSc experience many additional problems that can markedly impair their quality of life and general health [3, 14, 15]. Patients frequently experience pain that is multifactorial in nature, occurring as a result of, but not limited to, fingertip ulcers, Raynaud's phenomenon, skin inflammation, calcinosis, inflammatory arthritis, and muscle tenderness [16, 17]. A sometimes overlooked but common symptom of SSc is pruritus, which negatively impacts quality of life through several physical and psychosocial mechanisms, such as by affecting sleep cycles [18, 19]. The gastrointestinal tract can be a source of significant impairment as it becomes fibrotic, causing dysmotility and an inappropriately patent lower esophageal sphincter, resulting in gastroesophageal reflux disorder (GERD), dysphagia, choking, cramps, bloating, early satiety, gastric dumping, incontinence, diarrhea, and constipation [8, 16]. The lungs can be involved with interstitial lung disease (ILD) and pulmonary arterial hypertension (PAH), both of which can be lethal, and can cause symptoms of dyspnea and fatigue [8, 16]. ILD can be associated with cough and occasionally chest pain. There may be pleural or pericardial effusions, which can also cause chest pain. The kidneys may be affected with scleroderma renal crisis (SRC). There are several cardiac features in SSc including cardiomyopathy, arrhythmia, and constrictive pericarditis, further complicating the already complex systemic picture of SSc [16].

Personal, social, and work life are not only disrupted by the aggressive and widespread nature of SSc and its physically destructive complications, but also by other features including fatigue, difficulty sleeping, depressive symptoms, fear of progression and dying, body image issues, work disability, and sexual dysfunction that frequently occurs [8, 20–25]. In fact, the rate of work disability in SSc is higher than in rheumatoid arthritis [7]. Research by Bassel et al. demonstrated that fatigue was the most common symptom (89 %) SSc patients experienced, often with a moderate-to-severe impact on daily activities (72 %) [8]. Other notable symptoms in terms of frequency and impact were Raynaud's phenomenon, hand stiffness, joint pain, sleeping difficulties, poor hand function, and pain [8]. SSc impacts self-esteem by causing visible disfigurement on socially important areas of skin, such as the hands (e.g., digital ulcers or loss, contractures, and swollen fingers) and face (e.g., tight skin, telangiectasia, thin lips, loss of subcutaneous tissue, and increased wrinkles around the mouth as SSc regresses). No cure exists for SSc, and many features of SSc are physically prominent and worsen with time, further enhancing fears regarding their disease [24, 25]. See Fig. 11.1 for a visual depiction of some features of SSc.

Some symptoms can be managed to reduce their impact on patients; however, at present there is a paucity of proven effective disease-modifying agents and often a lack of recommendations for psychosocial management. Thus, SSc treatment typically requires a combination of organ-based symptomatic treatment and potentially disease-modifying agents. These treatments have possible side effects and risk to the patient and result in complex regimens of medications and frequent follow-up. By determining which treatments SSc patients find effective, high-quality instruments for measuring patient-reported outcomes (PROs) can help enrich and expand opti-

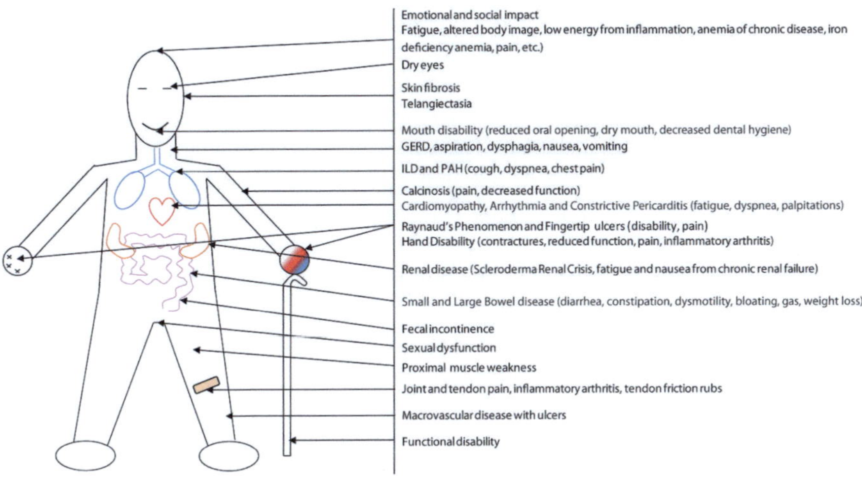

Fig. 11.1 A diagram depicting common features of systemic sclerosis (SSc). *GERD* gastroesophageal reflux disease, *ILD* interstitial lung disease, *PAH* pulmonary arterial hypertension

mal management of SSc. In addition, following patients with SSc is more complete in research cohorts and also clinical practice if some PROs are utilized.

Many organ-based complications of SSc have established outcome measurements that assess activity and severity of disease and response to treatment. These outcomes may have overlap with patient measures but are not identical. The patient viewpoint gives a different and more holistic perspective. Understanding what components of their disease the patient perceives as most important or debilitating is crucial to helping them cope with SSc. It is important to know if a treatment is concordant between the patient and physician, as a treatment that improves skin could have side effects that outweigh the benefits or have benefits that are not relevant to the patient. A physician would likely view significant organ involvement, even if asymptomatic, as a critically important aspect in the management of SSc, whereas a patient may consider symptomatic involvement, even if not life threatening, as their principle concern. As such, there is often a disconnect between what the physician and patient prioritize as the chief issues with respect to their condition [26]. Healthcare should improve health outcomes for patients, so effective methods of capturing the essence of illness experience across the many facets of life are important. Thus, the development and validation of tools measuring patient-reported outcomes in SSc are necessary.

Key Elements

SSc is chronic and multisystemic, thus impacting patients throughout many domains of their well-being. Measurement of PROs is needed to properly address emotional, functional, and social states. Such instruments are valuable tools that go beyond objective physical findings of disease. It is simple to count digital ulcers on physical exam, or to measure pulmonary function through testing, but the intricacies of human experience cannot be recorded from clinical assessment.

In order to confidently utilize tools that measure PROs, they should have validity, reliability, and sensitivity to change. If the measurement is to be trusted and used as a part of clinical management or research trials, it must be applicable to patients with certain features, have meaningful outcomes, and should be representative of its stated purpose. Appropriate study of the instruments is especially required in SSc, owing to its rarity in the general population and vast impact on the patient's quality of life and function.

The instruments should be accessible, easy to administer, and relevant to the population being assessed. SSc can affect individuals of varying age, culture, language, and education, so therefore the tools should be clear in their wording and comprehensibility. In general, scoring should be relatively quick, straightforward, and the score clear and meaningful.

Owing to the rarity and uniqueness of SSc, it is also important that some instruments used to measure patient outcomes are specific to SSc. For particular aspects of SSc, general instruments may not be sufficient, so SSc-specific PROs are also necessary. In order to compare the impact on health in SSc to other diseases, the generic instruments may suffice. Many PROs can be visual analog scales (VAS) or Likert scales (measuring change) and often they perform as well as long complicated questionnaires.

Patient-Reported Outcome Measures

Considering the many possible presentations of SSc, patients experience the effects of their disease throughout many domains of their well-being. Consequentially, there is a multitude of possible instruments to measure PROs. These measures are important for the evaluation and monitoring of patients with SSc and for clinical trials regarding SSc treatment. See Table 11.1 for a chronological list of some patient-reported outcome measures (PROMs) used in SSc.

General Measures of Functional Ability, Symptom Burden, and Quality of Life

Health Assessment Questionnaire

In 1980, Fries et al. published the Health Assessment Questionnaire (HAQ), a self-reported measurement tool structured around five core measurements: death, discomfort, disability, drug toxicity, and dollar cost [27]. It was one of the first measures of PROs for rheumatic disease.

Table 11.1 Patient-reported outcomes used in systemic sclerosis[a]

Score	Publication year	Authors	Measures	Specific to SSc?
Health Assessment Questionnaire (HAQ) and HAQ-Disability Index (HAQ-DI) [27]	1980	Fries et al.	Health-related quality of life (HRQoL) and functional status	
Borg Dyspnea Index [86]	1982	Borg et al.	Dyspnea	
Baseline Dyspnea Index (BDI) and Transition Dyspnea Index (TDI) [84]	1984	Mahler et al.	Dyspnea	
EuroQol-5D (EQ-5D) [35]	1990	The EuroQol Group	HRQoL and overall health	
Short-Form Health Survey (SF-36) [44]	1992	Ware et al.	HRQoL	
Cochin Hand Function Scale/Duruoz Hand Index [66]	1996	Duruoz et al.	Functional status of the hands	
Disabilities of the Arm, Shoulder, and Hand (DASH) [72]	1996	Hudak et al.	Functional status of the upper extremities	
SSc Health Assessment Questionnaire (SHAQ) [32]	1997	Steen and Medsger	HRQoL, functional status, GI, lung, and vascular disease, digital ulcers, pain, and overall disease severity	✔
ABILHAND [76]	1998	Penta et al.	Functional status of the hands	
Michigan Hand Questionnaire [78]	1998	Chung et al.	Functional status of the hands	
UK SSc Functional Score (UKFS) [52]	1998	Silman et al.	Functional assessment	✔
Short Form-6D (SF-6D) [49]	2002	Brazier et al.	HRQoL	
Raynaud's Condition Score [30]	2002	Merkel et al.	Frequency, duration, and severity and impact of RP attacks	
Functional Assessment of Chronic Illness Therapy (FACIT) [99]	2003	Webster et al.	HRQoL in chronic diseases (symptom—and disease-specific measures exist)	
Cambridge Pulmonary Hypertension Outcome Review (CAMPHOR) [91]	2006	McKenna et al.	HRQoL measure specific to PAH	
Mouth Handicap Scale in Systemic Sclerosis (MHISS) [79]	2007	Mouthon et al.	Mouth disability in SSc	✔

(continued)

Table 11.1 (continued)

Score	Publication year	Authors	Measures	Specific to SSc?
Patient-Reported Outcomes Measurement Information System (PROMIS) [98]	2007	National Institute of Health (Cella et al.)	Health status and symptoms in chronic conditions	
SSc Gastrointestinal Tract 1.0 (SSc-GIT 1.0) [59]	2007	Khanna et al.	Gastrointestinal disease in scleroderma	✔
University of California, Los Angeles, Scleroderma Clinical Trials Consortium Gastrointestinal Scale GIT 2.0 (UCLA SCTC GIT 2.0) [60]	2009	Khanna et al.	Reflux, diarrhea, fecal incontinence, distension and bloating, emotional well-being, constipation, and social functioning	✔
Symptom Burden Index (SBI) [51]	2010	Kallen et al.	Reflux, diarrhea, fecal incontinence, distension and bloating, emotional well-being, constipation, and social functioning	✔
Global Assessments			Disease or symptom activity, severity, and/or damage	

[a]These are examples and not meant to include all possible patient-reported outcome measures in SSc studies

The disability index section of the HAQ (HAQ-DI) measures patient-reported function in eight domains (dressing and grooming, eating, arising, walking, hygiene, grip, reach, and other common daily activities), and is one of the most widely used quality of life and disability measures in SSc [27, 28]. Originally designed for rheumatoid arthritis (RA), it has now been applied to multiple diseases.

The HAQ is inexpensive and scoring is quick and easy. Scores for each item ranges from 0 to 3, with the latter representing greater disability. If a device or aid is used for a specific category, an extra point is added to a maximum of three per domain in the usual scoring system. The scorer sums the disability score from each category and divides by the number of completed categories [27, 28]. The HAQ can also include a visual analog scale (VAS) for pain (discussed in the next paragraph) [29]. A review by Johnson et al. showed that the HAQ-DI appears reliable, responsive to change, and has good concurrent, construct, and predictive validity [28–30]. Furthermore, HAQ-DI scores are predictive of mortality in early diffuse SSc [31, 32] and low scores at baseline indicate a higher chance of an improvement in skin score over the next year in early dcSSc [33].

Although the HAQ-DI is used extensively in research and clinical practice, it may be outdated, not applicable to all patients (e.g., one domain assesses ability to open a milk carton) and seems to primarily focus on musculoskeletal-related disability [28]. There may also be concerns that adding points for the use of assistive devices overestimates disability and they should not be counted [34].

Scleroderma Health Assessment Questionnaire (SHAQ)

The HAQ is not disease specific. Although it was designed for RA, it is used in several types of inflammatory arthritis and some connective tissue diseases (CTDs), but it focuses mostly on upper extremity function. Steen and Medsger developed the Scleroderma HAQ (SHAQ), an adapted version of the HAQ to address concerns specific to SSc, with added visual analog scales (VAS) for gastrointestinal symptoms, lung symptoms, vascular problems, digital ulcers, pain, and overall disease severity [32]. These added scales assess common symptoms of SSc beyond functional impairment and pain. Patients mark on a 15 cm line how much they feel their symptoms or disease interfere with their activities, and a score is generated according to a translation of 1 cm to 0.2 points (or measuring the total in cm and dividing by 5 to convert the scale into 0–3). Like the HAQ, it is an inexpensive, fast, and easy-to-use tool. With the SHAQ, an aggregate score is generated, as in the HAQ-DI, but each VAS score is reported individually.

The SHAQ has demonstrated concurrent, convergent and predictive validity, reliability, and responsiveness to change [6, 28, 30, 32]. Comparing the two tools, the SHAQ has incremental content and face validity over the HAQ-DI; this is because the SHAQ assesses manifestations specific to SSc [29].

EuroQol-5D

Many general measures for health-related quality of life (HRQoL) beyond the HAQ have been used in SSc. Developed in 1987, the EuroQol-5D (EQ-5D) is a general measure of HRQoL, assessing health states related to the domains of self-care, pain/discomfort, mobility, anxiety/depression, and usual activities, based on the severity of problems [35, 36], for a total of 245 states. The EQ-5D also includes a VAS scale from 0 (worst imaginable health state) to 100 (best imaginable health state) for overall self-reported health [36]. The EQ-5D correlates well with the HAQ-DI, SHAQ, and SF-6D, as well as assessments of pain, dyspnea, weakness, fatigue, and other disease factors for SSc [37–40]. The EQ-5D has been found to have acceptable validity for patients with SSc [37, 40].

Global Assessments

Global assessments are helpful and important tools for examining many aspects of disease. They can be completed by the patient and/or physician and may be in the form of a VAS from 0 to 100 or a Likert scale ranging between a negative and positive value, with a lower number usually representing less disease activity, severity, or damage. The assessment can be just a single global assessment or may also contain several subscales for different manifestations. Scoring is easy and fast, and the result is helpful because it quantifies what the patient is experiencing and how they perceive the impact of their disease activity. The patient and physician may weigh the importance of certain aspects differently, and therefore there may be significant differences between physician and patient global assessment [41]. Although the actual questions asked for patient-rated global assessments are not standardized, they are valid and sensitive to change [33, 42, 43].

Short-Form Health Survey

Developed in 1992, the Short-Form Health Survey, or SF-36, examines the impact of disease on a patient's mental and physical well-being. It assesses eight domains that may be affected by disease: physical and social functioning, role limitations due to both physical health and emotional problems, physical pain, general mental health, energy/fatigue, and general health perceptions [44]. The domains are each scored on a multi-item scale, using the Likert method of summated ratings, and are further subcategorized into the Physical Component Summary (PCS) (0–100) and the Mental Component Summary (MCS) (0–100) [44, 45]. This tool was developed to be comprehensive, but shorter than previous questionnaires used to investigate the quality of life impact and burden of disease. The SF-36 assesses the influence of any disease on overall well-being, rather than specific manifestations of a rheumatic disease. One benefit of using such a general score is that it may detect an unexpected clinical event during a trial, which would otherwise be missed by measures that are more specific [43].

The SF-36 has been shown to be a reliable assessment of health-related quality of life in several rheumatic diseases [46]. Danieli et al. examined the use of the SF-36 for determining HRQoL in SSc and found that, when compared to findings in RA, the SF-36 appears to correlate well to HRQoL in SSc [46]. The SF-36 is strongly correlated with HAQ-DI scores in SSc [43, 47] Adequate validity of the SF-36, including satisfactory internal consistency, has been determined [43, 48]. Reliability of the SF-36 in SSc, however, has not been fully investigated [49]. When compared to the HAQ-DI for diffuse cutaneous SSc (dcSSc), the SF-36 appears to be more responsive to patient and physician global assessment, but less responsive to clinical measures, such as variation in skin score and percent forced vital capacity (FVC) predicted. The increased clinical responsiveness of the HAQ-DI may be because it is geared more toward musculoskeletal disease than the generic SF-36 [43].

Data from the SF-36 can been used to generate an indirect preference-based measure: the SF-6D [50]. Preference-based measures are often used in determining HRQoL for economic analysis. In SSc, the SF-6D has excellent test–retest reliability, and low floor and ceiling effects [51], and it is associated with the HAQ-DI and pain scores. As with the SF-36, the SF-6D lacks strong correlations with some SSc clinical measures such as change in skin and lung involvement [51].

Symptom Burden Index

Though the HAQ and the SF-36 have their merits, they are still relatively general. In an attempt to develop a scale more specific to scleroderma, Kallen et al. created the Symptom Burden Index (SBI), published in 2010 [52]. The SBI examines eight major domains in SSc. They include skin involvement, calcinosis, difficulties sleeping, hand mobility, dyspnea, eating, bowel involvement, and pain. Some of these are specific to SSc, compared to the HAQ. The patient assesses each question in the SBI on a Likert scale ranging from 0 to 10, with 10 indicating worse severity, frequency, or higher symptoms according to five questions per each domain, for a total of 40 questions [52]. Each scale is scored and an average burden score for each of the eight domains is calculated. The data from the SBI also can be used to indicate the proportion experiencing each SSc-related problem and the number of problems each patient experiences.

The SBI has good reliability between items, with moderate to high interitem and item-total score correlations per domain and high internal consistency reliability estimates. The SBI is correlated with the HAQ and the SF-36 for both physical and mental health [52]. The SBI has construct validity, but has not been investigated with regard to sensitivity to change [52]. Despite the existence of research demonstrating its strengths, the SBI has not been widely used in SSc trials.

The UK Scleroderma Functional Score

Like the SBI and the SHAQ, the UK Scleroderma Functional Score (UKFS) is a general measure made to examine elements of disease specific to SSc. The UKFS is an 11-item, 4-grade questionnaire used for functional assessment [53]. Eleven items for upper and lower extremity function and weakness are given a score of 0 (normal ability to perform a task) to 3 (impossible to perform) to produce an overall score between 0 and 33. In SSc, the UKFS is reliable and valid [6, 53, 54], with acceptable test–retest reliability and can differentiate between lcSSc and dcSSc. The UKFS correlates well with the HAQ-DI (r=0.90) and can demonstrate change in a longitudinal study [6, 55]. Like the SBI, the UKFS is meant to be an SSc-specific measure. However, like the SBI, the UKFS is not widely used.

Symptom and Organ-Specific Measures

Gastrointestinal Disease

In SSc, gastrointestinal (GI) organ involvement occurs in approximately 90 % of patients and is burdensome [56, 57]. The entire GI tract can be affected, leading to the possibility for a wide range of presentations and complications. The negative HRQoL can be difficult to capture due to the unique complexity and overlap of GI symptoms seen in SSc [58, 59].

In 2007, Khanna et al. noted the lack of GI instruments pertinent to SSc HRQoL. As a result, they developed the SSc Gastrointestinal Tract 1.0 (SSc-GIT 1.0) [60]. The SSc-GIT 1.0 was a comprehensive, reliable, and valid 52-item, self-reported measure of SSc-related GI disease [60]. Although thorough, it was found to take a lot of time to complete [61].

In 2009, Khanna et al. refined and improved upon the SSc-GIT 1.0 to create the University of California, Los Angeles, Scleroderma Clinical Trials Consortium Gastrointestinal Scale 2.0 (UCLA SCTC GIT 2.0) instrument. The UCLA SCTC GIT 2.0 contains 34 items under 7 multi-item scales: reflux, diarrhea, fecal soilage, distention/bloating, emotional well-being, constipation, and social functioning [61]. Each item is scored on a scale from 0 to 3, except for the constipation and diarrhea scales, which range from 0 to 2.5 and 0 to 2, respectively. Higher values indicate worse HRQoL [28, 49, 61]. A total score can be calculated by averaging the scores from 6 of the 7 scales (excluding constipation), which is then reported on a scale from 0 to 3—again with higher values indicating a worse HRQoL [28, 61].

The UCLA SCTC GIT 2.0 is feasible, quick, and has acceptable reliability (test–retest and internal consistency) and validity [28, 61, 62]. This PROM remains the only tool specific to SSc-related GI tract disease. Patients who described their GI disease as mild scored lower on all 7 scales. The total score is reliable and useful for describing overall disease burden and also enhances ability to discriminate between mild, moderate, and severe involvement [61]. It can differentiate between subjects with corresponding clinical gastrointestinal diagnoses and scores are responsive to change regarding patient-reported severity [49, 61, 63]. In the authors' opinion, the UCLA SCTC GIT 2.0 likely has a ceiling effect where someone with significant daily diarrhea or GERD can improve moderately and still not change their score.

The UCLA SCTC GIT 2.0 questionnaire can help in the clinical and experimental measurement of SSc-related GI disease. The GIT VAS from the SHAQ can also be used, but has not yet been compared to the UCLA SCTC GIT 2.0 scale. There are other scales that may be used, but are not specific to SSc, such as the Gastrointestinal Quality of Life Index [64].

Hand Function

Fibrosis of the skin of the hands, flexion deformities, and other musculoskeletal involvement commonly occur in SSc. Accordingly, hand function can be impaired, creating difficulties in daily activities. There are several questionnaires used to measure self-reported hand function in rheumatologic and musculoskeletal conditions. A detailed review of various scales has been published [65].

The Cochin Hand Function Scale (CHFS, or Duruoz Hand Index) is a self-reported scale used to measure functional disability of the hand with 18 items in various activity domains, such as kitchen, hygiene, dressing, office, and other [66]. The scales range from 0 (without difficulty) to 5 (impossible), which are then summed to produce a total disability score. It is easy to use and demonstrates content, construct, and convergent validity, and test–retest reliability [67, 68]. CHFS scores explained 75 % of the variance in HAQ scores and is a more SSc-specific assessment of hand function [68]. Its ability to detect change has been proven in RA and osteoarthritis, but has not yet been studied in SSc [69–71]. It was developed in 1996, so it may require an update reflecting contemporary uses of the hands, such as for using cell phones, texting, and typing on a computer keyboard [65].

The Disabilities of the Arm, Shoulder and Hand (DASH) is a PRO-measuring upper-extremity functional ability in musculoskeletal disease. Originally developed by Hudak et al., it consists of a 30-item symptom and function scale [72]. All items in the DASH are scored on a 5-point Likert scale, with 5 indicating extreme severity or lack of function [73]. There is an abbreviated version, the QuickDASH [74]. In SSc, the scale has been validated in Hungarian patients [75]. Both the DASH and QuickDASH correlate with the HAQ-DI and SF-36, confirming that much of the disability in SSc is from the upper extremities [75].

Another PRO adapted for use in SSc is the 57-item ABILHAND questionnaire [76]. The ABILHAND assesses the difficulty of a variety of manual activities, which the patient ranks from a scale of 0 to 5, with 0 indicating that the activity is impossible and 5 that it is very easy. Patients do not rate tasks that they have never performed [76]. Though it was originally developed in RA, it has been investigated in SSc by asking patients to rank manual activities as impossible, difficult, or easy [77]. The SSc-adapted ABILHAND was found to be reliable, valid, and reproducible, as well as linear and unidimensional [77].

The UK SSc Functional Score [53] and Michigan Hand Questionnaire [78] also assess hand function; however, the latter may have limited use in SSc [28]. Additionally, several questions of the HAQ-DI and the SHAQ measure impairment of the hands.

Mouth Disability

Many patients with SSc have oral problems, such as reduced oral opening, dry mouth, altered appearance, difficulty speaking, and impaired oral hygiene [28]. To address these common concerns, Mouthon et al. created the Mouth Handicap Scale in Systemic Sclerosis (MHISS) [79]. The MHISS has 12 self-reported items scored from 0 to 4, which are summed. The MHISS has excellent test–retest reliability, and good construct and divergent validity [79]. Three factors—reduced mouth opening, dryness, and appearance concerns—have been found to explain nearly two-thirds of the variance in scores [79]. MHISS scores also helped explain 36 % of HAQ score variance, which could be due to the fact that severe SSc can cause both reduced hand function and oral problems [79]. Thus, the assessment of oral disease in SSc is important. The MHISS is the only tool that measures patient-reported mouth disability in SSc. Further research may include this questionnaire, especially if oral health is being studied in SSc.

Pain

Pain in SSc is likely underrecognized, despite its occurrence in more than 80 % of patients. On average, patients reported their pain at 4 out of 10 [15]. Therefore, pain is an important outcome to measure. Pain in SSc is usually assessed by using VAS, Likert scales, or other change scales. The scales may assess global pain or problem-specific pain and can be a component of other assessments such as the SHAQ or SBI. Scoring depends on the type of scale used, but, for example, may be a 15 cm scale that is converted to a score from 0 to 3, where 1 cm equals 0.2 points, with 3 representing maximum pain [28]. Pain scales are valid alone or with other measures and correlate well with other disease manifestations [17, 30, 32]. They have good test–retest reliability [80] and are sensitive to change for certain effective treatments [81].

Pain in SSc is often multifactorial and can be the result of many disease processes. Therefore, if a patient is experiencing pain, it is important to discern the source in order to accurately utilize the outcome [28].

Fatigue

As with pain scales, there are no fatigue scales specific to SSc, despite the fact that it is one of the most common complaints in SSc [8, 15]. Several scales do exist, however, for the assessment of fatigue for general use. A review of other acceptable fatigue scales in various rheumatic diseases has been published [82]. Often a VAS scale performs as well in studies as a long fatigue questionnaire.

The SF-36 Vitality subscale and Functional Assessment of Chronic Illness Therapy (FACIT) Fatigue scale are commonly used tools to measure fatigue in rheumatic diseases [83]. The FACIT fatigue scale was found to provide a more complete coverage of the fatigue range in SSc and discriminates better than the SF-36 Vitality subscale at moderate-to-high ranges of fatigue [83]. For these reasons, the FACIT is suggested as the preferred measure of fatigue in SSc [83].

Dyspnea

Lung disease is a potential complication seen in scleroderma patients due to interstitial lung disease (ILD) and pulmonary arterial hypertension (PAH). These can result in dyspnea, affecting quality of life. There are no fully validated dyspnea questionnaires specific to SSc. However, the SHAQ and SBI have dyspnea subscales. Additionally, the questionnaire developed by Mahler et al., including the Baseline Dyspnea Index (BDI) and Transition Dyspnea Index (TDI), has been investigated for use in SSc [84, 85]. Moreover, the Borg Dyspnea Index, which measures the severity of dyspnea following a 6-min walk, has been partially validated in ILD and PAH [86].

The BDI and TDI are used to measure baseline severity and change in dyspnea over time, respectively. The BDI assesses the magnitude, effort, and impairment of varying tasks over a scale from 0 (severe) to 4 (unimpaired). These values are then summed to calculate a baseline score. Within the TDI, the patient rates from −3 (major deterioration) to +3 (major improvement), which is then summed to give a transition score [84]. The reliability has not been fully tested in SSc, but the construct and face validity of this instrument have been partially demonstrated [87, 88]. Validity was demonstrated for men with chronic obstructive pulmonary disease

[84]; however, predictive validity has not been examined in SSc. Both the TDI and BDI are able to detect change [89, 90].

There is disagreement about which scales should be used in SSc trails regarding dyspnea [28].

Pulmonary Arterial Hypertension

The Cambridge Pulmonary Hypertension Outcome Review (CAMPHOR) is the first pulmonary hypertension-specific instrument for assessing HRQoL using 3 scales with 65 items [91]. Though this instrument is specific to pulmonary arterial hypertension (PAH), it has not been validated specifically in SSc-associated PAH. The CAMPHOR assesses 25 items for impairment, 15 for function, and 25 for QOL, as well as the symptoms of energy, breathlessness, and mood through subscales [91]. The CAMPHOR has very good internal consistency, convergent and divergent validity, and good reproducibility when tested in idiopathic PAH [28, 91]. This instrument is also responsive to change and has been correlated with change in New York functional class [92, 93]. The CAMPHOR Utility Index and subscales are as responsive to change in class as the 6-min walking test (6MWT) [92]. Though the CAMPHOR has been tested for idiopathic PAH, it may not reflect all of the QOL aspects specific to SSc [28].

Raynaud's Condition Score and Digital Ulcers

Raynaud's phenomenon (RP) is a common and painful condition associated with SSc. The Raynaud's Condition Score (RCS) is a self-reported global assessment of RP activity in SSc patients [30]. The RCS uses a 0–10 ordinal scale to measure frequency, duration, severity, and impact of RP attacks. This information is used to calculate a composite score from daily measures over a defined period of time [30]. Research has indicated that the RCS is reliable [30, 94], with construct, content, criterion, and discriminant validity and is sensitive to change [30, 95]. Though this score is used in RP trials, its interpretation is sometimes uncertain and scoring may be confused as a visual analog scale [28].

Digital ulcers are a potential outcome in scleroderma and are associated with RP. The impact of digital ulcers can be measured from the SHAQ [32].

The Future of PROS in SSC: PROMIS and FACIT

With the emergence of better technologies, PROs have shifted toward more sophisticated computerized techniques. In the past, measuring PROs has relied on organ— or symptom-specific scales, which are not flexible or adaptive to specific patients. Some believe that continuing in this fashion is resource consumptive and inefficient because each scale needs to be developed and validated independently [96]. Moreover, the various PROs available make it difficult to compare results between studies [97]. In an attempt to find a solution for this problem, the National Institute of Health (NIH) began developing the Patient-Reported Outcomes Measurement Information System (PROMIS), starting in 2004 [98]. Their goal was to advance medical research by creating a comprehensive collection of item banks that are able to measure PROs and can be applied to a variety of chronic conditions [98].

The core areas addressed in the PROMIS are physical, social, and emotional health; fatigue; and pain. These areas reflect HRQoL. The PROMIS item banks are widely available, free, simple to use, and can be administered electronically and through Computerized Adaptive Testing (CAT). CAT works by selecting questions individualized to a patient based on their previous answers to gather data using a minimum number of questions while still maintaining precision [98]. The statistical method used to determine which question should be asked next is known as Item Response Theory (IRT). In contrast to PROMIS, scales such as the HAQ require patients to answer all questions, despite lack of relevance or applicability. In addition to the PROMIS item banks that can be administered through CAT, there are also static versions available.

Another adaptable tool that is compatible with the PROMIS network is the Functional Assessment of Chronic Illness Therapy (FACIT) measurement system. The FACIT consists of a set of questionnaires to determine the HRQoL in chronic conditions by measuring physical, social/family, emotional, and functional well-being [99]. Like PROMIS, the FACIT utilizes CAT to individualize questions to a specific patient [99]. Unlike PROMIS, however, the FACIT tends to be more disease-specific, rather than generic [96].

The PROMIS has been validated in a variety of diseases and has been found to be more precise than existing measures [96, 100–102]. In 2012, findings by Khanna et al. further supported the construct validity and feasibility of CAT-administered PROMIS in 11 health domains for SSc [103]. When administered in an SSc clinic with support staff, patients took an average time of up to 1.9 min to complete the CAT question bank, highlighting its efficiency and ease of use [103]. The generic global PROMIS-29 static scale and FACIT-dyspnea questionnaire are validated in SSc [97, 104]. In these studies, it was suggested that these tools may be of benefit over previously used instruments because of their ease of use and availability [97, 104]. However, for the evaluation of the functional impact of skin disease, longer PROMIS forms may be required [97, 104].

As we continue to realize the benefits of PROMIS and FACIT, further validation and calibration of these tools is important in SSc to better capture difficult to measure disease traits [96]. By using flexible and adaptive tools such as PROMIS and FACIT, we are able to more accurately capture PROs. Wider use of the PROMIS and FACIT systems can help standardize results for interstudy and interdisease analysis [96]. Although the use of CAT requires a computer, the benefits of this available and easy-to-use technology make it an appealing option to improve both translational research and clinical care.

Conclusion

SSc is a chronic connective tissue disease with many possible manifestations. The effects of SSc are often debilitating and tend to worsen with time, leading to functional, emotional, and social impairment. PROs are valuable tools to assess SSc patients, as they provide patients with the opportunity to concisely and quantitatively express their disease experience, which is different from physiologic parameters and measurements performed by a healthcare professional. Thus, this method of measuring disease aspects and symptoms goes beyond standard clinical assessments and is complementary to other outcome measurements. Due to the heterogeneous nature of SSc, there are consequentially many tools that can be used. These PROs may be either general (used in many diseases) or specific to SSc. Further, the tools may assess overall HRQoL or functional status, or they may be specific to certain disease manifestations, such as pain or dyspnea. One of the first and most commonly used assessments of functional status is the HAQ-DI. Although used extensively in SSc, it was originally designed for RA. On the other hand, tools such as the SHAQ, SBI, and UKFS were developed to measure functional status and HRQoL in SSc. Symptom-specific PROs designed for SSc include the MHISS and UCLA SCTC GIT 2.0 to measure mouth disability and gastrointestinal involvement, respectively. Many other PROs have been studied for use in SSc.

To effectively improve treatment for patients, it is important to understand what outcomes are meaningful to them. Therefore, in research trials and sometimes in clinical care, utilizing PROs allows us to determine which treatments make the greatest positive difference in patients' lives, or conversely, which are most detrimental to their well-being. Additional research is required to refine SSc PROs and investigate the validity of some measures within SSc. Due to the rarity and uniqueness of SSc, newer tools will be tested in SSc such as computer-based questionnaires that allow patients to skip areas that are irrelevant to their HRQoL such as use of the PROMIS questionnaire.

References

1. Pattanaik D, Brown M, Postlethwaite BC, Postlethwaite AE. Pathogenesis of systemic sclerosis. Front Immunol. 2015;6:272. doi:10.3389/fimmu.2015.00272.
2. Allanore Y, Avouac J, Kahan A. Systemic sclerosis: an update in 2008. Joint Bone Spine. 2008;75(6):650–5. doi:10.1016/j.jbspin.2008.07.003.
3. Johnson SR, Glaman DD, Schentag CT, Lee P. Quality of life and functional status in systemic sclerosis compared to other rheumatic diseases. J Rheumatol. 2006;33(6):1117–22.
4. Mayes MD, Lacey Jr JV, Beebe-Dimmer J, et al. Prevalence, incidence, survival, and disease characteristics of systemic sclerosis in a large US population. Arthritis Rheum. 2003;48:2246–55.
5. Paquette DL, Falanga V. Cutaneous concerns of scleroderma patients. J Dermatol. 2003;30:438–43.
6. Smyth AE, MacGregor AJ, Mukerjee D, Brough GM, Black CM, Denton CP. A cross-sectional comparison of three self-reported functional indices in scleroderma. Rheumatology (Oxford). 2003;42(6):732–8.

7. Ouimet JM, Pope JE, Gutmanis I, Koval J. Work disability in scleroderma is greater than in rheumatoid arthritis and is predicted by high HAQ scores. Open Rheumatol J. 2008;2:44–52. doi:10.2174/1874312900802010044.
8. Bassel M, Hudson M, Taillefer SS, et al. Frequency and impact of symptoms experienced by patients with systemic sclerosis: results from a Canadian National Survey. Rheumatology (Oxford). 2010;50:762–7.
9. Schnitzer M, Hudson M, Baron M, Steele R, Canadian Scleroderma Research Group. Disability in systemic sclerosis—a longitudinal observational study. J Rheumatol. 2011;38(4):685–92. doi:10.3899/jrheum.100635.
10. Leroy EC, Black C, Fleischmajer R, et al. Scleroderma (systemic sclerosis): classification, subsets and pathogenesis. J Rheumatol. 1988;15:202–5.
11. Seibold J. Connective tissue diseases characterized by fibrosis. In: Ruddy S, Harris Jr ED, Sledge CB, editors. Textbook of rheumatology. Philadelphia: WB Saunders; 2001. p. 1133–59.
12. Wigley F, Systemic SB. Clinical features. In: Klippel JH, editor. Primer on the rheumatic diseases. Atlanta: The Arthritis Foundation; 2001. p. 357–64.
13. Medsger Jr TA. Natural history of systemic sclerosis and the assessment of disease activity, severity, functional status, and psychologic well-being. Rheum Dis Clin North Am. 2003;29:255–73.
14. Hudson M, Thombs BD, Steele R, Panopalis P, Newton E, Baron M, Canadian Scleroderma Research Group. Quality of life in patients with systemic sclerosis compared to the general population and patients with other chronic conditions. J Rheumatol. 2009;36:768–72. doi:10.3899/jrheum.080281.
15. Sekhon S, Pope J, Canadian Scleroderma Research Group (CSRG), Baron M. The Minimally Important Difference (MID) for patient centered outcomes including Health Assessment Questionnaire (HAQ), Fatigue, Pain, Sleep, Global VAS and SF-36 in Scleroderma (SSc). J Rheumatol. 2010;37(3):591–8. doi:10.3899/jrheum.090375.
16. Varga J, Denton CP, Wigley FM, editors. Scleroderma: from pathogenesis to comprehensive management. New York: Springer; 2012. doi:10.1007/978-1-4419-5774-0_7.
17. Schieir O, Thombs BD, Hudson M, Boivin JF, Steele R, Bernatsky S, Hanley J, Baron M, Canadian Scleroderma Research Group. Prevalence, severity, and clinical correlates of pain in patients with systemic sclerosis. Arthritis Care Res (Hoboken). 2010;62(3):409–17. doi:10.1002/acr.20108.
18. El-Baalbaki G, Razykov I, Hudson M, Bassel M, Baron M, Thombs BD, Canadian Scleroderma Research Group. Association of pruritus with quality of life and disability in systemic sclerosis. Arthritis Care Res (Hoboken). 2010;62(10):1489–95. doi:10.1002/acr.20257.
19. Zucker I, Yosipovitch G, David M, Gafter U, Boner G. Prevalence and characterization of uremic pruritus in patients undergoing hemodialysis: uremic pruritus is still a major problem for patients with end-stage renal disease. J Am Acad Dermatol. 2003;49:842–6.
20. Thombs BD, Hudson M, Taillefer SS, Baron M, Canadian Scleroderma Research Group. Prevalence and clinical correlates of symptoms of depression in patients with systemic sclerosis. Arthritis Rheum. 2008;59(4):504–9. doi:10.1002/art.23524.
21. Jewett LR, Hudson M, Malcarne VL, Baron M, Thombs BD, Canadian Scleroderma Research Group. Sociodemographic and disease correlates of body image distress among patients with systemic sclerosis. PLoS One. 2012;7(3), e33281. doi:10.1371/journal.pone.0033281.
22. Knafo R, Thombs BD, Jewett L, Hudson M, Wigley F, Haythornthwaite JA. (Not) talking about sex: a systematic comparison of sexual impairment in women with systemic sclerosis and other chronic disease samples. Rheumatology (Oxford). 2009;48(10):1300–3. doi:10.1093/rheumatology/kep240.
23. Hudson M, Steele R, Lu Y, Thombs BD, Canadian Scleroderma Research Group, Baron M. Work disability in systemic sclerosis. J Rheumatol. 2009;36(11):2481–6. doi:10.3899/jrheum.081237.

24. Malcarne VL, Fox RS, Mills SD, Gholizadeh S. Psychosocial aspects of systemic sclerosis. Curr Opin Rheumatol. 2013;25:707–13. doi:10.1097/01.bor.0000434666.47397.c2.
25. Thombs BD, van Lankveld W, Bassel M, et al. Psychological health and well-being in systemic sclerosis: state of the science and consensus research agenda. Arthritis Care Res (Hoboken). 2010;62:1181–9. doi:10.1002/acr.20187.
26. Suarez-Almazor ME, Kallen MA, Roundtree AK, Mayes M. Disease and symptom burden in systemic sclerosis: a patient perspective. J Rheumatol. 2007;34(8):1718–26.
27. Fries JF, Spitz P, Kraines RG, Holman HR. Measurement of patient outcome in arthritis. Arthritis Rheum. 1980;23:137–45.
28. Pope J. Measures of systemic sclerosis (scleroderma). Arthritis Care Res. 2011;63(S11):S98–111. doi:10.1002/acr.20598.
29. Johnson SR, Hawker GA, Davis AM. The Health Assessment Questionnaire disability index and Scleroderma Health Assessment Questionnaire in Scleroderma Trials: an evaluation of their measurement properties. Arthritis Rheum. 2005;53:256–62.
30. Merkel PA, Herlyn K, Martin RW, Anderson JJ, Mayes MD, Bell P, et al. Measuring disease activity and functional status in patients with scleroderma and Raynaud's phenomenon. Arthritis Rheum. 2002;46:2410–20.
31. Clements PJ, Wong WK, Hurwitz EL, Furst DE, Mayes M, White B, et al. The disability index of the health assessment questionnaire is a predictor and correlate of outcome in the high-dose versus low-dose penicillamine in systemic sclerosis trial. Arthritis Rheum. 2001;44(3):653–61.
32. Steen VD, Medsger Jr TA. The value of the Health Assessment Questionnaire and special patient-generated scales to demonstrate change in systemic sclerosis patients over time. Arthritis Rheum. 1997;40:1984–91. doi:10.1002/art.1780401110.
33. Sultan N, Pope JE, Clements PJ, Scleroderma Trials Study Group. The health assessment questionnaire (HAQ) is strongly predictive of good outcome in early diffuse scleroderma: results from an analysis of two randomized controlled trials in early diffuse scleroderma. Rheumatology (Oxford). 2004;43:472–8.
34. Khanna D, Clements PJ, Postlethwaite AE, Furst DE. Does incorporation of aids and devices make a difference in the score of the health assessment questionnaire-disability index? Analysis from a scleroderma clinical trial. J Rheumatol. 2008;35:466–8.
35. The EuroQol Group. EuroQol-a new facility for the measurement of health-related quality of life. Health Policy. 1990;16:199–208.
36. Rabin R, de Charro F. EQ-SD: a measure of health status from the EuroQol Group. Ann Med. 2001;33:337–43.
37. Gualtierotti R, Scalone L, Ingegnoli F, Cortesi P, Lubatti C, Zeni S, et al. Health related quality of life assessment in patients with systemic sclerosis. Reumatismo. 2010;62(3):210–4.
38. Muller H, Rehberger P, Gunther C, Schmitt J. Determinants of disability, quality of life and depression in dermatological patients with systemic scleroderma. Br J Dermatol. 2011;166(2):343–53. doi:10.1111/j.1365-2133.2011.10624.x.
39. Strickland G, Pauling J, Cavill C, McHugh N. Predictors of health-related quality of life and fatigue in systemic sclerosis: evaluation of the EuroQol-5D and FACIT-F assessment tools. Clin Rheumatol. 2012;31:1215–22. doi:10.1007/s10067-012-1997-1.
40. Kwakkenbos L, Fransen J, Vonk MC, Becker ES, Jeurissen M, van den Hoogen FH, van den Ende CH. A comparison of the measurement properties and estimation of minimal important differences of the EQ-5D and SF-6D utility measures in patients with systemic sclerosis. Clin Exp Rheumatol. 2013;31(2 Suppl 76):50–6.
41. Hudson M, Impens A, Baron M, Seibold JR, Thombs BD, Walker JG, et al. Discordance between patient and physician assessments of disease severity in systemic sclerosis. J Rheumatol. 2010;37:2307–12. doi:10.3899/jrheum.100354.
42. Clements PJ, Hurwitz EL, Wong WK, Seibold JR, Mayes M, White B, et al. Skin thickness score as a predictor and correlate of outcome in systemic sclerosis: high-dose versus low-dose penicillamine trial. Arthritis Rheum. 2000;43:2445–54.

43. Khanna D, Furst DE, Clements PJ, Park GS, Hays RD, Yoon J, et al. Responsiveness of the SF-36 and the Health Assessment Questionnaire disability index in a systemic sclerosis clinical trial. J Rheumatol. 2005;32:832–40.
44. Ware Jr JE, Sherbourne CD. The MOS 36-Item Short Health Survey (SF-36) I. Conceptual framework and item selection. Med Care. 1992;30:473–83.
45. Ware Jr JE, Kosinki M, Keller S. SF-36 physical and mental health summary scales: a user's manual. Boston: New England Medical Center Health Institute; 1994.
46. Danieli E, Airo P, Bettoni L, Cinquini M, Antonioli CM, Cavazzana I, et al. Health-related quality of life measured by the short form in systemic sclerosis: correlations with indexes of disease severity, disability, and depressive symptoms. Clin Rheumatol. 2005;24:48–54. doi:10.1007/s10067-004-0970-z.
47. Cosutta R, Zeni S, Soldi A, Colombelli P, Belotti Masserini A, Fantini F. Evaluation of quality of life in patients with systemic sclerosis by the SR-36 questionnaire (In Italian). Rheum. 2002;54:122–7.
48. McHorney CA, Ware JE, Raczek AE. The MOS 36-item short-form health survey (SF-36): II. Psychometric and clinical validity in measuring physical and mental health constructs. Med Care. 1993;31(3):247–63.
49. Khanna D. Measuring disease activity and outcomes in clinical trials. In: Varga J, Denton CP, Wigley FM, editors. Scleroderma: from pathogenesis to comprehensive management. New York: Springer; 2012. p. 661–72.
50. Brazier L, Roberts J, Deverill M. The estimation of a preference-based measure of health from the SF-36. J Health Econ. 2002;21(2):271–92.
51. Khanna D, Furst DE, Wong WK, Tsevat J, Clements PJ, Park GS, Postlethwaite AE, Ahmed M, Ginsburg S, Hays RD, Scleroderma Collagen Type 1 Study Group. Reliability, validity and minimally important differences of the SF-6D in systemic sclerosis. Qual Life Res. 2007;16:1083–92. doi:10.1007/s11136-007-9207-3.
52. Kallen MA, Mayes MD, Kriseman YL, de Achaval SB, Cox VL, Suarez-Almazor ME. The symptom burden index: development and initial findings from use with patients with systemic sclerosis. J Rheumatol. 2010;37:1692–8. doi:10.3899/jrheum.090504.
53. Silman A, Akesson A, Newman J, Henriksson H, Sandquist G, Nihill M, Palfrey S, et al. Assessment of functional ability in patients with scleroderma: a proposed disability assessment instrument. J Rheumatol. 1998;25(1):79–83.
54. Poole JL, Brower L. Validity of the scleroderma functional assessment questionnaire. J Rheumatol. 2004;31:402–3.
55. Serednicka K, Smyth AE, Black CM, Denton CP. Using a self-reported functional score to assess disease progression in systemic sclerosis. Rheumatology (Oxford). 2007;46(7): 1107–10.
56. Sjogren RW. Gastrointestinal motility disorders in scleroderma [review]. Arthritis Rheum. 1994;37:1265–82.
57. Lock G, Holstege A, Lang B, Scholmerich J. Gastrointestinal manifestations of progressive systemic sclerosis. Am J Gastroenterol. 1997;92:763–71.
58. Nietert PJ, Mitchell HC, Bolster MB, Curran MY, Tilley BC, Silver RM. Correlates of depression, including overall and gastrointestinal functional status, among patients with systemic sclerosis. J Rheumatol. 2005;32:51–7.
59. Gliddon AE, Dore CJ, Maddison PJ, QUINS Trial Study Group. Influence of clinical features on the health status of patients with limited cutaneous systemic sclerosis. Arthritis Rheum. 2006;55:473–9.
60. Khanna D, Hays RD, Park GS, Braun-Moscovici Y, Mayes MD, McNearney TA, et al. Development of a preliminary scleroderma gastrointestinal tract 1.0 quality of life instrument. Arthritis Rheum. 2007;57:1280–6.
61. Khanna D, Hays RD, Maranian P, Seibold JR, Impens A, Mayes MD, et al. Reliability and validity of the University of California, Los Angeles Scleroderma Clinical Trial Consortium Gastrointestinal Tract Instrument. Arthritis Rheum. 2009;61:1257–63. doi:10.1002/art.24730.

62. Baron M, Hudson M, Steele R, Lo E. Canadian Scleroderma Research G. Validation of the UCLA Scleroderma Clinical Trial Gastrointestinal Tract Instrument version 2.0 for systemic sclerosis. J Rheumatol. 2011;38(9):1925–30. doi:10.3899/jrheum.110060.
63. Frech TM, Khanna D, Maranian P, Frech EJ, Sawitzke AD, Murtaugh MA. Probiotics for the treatment of systemic sclerosis-associated gastrointestinal bloating/distention. Clin Exp Rheumatol. 2011;29(2 Suppl 65):S22–5.
64. Eypasch E, Williams JI, Wood-Dauphinee S, Ure BM, Schmulling C, Neugebauer E, et al. Gastrointestinal quality of life index: development, validation and application of a new instrument. Br J Surg. 1995;82:216–22.
65. Poole JL. Measures of hand function. Arthritis Care Res (Hoboken). 2011;63:S189–99.
66. Duruoz MT, Poiraudeau S, Fermanian J, Menkes C, Amor B, Dougados M, et al. Development and validation of a rheumatoid hand functional disability scale that assesses functional handicap. J Rheumatol. 1996;23:1167–72.
67. Brower LM, Poole JL. Reliability and validity of the Duruoz Hand Index in persons with systemic sclerosis (scleroderma). Arthritis Rheum. 2004;51:805–9.
68. Rannou F, Poiraudeau S, Berezne A, Baubet T, Le-Guern V, Cabane J, et al. Assessing disability and quality of life in systemic sclerosis: construct validities of the Cochin Hand Function Scale, Health Assessment Questionnaire (HAQ), Systemic Sclerosis HAQ, and Medical Outcomes Study 36-Item Short Form Health Survey. Arthritis Rheum. 2007;57:94–102.
69. Poiraudeau S, Chevalier X, Conrozier T, Flippo RM, Liote F, Lefevre-Colau MM, et al. Reliability, validity, and sensitivity to change of the Cochin Hand Functional Disability Scale in hand osteoarthritis. Osteoarthritis Cartilage. 2001;9:570–7.
70. Lefevre-Colau MM, Poiraudeau S, Fermanian J, Etchepare F, Alnot JY, Le Viet D, et al. Responsiveness of the Cochin rheumatoid disability scale after surgery. Rheumatology (Oxford). 2001;40:843–50.
71. Poiraudeau S, Lefevre-Colau MM, Fermanian J, Revel M. The ability of the Cochin Rheumatoid Arthritis Hand Functional Scale to detect change during the course of disease. Arthritis Care Res. 2000;13:296–303.
72. Hudak PL, Amadio PC, Bombardier C. Development of an upper extremity outcome measure: the DASH (Disabilities of the Arm, Shoulder and Hand). Am J Ind Med. 1996;29:602–8.
73. Kennedy CA, Beaton DE, Solway S, McConnell S, Bombardier C. The DASH outcome measure user's manual. 3rd ed. Toronto: Institute for Work & Health; 2011.
74. Gabel CP, Yelland M, Melloh M, Burkett B. A modified QuickDASH-9 provides a valid outcome instrument for upper limb function. BMC Musculoskelet Disord. 2009;10:161. doi:10.1186/1471-2474-10-161.
75. Varju C, Balint Z, Solyom AI, Farkas H, Karpati E, Berta B, et al. Cross-cultural adaptation of the disabilities of the arm, shoulder, and hand (DASH) questionnaire into Hungarian and investigation of its validity in patients with systemic sclerosis. Clin Exp Rheumatol. 2008;26(5):776–83.
76. Penta M, Thonnard JL, Tesio L. ABILHAND: a Rasch-built measure of manual ability. Arch Phys Med Rehabil. 1998;79:1038–42.
77. Vanthuyne M, Smith V, Arat S, Westhovens R, De Keyser F, Houssiau FA, et al. Validation of a manual ability questionnaire in patients with systemic sclerosis. Arthritis & Rheum. 2009;61(5):695–703. doi:10.1002/art.24426.
78. Chung KC, Pillsbury MS, Walters MR, Hayward RA. Reliability and validity testing of the Michigan Hand Outcomes Questionnaire. J Hand Surg Am. 1998;23:575–87.
79. Mouthon L, Rannou F, Berezne A, Pagnoux C, Arene JP, Fois E, et al. Development and validation of a scale for mouth handicap in systemic sclerosis: the Mouth Handicap in Systemic Sclerosis scale. Ann Rheum Dis. 2007;66:1651–5.
80. Stevens A, Pope JE. Retest reliabilities and variability among scleroderma patients for 4 tests of disability: support for a better measure. Presented at the Canadian Rheumatology Association Meeting, 1995. J Rheumatol. 1995;22:1603.

81. Thompson AE, Shea B, Welch V, Fenlon D, Pope JE. Calcium channel blockers for Raynaud's phenomenon in progressive systemic sclerosis. Arthritis Rheum. 2001;44:1841–7.
82. Hewlett S, Dures E, Almeida C. Measures of fatigue. Arthritis Care Res (Hoboken). 2011;63:S263–86.
83. Harel D, Thombs BD, Hudson M, Baron M, Steele R, Canadian Scleroderma Research Group. Measuring fatigue in SSc: A comparison of the Short Form-36 vitality subscale and Functional Assessment of Chronic Illness Therapy-Fatigue scale. Rheumatology. 2012;51:2177–85. doi:10.1093/rheumatology/kes206.
84. Mahler DA, Weinberg DH, Wells CK, Feinstein AR. The measurement of dyspnea: contents, interobserver agreement and physiologic correlates of two new clinical indexes. Chest. 1984;85:751–8.
85. Tashkin DP, Elashoff R, Clements PJ, Goldin J, Roth MD, Furst DE, et al. Cyclophosphamide versus placebo in scleroderma lung disease. N Engl J Med. 2006;354:2655–66. doi:10.1056/NEJMoa055120.
86. Borg G. Psychophysical basis of perceived exertion. Med Sci Sports Exerc. 1982;14:377–81.
87. Khanna D, Clements PJ, Furst DE, Chon Y, Elashoff R, Roth MD, et al. Correlation of the degree of dyspnea with health-related quality of life, functional abilities, and diffusing capacity for carbon monoxide in patients with systemic sclerosis and active alveolitis: results from the Scleroderma Lung Study. Arthritis Rheum. 2005;52:592–600.
88. Khanna D, Yan X, Tashkin DP, Furst DE, Elashoff R, Roth MD, et al. Impact of oral cyclophosphamide on health-related quality of life in patients with active scleroderma lung disease: results from the scleroderma lung study. Arthritis Rheum. 2007;56:1676–84.
89. Khanna D, Tseng CH, Furst DE, Clements PJ, Elashoff R, Roth M, for Scleroderma Lung Study Investigators, et al. Minimally important differences in the Mahler's Transition Dyspnoea Index in a large randomized controlled trial: results from the Scleroderma Lung Study. Rheumatology (Oxford). 2009;48:1537–40.
90. Goldin J, Elashoff R, Kim HJ, et al. Treatment of scleroderma-interstitial lung disease with cyclophosphamide is associated with less progressive fibrosis on serial thoracic high-resolution CT scan than placebo: findings from the scleroderma lung study. Chest. 2009;136:1333–40.
91. McKenna SP, Doughty N, Meads DM, Doward LC, Pepke-Zaba J. The Cambridge Pulmonary Hypertension Outcome Review (CAMPHOR): a measure of health-related quality of life and quality of life for patients with pulmonary hypertension. Quality Life Res. 2006;15:103–15.
92. Meads DM, McKenna SP, Doughty N, Das C, Gin-Sing W, Langley J, et al. The responsiveness and validity of the CAMPHOR Utility Index. Eur Respir J. 2008;32:1513–9.
93. Gomberg-Maitland M, Thenappan T, Rizvi K, Chandra S, Meads DM, McKenna SP. United States validation of the Cambridge Pulmonary Hypertension Outcome Review (CAMPHOR). J Heart Lung Transplant. 2008;27:124–30.
94. Shenoy PD, Kumar S, Jha LK, Choudhary SK, Singh U, Misra R, et al. Efficacy of tadalafil in secondary Raynaud's phenomenon resistant to vasodilator therapy: a double-blind randomized cross-over trial. Rheumatology (Oxford). 2010;49:2420–8. doi:10.1093/rheumatology/keq291.
95. Khanna PP, Maranian P, Gregory J, Khanna D. The minimally important difference and patient acceptable symptom state for the Raynaud's condition score in patients with Raynaud's phenomenon in a large randomised controlled clinical trial. Ann Rheum Dis. 2010;69:588–91. doi:10.1136/ard.2009.107706.
96. Hinchcliff M, Cella D. Patient-reported outcomes. In: Varga J, Denton CP, Wigley FM, editors. Scleroderma: from pathogenesis to comprehensive management. New York: Springer; 2012. p. 673–8.
97. Hinchcliff M, Beaumont JL, Thavarajah K, Varga J, Chung A, Podlusky S, et al. Validity of two new patient-reported outcome measures in systemic sclerosis: Patient-Reported Outcomes Measurement Information System 29-item Health Profile and Functional Assessment of Chronic Illness Therapy-Dyspnea short form. Arthritis Care Res (Hoboken). 2011;63(11):1620–8. doi:10.1002/acr.20591.

98. Cella D, Yount S, Rothrock N, Gershon R, Cook K, Reeve B, Ader D, et al. The Patient-Reported Outcomes Measurement Information System (PROMIS): Progress of an NIH Roadmap Cooperative Group during its first two years. Med Care. 2007;45(5):S3–11.
99. Webster K, Cella D, Yost K. The Functional Assessment of Chronic Illness Therapy (FACIT) Measurement System: properties, applications, and interpretation. Health Qual Life Outcomes. 2003;1:79. doi:10.1186/1477-7525-1-79.
100. Fries JF, Krishnan E, Bruce B. Items, instruments, crosswalks, and PROMIS. J Rheumatol. 2009;36:1093–5.
101. Khanna D, Krishnan E, Dewitt EM, Khanna PP, Spiegel B, Hays RD. The future of measuring patient-reported outcomes in rheumatology: Patient-Reported Outcomes Measurement Information System (PROMIS). Arthritis Care Res. 2011;63:S486–90. doi:10.1002/acr.20581.
102. Cella D, Riley W, Stone A, et al. The Patient-Reported Outcomes Measurement Information System (PROMIS) developed and tested its first wave of adult self-reported health outcome item banks: 2005–2008. J Clin Epidemiol. 2010;63(11):1179–94. doi:10.1016/j.jclinepi.2010.04.011.
103. Khanna D, Maranian P, Rothrock N, Cella D, Gershon R, Khanna P, et al. Feasibility and construct validity of PROMIS and "legacy" instruments in an academic scleroderma clinic. Value Health. 2012;15:128–34.
104. Hinchcliff M, Beaumont JL, Carns MA, Podlusky S, Thavarajah K, Varga J, et al. Longitudinal evaluation of PROMIS-29 and FACIT-dyspnea short forms in systemic sclerosis. J Rheumatol. 2015;42(1):64–72. doi:10.3899/jrheum.140143.

Chapter 12
PROMs for Sjögren's Syndrome

Mohamed Osama Hegazi, Sally Youssef, and Yasser El Miedany

Introduction

Sjögren's (pronounced Show-grin's) syndrome (SS) is a chronic inflammatory condition characterized by affection of the exocrine lacrimal and salivary glands leading to dry eyes and dry mouth [1]. It is categorized as one of the systemic autoimmune disorders for a number of reasons. These include, but are not limited to, the presence of autoantibodies, the shared clinical manifestations (e.g., arthritis) with other autoimmune rheumatic diseases, and the association of SS with disorders such as systemic lupus erythematosus (SLE) and rheumatoid arthritis (RA) [2, 3]. SS is mainly classified as primary SS (pSS) if it occurs without another underlying or associated autoimmune disease, and as secondary SS (sSS) whenever it is associated with an autoimmune disorder such as RA, SLE, spondyloarthritis, and systemic sclerosis [1].

SS is a disease of adults with the mean age of onset usually in the fourth to fifth decade [3]. There are two peaks of the disease age of onset. The first peak occurs during the childbearing period in the mid 30s and a second peak in postmenopausal years during the mid 50s, although the condition can occur at virtually any age, including

M.O. Hegazi, M.R.C.P. (U.K.) (✉)
Medical Department, Al Adan Hospital, P.O. Box 262, Hadiya 52853, Kuwait
e-mail: drosama02@gmail.com

S. Youssef, M.D.
Rheumatology and Rehabilitation Department, Ain Shams University, Cairo, Egypt
e-mail: sallysayed70@yahoo.com

Y. El Miedany, M.D., F.R.C.P.
Honorary Senior Clinical Lecturer, King's College London, London, UK

Professor of Rheumatology and Rehabilitation, Ain Shams University, Cairo, Egypt

Department of Rheumatology, Darent Valley Hospital, Gravesend, Kent, UK
e-mail: drelmiedany@rheumatology4u.com

Y. El Miedany (ed.), *Patient Reported Outcome Measures in Rheumatic Diseases*,
DOI 10.1007/978-3-319-32851-5_12

in children as part of the spectrum of juvenile rheumatoid arthritis. In concordance with most of the inflammatory arthritic conditions, SS has a strong female propensity with a more than ten times female-to-male preponderance [3]. The prevalence of pSS was reported around 0.4 % among Caucasian women from Birmingham, UK [4]. An annual incidence of SS of approximately 4 per 100,000 people was found in a population-based study from Olmsted County, Minnesota [5]. Of the incident cases, 70 % were diagnosed as primary SS, and the remainder were associated with underlying illnesses [5]. Among other rheumatic disorders, RA was depicted to be the highest in its association with sSS [3].

Clinical Manifestations

SS characteristically manifests with dry eyes and dry mouth (sicca symptoms); however, systemic and extraglandular affection is not uncommon [1, 6]. Keratoconjunctivitis sicca (KCS) is the term that is occasionally used to describe corneal and conjunctival affection in dry eyes. The ocular symptoms include irritation, grittiness, and a foreign body sensation. In advanced cases, inflammation becomes progressive and visual disturbances ensue [1]. Oropharyngeal manifestations due to salivary hyposecretion include dry mouth, dysphagia, dental caries, and oral candidiasis, as well as salivary glands enlargement, which may occur through the disease course. The parotid gland enlargement that accompanies dry mouth is sometimes referred to as Mikulicz syndrome [1, 2]. Both dry eyes and dry mouth were shown to have a significant negative impact on the patient's quality of life (QOL) [7].

Patients with SS may additionally develop general systemic symptoms such as fatigue, malaise, or fever. Fatigue is one of the most common and disabling complaints in SS. The pathogenesis of fatigue is poorly understood; however, approximately 70 % of pSS patients suffer from a disabling fatigue [8]. Because of its high prevalence, fatigue was identified as one of the main causes of reduced health-related quality of life (HRQOL) in SS patients [8].

Though sicca symptoms represent the main disease manifestation, it can be said that almost every body organ or system is vulnerable. SS patients are prone to a diverse array of extraglandular manifestations, including the joints (arthralgia or arthritis), skin (e.g., vasculitis or skin rashes), muscles (myalgia or inflammatory myositis), lungs (e.g., interstitial lung disease), heart (e.g., pericarditis), liver (e.g., primary biliary cirrhosis), kidneys (interstitial nephritis), and nervous system [1]. The prevalence of nervous system involvement may exceed 20 % in SS patients [9]. There is a myriad of nervous system affection patterns including peripheral neuropathy, focal neurologic deficits due to central nervous system lesions, trigeminal neuralgia, seizures, dementia, aseptic meningitis, optic neuritis, and transverse myelitis [9].

Diagnosis

The diagnosis of SS is often challenging, hence it is not infrequently overlooked. Initially, the diagnosis requires a high index of suspicion with a focused enquiry about dry eyes and dry mouth. A thorough history and clinical scrutiny for extraglandular affection is also mandatory. Without a high index of suspicion, the nonspecific nature of symptoms may lead to a considerable delay of the diagnosis that averaged 7 years in one survey [10]. Tests to quantify lacrimal (e.g., Schirmer test) and salivary (e.g., sialometry) secretions are utilized to diagnose KCS and dry mouth [1]. Salivary gland ultrasonography, magnetic resonance angiography (MRA), and biopsy are also used in the diagnostic evaluation of dry mouth [1, 11]. Several non-specific laboratory markers of SS are described. These include the presence of anemia, leukopenia, eosinophilia, hypergammaglobulinemia, and elevated erythrocyte sedimentation rate (ESR) [1]. Testing for autoantibodies is mandatory in the workup of SS. Antibodies to SS antigen type A (SSA), also called anti-Ro, and/or antibodies to SS antigen type B (SSB), also called anti-La, are present in a considerable proportion of patients with pSS. Anti-Ro and/or anti-La may also be found in some of the sSS patients and occasionally in healthy individuals as well. Additionally, their absence does not rule out the diagnosis of SS. Antinuclear antibodies may test positive in pSS and in SS secondary to SLE. Rheumatoid factor may be detected in patients with pSS and RA-associated sSS as well. The diagnosis of SS should not be confused with other disorders that may lead to similar systemic symptoms (e.g., fibromyalgia and depression), glandular enlargement (lymphoma or sarcoidosis), and dry mouth (e.g. the use of drugs with anticholinergic side effects) [1, 3]. To improve diagnostic accuracy a number of diagnostic classification criteria have evolved to be used by professionals and researchers. The most widely accepted set of criteria are known as the American-European Consensus Group classification criteria (AECG) [12].

Treatment Modalities

Artificial tears eye drops and lubricating ointments are used to treat dry eyes. Cyclosporine 0.05 % eye drops are usually kept for severe cases. Saliva replacement products and sugar-free chewing gums may improve the dry mouth symptoms. Oral drugs that increase salivary secretions (sialogogues), for example, pilocarpine, were found effective also to treat xerostomia [13]. There is limited or no evidence for the benefit of systemic immunosuppressive/immunomodulatory drugs (mycophenolate, azathioprine, and cyclosporine) in the treatment of KCS and xerostomia [13]. Studies that evaluated the synthetic disease-modifying antirheumatic drugs (DMARDS)—methotrexate, leflunomide, and hydroxychloroquine—found only limited improvements in sicca symptoms [3, 13]. Trials on the tumor necrosis factor alpha inhibitors (anti-TNF)—infliximab and etanercept—also did not show significant improvements. Of the biologic DMARDS, the anti-B lymphocyte rituximab was the only remedy that showed promising results with improvements in both xerostomia/xerophthalmia and extraglandular features as well [8, 13].

Monitoring Response to Treatment

It is not enough to measure disease progression and response to treatment based on symptoms, objective physical findings, and laboratory criteria for each individual patient without a standardized scale. Additionally, the patients' self-reported responses are increasingly gaining significance and preference in the face of objective clinical and laboratory findings. The need for a unified SS disease activity index has been growing over the last few decades. In the year 2010, the EULAR Sjögren's Syndrome Disease Activity Index (ESSDAI) was published [14] (Appendix 1). It has been developed as a reference index to assess disease activity and response to therapy for both clinical practice and research purposes [14]. Giving more weight to the patient responses, the EULAR Sjögren's Syndrome Patient-Reported Index (ESSPRI) was generated in the year 2011 [15] (Appendix 2). ESSPRI is a very simple index designed to measure patients' symptoms in pSS [15]. It is validated for use as an outcome measure in clinical trials [15]. More details about the aforementioned indices will follow in this chapter (see "Disease Activity").

Prognosis and Impact on Quality of Life

Earlier studies revealed that dry eyes and dry mouth with or without the general systemic symptoms, such as fatigue, have a significant negative impact on patients' QOL [10, 16]. The development of extraglandular organ or system involvement also increases morbidity and further deteriorates the QOL. More details about QOL measures in SS will follow in this chapter (see section "Health-Related Quality of Life Measures in Sjögren's Syndrome"). In addition to the burden imposed by sicca symptoms and fatigue, SS patients could also be dreadfully at increased risk of both mortality and malignancy [6]. Some of the systemic organ-specific complications (e.g., glomerulonephritis or interstitial lung disease) of SS may approach a life-threatening severity [13]. In a study carried out in Spain, patients with pSS, who present at diagnosis with high systemic activity (ESSDAI $\geq$ 14) were shown to be at higher risk of death [6, 16]. Patients with SS and with severe involvement of the exocrine glands, vasculitis, and cryoglobulinemia were found to be at increased risk for developing non-Hodgkin's lymphoma [6]. In a series of 380 Spanish patients with pSS, 3 % had developed lymphoma during 9 years of observation [17]. It is prudent to identify SS patients with predictors for the development of lymphoma, who may need more vigilant screening and follow-up schedules.

Patient-Reported Outcome Measures in Sjögren's Syndrome

Patient-reported outcome measures (PROMs) are patient-self-completed questionnaires that assess different disease parameters including functional ability as well as quality of life. Some questionnaires are generic, hence can be used widely for different diseases, whereas others are specific, hence applicable only to specific disorders or patient groups. They have been used as an outcome measure tool in different situations including research trials, standard clinical practice as well as economic evaluations. The role of PROMs in chronic arthritic conditions has been endorsed recently by the new trend of the "patient-centered approach" [18]. Its value has been augmented in some chronic musculoskeletal conditions such as SS and fibromyalgia, which relies mainly on the patients' symptoms. In SS, PROMs has been used to assess different aspects of the disease such as disease activity, health-related quality of life (HRQOL), as well as fatigue.

SS has two main patterns (1) a slowly progressive pattern that affects mainly the exocrine glands (epithelial regions) and characterized clinically by sicca symptoms associated with systemic manifestations mainly in the form of fatigue and joint/musculoskeletal pains and (2) progressive systemic disorder, affecting exocrine glands, in addition to extraepithelial manifestations as well as serological markers of autoimmune activation. This highlighted the need for tools to define disease activity addressing such subjective symptoms as well as systemic and laboratory features. The EULAR SS Patient-Reported Index (ESSPRI) was developed to assess the first, and most common, disease pattern, including sicca complaints such as dryness, fatigue, and pain from the patients' perspective, which are the most important items from the patients' point of view. Another index, "EULAR SS Disease Activity Index (ESSDAI)," was developed to assess global disease activity in relation to the disease systemic features.

Disease Activity

The ESSPRI was developed as a questionnaire addressing the main primary SS patients' symptoms. Considering the patient global assessment as the gold standard (dependent variable), a multiregression analysis model was implemented to select the most relevant domains and their weights based on the patients' perception. This revealed three main features, namely dryness, pain, and fatigue (both mental and somatic). The questionnaire adopted the numerical (0–10) scale for each domain to assess for these features [15, 19]. The questionnaire gives a composite total score defined as the mean of the Likert scores (0–10) of dryness, fatigue and pain [15] (Appendix 2). The EULAR Sjögren's syndrome (SS) disease activity index (ESSDAI) is a clinical index that measures disease activity in primary Sjögren's syndrome. It includes 12 domains, namely organ systems: cutaneous, respiratory, renal, articular, muscular, peripheral nervous system (PNS), central nervous system

(CNS), hematological, glandular, constitutional, lymphadenopathic, and biological (Appendix 1). The ESSDAI is now in use as a gold standard, as the SLEDAI is in lupus. In addition, ESSDAI started to be used as an outcome measure in randomized controlled trials (RCTs) in SS, and even as the primary outcome measure in currently ongoing RCTs. Both ESSDAI and ESSPRI were reported sensitive to change in response to therapeutic interventions. Recently, the definition of disease activity levels and thresholds of minimal clinically important improvement (MCII) have been proposed for that tool: a moderately active disease being defined as an ESSDAI ≥ 5 and an MCII as a decrease of at least three points. These cut-offs have started to be used, respectively, as entry criteria and primary end points for RCTs. In this setting, enhancing the accuracy and the reliability of disease activity scoring to correctly classify patients at study entry but also at final evaluation is a crucial point to determine the efficacy of the drug under investigation [20].

Health-Related Quality of Life Measures in Sjögren's Syndrome

Health-related quality of life (HRQOL) handles the patients' physical and psychological well-being aspects as well as the impact of ill-health on the patient's social relationships. On the other hand, the term "quality of life" (QOL) is used to describe the general well-being of individuals and societies [21]. Therefore, QOL studies emphasize mainly the economic well-being. Assessment of HRQOL in SS is important as it addresses the unique contribution of sicca manifestations as well as oral health to more general measures of health and well-being, including activities of daily living and social functioning. Tools for HRQOL assessment can be stratified into either generic or specific tools:

Generic Tools

The World Health Organization (WHO) developed a generic questionnaire to assess QOL (the initial WHOQOL-100) [22]. This was further shortened into 26-items, the WHOQOL-BREF [23]. The WHOQOL-BREF is composed of four domains, namely: physical health, psychological, social relationships, and environment. In comparison to the control group, primary SS patients were found to have reduced QOL across the four WHOQOL-BREF domains [24]. In comparison to the other chronic musculoskeletal inflammatory conditions, while the pattern of affection in primary SS patients showed similar pattern to systemic lupus erythematosus patients, there were significant differences in contrast to the rheumatoid arthritis subgroup. RA patients had significantly lower scores on the physical function domain scale. The Short Form-36 (SF-36) [25] is another generic questionnaire that has been used widely in different chronic disorders. The WHOQOL-BREF physical scale scores correlated well with SF-36 vitality and physical domain scores.

Another generic tool is the Euro-QOL [26]. The tool comprises five domains: mobility, self-care, usual activities, pain/ discomfort, and anxiety/ depression as well as a global health status (using a 0–100 mm visual analogue scale). In concordance with the WHOQOL questionnaire, the Euro-QOL gives a single global score, in addition to individual domain scores. The Euro-QOL was assessed in patients with pSS in comparison to SF-36. Results revealed comparable reduction in the HRQOL scores in both tools [27]. In another study, a group of researchers from Sweden reported reduction of QOL in patients with pSS using the Gothenburg Quality of Life Instrument [28].

Disease-Specific Tools

For any given area of health, condition-specific instruments may have greater clinical appeal due to incorporation of content specific to the particular conditions, and the likelihood of increased responsiveness to interventions. In view of the fact that there is no single measure that can serve as a "gold standard" in all patients suffering from inflammatory arthritic conditions, mutual index of several measures has been recommended for assessment of disease activity and monitoring response to therapy. The most widely used indices in RA are the ACR Core Data Set, disease activity score (DAS-28), whereas ASDAS is commonly used in ankylosing spondylitis and SLEDAI for lupus patients [29]. In SS, the scenario might differ to some extent as there is no composite measure like the other chronic inflammatory conditions; hence, specific questionnaires were developed specifically to address the most important disease manifestations, namely dryness in the eye and mouth as well as fatigue. This is discussed in the following section.

Dry Mouth

Dryness of the oral mucosa and hyposalivation put SS patients at high risk for poor oral health. Therefore, maintaining oral health is a significant issue for this population. Patients can also experience changes in the composition of saliva that increases the susceptibility to dental caries and periodontal disease, increases incidence of oral candidiasis and ulceration, causes changes in taste sensation, and complicates wearing dentures. Patients frequently experience difficulty chewing and swallowing food, difficulty speaking, and suffer embarrassment or self-consciousness in social situations as a result of xerostomia. For SS patients, a number of questionnaires were developed focusing mainly on the oral and ocular symptoms. The Sicca Symptoms Inventory [30] assesses both ocular and oral dryness as well as other sicca symptoms. The Oral Health Impact Profile (OHIP) [31] was endorsed as a disease-specific HRQOL tool. This was attributed to its measurement of both oral sicca symptoms and the social impact of these symptoms. Furthermore, the tool measures aspects of quality of life directly related to oral health and function independent of the other problems associated with SS. The questionnaire is composed of 49 questions, stratified under seven domains: functional limitation (Q1–Q9), physical pain (Q10–Q18), psychological discomfort (Q19–Q23), physical disability (Q24–Q32), psychological disability (Q33–Q38), social disability (Q39–Q43), and handicap (Q44–Q49). The OHIP-49 questionnaire was shortened in another study to produce a shortened OHIP-14 version [32]. Studies carried out to assess primary SS patients revealed that OHIP is a powerful predictor of self-rated psychological variables such as depression, self-esteem, and overall life satisfaction. The results indicate that oral health and function have an independent influence on general quality of life in these patients [33]. Furthermore, the reduction in OHIP-49 scores was comparable to the reduction in SF-36 scores, whereas it was significantly lower than the control scores [7, 34]. Similarly, in another research, the OHIP-14 total score was significantly correlated with five of the eight SF-36 domain scores [35, 36]. These findings indicate that xerostomia and hypo-salivation have a considerably negative effect on activities of daily living and social relationships. This demonstrates how oral disease and poor oral function may have considerable social and psychological impacts.

Dry Eyes

The Dry Eye Workshop defined dry eye as a "multifactorial disease of the tears and ocular surface that results in symptoms of discomfort, visual disturbance, and tear film instability with potential damage to the ocular surface." [37] It is accompanied by detrimental impact on the patients' HRQOL [38–42]. Earlier published studies revealed that clinical tests and assessment can be poorly associated with the changes in symptoms and self-perceived severity of the condition particularly as the disease progresses [37, 43–47]. Thus, validated questionnaires that fully assess symptoms together with the effect of dry eye on daily living have been endorsed [48–50].

Patient-reported outcome measures, used to evaluate the discomfort (specific impact of the eye disease and vision on symptoms), functioning (the ability to carry out activities in daily living), and perceptions (concern about one's health), are referred to as vision-targeted health-related quality of life (VT-HRQ) instruments. Valid and reliable measurements of VT-HRQ have become mandatory to the assessment of disease status and treatment effectiveness in ocular disease [27]. There are two general categories of VT-HRQ instruments: generic, which are designed to be used for a broad spectrum of visual disorders and ocular disease; and disease-specific, which are tailored toward particular aspects of a specific ocular disorder. In general, disease-specific instruments tend to be more sensitive than generic ones in detecting the VT-HRQ impairments [51]; however, generic instruments enable comparisons across more diverse populations and diseases [52–55].

The 25-item National Eye Institute Visual Function Questionnaire (NEI-VFQ-25) [56] is a nondisease-specific (i.e., generic) instrument designed to measure the impact of ocular disorders on VT-HRQ. Depending on the item, responses to the NEI-VFQ pertain to either frequency or severity of a symptom or functioning problem. A recall period is not specified in the questionnaire. Responses to the NEI-VFQ scores can range from 0 to 100, with lower scores indicating more problems or symptoms. Subscale scores are assessed for general vision, ocular pain, near vision, distance vision, social functioning, mental functioning, role functioning, dependency, driving, color vision, and peripheral vision, as well as an overall score. Limitations of the NEI-VFQ-25 for assessing QOL in patients with dry eyes are that it is not disease-specific, needs further validity and reliability testing in a dry eye population, lacks a specified recall period, and requires 10 min to administer the questionnaire [53].

The Texas Eye Research and Technology Center (DEQ) is a 33-item questionnaire based on the original dry eye questionnaire that adds several components to the original dry eye questionnaire, including two questions on the disease effect on QOL [48, 54]. The questionnaire has undergone some validity testing and can discriminate between normal patients and patients with moderate dry eyes. Limitations of the questionnaire for measuring QOL in patients with dry eyes include the need for further test–retest reliability testing. In addition, only a small portion of the questionnaire is dedicated to QOL measures [55].

The Ocular Surface Disease Index (OSDI) [37] (provided by Allergan, Inc., Irvine, CA) was used to quantify the specific impact of dry eye on VTHRQ. This disease-specific questionnaire includes three subscales: ocular discomfort (OSDI-symptoms), which entails symptoms such as gritty or painful eyes; functioning (OSDI-function), which measures limitation in performance of common activities such as reading and working on a computer; and environmental triggers (OSDI-triggers), which measures the impact of environmental triggers, such as wind or drafts, on dry eye symptoms.

The questions are asked with reference to a 1-week recall period. Possible responses refer to the frequency of the disturbance: none of the time, some of the time, half of the time, most of the time, or all of the time. Responses to the OSDI were scored using the methods described by the authors [55]. Subscale scores were computed for OSDI symptoms, OSDI function, and OSDI triggers, as well as an overall averaged score. OSDI subscale scores can range from 0 to 100, with higher scores indicating more problems or symptoms.

The Impact of Dry Eye on Everyday Life (IDEEL) [57] is another disease-specific patient-reported outcomes (PRO) questionnaire for the assessment of the burden of dry eye on patients. The 57-item IDEEL questionnaire for the assessment of dry eye impact comprises three modules: dry eye symptom-bother; dry eye impact on daily life including impact on daily activities, emotional impact, impact on work; and dry eye treatment satisfaction, which includes satisfaction with treatment effectiveness and treatment-related bother/inconvenience. The psychometric analysis results indicated that the IDEEL met the criteria for item discriminant validity, internal consistency reliability, test–retest reliability, and floor/ceiling effects.

A review [55] carried out to analyze the currently available dry eye questionnaires in relation to the vision-related QOL in patients with dry eye disease revealed that the IDEEL, for its extensive development process and multiple QOL measures, offers a more thorough assessment of the effect of eye dryness on quality of life for clinical trials, whereas the OSDI may be the more convenient option for clinical use as a result of its shorter completion time. Other questionnaires used to assess quality of life in patients suffering from dryness of the eye (such as, 25-item National Eye Institute Visual Function Questionnaire and Texas Eye Research and Technology Center DEQ) were fairly limited in that assessment.

Fatigue

Fatigue is one of the main SS manifestations, reported by about 75 % of the patients, and is a key predictor of reduced social activities and work productivity [58–60]. Fatigue was identified as a predictor of SF-36 domain scores in a variety of studies. In a study that included 94 primary SS patients, pain, helplessness, and depression were predictors of physical and mental fatigue [42]. The best approach to assess fatigue has not yet been defined, visual/numerical analogue scales have been used in standard clinical practice as well as research studies. The ESSPRI contains two Likert scales (0–10) on fatigue (physical and mental) that can be used for patient assessment [20]. The Profile of Fatigue and Discomfort—Sicca Symptoms Inventory (PROFAD-SSI) questionnaire [61] was developed specifically to assess fatigue in primary SS patients. It includes 64 questions in eight domains (somatic fatigue, mental fatigue, arthralgia, vascular dysfunction, oral dryness, ocular dryness, cutaneous dryness, and vaginal dryness) scored on an 8-point (0–7) Likert scale. The domains are made up of one or more facets, which each contain one or more related questions. However, this long questionnaire is inconvenient for use in a clinical trial context, where several other questionnaires may also need to be completed. The somatic and mental fatigue domain scores can also be summated to form the Profile of Fatigue (PROF) score; the fatigue, arthralgia, and vascular dysfunction domains to form the PROFAD score; and the sicca domains to form the SSI score. A shorter version (PROFAD-SSI-SF) with 19 questions, each question reflecting a single facet of the long-form (PROFAD-SSI-LF), was developed to tackle this long version hurdle [59]. These 19 questions can still be grouped into the same eight domains and summary scores as above. The long form of the PROFAD-SSI questionnaire was compared to the short form. Furthermore, a comparison of the short form with a briefer ("brev") version comprising a series of visual analogue scales (VAS) representing the major domains of the PROFAD-SSI that may be particularly useful in clinical trials in PSS was carried out. The long- and short-form PROFAD-SSI questionnaires correlate closely, suggesting that the PROFAD-SF is valid as an outcome tool. Preliminary data also suggest that an even briefer form with compression of the domains into a single VAS is also feasible [62, 63].

Among other instruments used to assess fatigue in rheumatic disease studies, including SS, is the Fatigue Severity Scale (FSS), Functional Assessment of Chronic Illness Therapy-Fatigue (FACIT-F), and different VAS variants. FSS assesses functional issues during the preceding 2 weeks [64]. FACIT-F is a general fatigue measure with emphasis on daily life function [65]. In contrast, SF-36 assesses different health aspects during the preceding 4 weeks [25]. The vitality domain of

SF-36 has been used as a proxy measure of fatigue in several conditions. FSS and fatigue VAS are positive scales in that higher values mean higher fatigue levels, whereas FACIT-F and vitality have the opposite direction [66].

Challenges to Outcome Measures Assessment in Sjögren's Syndrome

The development of assessment tools in SS has faced several challenges. The first challenge is the lack of a gold standard for outcome measures. So far, there is no single or set of clinical and immune-pathogenic markers that can be reliably used to reflect adequately all aspects of outcomes in SS. This lack of common assessment criteria led to the application of various invalidated assessment tools in clinical trials, making comparison of the efficacy of treatment between studies extremely difficult. In addition, there is lack of knowledge of the nature and frequency of disease exacerbations or remissions. This is supported by the data documenting delays of 5–10 years after symptom onset prior to diagnosis [66, 67]. Furthermore, this partly silent and partly unknown clinical course of SS has made it difficult to define what characterizes active disease in SS and how to stratify clinical disease manifestations into features of activity and features of damage/chronicity. Such distinction has been proven valuable in other chronic inflammatory arthritic conditions.

Since the sicca symptoms are the hallmarks of the syndrome, they became the primary targets for objective assessment (such as Schirmer's test [36] and Saliva Ferning test [68]), as well as for assessment as outcome measures of management. On the other hand, though comorbidities have been reported in association with SS, there is not, so far, any tool for assessment. A multidimensional PROMs questionnaire remains an unmet demand, and most of the tools used currently were originally designed for other rheumatic diseases [69] or generic questionnaires [70]. Further work is still needed in this aspect.

Conclusion

PROMs questionnaires remain one of the best ways to measure the disease activity as well as its impact on the patient's daily living. In SS, patient-reported symptoms such as dryness or fatigue have been used as primary outcome measures in clinical trials. PROMs instruments in SS should not only focus on the ability to identify and diagnose the problem such as dry eye/mouth, measure the prevalence of the condition, and assess the severity as well as frequency of symptoms, but also enable the assessment of change of the patient's condition in response to management. From a clinician's perspective, this will help in setting realistic expectations and in monitoring the improvement level in individual patients.

Acknowledgment The authors

would like to express their sincere gratitude to *Annals of Rheumatic Diseases* for giving the kind permission to include both the "EULAR Sjögren's syndrome disease activity index" and the "EULAR Sjögren's syndrome patient-reported index" in the appendices of this chapter.

Appendix 1: EULAR Sjogren's Syndrome Disease Activity Index (ESSDAI)

The EULAR Sjögren's Syndrome Disease Activity Index (ESSDAI): Domain and item definitions and weights

Domain [weight]	Activity level	Description
Constitutional [3] *Exclusion of fever of infectious origin and voluntary weight loss*	No = 0	Absence of the following symptoms
	Low = 1	Mild or intermittent fever (37.5°–38.5 °C)/night sweats and/or involuntary weight loss of 5–10 % of body weight
	Moderate = 2	Severe fever (>38.5 °C)/night sweats and/or involuntary weight loss of >10 % of body weight
Lymphadenopathy [4] *Exclusion of infection*	No = 0	Absence of the following features
	Low = 1	Lymphadenopathy ≥ 1 cm in any nodal region or ≥ 2 cm in inguinal region
	Moderate = 2	Lymphadenopathy ≥2 cm in any nodal region or ≥3 cm in inguinal region, and/or splenomegaly (clinically palpable or assessed by imaging)
	High = 3	Current malignant B-cell proliferative disorder
Glandular [2] *Exclusion of stone or infection*	No = 0	Absence of glandular swelling
	Low = 1	Small glandular swelling with enlarged parotid (≥ 3 cm), or limited submandibular or lachrymal swelling
	Moderate = 2	Major glandular swelling with enlarged parotid (> 3 cm), or important submandibular or lachrymal swelling
Articular [2] *Exclusion of osteoarthritis*	No = 0	Absence of currently active articular involvement
	Low = 1	Arthralgias in hands, wrists, ankles, and feet accompanied by morning stiffness (>30 min)
	Moderate = 2	1–5 (of 28 total count) synovitis
	High = 3	≥ 6 (of 28 total count) synovitis
Cutaneous [3] *Rate as "No activity" stable long-lasting features related to damage*	No = 0	Absence of currently active cutaneous involvement
	Low = 1	Erythema multiforma
	Moderate = 2	Limited cutaneous vasculitis, including urticarial vasculitis, or purpura limited to feet and ankle, or subacute cutaneous lupus
	High = 3	Diffuse cutaneous vasculitis, including urticarial vasculitis, or diffuse purpura, or ulcers related to vasculitis

(continued)

Domain [weight]	Activity level	Description
Pulmonary [5] *Rate as "No activity" stable long-lasting features related to damage, or respiratory involvement not related to the disease (tobacco use, etc.)*	No = 0	Absence of currently active pulmonary involvement
	Low = 1	Persistent cough or bronchial involvement with no radiographic abnormalities on radiography Or radiological or HRCT evidence of interstitial lung disease with: No breathlessness and normal lung function test.
	Moderate = 2	Moderately active pulmonary involvement, such as interstitial lung disease shown by HRCT with shortness of breath on exercise (NHYA II) or abnormal lung function tests restricted to: $70\% > DL_{CO} \geq 40\%$ or $80\% > FVC \geq 60\%$
	High = 3	Highly active pulmonary involvement, such as interstitial lung disease shown by HRCT with shortness of breath at rest (NHYA III, IV) or with abnormal lung function tests: $DL_{CO} < 40\%$ or $FVC < 60\%$
Renal [5] *Rate as "No activity" stable long-lasting features related to damage, and renal involvement not related to the disease. If biopsy has been performed, please rate activity based on **histological** features first*	No = 0	Absence of currently active renal involvement with proteinuria <0.5 g/day, no hematuria, no leukocyturia, no acidosis, or long-lasting stable proteinuria due to damage
	Low = 1	Evidence of mild active renal involvement, limited to tubular acidosis without renal failure or glomerular involvement with proteinuria (between 0.5 and 1 g/day) and without hematuria or renal failure (GFR ≥ 60 mL/min)
	Moderate = 2	Moderately active renal involvement, such as tubular acidosis with renal failure (GFR <60 mL/min) or glomerular involvement with proteinuria between 1 and 1.5 g/day and without hematuria or renal failure (GFR ≥60 mL/min) or histological evidence of extramembranous glomerulonephritis or important interstitial lymphoid infiltrate
	High = 3	Highly active renal involvement, such as glomerular involvement with proteinuria >1.5 g/day or hematuria or renal failure (GFR <60 mL/min), or histological evidence of proliferative glomerulonephritis or cryoglobulinemia-related renal involvement
Muscular [6] *Exclusion of weakness due to corticosteroids*	No = 0	Absence of currently active muscular involvement
	Low = 1	Mild active myositis shown by abnormal EMG or biopsy with no weakness and creatine kinase (N < CK ≥ 2 N)
	Moderate = 2	Moderately active myositis proven by abnormal EMG or biopsy with weakness (maximal deficit of 4/5), or elevated creatine kinase (2 N < CK ≤4 N),
	High = 3	Highly active myositis shown by abnormal EMG or biopsy with weakness (deficit ≥ 3/5) or elevated creatine kinase (>4 N)

(continued)

Domain [weight]	Activity level	Description
PNS [5] *Rate as "No activity" stable long-lasting features related to damage or PNS involvement not related to the disease*	No = 0	Absence of currently active PNS involvement
	Low = 1	Mild active peripheral nervous system involvement, such as pure sensory axonal polyneuropathy shown by NCS or trigeminal (V) neuralgia
	Moderate = 2	Moderately active peripheral nervous system involvement shown by NCS, such as axonal sensory-motor neuropathy with maximal motor deficit of 4/5, pure sensory neuropathy with presence of cryoglobulinemic vasculitis, ganglionopathy with symptoms restricted to mild/moderate ataxia, inflammatory demyelinating polyneuropathy (CIDP) with mild functional impairment (maximal motor deficit of 4/5or mild ataxia), Or cranial nerve involvement of peripheral origin (except trigeminal (V) neuralgia)
	High = 3	Highly active PNS involvement shown by NCS, such as axonal sensory-motor neuropathy with motor deficit ≤3/5, peripheral nerve involvement due to vasculitis (mononeuritis multiplex, etc.), severe ataxia due to ganglionopathy, inflammatory demyelinating polyneuropathy (CIDP) with severe functional impairment: motor deficit ≤3/5 or severe ataxia
CNS [5] *Rate as "No activity" stable long-lasting features related to damage or CNS involvement not related to the disease*	No = 0	Absence of currently active CNS involvement
	Low = 1	Moderately active CNS features, such as cranial nerve involvement of central origin, optic neuritis, or multiple sclerosis-like syndrome with symptoms restricted to pure sensory impairment or proven cognitive impairment
	High = 3	Highly active CNS features, such as cerebral vasculitis with cerebrovascular accident or transient ischemic attack, seizures, transverse myelitis, lymphocytic meningitis, multiple sclerosis-like syndrome with motor deficit
Hematological [2] *For anemia, neutropenia, and thrombopenia, only auto-immune cytopenia must be considered Exclusion of vitamin or iron deficiency, drug-induced cytopenia*	No = 0	Absence of autoimmune cytopenia
	Low = 1	Cytopenia of autoimmune origin with neutropenia (1000 < neutrophils < 1500/mm^3), and/or anemia (10 < hemoglobin < 12 g/dL), and/or thrombocytopenia (100,000 < platelets < 150,000/mm^3) Or lymphopenia (500 < lymphocytes < 1000/mm^3)
	Moderate = 2	Cytopenia of auto-immune origin with neutropenia (500 ≤ neutrophils ≥ 1000/mm^3), and/or anemia (8 ≤ hemoglobin ≥ 10 g/dL), and/or thrombocytopenia (50,000 ≥ platelets ≥ 100,000/mm^3) Or lymphopenia (≥ 500/mm^3)
	High = 3	Cytopenia of auto-immune origin with neutropenia (neutrophils < 500/mm^3), and/or or anemia (hemoglobin < 8 g/dL) and/or thrombocytopenia (platelets <50,000/mm^3)

(continued)

Domain [weight]	Activity level	Description
Biological [1]	No=0	Absence of any of the following biological feature
	Low=1	Clonal component and/or hypocomplementemia (low C4 or C3 or CH50) and/or hypergammaglobulinemia or high IgG level between 16 and 20 g/L
	Moderate=2	Presence of cryoglobulinemia and/or hypergammaglobulinemia or high IgG level > 20 g/L, and/or recent onset hypogammaglobulinemia or recent decrease of IgG level (<5 g/L)

Reprinted with permission from Seror R, Ravaud P, Bowman SJ, Baron G, Tzioufas A, Theander E, et al; EULAR Sjögren's Task Force. EULAR Sjögren's syndrome disease activity index: development of a consensus systemic disease activity index for primary Sjögren's syndrome. Ann Rheum Dis. 2010 Jun; 69(6): 1103–1109

CIDP chronic inflammatory demyelinating polyneuropathy, *CK* creatine kinase, *CNS* central nervous system, *DLCO* diffusing CO capacity, *EMG* electromyogram, *FVC* forced vital capacity, *GFR* glomerular filtration rate, *Hb* hemoglobin, *HRCT* high-resolution computed tomography, *IgG* immunoglobulin G, *NCS* nerve conduction studies, *NHYA* New York heart association classification, *Plt* platelet, *PNS* peripheral nervous system

1. Vivino FB, Al-Hashimi I, Khan Z, LeVeque FG, Salisbury PL, 3rd, Tran-Johnson TK, et al. Pilocarpine tablets for the treatment of dry mouth and dry eye symptoms in patients with Sjogren syndrome: a randomized, placebo-controlled, fixed-dose, multicenter trial. P92-01 Study Group. Arch Intern Med. 1999;159: 174–81.
2. Drosos AA, Skopouli FN, Costopoulos JS, Papadimitriou CS, Moutsopoulos HM. Cyclosporin A (CyA) in primary Sjogren's syndrome: a double blind study. Ann Rheum Dis. 1986;45:732–5.
3. Kruize AA, Hene RJ, Kallenberg CG, van Bijsterveld OP, van der Heide A, Kater L, et al. Hydroxychloroquine treatment for primary Sjogren's syndrome: a two year double blind crossover trial. Ann Rheum Dis. 1993;52:360–4.
4. Price EJ, Rigby SP, Clancy U, Venables PJ. A double blind placebo controlled trial of azathioprine in the treatment of primary Sjogren's syndrome. J Rheumatol. 1998;25:896–9.
5. Mariette X, Ravaud P, Steinfeld S, Baron G, Goetz J, Hachulla E, et al. Inefficacy of infliximab in primary Sjogren's syndrome: results of the randomized, controlled Trial of Remicade in Primary Sjogren's Syndrome (TRIPSS) Arthritis Rheum. 2004;50:1270–6.
6. Sankar V, Brennan MT, Kok MR, Leakan RA, Smith JA, Manny J, et al. Etanercept in Sjogren's syndrome: a twelve-week randomized, double-blind, placebo-controlled pilot clinical trial. Arthritis Rheum. 2004;50:2240–5.

Appendix 2: EULAR Sjogren's Syndrome Patient-Reported Index (ESSPRI)

Reprinted with permission from Seror R, Theander E, Brun JG, Ramos-Casals M, Valim V, Dörner T, et al; EULAR Sjögren's Task Force. Validation of EULAR primary Sjögren's syndrome disease activity (ESSDAI) and patient indexes (ESSPRI). Ann Rheum Dis. 2015; 74: 859–866 from BMJ Publishing Group Ltd

1) How severe has your dryness been during the last 2 weeks ?

No dryness	☐ 0	☐ 1	☐ 2	☐ 3	☐ 4	☐ 5	☐ 6	☐ 7	☐ 8	☐ 9	☐ 10	Maximal imaginable dryness

2) How severe has your fatigue been during the last 2 weeks ?

No fatigue	☐ 0	☐ 1	☐ 2	☐ 3	☐ 4	☐ 5	☐ 6	☐ 7	☐ 8	☐ 9	☐ 10	Maximal imaginable fatigue

3) How severe has your pain (joint or muscular pains in your arms or legs) been during the last 2 weeks ?

No pain	☐ 0	☐ 1	☐ 2	☐ 3	☐ 4	☐ 5	☐ 6	☐ 7	☐ 8	☐ 9	☐ 10	Maximal imaginable pain

References

1. Kassan SS, Moutsopoulos HM. Clinical manifestations and early diagnosis of Sjögren syndrome. Arch Intern Med. 2004;164:1275–84.
2. Brito-Zerón P, Ramos-Casals M, EULAR-SS task force group. Advances in the understanding and treatment of systemic complications in Sjögren's syndrome. Curr Opin Rheumatol. 2014;26:520–7.
3. Patel R, Shahane A. The epidemiology of Sjögren's syndrome. Clin Epidemiol. 2014;6:247–55.
4. Bowman SJ, Ibrahim GH, Holmes G, et al. Estimating the prevalence among Caucasian women of primary Sjögren's syndrome in two general practices in Birmingham, UK. Scand J Rheumatol. 2004;33:39–43.
5. Pillemer SR, Matteson EL, Jacobsson LT, et al. Incidence of physician-diagnosed primary Sjögren syndrome in residents of Olmsted County, Minnesota. Mayo Clin Proc. 2001;76:593–9.
6. Voulgarelis M, Tzioufas AG, Moutsopoulos HM. Mortality in Sjögren's syndrome. Clin Exp Rheumatol. 2008;26:S66–71.
7. Lopez-Jornet P, Camacho-Alonso F. Quality of life in patients with Sjogren's syndrome and sicca complex. J Oral Rehabil. 2008;35:875–81.

8. Ng WF, Bowman SJ. Primary Sjogren's syndrome: too dry and too tired. Rheumatology (Oxford). 2010;49:844–53.
9. Soliotis FC, Mavragani CP, Moutsopoulos HM. Central nervous system involvement in Sjogren's syndrome. Ann Rheum Dis. 2004;63:616–20.
10. Segal B, Bowman SJ, Fox PC, et al. Primary Sjögren's syndrome: health experiences and predictors of health quality among patients in the United States. Health Qual Life Outcomes. 2009;7:46.
11. El Miedany YM, Ahmed I, Mourad HG, et al. Quantitative ultrasonography and magnetic resonance imaging of the parotid gland: can they replace the histopathologic studies in patients with Sjogren's syndrome? Joint Bone Spine. 2004;71:29–38.
12. Vitali C, Bombardieri S, Jonsson R, European Study Group on Classification Criteria for Sjögren's Syndrome, et al. Classification criteria for Sjögren's syndrome: a revised version of the European criteria proposed by the American-European Consensus Group. Ann Rheum Dis. 2002;61:554–8.
13. Ramos-Casals M, Tzioufas AG, Stone JH, et al. Treatment of primary Sjögren syndrome: a systematic review. JAMA. 2010;304:452–60.
14. Seror R, Ravaud P, Bowman SJ, EULAR Sjögren's Task Force, et al. EULAR Sjogren's syndrome disease activity index: development of a consensus systemic disease activity index for primary Sjogren's syndrome. Ann Rheum Dis. 2010;69:1103–9.
15. Seror R, Ravaud P, Mariette X, et al. EULAR Sjogren's syndrome patient reported index (ESSPRI). Development of consensus patient complex for primary Sjogren's syndrome. Ann Rheum Dis. 2011;70:968–72.
16. Brito-Zerón P, Kostov B, Solans R, SS Study Group, Autoimmune Diseases Study Group (GEAS), Spanish Society of Internal Medicine (SEMI), et al. Systemic activity and mortality in primary Sjögren syndrome: predicting survival using the EULAR-SS Disease Activity Index (ESSDAI) in 1045 patients. Ann Rheum Dis. 2016;75(2):348–55.
17. Ramos-Casals M, Font J, Garcia-Carrasco M, et al. Primary Sjögren syndrome: hematologic patterns of disease expression. Medicine (Baltimore). 2002;81:281–92.
18. El Miedany Y. PROMs in inflammatory arthritis: moving from static to dynamic. Clin Rheumatol. 2013;32:735–42.
19. Bowman SJ, Booth DA, Platts RG. Measurement of fatigue and discomfort in primary Sjogren's syndrome using a new questionnaire tool. Rheumatology (Oxford). 2004;43:758–64.
20. Meiners PM, Arends S, Brouwer E. Responsiveness of disease activity indices ESSPRI and ESSDAI in patients with primary Sjogren's syndrome treated with rituximab. Ann Rheum Dis. 2012;71:1297–302.
21. Seror R, Mariette X, Bowman S, et al. Accurate detection of changes in disease activity in primary Sjogren's syndrome the European League Against Rheumatism Sjogren's syndrome Disease Activity Index. Arthritis Care Res. 2010;62:551–8.
22. Carr AJ, Thompson PW, Kirwan JR. Quality of life measures. Br J Rheumatol. 1996;35:275–81.
23. WHOQOL Group. Development of the QHOQOL: rationale and current status. Int J Ment Health. 1994;23:24–56.
24. WHOQOL Group. Development of the World Health Organization WHOQOL-BREF quality of life assessment. Psychol Med. 1998;28:551–8.
25. Ware JE, Sherbourne CD. The MOS 36-item short-form health survey (SF-36): conceptual framework and item selection. Med Care. 1992;30:473–83.
26. EuroQoL Group. Euro-QoL—a new facility for the measurement of health related quality of life. Health Policy. 1990;16:199–208.
27. Rajagopalan K, Abetz L, Merzanis P. Comparing the discriminate validity of two generic and one disease specific health related quality of life measures in a sample of patients with dry eye. Value Health. 2005;8:168–74.
28. Valtysdottir ST, Gudbjornsson B, Lindqvist U. Anxiety and depression in patients with primary Sjogren's syndrome. J Rheumatol. 2000;27:165–9.

29. El Miedany Y. Patient reported outcome measures: from generic to specific. Clin Rheumatol. 2014;32:S40–6.
30. Bowman SJ, Booth DA, Platts RG, Field A, Rostron J, UK Sjögren's Interest Group. Validation of the Sicca symptoms Inventory for clinical studies of Sjögren's syndrome. J Rheumatol. 2003;30:1259–66.
31. Slade GD, Spencer AJ. Development and evaluation of the Oral Health Impact Profile. Community Dent Health. 1994;11:3–11.
32. Iacopino AM. Relationship between periodontal disease and general health: role of inflammation. J Can Dent Assoc. 2008;74:695–6.
33. Locker D, Matear D, Stephens M, et al. Comparison of the GOHAI and OHIP-14 as measures of the oral health related quality of life of the elderly. Community Dent Oral Epidemiol. 2001;29:373–81.
34. McMillan AS, Leung KC, Leung WK, et al. Impact of Sjogren's syndrome on oral health-related quality of life in southern Chinese. J Oral Rehabil. 2004;31:653–9.
35. Larsson P, List T, Lundstrom I, et al. Reliability and validity of a Swedish version of the Oral Health Impact Profile (OHIP-S). Acta Odontol Scand. 2004;62:147–52.
36. Allen PF, McMillan AS, Walshaw D, Locker D. A comparison of the validity of generic and disease specific measures in the assessment of oral health related quality of life. Community Dent Oral Epidemiol. 1999;27:344–52.
37. Schiffman RM, Christianson MD, Jacobsen G. Reliability and validity of the Ocular Surface Disease Index. Arch Ophthalmol. 2000;118:615–21.
38. Vitale S, Goodman LA, Reed GF, Smith JA. Comparison of the NEI-VFQ and OSDI questionnaires in patients with Sjogren's syndrome related dry eye. Health Qual Life Outcomes. 2004;2:44–9.
39. Dry eye workshop: the definition and classification of dry eye disease: report of the Definition and Classification Subcommittee of the International Dry Eye WorkShop (2007). Ocul Surf. 2007; 5:75–92.
40. Goto E, Yagi Y, Matsumoto Y, Tsubota K. Impaired functional visual acuity of dry eye patients. Am J Ophthalmol. 2002;133:181–6.
41. Friedman NJ. Impact of dry eye disease and treatment on quality of life. Curr Opin Ophthalmol. 2010;21:310–6.
42. Mertzanis P, Abetz L, Rajagopalan K, Espindle D, Chalmers R, Snyder C, Caffery B, Edrington T, Simpson T, Nelson JD, et al. The relative burden of dry eye in patients' lives: comparisons to a U.S. normative sample. Invest Ophthalmol Vis Sci. 2005;46:46–50.
43. Nichols KK, Mitchell GL, Zadnik K. Performance and repeatability of the NEI-VFQ-25 in patients with dry eye. Cornea. 2002;21:578–83.
44. Begley CG, Chalmers RL, Abetz L, Venkataraman K, Mertzanis P, Caffery BA, Snyder C, Edrington T, Nelson D, Simpson T. The relationship between habitual patient-reported symptoms and clinical signs among patients with dry eye of varying severity. Invest Ophthalmol Vis Sci. 2003;44:4753–61.
45. McCarty CA, Bansal AK, Livingston PM, Stanislavsky YL, Taylor HR. The epidemiology of dry eye in Melbourne, Australia. Ophthalmology. 1998;105:1114–9.
46. McMonnies CW. Key questions in a dry eye history. J Am Optom Assoc. 1986;57:512–7.
47. Schein OD, Munoz B, Tielsch JM, Bandeen-Roche K, West S. Prevalence of dry eye among the elderly. Am J Ophthalmol. 1997;124:723–8.
48. Guillemin I, Begley C, Chalmers R, et al. Appraisal of patient-reported outcome instruments available for randomized clinical trials in dry eye: revisiting the standards. Ocul Surf. 2012;10:84–99.
49. Chalmers RL, Begley CG, Edrington T, Caffery B, Nelson D, Snyder C, Simpson T. The agreement between self-assessment and clinician assessment of dry eye severity. Cornea. 2005;24:804–10.
50. Sullivan BD, Whitmer D, Nichols KK, Tomlinson A, Foulks GN, Geerling G, Pepose JS, Kosheleff V, Porreco A, Lemp MA. An objective approach to dry eye disease severity. Invest Ophthalmol Vis Sci. 2010;51:6125–30.

51. Vitale S, Schein OD. Qualitative research in functional vision. Int Ophthalmol Clin. 2003;43:17–30.
52. Damiano AM, Steinberg EP, Cassard SD, Bass EB, Diener-West M, Legro MW, Tielsch J, Schein OD, Javitt J, Kolb M. Comparison of generic versus disease-specific measures of functional impairment in patients with cataract. Med Care. 1995;33:AS120–30.
53. Patrick DL, Deyo RA. Generic and disease-specific measures in assessing health status and quality of life. Med Care. 1989;27:S217–32.
54. Narayanan S, Miller WL, Prager TC, et al. The diagnosis and characteristics of moderate dry eye in non-contact lens wearers. Eye Contact Lens. 2005;31:96–104.
55. Grubbs Jr J, Tolleson-Rinehart S, Huynh K, Davis R. A review of quality of life measures in Dry Eye questionnaires. Cornea. 2014;33:215–8.
56. Mangione CM, Lee PP, Gutierrez PR, et al. Development of the 25-item National Eye Institute Visual function Questionnaire. Arch Ophthalmol. 2001;119:1050–8.
57. Abetz L, Rajagopalan K, Mertzanis P, Begley C, Barnes R, Chalmers R, Impact of Dry Eye on Everyday life (IDEEL) Study Group. Development and validation of the Impact of Dry Eye on Everyday Life (IDEEL) questionnaire, a patient-reported outcomes (PRO) measure for the assessment of the burden of dry eye on patients. Health Qual Life Outcomes. 2011;9:111.
58. Segal B, Thomas W, Rogers T. Prevalence, severity and predictors of fatigue in subjects with primary Sjogren's syndrome. Arthritis Rheum. 2008;59:1780–7.
59. Bowman SJ, Booth DA, Platts RG; the UK Sjogren's Interest Group. Measurement of fatigue and discomfort in primary Sjogren's syndrome using a new questionnaire tool. Rheumatology. 2004; 43:758–64.
60. Lwin CT, Bishay M, Platts RG. Measurement of fatigue and discomfort in primary Sjogren's syndrome. Scand J Rheumatol. 2003;32:33–7.
61. Goodchild CT, Treharne GJ, Booth DA, et al. Measuring fatigue among women with Sjogren's syndrome or rheumatoid arthritis. A comparison of the Profile of Fatigue (ProF) and the multidimensional fatigue Inventory (MFI). Musculoskeletal Care. 2008;6:31–48.
62. Bowman S, Hamburger J, Richards A, Barry R, Rauz S. Patient-reported outcomes in primary Sjogren's syndrome: comparison of the long and short versions of the Profile of Fatigue and Discomfort—Sicca Symptoms Inventory. Rheumatology. 2009;48:140–3.
63. Dass S, Bowman SJ, Vital EM, et al. Reduction of fatigue in Sjogren's syndrome with rituximab: results of a randomised, double-blind, placebo controlled pilot study. Ann Rheum Dis. 2008;67:1541–4154.
64. Krupp LB, LaRocca NG, Muir-Nash J, Steinberg AD. The fatigue severity scale. Application to patients with multiple sclerosis and systemic lupus erythematosus. Arch Neurol. 1989;46:1121–3.
65. Cella D, Yount S, Sorensen M, Chartash E, Sengupta N, Grober J. Validation of the Functional Assessment of Chronic Illness Therapy Fatigue Scale relative to other instrumentation in patients with rheumatoid arthritis. J Rheumatol. 2005;32:811–9.
66. Asmussen K, Bowman S. Outcome measures in Sjogren's syndrome. Rheumatology. 2001;40:1085–8.
67. Hay EM, Thomas E, Pal B, Hajeer A. Weak association between subjective symptoms and objective testing for dry eyes and dry mouth: results from a population based study. Ann Rheum Dis. 1998;57:20–4.
68. El-Miedany YM, El-Hady SM, El-Baddin MA. Validity of the saliva Ferning test for the diagnosis of dry mouth in Sjögren's syndrome. Rev Rhum Engl Ed. 1999;66:73–8.
69. El Miedany Y, El Gaafary M, Youssef S, Palmer D. Incorporating patient reported outcome measures in clinical practice: development and validation of a questionnaire for inflammatory arthritis. Clin Exp Rheumatol. 2010;28:734–44.
70. Pincus T, Yazici Y, Bergman M. Development of a multi-dimensional health assessment questionnaire (MDHAQ) for the infrastructure of standard clinical care. Clin Exp Rheumatol. 2005;23:S19–28.

Chapter 13
PROMs for Carpal Tunnel Syndrome

Yasser El Miedany

Introduction

Carpal tunnel syndrome (CTS), first reported by Phalen [1], is one of the most common compression peripheral mono-neuropathies, which occurs due to localized entrapment of the median nerve (MN) as it passes through the carpal tunnel. CTS is a common clinical condition presenting with numbness, paresthesia, and sometimes pain or weakness of the hand muscles. Whilst symptoms severity may vary from one person to another, if left untreated, it may lead to permanent "median nerve damage," causing irreversible numbness, muscle wasting, and weakness of the affected hand. Earlier studies revealed it has an overall prevalence of 3.0–5.8 % among women and 0.6–2.1 % among men in general population samples [2, 3]. The vast expanding use of new technology gadgets led to widening of the age range of people suffering from CTS symptoms and a significant increase in the condition prevalence. Recent reports depicted that CTS account for up to 90 % of all entrapment neuropathies [4–6].

Whilst its onset in most of the cases is insidious and progressive, a growing body of evidence indicates that the common pathway for CTS development is increased pressure within the carpal canal. Experimental studies reported that the changes in the CTS are linked to the amount and duration of the increased interstitial fluid pressure and could be reversible up to a point with management [7]. Therefore, understanding the pathophysiological changes in the carpal tunnel and its effect on the median nerve would have a positive impact not only on the diagnosis but also on the management of the condition. Earlier reports revealed that CTS pathophysiology is

Y. El Miedany (✉)
Honorary Senior Clinical Lecturer, King's College London, London, UK

Professor of Rheumatology and Rehabilitation, Ain Shams University, Cairo, Egypt

Department of Rheumatology, Darent Valley Hospital, Dartford, Kent, UK
e-mail: drelmiedany@rheumatology4u.com

Y. El Miedany (ed.), *Patient Reported Outcome Measures in Rheumatic Diseases*,
DOI 10.1007/978-3-319-32851-5_13

multifactorial, including anatomic, physiologic, biochemical, mechanical, histologic, as well as pathological components, which integrate to explain and characterize this syndrome [8].

Meta-analysis and systematic literature review reveal that no one test could be identified as a "gold standard" for carpal tunnel syndrome diagnosis. Currently available evidence showed that neither clinical tests for CTS nor nerve conduction tests alone could reliably diagnose CTS. Though some studies reported that when both clinical tests and neurophysiologic tests were combined, this composite had a statistically significant correlation with positive postsurgical outcomes in CTS patients; there is no definitive conclusion available about which combination of clinical and neurophysiologic tests could provide the best performance [9].

Patient reported outcome measures (PROMs) are critical measures of management efficacy as the "patient perceived benefit" is considered the ultimate treatment goal. Therefore, they should be considered as supplement to data derived from physical examination as they provide the context of the impact on the patient's ability to carry out activities of daily living as well as quality of life. Over the past years, PROMs have attained further reputation following the recent recommendations of taking a patient-centered approach in standard clinical practice [10]. The lack of a gold standard in the CTS diagnosis and management highlighted the need for a common consensus regarding the assessment of the patient's condition as well as reporting of treatment outcomes. Utilizing a validated set of commonly accepted outcome measures reported by the patient has been implemented in several studies to assess for the natural history of the disease as well as monitoring of response to treatment.

This chapter will discuss the different patient reported outcome measures tools available for CTS and outline their role in the diagnosis and management of CTS. It aims at improving the quality and efficiency of the patients' care in standard practice.

Challenges in Carpal Tunnel Syndrome

Diagnosis and Evaluation of the Cases

The CTS diagnosis is based on a mix of clinical subjective criteria. The American Academy of Neurology proposed that: paresthesia, swelling, pain, weakness or clumsiness of the hand, provoked or worsened by sleep, sustained hand or arm position, repetitive action of the hand or wrist that is alleviated by changing posture or by shaking of the hand, sensory deficit in the median nerve innervated part of the hand, as well as motor deficit of the median nerve innervated thenar muscles represent the characteristic CTS manifestations [11]. Evaluation of patients presenting with CTS manifestations has long relied on their clinical symptoms as well as neurophysiological assessment [12]. However, although standard CTS symptoms and positive provocative testing may enable the diagnosis in some cases, the subjectivity and sensitivity of these measures resulted in very poor reliability and diagnostic accuracy [13–16]. Similarly, though earlier studies revealed sensitivity and specificity data in favor of electrodiagnostic testing for the CTS diagnosis [17–19], abnormal nerve conduction study results do not necessarily equate to the correct diagnosis. Furthermore, earlier reports showed that nerve conduction testing can be normal in early cases [20]. In concordance with these findings, other studies revealed that neurophysiological measures of the median nerve in CTS were "nonsensitive" to change or management, hence, a poor predictor of treatment outcomes [21, 22]. This dissociation between clinical-neurophysiological outcomes and patients' symptoms paved the way for most of the recent research studies on CTS to rely on patient symptoms analysis. Studies revealed that patient reported outcomes were able to measure outcome dimensions not captured by traditional objective evaluations of median nerve impairment [23, 24].

Status and Response Measures in Carpal Tunnel Syndrome

When assessing patients with CTS, it is important to differentiate between two concepts: "status" and "response" measures. Whilst "status measures" assess the disease severity at a specific point in time, "response measures" assess how disease status changes over time, for example, response to management whether conservative or surgical. Therefore, remission is considered to be a status measure [25]. These measures are important when the treating health care professional evaluates treatment strategies in individual CTS patients. Furthermore, as response measures evaluate change in clinical status over time, it can be used, not only to determine efficacy but it can also be implemented in longitudinal observational studies to evaluate clinical change over time.

Outcome Measures

The evidence-based medicine is moving swiftly toward outcome-driven practice. Data and consequent outcome analysis attained from various treatment protocols are expected to facilitate the assessment of quality of the management provided and potentially may help to modify our practice. Outcomes from carpal tunnel management have been evaluated in several ways, including objective neurophysiological assessment, clinical measures of sensory and muscle affection, patient-perceived symptoms and functional ability, as well as the impact on activities of daily living and work. Broadly, there is a lack of consensus among researchers over what could be the most reliable, valid, and responsive tool to assess outcomes in CTS management [26–28]. However, in general, there is an agreement on three domains that can be used to describe the long- and short-term CTS consequences and should be considered in defining remission: clinical symptoms and signs, functional impairment, and structural nerve damage (muscle wasting or weakness/sensory deficit) [21, 22].

Patient Reported Outcome Measures Tools in Carpal Tunnel Syndrome

Patient Empowerment—i.e., involving CTS patients in the decision-making regarding their condition and its management—paved the way for further research, initially to identify tools to assess the patient's symptoms and its severity and later on to assess its responsiveness to change. This included validity and reproducibility of these scales. Results from follow-up studies showed that these scales are considerably more responsive to clinical improvement than traditional measures [24]. Furthermore, patient reported outcome measures were also found able to predict response to conservative treatment and thereby predict probability of undergoing surgery [25]. These data highlighted the important role of patient reported outcome measure assessment in CTS as a potential bridge between research and good practice in CTS patients.

Reviewing the literature revealed several patient-reported-based questionnaires for CTS. These can be categorized into three main groups:

1. Questionnaires to screen and assess for the possibility of having CTS, i.e., diagnosis. These can be either Web-based or in paper format.
2. Questionnaires to assess for the severity of CTS symptoms.
3. Questionnaires to assess for the patients' functional ability as well as the impact of the condition on their work, life, and leisure.

These PROMs questionnaires can be also classified into (Table 13.1) [29, 30]: generic health status, and condition- or population-specific measures. (There is a third category, called "preference-based measures," which is also broad in content, however, it also provides utilities or values regarding health for use in, for example, cost-utility analyses of interventions.) Generic instruments encompass items relevant to the widest range of patient conditions/general population. Condition-specific instruments tend to be more focused on a particular disease or health condition (e.g., rheumatoid arthritis or CTS), a patient population (e.g., older people), a specific problem or symptom (e.g., pain), or a described function (e.g., activities of daily living). For any given area of health in standard clinical practice, condition-specific instruments usually have greater clinical appeal due to the inclusion of content specific to a particular condition, and the likelihood of increased responsiveness to interventions. Examples of these specific tools for assessment of CTS patients include the following.

The Boston Carpal Tunnel Questionnaire (BCTQ)

The questionnaire (BCTQ), developed in 1993 [31], is a patient-based outcome measure questionnaire that has been developed specifically for CTS patients. Though it is well known for its current name (BCTQ), it can be also referred to as

Table 13.1 Patient reported outcome measures in carpal tunnel syndrome

Tool	Items (number of items)	Response	Score
Specific tools			
BCTQ 5= severe	Symptoms severity (11)	5 Point Likert scale	Mean of each scale items scores
	Functional status (8)		1 Point = best score
Modified BCTQ	Functional status (10)	5 Point Likert scale	Mean of the 10 items scores
			1 = Best outcome
			5 = Severe
MHQ	Six domains (37 items)	5 Point Likert scale	Pain score: higher score = greater pain
	Overall hand function, activities of daily living, pain, work performance, aesthetics, patient satisfaction with hand function		Other 5 scales: higher score = better performance
CTS-6 items	Symptoms scale (6 items)	5 Point Likert scale	Mean of the 6 items scores
			1 = Best outcome
			5 = Severe
PEM	3 Subscales (18 items)	7 Point Likert scale	Lower scores Better QoL
	Treatment 5, How my hand is now (10), Overall assessment (3)		
Kamath and Stothard	9 Questions	Yes/no	Score ≥ 3 = analysis in comparison to Nerve conduction testing
			Score ≥5 = can replace Nerve conduction testing
CTS-PROMs Symptom Scale	5 Symptom scales (11 questions)	Yes/no	Answer yes to question 1 about paresthesia in the median nerve distribution + any other 2 questions is diagnostic of CTS
CTS-PROMs Severity scale	Severity scale (6 items)	VAS: 0–100	Carpal tunnel response calculated (CT-response 20/70/90)
Discrete tool			
DASH	Two domains (30 items)	5–7 Point Likert scales	0–100
	Symptoms (5 scales)	100 = Maximum disability	0 = No disability; 100 = maximum Disability
	Function (3 scales)		

(continued)

Table 13.1 (continued)

Tool	Items (number of items)	Response	Score
Generic tool			
The Short Form Health Survey (36) (SF-36) [29]	– Physical functioning (10)	Categorical: 2–6 options	0–100, (100 best health)
	– Role limitation-physical (4)		
	– Bodily pain (2)		
	– General health (5)		
	– Vitality (4)		
	– Social functioning (2)		
	– Role limitation-emotional (3)		
	– Mental health (5)		
	– Health transition (1)		
Nottingham Health Profile (NHP) [30]	– Bodily pain (8)	Yes/no	0–100, (100 is maximum limitation)
	– Emotional reactions (9)		
	– Energy (E) (3)		
	– Physical mobility (8)		
	– Sleep (5)		
	– Social isolation (5)		

BCTQ Boston Carpal Tunnel Questionnaire, *MHQ* Michigan Hand Outcomes Questionnaire, *CTS-6* Six-Item CTS Symptoms Scale, *PEM* Patient Evaluation Measure, *CTS-PROMS* Carpal Tunnel Syndrome-Patient Reported Outcome Measures, *DASH* Disabilities of the Arm, Shoulder and Hand

the Levine scale, Brigham and Women's Carpal Tunnel Questionnaire, and Carpal Tunnel Syndrome Instrument. The questionnaire has two distinct scales: (1) the "Symptom Severity Scale," which includes 11 questions and uses a 5-point Likert rating scale and (2) the "Functional Status Scale" containing eight items that rate the degree of difficulty on a 5-point scale. Each scale generates a final score (sum of individual scores divided by number of items), which ranges from 1 to 5, with a higher score indicating symptoms severity or greater disability. The BCTQ has been used as an outcome measure in several clinical studies, and has also undergone extensive testing for validity, reliability, and responsiveness [32, 33]. A systematic review of the psychometric properties of the Boston Carpal Tunnel Questionnaire [35] revealed that the two sub-scales of the questionnaire measuring symptoms severity as well as functional status were reliable and valid, being the most important reasons for seeking medical advice.

Convergent validity of the BCTQ has been demonstrated by moderate correlations between the symptoms severity scale scores and grip measures, pinch as well as strength. Similarly there was moderate correlation between functional status scores and the same parameters (pinch, grip, and strength) [31, 35]. All correlations were in the predicted direction; worse status is associated with worse impairment. Higher satisfaction with postoperative results was associated with greater improvement in both the symptoms severity and functional status scores. Pain scores in the symptoms severity domain correlated significantly with the functional ability score, indicating more functional impairment as pain is increased [36]. Moreover, the mean baseline symptoms severity and functional status scores were reported to be significantly higher for patients who later (1 year follow-up) had carpal tunnel decompression, indicating strong predictive validity. In concordance, responsiveness has been demonstrated for both dimension of the BCTQ after carpal tunnel release surgery [23]. In another study [37], both symptom severity and functional status domains of the BCTQ were found to be 2–4 times more responsive to clinical improvement than measures of neuromuscular impairment.

However, the questionnaire was criticized for two main points. The first one (bearing in mind the questionnaire was developed in 1993) is that, whilst the functional status scale covers activities usually performed by a broad range of CTS patients, it does not include other items of relevance to specific groups such as workers or computer/gadget-related activities, which have been recently reported as the commonest causes for CTS symptoms. Secondly, Atroshi et al. [38] reported that the BCTQ scales were initially developed without assessing the questionnaire item structure such as for factor analysis. This was supported by the results of a study [39] investigating the symptom severity and functional status scales using modern measurement methodology in a stepwise process. Results revealed that four items did not fit well in the symptom severity scale whereas it was possible to merge two other items in that scale.

The Modified Boston Carpal Tunnel Questionnaire

The modified BCTQ was developed in 2006 aiming at enclosure of the missing items relevant to specific groups such as workers or computer/gadget-related activities [40] (Appendix 1). It was developed specifically to assess functional ability in CTS patients. Two questions were added to the original BCTQ [31] that represent the current most common forms of repetitive stress injury (computer work/typing and driving). The questionnaire contains ten items that rate the degree of functional ability on a 5-point scale. The final score (sum of individual scores divided by number of items) ranges from 1 to 5, with a higher score indicating greater disability. The modified BCTQ can be self-, interview-, or telephone-administered.

The modified questionnaire was tested in the original study [40] for internal consistency, reliability, and construct validity by correlating the yield of the questionnaire with other disease testings, namely the Boston carpal tunnel severity self-administered questionnaire, nerve conduction study, and ultrasonography of the carpal tunnel findings. Appropriateness of the two added items was evaluated by principal component analysis in comparison to the correlation of the other eight items with the principal component. Test–retest analysis showed strong reliability with high percentage of agreement and high rates for kappa (0.94–0.981). Internal consistency showed a high value for standardized alpha (Cronbach) 0.973. The modified questionnaire has shown a strong validity on correlating its results with other disease parameters, nerve conduction, and ultrasonography testing. All ten items had similar correlation coefficient with the principal component (0.71–0.84). The authors concluded that the modified BCTQ was found to be a reliable and valid instrument that can be self-administered to evaluate the functional disability of patients presenting with carpal tunnel syndrome manifestations.

The Michigan Hand Outcomes Questionnaire (MHQ)

The questionnaire was developed in 1998 for use in the assessment of outcome for various hand disorders [41]. Content was guided by several established questionnaires including items from the SF-36 and the Arthritis Impact Measurement Scale, which were for dimensions relating to work performance and physical function, whilst items from the McGill Pain Scale and Carpal Tunnel Questionnaire were used for the development of questions for the pain domain. Additional items were generated by a group of patients.

The instrument has 37 items and consists of 6 domains: (1) overall hand function, (2) activity of daily living, (3) pain, (4) work performance, (5) aesthetics, and (6) patient satisfaction with hand function.

All items are in the form of questions ranked on a scale of 1–5. In the pain scale, high scores indicate greater pain; while in the other 5 scales, high scores denote better hand performance.

The raw scale score for each of the 6 scales is the sum of the responses of each scale item. The raw score is converted to a score ranging from 0 to 100. The instrument may be self-, interview-, or telephone-administered.

Several aspects of validity have been demonstrated by the authors of the original evaluation of the MHQ [42]. Significantly improved MHQ scores have been shown after surgery for all dimensions, with pain being the most responsive dimension. Kotsis et al. [43] reported that MHQ was more responsive to change than the Disabilities of the Arm, Shoulder and Hand (DASH) outcome questionnaire (see later) in CTS patients undergoing carpal tunnel decompression surgery. In contrast, in another study [44], which included 53 CTS patients undergoing carpal tunnel decompression surgery, significant improvements were reported only in three of six domains (function, work, and pain) when related to patient satisfaction.

The Six-Item CTS Symptoms Scale (CTS-6)

The questionnaire was developed in 2009 [39] as a brief outcome measure of symptoms in CTS. It was developed based on the 11-item Symptom Severity Scale suggested by Levine et al. [31]. The questionnaire is composed of six tests varying from history and physical exam, namely: (1) numbness in the hand and fingers supplied by the median nerve, (2) muscle atrophy and/or weakness, (3) a positive Phalen's test (standard clinical test used to diagnose carpal tunnel syndrome), (4) loss of 2-point discrimination (feeling 2 separate points touched on the skin), (5) numbness at night that wakes the patient up, and (6) a positive Tinel's sign (another standard clinical test used to diagnose carpal tunnel syndrome). The CTS-6 is scored with conventional scoring (similar to that used for the 11-item symptom severity scale); each item was scored on a scale of 1 (no symptom) to 5 (most severe symptom). For each patient, a CTS-6 score was calculated as the mean of the items answered by the patient, with only 1 missing item response allowed, and would thus range from 1 (best) to 5 (worst).

The original study carried out by Atroshi et al. [39] revealed that the 6-item CTS symptoms scale demonstrated good internal consistency, test–retest reliability, and validity compared with the 11-item symptom severity scale and did not exhibit differential item functioning with regard to gender. In another study [45], the CTS-6 was reported to be highly responsive to change in symptoms, and has been recommended by the authors (who originally developed the questionnaire) as a tool for evaluating primary and secondary outcomes measures in clinical trials studying carpal tunnel syndrome. Because the CTS-6 has previously shown good agreement with the 11-item symptom severity score, is scored on similar scale, and the fact the CTS-6 is shorter with improved layout, the authors suggested using the CTS-6 as an alternative to the 11-item symptom severity scale. John et al. [44] compared changes in the 6-item CTS symptoms scale and portable nerve conduction study parameters as outcome tools in CTS patients treated with steroid injections. There was a statistically significant difference between the CTS-6 scores before and after injection. There were also statistically significant changes in five of the nerve conduction testing parameters. However, none of the correlations between the CTS-6 and the nerve conduction study parameters were statistically significant.

Patient Evaluation Measure (PEM)

The questionnaire, developed in 1995 by Macey et al. [46], consists of three domains: patients' opinion on delivery of care, hand health profile, and overall assessment. The instrument has a total of 18 items that are scored using a 7-point scale. In all scales, low scores indicate positive outcomes. The authors did not report on item generation and item reduction. Similarly, there was no report on other aspects of the instrument development. The instrument may be self-, interview-, or telephone-administered.

Support for construct validity was revealed in a study carried out by Forward et al. [47], which reported significant correlation between the objective measures (PEM scores) and the subjective measures (e.g., increased grip strength). Convergent validity was demonstrated by strong significant correlations between PEM and DASH scores both pre- and postoperatively in CTS patients [48]. In concordance, there was a significant reduction in PEM scores in a sample of 97 patients undergoing carpal tunnel decompression surgery. This was recorded at 6 weeks as well as 6 months postsurgery.

Kamath and Stothard Questionnaire

A clinical questionnaire developed in 2003 [49] for the diagnosis of CTS and to assess whether the patients presenting with CTS symptoms should go for surgery. The questionnaire consists of nine questions based on the work of Levine et al. [31].

The questionnaire has been validated in secondary care for the diagnosis of CTS by Kamath and Stothard [49]. In their study, patients diagnosed as having CTS by either the questionnaire, nerve conduction testing, or both, underwent decompression surgery. Symptom improvement was considered as the "gold standard" for true CTS. The results revealed a sensitivity of 85 % for the scored questionnaire and 92 % for nerve conduction testing with a positive predictive value of 90 % for the scored questionnaire and 92 % for neurophysiological assessment. Therefore, it was concluded that a scored questionnaire can replace nerve conduction studies in the initial assessment of whether patients presenting with dysesthesia in the fingers should undergo surgery.

CTS-PROMs Questionnaire

The questionnaire, developed in 2006, is a composite patient-based outcome measure questionnaire developed specifically for CTS patients. One questionnaire was designed for CTS diagnosis [49] (Appendix 2), whereas the other questionnaire (CTS-PROMs Severity Scale Appendix 3) was for global assessment of symptoms severity and functional status of CTS patients [50]. Both physicians and patients were involved in the item generation process. After developing an item pool and a list of the main clinical presenting symptoms was compiled, the CTS-PROMs for diagnosis questionnaire was developed including 11 questions split over 5 scales: paresthesia, nocturnal pain, diurnal pain, weakness, and repetitive stress injury symptoms. This was the first questionnaire to include specific three questions about repetitive stress, which is the most important current underlying case for CTS. Answering "yes" to the first question about paresthesia in the median nerve distribution plus any other two questions was considered diagnostic of CTS.

Support for construct validity was demonstrated in the study carried out by El Miedany et al. [51], which included 233 patients presenting with CTS symptoms. The results of the scale were compared to the results of other validated measurements including: (1) the Boston Carpal Tunnel Questionnaire, (2) the clinical assessment, (3) the neurophysiological study (NCS), and (4) ultrasound (US) evaluation for both carpal tunnel and tendonitis. Comprehensibility and reproducibility of the model were also assessed. Results revealed that overall scale and each domain were internally consistent (Cronbach alpha, 0.86–0.94), and correlated significantly to other parameters. Reproducibility of the overall questionnaire and individual domains was excellent (Spearman–Brown index, 0.94–0.98).

The CTS-PROMs severity scale [52] is another self-administered questionnaire for global assessment of symptoms severity and the functional status (global severity score: GSS). The questionnaire consists of multi-item scales including the following domains: paresthesia, nocturnal pain, diurnal pain, weakness/clumsiness, repetitive stress pain, and global functional assessment. Each domain was graded separately and the patients were asked to rate their symptoms on a visual analogue scale of 0–10, where 0 = no symptoms and 10 = severe symptoms. Mean of the total score was calculated; consequently the relative severity measure for each domain was calculated by dividing the patient's rating for that symptom by the patient's total symptom severity mean score. A score >1 would indicate the relevance of this symptom and its value in monitoring the patient's condition as well as outcome of management.

Validity studies revealed that the scale was internally consistent (Cronbach alpha, 0.93 and 0.91 for severity of symptoms and functional status, respectively). Reproducibility of the overall questionnaire and individual domains was excellent (Spearman–Brown index, 0.94–0.98). Responsiveness to management was assessed in a third study [53], which included 106 patients treated either conservatively (55 patients) or surgically (51 patients). This study represented a step forward toward "optimizing outcomes in CTS patients" with inadequate responses to management whether treated conservatively or surgically. Response to therapy (*CTS-response*) was considered to separate patients into non-overlapping groups according to their responses to treatment. Results of the work revealed that CTS-response 20, 50, and 70 enabled the treating health care professional to interpret and quantitate treatment outcomes.

The Disabilities of the Arm, Shoulder and Hand (DASH) Outcome Questionnaire

The DASH outcome instrument is not specific to CTS. It was developed in 1996 as a joint initiative of the American Academy of Orthopaedic Surgeon (AAOS), the council of Musculoskeletal Specialty Societies (COMSS), and the Institute for Work and Health (Toronto, Ontario, Canada) [54]. It can be used to measure function in people with musculoskeletal disorders of the upper limb. The final version of the DASH is a 30-item scale and consists of 2 dimensions: (1) Physical Functioning and Symptoms, which include three scales under physical function (physical, social, and psychological) and (2) five scales within symptoms (pain, weakness, tingling and numbness, and stiffness). The questionnaire items focus on the upper-extremity activities and are intended to assess disability. The DASH questionnaire can be self-, interview-, or telephone-administered.

Assessment for construct validity of DASH revealed significant correlation with BCTQ score [55] as well as the Patient Evaluation Measure score both before and after carpal tunnel decompression surgery [48]. In concordance, significantly improved scores have been reported for both DASH domains at 3 months [56] and at 6 months follow-up post-CT decompression surgery [57]. In another study, which included 40 patients undergoing carpal tunnel decompression surgery, Gay et al. [32] found DASH to have greater responsiveness than the Short Form Health Survey 36 (SF-36) but not BCTQ. In another study, Kotsis et al. [43] reported moderate responsiveness for DASH after carpal tunnel release surgery. However, two dimensions of the Michigan Hand Outcome questionnaire (Pain and Satisfactions) were found to be more responsive than the DASH. In contrast, Heebner and Roddey [58], in a randomized controlled trial of CTS patients, recorded that the DASH was not able to detect any significant changes between the standard treatment group and the intervention group. However, this could be as a result of the effectiveness of the intervention, rather than the responsiveness of the DASH.

Patient Reported Outcome Measures and Quality of Care in Carpal Tunnel Syndrome Management

Patient-reported outcomes measures are a critical component of assessing whether the patients' health is improving in response to management provided by health care professionals. In contrast to standard process measures, which capture the clinician's productivity and adherence to the guidelines of recommended care, or patient experience measures, which focus on the patients' journey and aspects of care delivery, PROMs attempt to capture whether the services provided actually improved patients' health and sense of well-being. Figure 13.1 shows aspects where PROMs can play a role in the management of CTS patients. This includes:

PROMs as Predictors of CTS Underlying Pathology

The diagnosis of CTS is based primarily on clinical manifestations elicited on both taking history and physical examination. The commonest symptom is paresthesia in the median nerve distribution (mainly lateral fingers of the hand). Other symptoms include clumsiness and weakness in the affected hand, which tend to get worse with activity. However, symptoms may vary according to the underlying pathology. Proximal radiation of pain or paresthesia to the elbow usually indicates tenosynovitis of the flexors of the hand (Fig. 13.2). This usually occurs in combination with worsening of pain and paresthesia at night, which may wake up the patient from sleep. These symptoms reflect the state of engorgement and relative venostasis in the small blood vessels within the flexor tendons synovial sheath, producing swelling, and further compression on the nerve within the tunnel (Fig. 13.3) [1, 21]. Active movement of the fingers and wrist or shaking the hands decreases venous engorgement and relieves pain, a phenomenon commonly reported in several

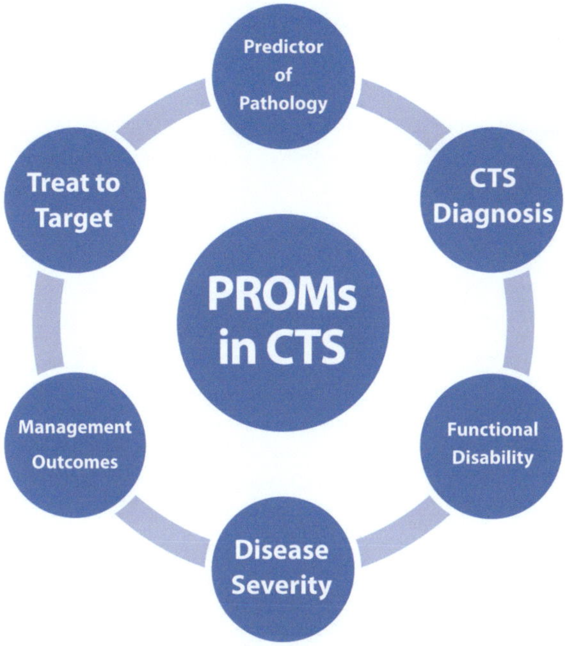

Fig. 13.1 Role of PROMs in the quality of care provided to carpal tunnel syndrome patients

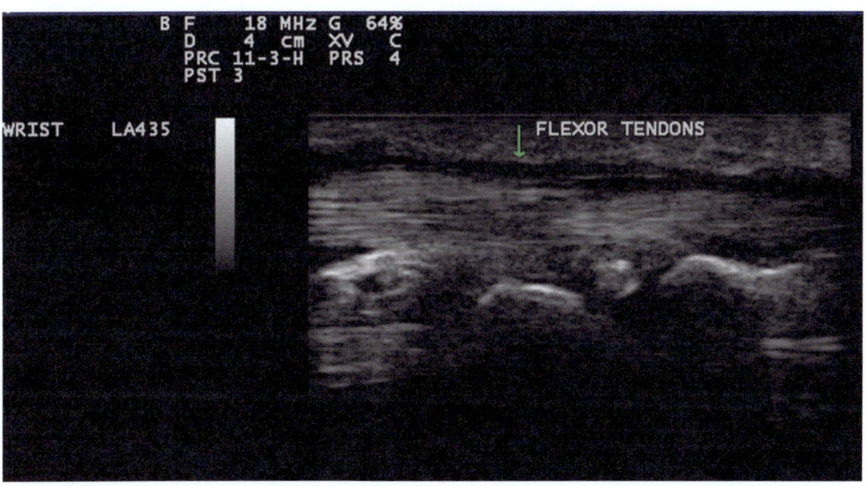

Fig. 13.2 Grayscale ultrasound using Esaote Mylab 25 system. Palmar longitudinal view at the proximal inlet of the carpal tunnel showing tenosynovitis flexors of the hand (US)

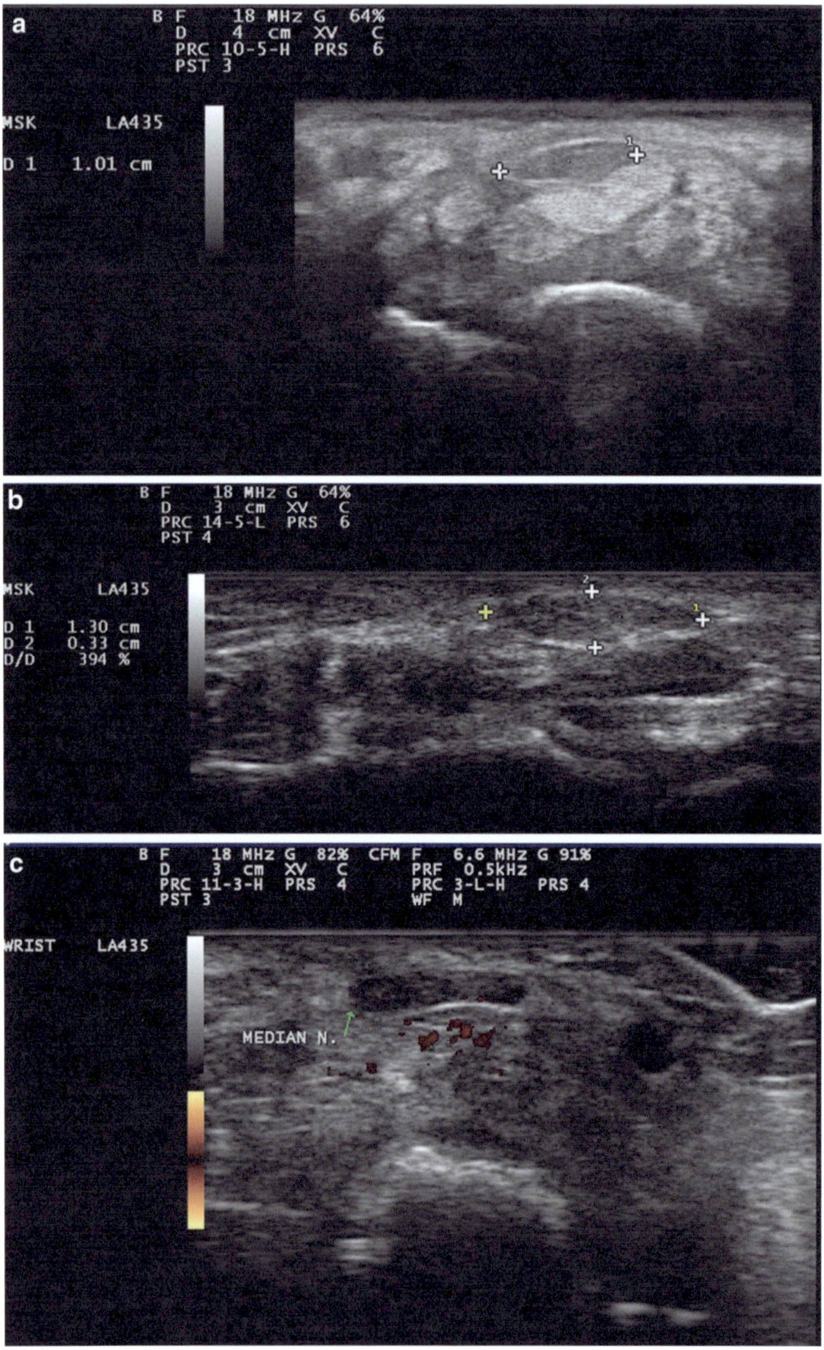

Fig. 13.3 Grayscale ultrasound using Esaote Mylab 25 system. Palmer transverse view at the proximal inlet of the carpal tunnel, showing (*highlighted* by the cursors): (**a**) Normal elliptical median nerve. (**b**) Median nerve swelling manifested by increased median nerve cross section area. (**c**) Flattening of the median nerve, which appears in late stages of median nerve compression. MN: median nerve; Flex Tendons: Flexor tendons

patients' histories. It is an interesting theory that emphasizes the vascular etiology of the disorder. Alternatively, it may be that patients hold their wrists flexed while sleeping, thus increasing the pressure on the median nerve and causing pain. Therefore, preventing wrist flexion would be expected to decrease symptoms, and may be why many patients find it beneficial to wear neutral-position wrist splints at night. Alternatively, in patients who do not have significant inflammatory changes within the carpal tunnel, thenar muscle atrophy or significant sensory impairment, which reflect an advanced CTS state of long-standing duration, tend to develop without any nocturnal symptoms. This usually occurs in older adults [59].

Considering the patients' symptoms and the possible underlying pathology, sounds attractive to the treating doctors when the appropriate treatment approach is set. Questionnaires helping to diagnose the condition as well as the possible predisposing factors in one go would be the most preferred in standard clinical practice. Questionnaires such as the BCTQ, CTS-6 items, and CTS-PROMs would be of help in this aspect. The outcome of these questionnaires had shown significant correlations when setting up the treatment algorithm for the patient. Outcomes of the CTS-PROMs Severity Scale study [51] revealed that relative severity assessment helped to identify the attributable risk factors, e.g., tendonitis. There was positive significant association between repetitive stress pain and diurnal pain. Similarly, there was a positive significant association between paresthesia and nocturnal pain.

PROMs and CTS Diagnosis

Several attempts have been made at formalizing diagnostic criteria for CTS, yet there has not been a clear-cut consensus on the best diagnostic criteria for the syndrome. In view of this and in an attempt to find an alternative diagnostic tool, mathematical approaches based upon the degree of association between clinical features and diagnosis have been suggested. In this approach for any clinical feature, which is either present or absent, the association with the diagnosis can be expressed as sensitivity and specificity, or positive and negative predictive values. Several diagnostic tools have been assessed, some of them Web-based aiming at screening people and the others are used for diagnostic purposes. An example is the questionnaire developed by Kamath and Stothard [49], which is a scored clinical questionnaire for the initial assessment of patients presenting with CTS symptoms. The questionnaire was proposed to replace nerve conduction studies, and was validated in secondary care for the diagnosis of CTS. A score of 5 or more was recommended for use as a diagnostic screening tool to replace nerve conduction studies, whereas a score of 3 or more has been submitted to analysis in comparison to nerve conduction studies. The CTS-6 is another diagnostic scale for carpal tunnel syndrome, suggested to estimate the likelihood that carpal tunnel syndrome is present. A total score of 12 or more suggests a strong probability (80 % chance) that the patient has carpal tunnel syndrome. A total score less than 5 indicates a very small chance (25 %) that the patient has carpal tunnel syndrome. Comparing the results of the CTS-6 test with the results of the nerve conduction velocity test, the authors reported the added information from the electrodiagnostic test was not enough to change the diagnosis. Furthermore, the authors concluded that there was not much value added by the electrodiagnostic test—not enough to support the cost and discomfort to the patient [60].

PROMs for Assessment of Functional Disability in CTS Patients

Traditionally, outcome assessment in hand therapy tended to focus on measures of range of motion, strength, and sensation. However, in the last decade the focus has shifted toward a patient-centered approach assessing health at the activity and participation levels [61, 62]. Specific patient-completed questionnaires were reported to be the most efficient way of collecting information on progress of cases or outcome of management, for routine use, in cases such as inflammatory arthritis or CTS [63, 64]. Reviewing the literature for assessment tools for functional ability in CTS patients revealed two main questionnaire categories:

1. SF-36 and the Nottingham Health Profile, which are generic tools assessing the patient's whole state.
2. BCTQ and the modified-BCTQ, which are tools designed specific for CTS patients.

Questionnaire such as DASH (Disabilities of the Arm, Shoulder and Hand) is considered as discrete. A systematic review of the psychometric properties of the BCTQ [35] revealed that the two sub-scales of the questionnaire, namely severity of symptoms and functional status, are considered the most important reasons for seeking treatment. The analysis of the relationship between patient satisfaction with the overall results of surgery and the BCTQ Functional Status Scales showed significant correlation with worse scores for functional ability in patients with lower degree of satisfaction. Katz et al. [37] compared satisfaction with change in both BCTQ functional status and symptom severity scores, perceived improvement in quality of life, and perceived improvement in symptoms severity between recipients and non-recipients of workers' compensation. As hypothesized, there was evidence of a difference between the two groups of patients for the BCTQ Functional Status Scale and the Symptom Severity Scale. The modified BCTQ [41] include items relevant to specific groups, such as workers prone to repetitive stress injury. In addition to being reliable and valid instrument, it was reported also relevant to the patients' current functional status and work abilities.

PROMs for Assessment of Disease Severity

Anything that compromises the space available for the median nerve within the carpal tunnel can induce CTS symptoms. Focal structural changes or swellings at the wrist are known predisposing factors, including fracture of distal radius, hemorrhage and swelling secondary to blunt trauma, and swellings such as ganglion cysts or lipomas. However, the commonest cause in recent years has been identified as inflammatory changes in the hand's flexors muscle tendon sheath, attributed to the expanding use of electronic gadgets such as mobile phones, tablets, and computers. In addition, a wide variety of metabolic diseases, systemic illnesses, and aberrant anatomic structures also have been described as causes of CTS.

However, the patients' symptoms and disease severity remain the same and can be linked to the pathophysiologic changes occurring in the median nerve in response to compression [65, 66]. The initial impact is reduction in the epineural blood flow, which occurs at 20–30 mmHg compression. In CTS patients, the least intracarpal canal pressure recorded was 33 mmHg and with wrist extension it can go up to 110 mmHg [67]. Persistent or increased pressure ultimately causes edema in the epineurium as well as endoneurium. If pressure of 50 mmHg has been applied for 2 h, it will cause epineural edema, and if applied for 8 h, it will lead to increase in peri-neural congestion (Fig. 13.4) and consequently increase in endoneural fluid pressure up to fourfold, which eventually will block axonal transport [37]. As further injury occurs to the capillary endothelium, more protein leaks out into the tissues, which gets more edematous, and a vicious cycle starts. The effects are most pronounced within the endoneurium, since more exudate and edema accumulate there, being unable to diffuse across the perineurium. The perineurium resists pressure changes because of its higher tensile strength and acts as a diffusion barrier creating in effect a "compartment syndrome" within the nerve [68]. These pathophysiologic changes mirror the patient's symptoms severity as well as neurological findings that range from tingling, numbness, and pain, down to loss of sensation.

As it is difficult to assign severity on the basis of the symptoms, questionnaires offered a way to calibrate the severity of CTS. The BCTQ Severity Scale is the most common tool used to assess the global severity. A systematic review [16] of the Boston CTS questionnaire revealed moderate correlations reported with measures of symptom severity as well as post-management relief, generic measures of health status, quality of life, and satisfaction [69, 70]. The CTS-PROMs severity scale is the only questionnaire to raise the relative severity measure for each domain assessed. Attaining a high relative score (>1) indicates that this symptom was prominent relative to the other symptoms. This should be taken into consideration on assessment of the possible underlying pathology or setting up the treatment plan.

PROMs and Management Outcomes

Treatment options available for CTS patients include either conservative or surgical interventions. However, it is not known which patients are more likely to benefit from what treatment. Also the rate to what extent the patient has improved is also important, not only as quantity but also as a quality measure. In view of the absence of the "gold standard" to diagnose or monitor CTS patients, patient reported

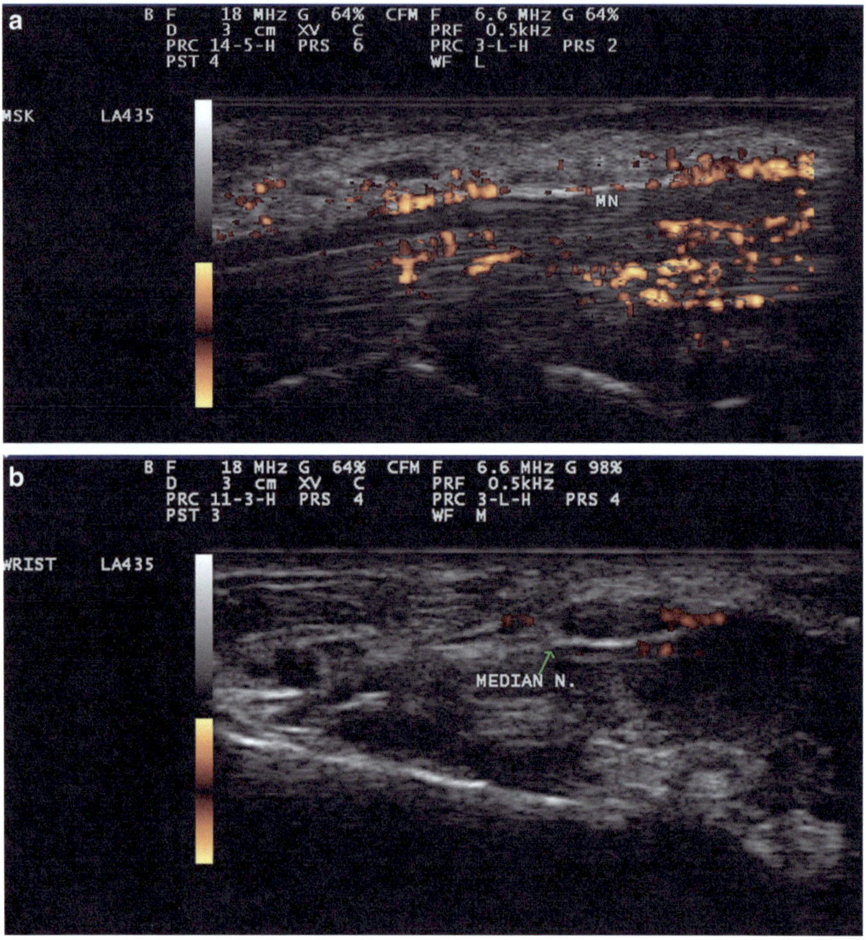

Fig. 13.4 Power Doppler ultrasound scan of the wrist in a patient presenting with carpal tunnel syndrome symptoms using Esaote Mylab 25 system. (**a**) Palmar longitudinal view at the proximal inlet of the carpal tunnel showing perineurial enhanced vascularity of the median nerve. (**b**) Palmar transverse view at the proximal inlet of the carpal tunnel showing perineurial enhanced vascularity of the median nerve secondary to tenosynovitis

outcome measures booked its place as the best tool for this task. Using a responsive outcome measure will facilitate the detection of moderate treatment effects in both standard clinical practice and clinical research. Furthermore, the results of a recent systematic review of surgical and non-surgical CTS treatments highlighted the need to focus on "prognostic studies" that lead to better patient characterization and the identification of predictive factors indicating likely response to specific treatments [71]. This gave clues for other studies to be carried out to assess PROMs as a predictor of management outcome. A study carried out by Kaye and Reynolds [24] to assess the ability of self-reported measures to predict treatment response in CTS patients revealed that the patients who had higher self-reported symptom severity scores at initial evaluation, as assessed by BCTQ, were significantly more likely to fail conservative treatment and undergo surgery during the next 2-year period. Therefore, the symptom severity questionnaire was reported as useful not only in evaluating response to therapy but also in predicting response to therapy. In another systematic review [26], responsiveness of the BCTQ to clinical change was assessed. The data on effect sizes and standard response means demonstrated that the Symptom Severity Scale and Functional Status Scales were able to detect clinically meaningful change resulting from the CTS treatment and yielded large effect sizes over a 6-month interval.

One study [52] was carried out to assess the ability of CTS-PROMs Severity Scoring System to identify outcome response (symptoms severity as well as functional status) in response to management in patients presenting with carpal tunnel syndrome. Response to therapy (CTS-response) was considered if there has been an improvement achieved by >20 % of the following: (1) score of paresthesia as well as scores of two out of the four domains (nocturnal pain, diurnal pain, weakness, and repetitive stress pain), in addition to (2) >20 % improvement of the functional status score (CTS-response 20). To evaluate sensitivity to change in clinical status, each patient was assigned to one of the following groups: <20 % improvement in the CTS-response, 20–49 % improvement, 50–69 % improvement, and >70 % improvement. Results revealed that the definitions of improvement were valid and were significantly correlated with changes in NCS and/or US findings. In addition, they have the advantage of quantifying the outcome measures. The GSS showed significant sensitivity to change after 1, 3, and 6 months and was significantly correlated with the nerve conduction studies and ultrasound findings (standardized effect size was 2.12, 2.41, and 2.47 after 1, 3, and 6, months, respectively).

PROMs and Treat-to-Target in Carpal Tunnel Syndrome

Searching for markers identifying key targets for the valuation of major outcomes in musculoskeletal diseases has become one of the hot issues in rheumatology. Possible markers should be objectively measured, indicatory of normal biology as well as the pathologic process, indicator of response to therapy and prognosis. It should also be a good indicator of modification of the pathological process and help to identify (in early cases) the patients who are going to respond quickly to therapy with the vision of tailoring the management to the individual patient's status [72, 73]. So far this target has not been achieved in CTS. Earlier study revealed that CTS management can be tailored to the patient underlying pathology [74]. Another recent study [21], carried out to assess the use of US as a biomarker for a treat-to-target approach in CTS patients, was set up based on the analysis of the baseline parameters in association with the clinical as well as patient-reported management outcomes, and relied on improvement of the patient reported outcome measures as a primary end point. A multidimensional model of predictors was implemented including patient-reported management outcomes, severity of symptoms, functional disability, as well as patients' satisfaction. Results of this work showed that the patient reported outcome measures, which represent the key indicators of successful management approach from the patient's point of view, were sensitive to change and correlated significantly to changes in the US outcome measures starting from the first week after treatment. Underlying pathology such as tenosynovitis of the flexors of the hands was in favor of conservative management with successful outcomes, whereas good postsurgical outcomes were reported in other conditions such as metabolic disorders and focal swellings.

Which Questionnaire to Use

Several studies were carried out to compare the variable questionnaires on their capacity to assess the CTS patients' subjective symptoms. Most of the published research revealed that BCTQ had the best characteristics as an assessment tool for function as well as symptoms. In comparison to generic questionnaires, BCTQ had significantly better sensitivity and specificity ratios. The modified BCTQ was published recently addressing some domains, closely linked to the condition pathogenesis, which were not present when the original questionnaire was developed. A possible alternative to the BCTQ is the CTS-PROMs questionnaire, which offers a symptom scale for the diagnosis as well as a severity scale to assess the severity of the condition and to monitor response to therapy. It has been utilized in CTS patients treated conservatively as well as those undergoing carpal tunnel surgery and has proven to be reliable, valid, and responsive. The option of Carpal Tunnel Response "CTS-response 20/70/90" represents a forward move in the calibration of the treatment outcomes.

The DASH questionnaire (Disability Arm Shoulder and Hand questionnaire) can be categorized as a "discrete or district questionnaire." This classification was considered as it assesses only one bodily district of the body (upper limb); therefore, it represents a midway between specific and generic questionnaires. In contrast, SF-36 in CTS received initially a lot of attention, in particular toward the analysis of this tool in orthopedics (which applies to CTS too). However, its limitations were highlighted in some research studies [75–78]. Another study revealed its poor efficacy as well as inconsistent responsiveness in CTS. This gave SF-36 a secondary role in CTS assessment [79].

Conclusion

CTS is the most well-known and frequent form of median nerve entrapment, and accounts for 90 % of all entrapment neuropathies. Patient reported outcome measures play an important role in the diagnosis, assessment of disease severity, as well as in monitoring the response to management. Several questionnaires are available, with a general good validity, reliability, as well as responsiveness. Implementation in standard daily practice is highly recommended not only to assess the patients clinically, but also to set up a treatment plan tailored to the patient's condition.

Acknowledgement Special thanks to Dr. Kirstin Weyrich, Consultant Neurologist, Darent Valley Hospital, Kent, England, for peer reviewing this chapter.

Appendix 1: Modified Boston Carpal Tunnel Questionnaire

On a typical day during the past 2 weeks, have the hand or wrist symptoms caused you to have difficulty doing any of the activities listed below? Please circle one number that best describes your ability to do the activity.

Activity	No difficulty	Mild difficulty	Moderate	Severe	Can not do it	Not applicable
Writing	1	2	3	4	5	
Buttoning of clothes	1	2	3	4	5	
Holding a book while reading	1	2	3	4	5	
Gripping a telephone receiver	1	2	3	4	5	
Opening of jars	1	2	3	4	5	
Household chores	1	2	3	4	5	
Carrying of grocery bags	1	2	3	4	5	
Bathing and Dressing	1	2	3	4	5	
Computer/Typing	1	2	3	4	5	
Driving	1	2	3	4	5	

El Miedany et al. Arthritis Rheumatism 2006; 54(9): S650

Appendix 2: Carpal Tunnel PROMs diagnosis questionnaire

Carpal Tunnel PROMs Questionnaire - Diagnosis

Please tick the most appropriate box that best describes your case

Symptom	Question	Rt. Hand	Lt. Hand
Paraesthesia	Do you have tingling/numbness (loss of sensation) in your hand/ thumb, index or middle fingers?	Yes: ☐ ☐ No: ☐ ☐	Yes: ☐ ☐ No: ☐ ☐
	Do you have tingling/numbness (loss of sensation) in your hand/thumb, index or middle fingers?	Yes: ☐ ☐ No: ☐ ☐	Yes: ☐ ☐ No: ☐ ☐
	Do your numbness/tingling get better on shaking your hands?	Yes: ☐ ☐ No: ☐ ☐	Yes: ☐ ☐ No: ☐ ☐
Nocturnal Pain	Do you feel numbness (loss of sensation) or tingling in your hand at night?	Yes: ☐ ☐ No: ☐☐	Yes: ☐ ☐ No: ☐ ☐
	Does your hand numbness or tingling wake you up from sleep during night?	Yes: ☐☐ No: ☐☐	Yes: ☐ ☐ No: ☐ ☐
Diurnal Pain	Do you feel tingling/numbness in your hand when you wake up in the morning?	Yes: ☐☐ No: ☐	Yes: ☐ ☐ No: ☐
	Does your hand tingling/numbness get worse during day time?	Yes: ☐ ☐ No: ☐ ☐	Yes: ☐ ☐ No: ☐ ☐
Weakness	Do you have weakness in your hand or wrist?	Yes: ☐ ☐ No: ☐ ☐	Yes: ☐ ☐ No: ☐ ☐
RSI	Does your affected hand(s) or forearm feel fatty or swollen?	Yes: ☐ ☐ No: ☐☐	Yes: ☐ ☐ No: ☐ ☐
	Do your symptoms get worse with driving, typing, or grasping and use of small objects such as keys/pens?	Yes: ☐☐ No: ☐ ☐	Yes: ☐ ☐ No: ☐ ☐
	Do you feel your hand pain radiates up to your forearm?	Yes: ☐ ☐ No: ☐	Yes: ☐ ☐ No: ☐ ☐

El Miedany et al. Ann Rheum Dis 2006; 65 (SII): 259

Appendix 3: Carpal Tunnel Severity Index

Carpal Tunnel Severity Index

Please put a no. from 0 to 10 that best describes the severity of your symptoms over the past week

How severe is the numbness (loss of sensation) or tingling you feel in your hand / finger(s)?

Lt. Hand | None ... Severe | Rt. Hand

0.5 2.5 1.5 3.5 4.5 5.5 6.5 7.5 8.5 9.5

0 1 2 3 4 5 6 7 8 9 10

How often does your hand numbness (loss of sensation) or tingling wake you up during a typical night in the past week?

Lt. Hand | Not at all ... Often | Rt. Hand

0.5 2.5 1.5 3.5 4.5 5.5 6.5 7.5 8.5 9.5

0 1 2 3 4 5 6 7 8 9 10

How often do you have numbness or tingling in your hands during the daytime?

Lt. Hand | Never ... Often | Rt. Hand

0.5 2.5 1.5 3.5 4.5 5.5 6.5 7.5 8.5 9.5

0 1 2 3 4 5 6 7 8 9 10

How would you rate the weakness you feel in your hand(s)?

Lt. Hand | No weakness ... Severe weakness | Rt. Hand

0.5 2.5 1.5 3.5 4.5 5.5 6.5 7.5 8.5 9.5

0 1 2 3 4 5 6 7 8 9 10

How would you rate the pain you feel in your hand/wrist or forearm when you grasp or use a small object?

Lt. Hand | No pain ... Severe pain | Rt. Hand

0.5 2.5 1.5 3.5 4.5 5.5 6.5 7.5 8.5 9.5

0 1 2 3 4 5 6 7 8 9 10

In general, How would you rate the functional impairment you got because of your hand symptoms over the past week?

References

1. Phalen GS. The carpal-tunnel syndrome: seventeen years' experience in diagnosis and treatment of six hundred fifty-four hands. J Bone Joint Surg Am. 1966;48:211–28.
2. de Krom MC, Knipschild PG, Kester AD, Thijs CT, Boekkooi PF, Spaans F. Carpal tunnel syndrome: prevalence in the general population. J Clin Epidemiol. 1992;45:373–6.
3. Atroshi I, Gummesson C, Johnsson R, Ornstein E, Ranstam J, Rosen I. Prevalence of carpal tunnel syndrome in a general population. JAMA. 1999;282:153–8.
4. Aroori S, Spence RA. Carpal tunnel syndrome. Ulster Med J. 2008;77:6–17.
5. Mohammadi A, Afshar A, Etemadi A, Masoudi S, Baghizadeh A. Diagnostic value of cross-sectional area of median nerve in grading severity of carpal tunnel syndrome. Arch Iran Med. 2010;13:516–21.
6. El Miedany Y, Aty S, Ashour S. Ultrasonography versus nerve conduction study in patients with carpal tunnel syndrome: substantive or complementary tests? Rheumatology (Oxford). 2004;43:887–95.
7. Mackinnon SE. Pathophysiology of nerve compression. Hand Clin. 2002;18(2):231–41.
8. El Miedany Y. US in carpal tunnel syndrome. In: El Miedany Y, editor. US in rheumatic diseases. Switzerland: Springer publisher; 2015.
9. Keith M, Mascar V, Chung K. et al. Clinical practice guidelines on the diagnosis of carpal tunnel syndrome. 2007. http://www.aaos.org/research/guidelines/CTS_guideline.pdf. Accessed 3 July 2015.
10. Palmer D, El Miedany Y. PROMs: a novel approach to arthritis self-management. Br J Nurs. 2012;21(10):601–7.
11. American Academy of Neurology. Practice parameter for carpal tunnel syndrome (summary statement). Neurology. 1993;43(11):2406–9.
12. Jablecki CK, Andary MT, Floeter MK, Miller RG, Quartly CA, Vennix MJ, Wilson JR, American Association of Electrodiagnostic Medicine, American Academy of Neurology, American Academy of Physical Medicine and Rehabilitation. Practice parameter: electrodiagnostic studies in carpal tunnel syndrome. Report of the American Association of Electrodiagnostic Medicine, American Academy of Neurology, and the American Academy of Physical Medicine and Rehabilitation. Neurology. 2002;58:1589–92.
13. Salerno DF, Franzblau A, Werner RA, et al. Reliability of physical examination of the upper extremity among keyboard operators. Am J Ind Med. 2000;37:423–30.
14. Kuhlman KA, Hennessey WJ. Sensitivity and specificity of carpal tunnel syndrome signs. Am J Phys Med Rehabil. 1997;76:451–7.
15. Mondelli M, Passero S, Giannini F. Provocative tests in different stages of carpal tunnel syndrome. Clin Neurol Neurosurg. 2001;103:178–83.
16. El Miedany Y, Ashour S, Youssef S, Mehanna A, Meky F. Clinical diagnosis of carpal tunnel syndrome: old tests–new concepts. Joint Bone Spine. 2008;75:451–7.
17. Jordan R, Carter T, Cummins C. A systematic review of the utility of electrodiagnostic testing in carpal tunnel syndrome. Br J Gen Pract. 2002;52:670–3.
18. Strickland JW, Gozani SN. Accuracy of in-office nerve conduction studies for median neuropathy: a meta-analysis. J Hand Surg Am. 2011;36:52–60.
19. El Miedany Y, Ashour S, Youssef S, Mehanna A, et al. Sensitivity to change of the carpal tunnel syndrome global severity scoring index. A prospective study. Rheumatology (Oxford). 2007;46 Suppl 1:i142.
20. Evans K, Roll S, Volz K, Freimer M. Relationship between intraneural vascular flow measured with sonography and carpal tunnel syndrome diagnosis based on electrodiagnostic testing. Ultrasound Med. 2012;31:729–36.
21. El Miedany Y, El Gaafary M, Youssef S, Ahmed I, Nasr A. Ultrasound assessment of the Median Nerve: a biomarker that can help in setting a Treat to Target approach tailored for Carpal Tunnel Syndrome patients. Springerplus. 2015;4:13. doi:10.1186/s40064-014-0779-4.
22. Amadio PC. Outcomes measurements. J Bone Joint Surg Am. 1993;75:1583–4.

23. Katz JN, Gelberman RH, Wright EA, Lew RA, Liang MH. Responsiveness of self-reported and objective measures of disease severity in carpal tunnel syndrome. Med Care. 1994;32:1127–33.
24. Kaye J, Reynolds J. Carpal Tunnel Syndrome: Using self-report measures of disease to predict treatment response. Am J Orthop. 2007;36(4):E59–62.
25. Singh JA, Solomon DH, Dougados M, et al. Development of classification and response criteria for rheumatic diseases. Arthritis Rheum. 2006;55:348–52.
26. Gerritsen AA, de Vet HC, Scholten RJ, van Tulder MW, Bouter LM. Enabling meta-analysis in systematic reviews on carpal tunnel syndrome. J Hand Surg. 2002;27A(5):828–32.
27. Scholten RJ, Gerritsen AA, Uitdehaag BM, van Geldere D, de Vet HC, Bouter LM. Surgical treatment options for carpal tunnel syndrome. Cochrane Database Syst Rev. 2004;4, CD003905.
28. O'Connor D, Marshall S, Massy-Westropp N. Non-surgical treatment (other than steroid injection) for carpal tunnel syndrome. Cochrane Database Syst Rev. 2003;1, CD003219.
29. Ware JE, Sherbourne CD. The MOS 36-item short-form health survey (SF-36). Med Care. 1992;30(6):473–83.
30. Hunt SM, McKenna SP, McEwen J, Williams J, Papp E. The Nottingham health profile: Subjective health status and medical consultations. Soc Sci Med A. 1981;15(3):221–9.
31. Levine DW, Simmons BP, Koris MJ, et al. A self-administered questionnaire for the assessment of severity of symptoms and functional status in carpal tunnel syndrome. J Bone Joint Surg Am. 1993;75:1585–92.
32. Jarvik JG, Comstock BA, Heagerty PJ, et al. Magnetic resonance imaging compared with electrodiagnostic studies in patients with suspected carpal tunnel syndrome: predicting symptoms, function, and surgical benefit at 1 year. J Neurosurg. 2008;108:541–50.
33. Turner JA, Franklin G, Heagerty PJ, et al. The association between pain and disability. Pain. 2004;112(3):307–14.
34. Leite J, Jerosch-Herold C, Song F. A systematic review of the psychometric properties of the Boston Carpal Tunnel Questionnaire. BMC Musculoskelet Disord. 2006;7:78. doi:10.1186/1471-2474-7-78.
35. Guyette TM, Wilgis EF. Timing of improvement after carpal tunnel release. J Surg Orthop Adv. 2004;13:206–9.
36. Katz JN, Punnett L, Simmons BP, Fossel AH, Mooney N, Keller RB. Workers' compensation recipients with carpal tunnel syndrome: the validity of self-reported health measures. Am J Public Health. 1996;86:52–6.
37. Atroshi I, Lyrén P, Ornstein E, Gummesson C. The Six-item CTS symptoms scale and palmar pain scale in carpal tunnel syndrome. J Hand Surg. 2011;36A:788–94.
38. Atroshi I, Lyren PE, Gummesson C. The 6-item CTS symptoms scale: a brief outcomes measure for carpal tunnel syndrome. Qual Life Res. 2009;18:347–58.
39. El Miedany Y, Ashour S, Youssef S, Mehanna A, El Gaafary M. Validation of the modified self-administered questionnaire for assessment of functional status in patients with carpal tunnel syndrome. Arthritis Rheum. 2006;54(9):S650.
40. Chung KC, Pillsbury MS, Walters MR, Hayward RA. Reliability and validity testing of the Michigan Hand Outcomes Questionnaire. J Hand Surg. 1998;23:575–87.
41. Shauver MJ, Chung KC. The minimal clinically important difference of the Michigan hand outcomes questionnaire. J Hand Surg Am. 2009;34:509–14.
42. Kotsis SV, Chung KC. Responsiveness of the Michigan Hand Outcomes Questionnaire and the Disabilities of the Arm, Shoulder and Hand questionnaire in carpal tunnel surgery. J Hand-Surg. 2005;30:81–6.
43. Craw JR, Church DJ, Hutchison RL. Prospective comparison of the six-item carpal tunnel symptoms scale and portable nerve conduction testing in measuring the outcomes of treatment of carpal tunnel syndrome with steroid injection. Hand. 2015;10(1):49–53.
44. Atroshi I, Lyrén P, Ornstein E, Gummesson C. The Six-item CTS symptoms scale and palmar pain scale in carpal tunnel syndrome. J Hand Surg Am. 2011;36(5):788–94.

45. Macey AC, Burke FD. Outcomes of hand surgery. J Hand Surg. 1995;20-B:841–55.
46. Forward DP, Singh AK, Lawrence TM, Sithole JS, Davis TR, Oni JA. Preservation of the ulnar bursa within the carpal tunnel: does it improve the outcome of carpal tunnel surgery? A randomized, controlled trial. J Bone Joint Surg Am. 2006;88:2432–8.
47. Hobby JL, Venkatesh R, Motkur P. The effect of psychological disturbance on symptoms, self-reported disability and surgical outcome in carpal tunnel syndrome. J Bone Joint Surg. 2005;87B:196–200.
48. Kamath V, Stothard J. A clinical questionnaire for the diagnosis of carpal tunnel syndrome. J Hand Surg Br. 2003;28(5):455–9.
49. El Miedany Y, Ashor S, Youssef S. Development and validation of a new self-administered questionnaire for clinical diagnosis of carpal tunnel syndrome. Ann Rheum Dis. 2006;65(SII):259. abstract 476.
50. El M, Ashor S, Youssef S, El Gaafary M. A new self-administered questionnaire for global assessment of symptoms severity and functional status of patients with carpal tunnel syndrome. Ann Rheum Dis. 2006;65(SII):259. abstract 475.
51. El Miedany Y, Ashor S, Youssef S, Mehanna A, El Gaafary M. Sensitivity to change of the carpal tunnel syndrome global severity scoring system: a prospective study. Rheumatology (Oxford). 2007;46(S1):i123.
52. El M, Ashor S, Youssef S, El Gaafary M. Diagnosis of carpal tunnel syndrome: how far can we rely on clinical assessment. Arthritis Rheum. 2006;54(9):S651.
53. Hudak PL, Amadio PC, Bombardier C. Development of an upper extremity outcome measure: the DASH (disabilities of the arm, shoulder and hand) [corrected]. The Upper Extremity Collaborative Group (UECG). Am J Ind Med. 1996;29:602–8.
54. Beaton DE, Katz JN, Fossel AH, Wright JG, Tarasuk V, Bombardier CH. Measuring the whole or the parts? Validity, reliability, and responsiveness of the Disabilities of the Arm, Shoulder and Hand outcome measure in different regions of the upper extremity. J Hand Ther. 2001;14:128–46.
55. Appleby MA, Neville-Smith M, Parrott MW. Functional outcomes post carpal tunnel release: a modified replication of a previous study. J Hand Ther. 2009;22:240–8.
56. Kadzielski J, Malhotra LR, Zurakowski D, Lee SG, Jupiter JB, Ring D. Evaluation of preoperative expectations and patient satisfaction after carpal tunnel release. J Hand Surg Am. 2008;33:1783–8.
57. Gay RE, Amadio PC, Johnson JC. Comparative responsiveness of the Disabilities of the Arm, Shoulder, and Hand; the Carpal Tunnel Questionnaire; and the SF-36 to clinical change after carpal tunnel release. J Hand Surg. 2003;28:250–4.
58. Heebner ML, Roddey TS. The effects of neural mobilization in addition to standard care in persons with carpal tunnel syndrome from a community hospital. J Hand Ther. 2008;21:229–40.
59. Phalen GS. The carpal-tunnel syndrome. clinical evaluation of 598 hands. Clin Orthop. 1972;83:29–40.
60. Graham B. The value added by electrodiagnostic testing in the diagnosis of carpal tunnel syndrome. J Bone Joint Surg. 2008;90A(12):2587–93.
61. Chan J, Spencer J. Adaptation to hand injury: an evolving experience. Am J Occup Ther. 2004;58:128–39.
62. Keller RB, Rudicel SA, Liang MH. Outcomes research in orthopaedics. Instr Course Lect. 1994;43:599–611.
63. El M. Adopting Patient Centered Care in standard practice: PROMs moving toward disease specific era. Clin Exp Rheumatol. 2014;32(5 Suppl 85):S-40-6.
64. Miedany E. PROMs in inflammatory arthritis: moving from static to dynamic. Clin Rheumatol. 2013;32:735–42.
65. Gelberman RH, Rydevik BL, Pess GM, et al. Carpal tunnel syndrome: a scientific basis for clinical care. Orthop Clin North Am. 1988;19:115–24.
66. Sunderland S. The nerve lesion in the carpal tunnel syndrome. J Neurol Neurosurg Psychiatry. 1976;39:615–26.

67. Gelberman RH, Hergenroeder PT, Hargens AR, et al. The carpal tunnel syndrome: a study of carpal canal pressures. J Bone Joint Surg Am. 1981;63:380–4.
68. Lundborg G, Myers R, Powell H. Nerve compression injury and increased endoneurial fluid pressure a "miniature compartment syndrome.". J Neurol Neurosurg Psychiatry. 1983;46:1119–24.
69. Gay RE, Amadio PC, Johnson JC. Comparative responsiveness of the Disabilities of the Arm, Shoulder and Hand, the Carpal Tunnel Questionnaire and the SF-36 to clinical change after carpal tunnel release. J Hand Surg Am. 2003;28A:250–4.
70. Amadio PC, Silverstein MD, Ilstrup DM, Schleck CD, Jensen LM. Outcome assessment for carpal tunnel surgery: the relative responsiveness of generic, arthritis-specific, disease-specific, and physical examination measures. J Hand Surg. 1996;21A:338–46.
71. Shi Q, MacDermid JC. Is surgical intervention more effective than non-surgical treatment for carpal tunnel syndrome? A systematic review. J Orthop Surg Res. 2011;6:1–9.
72. Ferraccioli G, Alivernini S, Gremese E. Biomarkers of joint damage in rheumatoid arthritis: where Are We in 2013? J Rheumatol. 2013;40:1244–6.
73. Bessette L, Keller RB, Fossel AH, Mooney N, Katz JN. Patients' preferences and satisfaction following carpal tunnel release. J Hand Surg Am. 1997;22:613–20.
74. Katz JN, Gelberman RH, Wright EA, Abrahamsson S, Lew RA. A preliminary scoring system for assessing the outcome of carpal tunnel release. J Hand Surg Am. 1994;19:531–8.
75. El Miedany Y, El Gaafary M, Ahmed I, Mehanna A, Youssef S. Massage in carpal tunnel syndrome: a rational approach. J Rheumatol (Oxford). 2009;48 suppl 1:i94–5.
76. Busija L, Osborne R, Nilsdotter A, Buchbinder R, Roos E. Magnitude and meaningfulness of change in SF-36 scores in four types of orthopedic surgery. Health Qual Life Outcomes. 2008;6:55.
77. Vaile JH, Mathers DM, Ramos RC, Russell AS. Generic health instruments do not comprehensively capture patient perceived improvement in patients with carpal tunnel syndrome. J Rheumatol. 1999;26:1163–6.
78. Ettema AM, Amadio PC, Cha SS, Harrington JR, Harris AM, Offord KP. Surgery versus conservative therapy in carpal tunnel syndrome in people aged 70 years and older. Plast Reconstr Surg. 2006;118:947–58.
79. Jarvik JG, Comstock BA, Kliot M, et al. Surgery versus non-surgical therapy for carpal tunnel syndrome: a randomised parallel-group trial. Lancet. 2009;374:1074–81.

Chapter 14
PROMs for Polymyalgia Rheumatica

Isabel Castrejon

Introduction

Polymyalgia rheumatica (PMR) is a common inflammatory disease of elderly patients affecting from 0.1 to 0.5 % of the over-50-year-old population [1]. PMR is characterized by proximal pain, especially in the shoulder and pelvic girdle, and morning stiffness with high acute-phase reactants. Even though an elevation of acute-phase reactants may be not present, this does not necessarily indicate lesser severity or better prognosis [2]. The initial presentation may also mimic other rheumatic conditions—explaining the difficulty of diagnosis and a lack of agreement between physicians [3]. Because of the heterogeneity in the disease course and the lack of diagnostic laboratory test, physicians mainly rely on the clinical picture supported by a rapid response to glucocorticoids to make the diagnosis.

Glucocorticoids are the preferred treatment, leading to a rapid and dramatic improvement, but they may be required for several years in some patients [4]. PMR is a common indication for long-term steroid use in the community associated with serious adverse effects such as diabetes, osteoporosis, and infections [5].

A rapid resolution of symptoms after glucocorticoids is therefore a diagnostic hallmark, but there is no consensus on what constitutes an appropriate response and which outcomes should be monitored. The lack of reliable and sensitive measures to evaluate disease activity and the lack of standardized classification criteria to identify patients with PMR may explain the limited evidence for efficacy of any treatment different from glucocorticoids [6].

Current clinical guidelines recommend monitoring patients treated for PMR on the basis of symptoms since, as previously noted, conventional inflammatory

I. Castrejon, M.D., Ph.D. (✉)
Division of Rheumatology, Rush University Medical Center, Chicago, IL, USA
e-mail: isabelcastrejonf@gmail.com; isabel_castrejon@rush.edu

Y. El Miedany (ed.), *Patient Reported Outcome Measures in Rheumatic Diseases*,
DOI 10.1007/978-3-319-32851-5_14

markers can be misleading [6]. Reliable and comparable outcomes are required to balance the benefits and adverse events of long-term steroids therapy and to evaluate the use of corticosteroids sparing agents.

Patient reported outcomes (PROs), defined as outcomes that are completed by patients, have been increasingly recognized as important measures over the past few years. They incorporate the patient's perspective of the disease, capturing the impact of the disease in patients' lives, and they perform well in assessing disease activity in patients with PMR [7]. Different PROs, such as pain, morning stiffness, or physical function, have been proposed as recommended outcome measures to be used in practice and clinical trials [8]. In addition, most remission or flare definitions include at least one self-reported variable from the medical history [9].

This review summarizes the use of PROs in clinical trials of patients with PMR and the inclusion of PROs in diagnostic criteria or the evaluation of disease activity. In addition, data are presented concerning the performance of a multidimensional health assessment questionnaire (MDHAQ), only including PROs, to document improvement over time in patients with PMR seen in routine care.

Literature Review of PROs Used in Trials of PMR

A systematic review was performed in PubMed (up to April 2015) to obtain all published articles reporting any type of PROs in PMR [10]. Of 118 publications identified by the literature search, 20 met the selection criteria: 10 randomized controlled trials, 8 prospective cohorts, 1 case control study, and 1 pilot observational study. Patients included were typical for PMR populations, with a mean age between 62.5 and 76.6.

Pain was the most frequently reported domain, described as an outcome in the majority of the studies (90 %). Of these, 61 % used a visual analogue scale (VAS) to evaluate pain with no defined stem anchors, and the remainder used different grades or presence versus absence of pain. In some studies, pain was evaluated as an outcome to compare treatment groups [11–16], or to evaluate disease activity differences according to gender [17], or as a potential predictor of vertebral fractures [18].

Morning stiffness was recorded in 17 (85 %), with no consistency about how this was defined or collected. It was most frequently evaluated by morning stiffness duration in minutes without any grades (53 %); some studies graded morning stiffness from 0 to 3 or 4, and 2 studies only evaluated the presence or absence of morning stiffness. Function was only reported in 25 % of the studies, more frequently in cohorts than in randomized controlled trials (RCTs). The most frequent tool for this domain was the Health Assessment Questionnaire (HAQ) [19], and the modified HAQ (MHAQ), which is a modified shorter version of the original HAQ [20]. Both are self-reported questionnaires developed initially for rheumatoid arthritis (RA) that comprise eight categories of functioning including dressing, rising, eating, walking, self-hygiene, and other daily activities.

Other less frequently evaluated domains were patient global assessment (15 %), fatigue (15 %), and quality of life through a generic form, the Short-Form Health Survey (SF-36) (10 %) [21]. In addition, anxiety and depression were included in one of the studies aiming to evaluate outcomes of importance to patients without any specific information about how to measure these two domains [8].

In summary, pain on a visual analogue scale, morning stiffness in minutes, and physical function by HAQ were the three most frequently reported domains in published studies. Other domains such as patient global assessment, fatigue, quality of life, anxiety, and depression were infrequently reported in PMR studies, though they appear important from the patient's point of view [8].

PROs as Part of Diagnostic/Classification Criteria and to Assess Disease Activity

A variety of clinical diagnostic criteria sets have been proposed in the last years, but to date there has been no formal consensus in which one should be used in a regular basis. A comparison of the sensitivity of diagnostic criteria was performed in 2004, and the authors concluded that Bird 1979 and Hunder 1982 criteria should be used based on a higher sensitivity in the diagnosis of PMR [22]. More recently, classification criteria for PMR were proposed by a European League Against Rheumatism/American College of Rheumatology (EULAR/ACR) collaborative initiative [23]. These new classification criteria were proposed essentially to provide a basic framework for developing clinical trials of novel therapies. A summary of these diagnostic and classification criteria is presented in Table 14.1. There are two PROs that are included in most of these criteria: pain assessment and morning stiffness. The evaluation of pain has been included in each one of these criteria as pain/aching or tenderness in shoulder or pelvic girdle area, in shoulders, upper arm, hips or pelvis, and thighs. Pain is a very important and overwhelming symptom for patients with PMR. It is often not well localized to the joints but tended to be more responsive to medication in comparison to other symptoms such as morning stiffness [24]. In contrast, morning stiffness was included only in three of these criteria. Although morning stiffness is also considered an important diagnostic clue in PMR, it is difficult to evaluate and measure accurately. Duration of morning stiffness has been reported to show poor test–retest reliability in PMR [7], probably because of the fluctuation of this symptom during the day. From the patient's perspective, morning stiffness is defined as a restriction of movement, and patients, in general, experience this symptom as poorly responsive to treatment.

PROs have been also useful to define remission and relapse in PMR. In a recent review of relevant studies including definitions of PMR remission and relapse, two

Table 14.1 Included items and sensitivity of different diagnostic and classification criteria for polymyalgia rheumatica

	Bird/Wood criteria (1979)	Jones/Hazleman criteria (1981)	Hunder criteria (1982)	Nobunaga criteria (1989)	EULAR/ACR classification (2012)
Age	>65 years	–	>50 years	–	≥50 years
Duration onset	<2/52	>2/12	≥1 month	≥2 weeks	≥2 weeks
Pain/aching/tenderness	• Bilateral shoulder pain/stiffness	Shoulder/pelvic girdle pain	Bilateral: neck or torso; shoulders or upper arms; hips or thighs	Bilateral muscles pain in > 2: neck, shoulders, upper arm, hips/pelvis, thighs	Bilateral shoulder and/or pelvic girdle pain
	• Bilateral upper arm tenderness				Hip pain/limited range of motion (1 point)
Morning stiffness	>1 h	>1 h	–	–	>45 min (2 points)
ESR/CRP	>40 mm/h	>30 mm/h/> 6 μ(mu)g/mL	>40 mm/h	>40 mm/h	Elevated
Other	Depression and/or weight loss	–	–	–	Rapid corticosteroid response
Exclusion of other diagnosis	–	Absence of RA and muscle disease	Exclusion of other diagnoses	Normal myogenic enzymes	Absence of: RF/anti-CCP (2 points)
				No swelling hand joints	Peripheral joint pain (1 point)
Sensitivity	3 or more	All criteria	All criteria	All criteria	Score ≥ 4 points
	99.5 %	**84.9 %**	**93.3 %**	**67.8 %**	**68 %**

EULAR European League Against Rheumatism, *ACR* American College of Rheumatology, *RF* rheumatoid factor, *anti-CCP* anti-citrullinated protein antibody

PROs were identified as commonly included: assessment of patient's pain and morning stiffness [9]. Furthermore, using these clinical symptoms, pain and morning stiffness, was considered to be important by experts to define improvement or flare. Although including morning stiffness achieved the highest level of agreement (94.7 % to define remission and relapse), this group of experts previously questioned its value [25]. Additionally, many older patients with rheumatic conditions rarely consider themselves to be completely free from pain and stiffness, making the evaluation of remission more difficult in these patients. But other measures, as laboratory data, may have also exhibited some limitations to evaluate remission/flare. A relapse of PMR can occur with normal C-reactive protein (CRP) and/or erythrocyte sedimentation rate (ESR) and these acute phase reactants are not specific for PMR.

In 2003, the European Collaborating PMR group proposed the first response criteria for PMR based on a core set of 5 variables [26]. Pain on a VAS was selected as the central measure for disease activity, being the only one mandatory in this core set. The selection was based on the dominant role of pain in patients' symptoms and the proved sensitivity to change in pain on a VAS. Morning stiffness was also included in this response criteria core set with CRP, elevation of upper limbs, and the doctor's global assessment, but only a change in 3 of these 4 is required to reflect a change in disease activity. Having 2 PROs included in a set of only 5 variables for response highlights the importance of patient self-evaluation in PMR.

Based on the EULAR response criteria and in analogy with a simplified disease activity index (SDAI) for RA, a disease activity index for PMR has been proposed [27]. This composite index, the PMR activity score (PMR-AS), includes pain on a VAS and morning stiffness in minutes multiple by 0.1 to avoid a high weighting of this specific symptom. PMR-AS shows a high correlation not only with a patient's global assessment, but also with patient satisfaction.

In general, using a composite index helps describe the clinical situation better, adding feasibility. Furthermore, having a score as an absolute number helps in much more easily comparing patients. Composite indices may be useful also to establish disease activity categories, a crucial task to evaluate improvement/worsening or the presence of flares, which occur frequently during the course of PMR [28].

Patient Reported Outcome Measures to Evaluate Improvement in Patients with PMR in Routine Care

In consonance with the evaluation of disease activity in PMR through a composite index and to evaluate the performance of patient reported outcome measures (PROMs) to document improvement in clinical status, a study was conducted at Rush University Medical Center [29]. Quantitative assessment in rheumatic diseases is complicated by the absence of a single measure that can be applied to all individual patients with a specific diagnosis. Composite indices developed for a specific diagnosis are used widely in clinical trials and other clinical research, but appear impractical for usual care. Indeed, the only quantitative clinical data in the medical records of most patients seen by rheumatologists are laboratory tests, which, as we have previously seen, can be normal or not specific for a PMR flare.

Every patient, regardless of diagnosis, seen at this academic rheumatology center completes a multidimensional health assessment questionnaire (MDHAQ) (Appendix 1). The MDHAQ has been developed to provide quantitative data, rather than "gestalt" clinical impressions, in usual rheumatology care [30]. Although it was developed initially to assess disease status and changes over time in patients with RA, MDHAQ has been found informative in patients with other diagnoses [31]. The MDHAQ is a 2-page, single-sheet instrument, adapted from the standard Health Assessment Questionnaire (HAQ) to add information concerning a self-report joint count (including hips and shoulder, which are typically affected in PMR patients), review of symptoms, visual analogue scales for pain, patient global estimate, and fatigue, and also includes an evaluation of morning stiffness and demographic data. Laboratory data, mainly acute-phase reactants, and prednisone dose were retrospectively collected through chart review. PMR patients with complete data seen between 2010 and 2014 were included in this analysis and a baseline visit and the most recent visit were compared to evaluate improvement through PROs in comparison with prednisone doses and laboratory data. Thirty-four patients with PMR were analyzed. Patient characteristics were typical of PMR populations (59 % females and mean age 71.6 years). The mean duration from the baseline visit to a most recent visit was 15.5 months. At initial presentation, Routine Assessment of Patient Index Data 3 (RAPID3) was 12.2, FN 2.2, pain 5.3, and PATGL 4.7, fatigue 3.9, and morning stiffness 63.1 min; 64.7 % of the patients had painful hips, 79.4 % had painful shoulders, 73.5 % had abnormal ESR, and 70.6 % had abnormal CRP. Significant improvement was seen between baseline and last visit in mean level of RAPID3 and all other MDHAQ measures, except in the fatigue score ($p<0.05$), as well as ESR and CRP (Table 14.2). The most remarkable improvement was seen in morning stiffness and hip involvement. The mean dose of prednisone was decreased from 12.2 mg at first visit to 4.3 mg at most recent visit in agreement with the clinical improvement seen in these patients. In conclusion, improvement was seen according to MDHAQ/RAPID3 scores in a similar range to ESR and CRP, documenting effective response to prednisone.

Disease-specific questionnaires or measures, as the specific disease activity index for PMR, may be optimal for clinical trials and other research studies, but it is not feasible to have patients complete different self-report evaluations or questionnaires in busy clinical settings. MDHAQ completed by the patient in the waiting area not only provides data at the onset of the visit, rather than acquired during a visit, it also helps the patient prepare for the visit and may improve doctor–patient communication.

Table 14.2 Mean MDHAQ/RAPID3 scores, laboratory measures, and medication at baseline and most recent visit in 34 patients with PMR

	PMR patients ($n = 34$)				
	Baseline	Most recent visit	*P* value	Mean change	% Improvement
MDHAQ: Patient self-reported measures					
RAPID3, mean (SD)	12.2 (7.0)	8.5 (7.2)	0.02	3.7	30.7 %
MDHAQ-Function, mean (SD)	2.2 (2.1)	1.5 (1.7)	0.03	0.6	27.2 %
MDHAQ-Pain, mean (SD)	5.3 (2.9)	3.4 (3.4)	0.002	1.9	35.8 %
MDHAQ-PATGL, mean (SD)	4.7 (2.9)	3.1 (3.1)	0.01	1.6	34.0 %
RADAI-painful hip, *n* (%)	22 (64.7 %)	12 (35.3 %)	0.02	29.4	45.4 %
RADAI-painful shoulder, *n* (%)	27 (79.4 %)	17 (50 %)	0.02	10	37.0 %
MDHAQ-Fatigue, mean (SD)	3.9 (3.6)	3.5 (3.3)	0.54	0.4	10.5 %
Morning stiffness duration, minutes, mean (SD)	63.1 (97.7)	19.1 (34.1)	0.05	43.9	69.5 %
Laboratory measures					
Abnormal ESR, *n* (%)	25 (73.5 %)	14 (41.1 %)	0.007	32	43.5 %
Abnormal CRP, *n* (%)	24 (70.6 %)	13 (38.2 %)	0.007	32	45.3 %
Medication					
Prednisone dosage, mg, mean (SD)	12.2 (6.8)	4.3 (3.5)	<0.001	7.9	64.7 %

Conclusion

The Use of PROMs in PMR

PMR is a very heterogeneous disease with an important impact on patients' lives. There seems to be little evidence as to which set of criteria provides a reliable diagnosis or which outcomes are the most relevant to evaluate the most appropriate treatment. In an effort to propose new outcome measures, PROs may play an important role. The use of PROs is dramatically increasing in rheumatology. Most core outcome sets or minimum domains to be measured in clinical trials include at least one PRO [32].

PROs have been proven to show responsiveness [33] and distinguish routine care from treat-to-target strategies as effectively as other measures in clinical trials of RA patients [34]. In addition, the use of PROs may encourage the patient to have an active role to help manage his or her own illness.

In PMR, an Outcome Measures in Rheumatology (OMERACT) special interest group is working toward the development of a core set of outcomes, but pain, morning stiffness, fatigue, sleep disturbance, function, anxiety, and depression have been initially identified of interest [8]. In general, 3 PROs are commonly used across the majority of rheumatic diseases and included in most core data sets: pain, physical function, and the patient global assessment of disease activity [32]. In the systematic review previously presented, pain, morning stiffness, and physical function were the PROs most frequently reported in PMR studies.

Pain is the most important symptom in patients with PMR and plays a crucial role during the course of the disease. Pain is the principal feature of all diagnostic criteria for PMR published so far [35–38] and it has been included as a central measure in multiple remission/flare definition [9]. Pain is also the only mandatory criteria in the EULAR response criteria for PMR [26].

Morning stiffness is also considered an important diagnostic clue in PMR, but it is difficult to measure accurately, especially when using duration of morning stiffness that has been reported to show poor test–retest reliability in PMR [7]. From the patient's perspective, morning stiffness is better described as what it prevents them from doing, in relation to physical function, and it is less responsive to glucocorticoids in comparison to pain [24]. Morning stiffness has also been included in different diagnostic criteria—lasting for more than 1 h [35, 36]—as part of the response criteria previously described [26], and in the PMR-AS [27].

Function through HAQ or MHAQ was only reported in 25 % of the articles from the systematic review. This is a surprisingly low percentage, having taken into account that both are generic instruments that can be used in any rheumatic diagnosis [39]. Function correlates with other measures of disease activity in PMR and is responsive to change [40, 41]. Moreover, function is a strong predictor of mortality not only in patients with RA [42], but also in the general population [43].

For patients with PMR being able to perform common activities of daily living was described as the most important aspect of their disease that would indirectly reflect their morning stiffness [24].

Other domains such as patient global assessment, fatigue, quality of life, anxiety, and depression were infrequently reported in PMR studies, though they appear important from the patient's point of view [8]. Although the domains "pain" and "function" are relatively straightforward, the patient global assessment is more difficult to interpret [32]. This measure was initially developed in RA but is now commonly utilized in other rheumatic diagnoses with different formulations. Differences in formulation and interpretation may influence the poor concordance seen between patient and physician global assessments documented in many rheumatic diseases [44], which have been associated with poorer outcomes [45].

PMR has an important impact in patients' quality of life (QOL). Changes in pain and morning stiffness have been strongly associated with changes in the physical aspect of the SF-36, whereas changes in acute-phase reactants markers have been shown to be strongly associated with changes in the mental component [41]. The impaired mental QOL and depression commonly seen in PMR patients could be related to the neurologic effects of circulating cytokines, such as interleukin-6, which is elevated in PMR and may have significant effects on the central nervous system [46].

Assessment of a patient with PMR requires a careful history and physical examination, as well as relevant laboratory tests, including ESR and CRP, to formulate an optimal treatment plan for each individual patient. Quantitative PROs may add to clinical decisions, and to documentation of clinical improvement in individual patients with PMR. The MDHAQ appears to be a valuable tool to collect PROs in routine care, being suitable not only for PMR but also for any rheumatic condition.

In summary, PROs can be useful for better monitoring of disease activity and evaluating treatment response in PMR. Pain is the most important domain in patients with PMR and it has been systematically included in diagnostic criteria and the evaluation of disease activity. While morning stiffness is an important symptom for patients, there is no consistency about how it should be measured and presents several limitations. Multiple domains that are important for the patients are not routinely evaluated. Further work is needed to obtain a better insight of which outcomes should be necessary to incorporate the patient's perspective.

Appendix 1: MDHAQ

Multi-Dimensional Health Assessment Questionnaire (MDHAQ™)(R890-NP2R)

This questionnaire includes information not available from blood tests, X-rays, or any source other than you. Please try to answer each question, even if you do not think it is related to you at this time. Try to complete as much as you can yourself, but if you need help, please ask. There are no right or wrong answers. Please answer exactly as you think or feel. Thank you.

1. Please check (√) the ONE best answer for your abilities at this time:

OVER THE PAST WEEK, were you able to:	Without **ANY** difficulty	With **SOME** difficulty	With **MUCH** difficulty	**UNABLE** to do
a. Dress yourself, including tying shoelaces and doing buttons?	☐ 0	☐ 1	☐ 2	☐ 3
b. Get in and out of bed?	☐ 0	☐ 1	☐ 2	☐ 3
c. Lift a full cup or glass to your mouth?	☐ 0	☐ 1	☐ 2	☐ 3
d. Walk outdoors on flat ground?	☐ 0	☐ 1	☐ 2	☐ 3
e. Wash and dry your entire body?	☐ 0	☐ 1	☐ 2	☐ 3
f. Bend down to pick up clothing from the floor?	☐ 0	☐ 1	☐ 2	☐ 3
g. Turn regular faucets on and off?	☐ 0	☐ 1	☐ 2	☐ 3
h. Get in and out of a car, bus, train, or airplane?	☐ 0	☐ 1	☐ 2	☐ 3
i. Walk two miles or three kilometers, if you wish?	☐ 0	☐ 1	☐ 2	☐ 3
j. Participate in recreational activities and sports as you wish?	☐ 0	☐ 1	☐ 2	☐ 3
k. Get a good night's sleep?	☐ 0	☐ 1.1	☐ 2.2	☐ 3.3
l. Deal with feelings of anxiety or being nervous?	☐ 0	☐ 1.1	☐ 2.2	☐ 3.3
m. Deal with feelings of depression or feeling blue?	☐ 0	☐ 1.1	☐ 2.2	☐ 3.3

**2. How much pain have you had because of your condition OVER THE PAST WEEK?
Please indicate below how severe your pain has been:**

NO PAIN ○ PAIN AS BAD AS IT COULD BE
0 0.5 1.0 1.5 2.0 2.5 3.0 3.5 4.0 4.5 5.0 5.5 6.0 6.5 7.0 7.5 8.0 8.5 9.0 9.5 10

3. Please place a check (√) in the appropriate spot to indicate the amount of pain you are having today in each of the joint areas listed below:

	None	Mild	Moderate	Severe		None	Mild	Moderate	Severe
a. LEFT FINGERS	☐ 0	☐ 1	☐ 2	☐ 3	i. RIGHT FINGERS	☐ 0	☐ 1	☐ 2	☐ 3
b. LEFT WRIST	☐ 0	☐ 1	☐ 2	☐ 3	j. RIGHT WRIST	☐ 0	☐ 1	☐ 2	☐ 3
c. LEFT ELBOW	☐ 0	☐ 1	☐ 2	☐ 3	k. RIGHT ELBOW	☐ 0	☐ 1	☐ 2	☐ 3
d. LEFT SHOULDER	☐ 0	☐ 1	☐ 2	☐ 3	l. RIGHT SHOULDER	☐ 0	☐ 1	☐ 2	☐ 3
e. LEFT HIP	☐ 0	☐ 1	☐ 2	☐ 3	m. RIGHT HIP	☐ 0	☐ 1	☐ 2	☐ 3
f. LEFT KNEE	☐ 0	☐ 1	☐ 2	☐ 3	n. RIGHT KNEE	☐ 0	☐ 1	☐ 2	☐ 3
g. LEFT ANKLE	☐ 0	☐ 1	☐ 2	☐ 3	o. RIGHT ANKLE	☐ 0	☐ 1	☐ 2	☐ 3
h. LEFT TOES	☐ 0	☐ 1	☐ 2	☐ 3	p. RIGHT TOES	☐ 0	☐ 1	☐ 2	☐ 3
q. NECK	☐ 0	☐ 1	☐ 2	☐ 3	r. BACK	☐ 0	☐ 1	☐ 2	☐ 3

4. Considering all the ways in which illness and health conditions may affect you at this time, please indicate below how you are doing:

VERY WELL ○ VERY POORLY
0 0.5 1.0 1.5 2.0 2.5 3.0 3.5 4.0 4.5 5.0 5.5 6.0 6.5 7.0 7.5 8.0 8.5 9.0 9.5 10

FOR OFFICE USE ONLY

1.a-j FN (0-10): ☐

1=0.3	16=5.3
2=0.7	17=5.7
3=1.0	18=6.0
4=1.3	19=6.3
5=1.7	20=6.7
6=2.0	21=7.0
7=2.3	22=7.3
8=2.7	23=7.7
9=3.0	24=8.0
10=3.3	25=8.3
11=3.7	26=8.7
12=4.0	27=9.0
13=4.3	28=9.3
14=4.7	29=9.7
15=5.0	30=10

2.PN (0-10): ☐

4.PTGL (0-10): ☐

RAPID 3™ (0-30) ☐

Cat:
HS = >12
MS = 6.1-12
LS = 3.1-6
R = ≤3

5. Please check (√) if you have experienced any of the following over the last month:

__Fever
__Weight gain (>10 lbs)
__Weight loss (>10 lbs)
__Feeling sickly
__Headaches
__Unusual fatigue
__Swollen glands
__Loss of appetite
__Skin rash or hives
__Unusual bruising or bleeding
__Other skin problems
__Loss of hair
__Dry eyes
__Other eye problems
__Problems with hearing
__Ringing in the ears
__Stuffy nose
__Sores in the mouth
__Dry mouth
__Problems with smell or taste
__Lump in your throat
__Cough
__Shortness of breath
__Wheezing
__Pain in the chest
__Heart pounding (palpitations)
__Trouble swallowing
__Heartburn or stomach gas
__Stomach pain or cramps
__Nausea
__Vomiting
__Constipation
__Diarrhea
__Dark or bloody stools
__Problems with urination
__Gynecological (female) problems
__Dizziness
__Losing your balance
__Muscle pain, aches, or cramps
__Muscle weakness
__Paralysis of arms or legs
__Numbness or tingling of arms or legs
__Fainting spells
__Swelling of hands
__Swelling of ankles
__Swelling in other joints
__Joint pain
__Back pain
__Neck pain
__Use of drugs not sold in stores
__Smoking cigarettes
__More than 2 alcoholic drinks per day
__Depression - feeling blue
__Anxiety - feeling nervous
__Problems with thinking
__Problems with memory
__Problems with sleeping
__Sexual problems
__Burning in sex organs
__Problems with social activities

FOR OFFICE USE ONLY
5. ROS: ☐

Please check (√) here if you have had none of the above over the last month: _______.

6. When you awakened in the morning OVER THE LAST WEEK, did you feel stiff? ☐ No ☐ Yes
If "No," please go to Item 7. If "**Yes," please indicate the number of minutes_______, or hours ______**
until you are as limber as you will be for the day.

7. How do you feel TODAY compared to ONE WEEK AGO? Please check (✓) only one.
M**uch B**etter ☐ (1), **B**etter ☐ (2), the **S**ame ☐ (3), **W**orse ☐ (4), M**uch W**orse ☐ (5) than one week ago

8. How often do you exercise aerobically (sweating, increased heart rate, shortness of breath) **for at least one-half hour** (30 minutes)**? Please check (✓) only one.**
☐ 3 or more times a week (3) ☐ 1-2 times per month (1)
☐ 1-2 times per week (2) ☐ Do not exercise regularly (0) ☐ Cannot exercise due to disability/ handicap (9)

9. How much of a problem has UNUSUAL fatigue or tiredness been for you OVER THE PAST WEEK?

FATIGUE IS NO PROBLEM	○ 0	○ 0.5	○ 1.0	○ 1.5	○ 2.0	○ 2.5	○ 3.0	○ 3.5	○ 4.0	○ 4.5	○ 5.0	○ 5.5	○ 6.0	○ 6.5	○ 7.0	○ 7.5	○ 8.0	○ 8.5	○ 9.0	○ 9.5	○ 10	FATIGUE IS A MAJOR PROBLEM

10. Over the last 6 months have you had: [Please check (√)]
☐No ☐Yes An operation or new illness
☐No ☐Yes Medical emergency or stay overnight in hospital
☐No ☐Yes A fall, broken bone, or other accident or trauma
☐No ☐Yes An important new symptom or medical problem
☐No ☐Yes Side effect(s) of any medication or drug
☐No ☐Yes Smoke cigarettes regularly
☐No ☐Yes Change(s) of arthritis or other medication
☐No ☐Yes Change(s) of address
☐No ☐Yes Change(s) of marital status
☐No ☐Yes Change job or work duties, quit work, retired
☐No ☐Yes Change of medical insurance, Medicare, etc.
☐No ☐Yes Change of primary care or other doctor

Please explain any "Yes" answer below, or on a separate page.

____

11. Do you think that you have suffered from a flare of your condition during the PAST 6 months?
☐ No, ☐ Yes, If "No," you have completed the questionnaire. If "Yes," please answer the questions below:
12. If yes, how many flares have you had in the PAST 6 MONTHS?
☐ 1 ☐ 2-3 ☐ 4-5 ☐ >5
13. In general, how long did your flare(s) last? (Please check all that apply)
☐ Less than 1 day, ☐ 1-3 days, ☐ 4-6 days, ☐ 1-2 weeks, ☐ More than 2 weeks
14. How did you treat your flares? (Please check all that apply).
☐ New medication (please specify)_______________________,
☐ Increased medication dose (please specify)_______________
☐ Other treatment (please specify) ____________________ ☐ No treatment.
15. Has your arthritis returned to your pre-flare status? ☐ Yes ☐ No

Page 2 of 2 Thank you for completing this questionnaire to help keep track of your medical care. R890NP2R

References

1. Cimmino MA, Zaccaria A. Epidemiology of polymyalgia rheumatica. Clin Exp Rheumatol. 2000;18(4 Suppl 20):S9–11.
2. Proven A, Gabriel SE, O'Fallon WM, Hunder GG. Polymyalgia rheumatica with low erythrocyte sedimentation rate at diagnosis. J Rheumatol. 1999;26(6):1333–7.
3. Gamez-Nava JI, Gonzalez-Lopez L, Davis P, Suarez-Almazor ME. Referral and diagnosis of common rheumatic diseases by primary care physicians. Br J Rheumatol. 1998; 37(11):1215–9.
4. Narvaez J, Nolla-Sole JM, Clavaguera MT, Valverde-Garcia J, Roig-Escofet D. Longterm therapy in polymyalgia rheumatica: effect of coexistent temporal arteritis. J Rheumatol. 1999;26(9):1945–52.
5. Gabriel SE, Sunku J, Salvarani C, O'Fallon WM, Hunder GG. Adverse outcomes of antiinflammatory therapy among patients with polymyalgia rheumatica. Arthritis Rheum. 1997;40(10):1873–8.
6. Dasgupta B, Borg FA, Hassan N, Barraclough K, Bourke B, Fulcher J, Hollywood J, Hutchings A, Kyle V, Nott J, et al. BSR and BHPR guidelines for the management of polymyalgia rheumatica. Rheumatology (Oxford). 2010;49(1):186–90.
7. Matteson EL, Maradit-Kremers H, Cimmino MA, Schmidt WA, Schirmer M, Salvarani C, Bachta A, Dejaco C, Duftner C, Slott Jensen H, et al. Patient-reported outcomes in polymyalgia rheumatica. J Rheumatol. 2012;39(4):795–803.
8. Mackie SL, Arat S, da Silva J, Duarte C, Halliday S, Hughes R, Morris M, Pease CT, Sherman JW, Simon LS, et al. Polymyalgia Rheumatica (PMR) Special Interest Group at OMERACT 11: outcomes of importance for patients with PMR. J Rheumatol. 2014;41(4):819–23.
9. Dejaco C, Duftner C, Cimmino MA, Dasgupta B, Salvarani C, Crowson CS, Maradit-Kremers H, Hutchings A, Matteson EL, Schirmer M, et al. Definition of remission and relapse in polymyalgia rheumatica: data from a literature search compared with a Delphi-based expert consensus. Ann Rheum Dis. 2011;70(3):447–53.
10. Huang A, Castrejon I: Patient-reported outcomes in trials of patients with polymyalgia rheumatica: a systematic literature review. *Rheumatology international* 2016. Jan 14. [Epub ahead of print].
11. Lund B, Egsmose C, Jorgensen S, Krogsgaard MR. Establishment of the relative antiinflammatory potency of deflazacort and prednisone in polymyalgia rheumatica. Calcif Tissue Int. 1987;41(6):316–20.
12. Di Munno O, Beghe F, Favini P, Di Giuseppe P, Pontrandolfo A, Occhipinti G, Pasero G. Prevention of glucocorticoid-induced osteopenia: effect of oral 25-hydroxyvitamin D and calcium. Clin Rheumatol. 1989;8(2):202–7.
13. Di Munno O, Imbimbo B, Mazzantini M, Milani S, Occhipinti G, Pasero G. Deflazacort versus methylprednisolone in polymyalgia rheumatica: clinical equivalence and relative antiinflammatory potency of different treatment regimens. J Rheumatol. 1995;22(8):1492–8.
14. Krogsgaard MR, Lund B, Johnsson B. A long term prospective study of the equipotency between deflazacort and prednisolone in the treatment of patients with polymyalgia rheumatica. J Rheumatol. 1995;22(9):1660–2.
15. Salvarani C, Cantini F, Olivieri I, Barozzi L, Macchioni L, Boiardi L, Niccoli L, Padula A, Pulsatelli L, Meliconi R. Corticosteroid injections in polymyalgia rheumatica: a double-blind, prospective, randomized, placebo controlled study. J Rheumatol. 2000;27(6):1470–6.
16. Kreiner F, Galbo H. Effect of etanercept in polymyalgia rheumatica: a randomized controlled trial. Arthritis Res Ther. 2010;12(5):R176.
17. Cimmino MA, Parodi M, Caporali R, Montecucco C. Is the course of steroid-treated polymyalgia rheumatica more severe in women? Ann N Y Acad Sci. 2006;1069:315–21.
18. Calvo L, Pistone G, Arnone S, Colomba D, Amico S, Giacalone A, Vitale P, Nicosia C, Barone E, Scaglione R, et al. Polymyalgia rheumatica and vertebral fractures: a 1-year pilot controlled study. Rheumatol Int. 2010;30(9):1245–7.

19. Fries JF, Spitz PW, Young DY. The dimensions of health outcomes: the health assessment questionnaire, disability and pain scales. J Rheumatol. 1982;9(5):789–93.
20. Pincus T, Summey JA, Soraci Jr SA, Wallston KA, Hummon NP. Assessment of patient satisfaction in activities of daily living using a modified Stanford Health Assessment Questionnaire. Arthritis Rheum. 1983;26(11):1346–53.
21. McHorney CA, Ware Jr JE, Lu JF, Sherbourne CD. The MOS 36-item Short-Form Health Survey (SF-36): III. Tests of data quality, scaling assumptions, and reliability across diverse patient groups. Med Care. 1994;32(1):40–66.
22. Bird HA, Leeb BF, Montecucco CM, Misiuniene N, Nesher G, Pai S, Pease C, Rovensky J, Rozman B. A comparison of the sensitivity of diagnostic criteria for polymyalgia rheumatica. Ann Rheum Dis. 2005;64(4):626–9.
23. Dasgupta B, Cimmino MA, Maradit-Kremers H, Schmidt WA, Schirmer M, Salvarani C, Bachta A, Dejaco C, Duftner C, Jensen HS, et al. 2012 provisional classification criteria for polymyalgia rheumatica: a European League Against Rheumatism/American College of Rheumatology collaborative initiative. Ann Rheum Dis. 2012;71(4):484–92.
24. Mackie SL, Hughes R, Walsh M, Day J, Newton M, Pease C, Kirwan J, Morris M. "An impediment to living life": why and how should we measure stiffness in polymyalgia rheumatica? PLoS One. 2015;10(5), e0126758.
25. Dasgupta B, Salvarani C, Schirmer M, Crowson CS, Maradit-Kremers H, Hutchings A, Matteson EL, members of the American College of Rheumatology Work Group for Development of Classification Criteria for PMR. Developing classification criteria for polymyalgia rheumatica: comparison of views from an expert panel and wider survey. J Rheumatol. 2008;35(2):270–7.
26. Leeb BF, Bird HA, Nesher G, Andel I, Hueber W, Logar D, Montecucco CM, Rovensky J, Sautner J, Sonnenblick M. EULAR response criteria for polymyalgia rheumatica: results of an initiative of the European Collaborating Polymyalgia Rheumatica Group (subcommittee of ESCISIT). Ann Rheum Dis. 2003;62(12):1189–94.
27. Leeb BF, Bird HA. A disease activity score for polymyalgia rheumatica. Ann Rheum Dis. 2004;63(10):1279–83.
28. Cantini F, Salvarani C, Olivieri I, Macchioni L, Ranzi A, Niccoli L, Padula A, Boiardi L. Erythrocyte sedimentation rate and C-reactive protein in the evaluation of disease activity and severity in polymyalgia rheumatica: a prospective follow-up study. Semin Arthritis Rheum. 2000;30(1):17–24.
29. Castrejon I, Huang A, Everakes SL, Nika A, Sequeira W, Pincus T. Documentation of clinical improvement in patient with polymyalgia rheumatica according to MDHAQ/RAPID3 (Multidimensional Health Assessment Questionnaire/Routine Assessment of Patient Index Data): a longitudinal analysis from routine care. Arthritis Rheum. 2015;67 Suppl 10.
30. Pincus T, Sokka T, Kautiainen H. Further development of a physical function scale on a MDHAQ [corrected] for standard care of patients with rheumatic diseases. J Rheumatol. 2005;32(8):1432–9.
31. Castrejon I, Bergman MJ, Pincus T. MDHAQ/RAPID3 to recognize improvement over 2 months in usual care of patients with osteoarthritis, systemic lupus erythematosus, spondyloarthropathy, and gout, as well as rheumatoid arthritis. J Clin Rheumatol. 2013;19(4):169–74.
32. van Tuyl LH, Boers M. Patient-reported outcomes in core domain sets for rheumatic diseases. Nat Rev Rheumatol. 2015;11(12):705–12.
33. Wells G, Li T, Maxwell L, Maclean R, Tugwell P. Responsiveness of patient reported outcomes including fatigue, sleep quality, activity limitation, and quality of life following treatment with abatacept for rheumatoid arthritis. Ann Rheum Dis. 2008;67(2):260–5.
34. Castrejon I, Pincus T. Patient self-report outcomes to guide a treat-to-target strategy in clinical trials and usual clinical care of rheumatoid arthritis. Clin Exp Rheumatol. 2012;30 Suppl 73:S50–5.
35. Bird HA, Esselinckx W, Dixon AS, Mowat AG, Wood PH. An evaluation of criteria for polymyalgia rheumatica. Ann Rheum Dis. 1979;38(5):434–9.

36. Jones JG, Hazleman BL. Prognosis and management of polymyalgia rheumatica. Ann Rheum Dis. 1981;40(1):1–5.
37. Chuang TY, Hunder GG, Ilstrup DM, Kurland LT. Polymyalgia rheumatica: a 10-year epidemiologic and clinical study. Ann Intern Med. 1982;97(5):672–80.
38. Nobunaga M, Yoshioka K, Yasuda M, Shingu M. Clinical studies of polymyalgia rheumatica. A proposal of diagnostic criteria. Jpn J Med. 1989;28(4):452–6.
39. White DK, Wilson JC, Keysor JJ. Measures of adult general functional status: SF-36 Physical Functioning Subscale (PF-10), Health Assessment Questionnaire (HAQ), Modified Health Assessment Questionnaire (MHAQ), Katz Index of Independence in activities of daily living, Functional Independence Measure (FIM), and Osteoarthritis-Function-Computer Adaptive Test (OA-Function-CAT). Arthritis Care Res. 2011;63 Suppl 11:S297–307.
40. Kalke S, Mukerjee D, Dasgupta B. A study of the health assessment questionnaire to evaluate functional status in polymyalgia rheumatica. Rheumatology (Oxford). 2000;39(8):883–5.
41. Hutchings A, Hollywood J, Lamping DL, Pease CT, Chakravarty K, Silverman B, Choy EH, Scott DG, Hazleman BL, Bourke B, et al. Clinical outcomes, quality of life, and diagnostic uncertainty in the first year of polymyalgia rheumatica. Arthritis Rheum. 2007;57(5):803–9.
42. Pincus T, Callahan LF, Sale WG, Brooks AL, Payne LE, Vaughn WK. Severe functional declines, work disability, and increased mortality in seventy-five rheumatoid arthritis patients studied over nine years. Arthritis Rheum. 1984;27(8):864–72.
43. Sokka T, Hakkinen A, Krishnan E, Hannonen P. Similar prediction of mortality by the health assessment questionnaire in patients with rheumatoid arthritis and the general population. Ann Rheum Dis. 2004;63(5):494–7.
44. Castrejon I, Yazici Y, Samuels J, Luta G, Pincus T. Discordance of global estimates by patients and their physicians in usual care of many rheumatic diseases: association with 5 scores on a Multidimensional Health Assessment Questionnaire (MDHAQ) that are not found on the Health Assessment Questionnaire (HAQ). Arthritis Care Res. 2014;66(6):934–42.
45. Starfield B, Wray C, Hess K, Gross R, Birk PS, D'Lugoff BC. The influence of patient-practitioner agreement on outcome of care. Am J Public Health. 1981;71(2):127–31.
46. Dasgupta B, Panayi GS. Interleukin-6 in serum of patients with polymyalgia rheumatica and giant cell arteritis. Br J Rheumatol. 1990;29(6):456–8.

Chapter 15
Electronic Patient-Reported Outcome Measures (ePROMs) in Rheumatology

Jutta Richter, Christina Kampling, and Matthias Schneider

Introduction

In rheumatology, diagnosis, management, and prognosis rely on standardized physician and patient-reported outcome measures (PROMs) [1]. Generic and disease-related, uni- and multidimensional indices respectively PROMs influence individual treatment plans and determine follow-up intervals [2]. Translations of known PROMs in different languages and new PROMs are still under development, and evaluations of the latter might address yet unmet needs, be faster to complete, or easier to administer [3].

With the recognition of patients' perspectives as key outcome measures and indispensable prerequisites for improving the quality of care, inclusion of PROMs in the process of healthcare came to the fore [4, 5]. In addition to traditionally accepted treatment influencing factors, psychosocial and occupational conditions, individual fatigue and stress levels, as well as other patient-centered parameters that might be addressed by PROMs gained more attention [6, 7].

For clinical purposes, PROMs may support the assessment of clinical and related problems as well as the effects of treatment [8, 9]. They facilitate the immediate patient–physician communication, promote the model of shared decision making, improve patient satisfaction and knowledge, and contribute to the monitoring of quality of care [8, 9]. PROMs proved to be beneficial not only for clinical decision

J. Richter, M.D. (✉) • M. Schneider, M.D.
Policlinic for Rheumatology and Hiller Research Centre for Rheumatology, University Clinic Duesseldorf, Medical Faculty, Heinrich-Heine-University Duesseldorf, Moorenstr. 5, Duesseldorf, Germany
e-mail: richter@rheumanet.org; schneider@rheumanet.org

C. Kampling, M.D.
Policlinic for Rheumatology and Hiller Research Centre for Rheumatology, University Clinic Duesseldorf, Heinrich-Heine-University Duesseldorf, Duesseldorf, Germany
e-mail: christina.kampling@uni-duesseldorf.de

Y. El Miedany (ed.), *Patient Reported Outcome Measures in Rheumatic Diseases*,
DOI 10.1007/978-3-319-32851-5_15

making, but also on aggregate levels (e.g., for performance measures, in cohort studies for comparative effectiveness research, and registries that are used to deliver on-market data) [10–14]. They have been applied in population-based monitoring [10–14]. Furthermore, the use of disease-specific PROMs as (primary) outcome parameters of clinical trials in drug development has evolved and is now demanded by the European Medicines Agency [15] and the US Food and Drug Administration [16]. PROMs have even been used for health-economic studies and hence allow to substantiate health policy decisions [17]. PROMs are available from various websites in a diverse manner (see Table 15.1).

Paper-based assessments of PROMs are usually easily handled by patients or their accompanying relatives/friends, but their incorporation into clinical use, decision making, or scientific purposes is time-consuming [18, 19]. Thus, paper-based

Table 15.1 Link list of ePROMs

Link	Annotation
http://dgrh.de/klassifikationskrite.html	Provision of PDFs of PROMs for German-speaking countries
http://www.medal.org	Provision of multilanguage PROMs
http://www.nihpromis.org/?AspxAutoDetectCookieSupport=1#2	System that allows assessments of PROMs as health status (physical, mental, and social well-being)
http://oml.eular.org/	Comprehensive database of validated patient-reported instruments (indices, questionnaires, scales, or others) used in rheumatology (European League Against Rheumatism)
http://www.rheumatology.org/Practice-Quality/Clinical-Support/Quality-Measurement/Disease-Activity-Functional-Status-Assessments	Quality measures the American College of Rheumatology approved for use in clinical practice and research
https://www.assessmentcenter.net/	An Internet site that provides a tool for online data collection, includes instruments from PROMIS (The Patient-Reported Outcome Measurement Information System)
http://www.rheuma-online.de/selbsthilfe/online-monitoring/online-monitoring-der-rheumatoiden-arthritis/online-monitoring-der-krankheitsaktivitaet-einer-chronischen-polyarthritis-rheumatoiden-arthritis-der-elektronische-disease-activity-score-online-edas-online.html	Online self-monitoring rheumatoid arthritis
http://www.rheumatologie-berlin.de/aerzte/assessment.html	German Online-Assessments, for example, BASDAI, ASDAS, BASFI, and DAS28
http://www.meteorfoundation.com/	Free online tool to assess Rheumatoid Arthritis Disease Activity in clinical practice

ASDAS Ankylosing Spondylitis Disease Activity Score, *BASDAI* Bath Ankylosing Spondylitis Disease Activity Index, *BASFI* Bath Ankylosing Spondylitis Disease Functional Index, *DAS28* Disease Activity Score 28

PROMs are mostly regarded as costly and inefficient [20]. Even if all questionnaire items are filled out, scores are usually hard to calculate without a (special) pocket calculator, and can therefore barely be used in clinical practice when fast decision making is needed [1]. Among other reasons the paper-based assessments' inherent administrative burden is the leading reasons found for physicians' reluctance on PROMs' routine assessments [2, 21–25].

In the last decades, the technological facilities changed dramatically. Thus, electronic assessments of PROMs (so-called ePROMs) have been realized and their evaluations have been performed (see later). Electronic health/medical records (EHR/EMR) and (Web-based) applications running on various hardware devices have been developed. They include ePROMs as well as other care quality measures. In addition, ePROMs have been incorporated into computer applications that gather data for registries [12, 26]. The next generation of mobile information technology (IT)-supported registers has yet been positively noticed as they allow patients themselves to make real-time adjustments to their treatments and lifestyle, for example, by filling ePROMs [26]. Recently, even an Internet platform has been implemented and used for adaption and validation of an ePROM [27]. In addition, there is an ongoing discussion on the use of social media to collect data to support the content validity of patient-reported outcome instruments in drug development processes [28]. These new developments and opportunities reflect the fundamental change from paper-based PROMs to ePROMs.

Advantages of Electronic Data Capture and ePROMs

The technological infrastructures facilitate real-time and long-term systematic patient-centered data collection as integral components of care [5, 29, 30]. Today's information technologies allow intelligent orchestration of PROMs data collection, analyses, and reporting and thus provide a wide array of exciting challenges and opportunities not only for routine patient care but also medical research [31]. Various (non)proprietary applications simplify data acquisition and accelerate information transfer between patients and physicians by eliminating intermediate data collection and processing steps (e.g., double data entry), increase flexibility of data capture (e.g., frequencies and locations), facilitate clinical decisions, and can thus improve the efficiency of clinical workflow [30, 32–37]. Changing specific personal or disease-specific needs, treatment regimens, or phases might require different assessments. ePROMs might simplify context-based customization of the assessments [38]. They allow real-time flagging of important, clinically relevant symptoms. Frequent monitoring and reviewing of patient-centered issues and needs is enabled; thus, ePROMs offer an ability to enhance clinical care and quality assurance [29, 33]. Multiple follow-ups of definable time periods may be seen at a glance and/or compared with control groups, allowing adaptation of treatment plans and processes without the need for additional staff or equipment [39, 40]. As ePROMs improve the accuracy of data collection of symptoms indicating poor conditions and outcomes, they might even help to triage patients who need more extensive care, for example, in terms of evaluation and (non)medical interventions [2, 20, 30]. Electronic patient-centered monitoring may also facilitate patients' management across care transitions [41]. ePROMs can enhance cost-efficiencies [20]. More ePROMs in EHRs could even widen the capacity to undertake population-based research [42].

Assessments with the help of ePROMs (e.g., in electronic diaries) allow to document time-stamped entries and thereby might positively influence compliance [43]. Visual feedback for patients—integrated into the Electronic Recording of Outcome Measures for Inflammatory arthritis and Ankylosing spondylitis (EROMIA) system—had a positive and significant impact on the disease activity control [44]. Recently, a strong correlation was reported between the use of a software application (Rheum-PACER) and disease control [45]. ePROMs give the opportunity to obtain a broadened view on disease courses and patterns also for the empowered patients who proactively participate in the management of the course of their disease [46]. In contrast to initial beliefs, patients have a positive attitude toward the use of PROMs in computerized systems [33]. As the public and thereby the patients become more experienced and familiar in the use of new technologies, ePROMs gain higher acceptability and are commonly preferred by patients over paper-based versions [33, 40, 47, 48]. However, recently active ePROM use in a Web portal was only performed by less than half of the patients [49].

Not only advantages (pros) but also disadvantages (cons) of ePROMs are summarized in Table 15.2.

Table 15.2 Advantages (pros) and disadvantages (cons) for ePROMs (adapted from Schick-Makaroff) [93]

PROs	CONs
Real-time assessments with immediate access to the data and scoring	Need for IT system that might be costly
Rapid, time-saving	Validation studies necessary
Facilitate the immediate patient–physician communication	Integration in workflow need effort
Data entry by the patients themselves	Necessity of training of clinical staff and patients
Reduces human-dependent steps in data acquisition	Technical problems might lead to loss of data
Improved data quality by prevention of data entry errors	Linkage to EHR might need programming
More valid data	Users' resistance to technology
View of long-term follow-up data at a glance	Regular adoptions to software updates necessary
Depending on the system: use of different devices	
Link to electronic health records/patient documentation systems allowed	
Batched, stamped, and real-time data transactions	
Cost-efficiency in the long-term	
Automated alerts when problems are identified	
Patient and physician satisfaction	
PROs can be tailored to patient's specific needs	
Facilitate patient management in care transitions	

IT information technology, *EHR* electronic health records, *PROs* patient-reported outcomes

Prerequisites for ePROM Development and Their Assessments in Routine Care

Before broad introduction of ePROMs into clinical routine, careful comparison of data obtained by paper–pencil and computerized versions of the assessments was and is crucial, because equivalence of data obtained by the two acquisition methods cannot be taken for granted [18, 19, 36, 50, 51]. Detectable (test–retest) correlations between the modes of administration need to meet methodological requirements for demonstrating reliability and validity [50, 51]. Assessments on electronic devices need to be able to detect changes over time [17]. Coons et al. published a general framework for the transfer of paper-based PROs to electronic devices [52].

Meanwhile many traditional scales have been evaluated [5]. Gwaltney et al. showed in their meta-analysis that computer and paper measures produce equivalent scores. Subjects' computer experience and age did not influence this result when "small mean differences" were not regarded as clinically relevant [50]. Similarly, Campbell et al. published a review that summarizes 55 studies investigating 79 instruments. It provides a good overview for rheumatology and other disciplines [47]. The authors stated that paper-based and electronic formats are usually rated to be equivalent, and that study participants prefer electronic assessments [47]. However, they recommend further validations of electronic versions, taking into account that data assessed electronically should produce figures that are equivalent or superior to those retrieved via paper-based versions [47, 52].

ePROMs Application Systems

Electronic PROMs are available not only in EHRs and rheumatology-specific patient documentation systems, but also in (online) registries and other partly "registered user-restricted" online applications developed in a number of countries worldwide (e.g., http://www.medal.org and http://www.nihpromis.org/?AspxAutoDetectCookieSupport=1#2; [12, 32, 33, 44]). In addition, (non)profit organizations have implemented systems that allow ePROMs assessments (e.g., http://c-path.org/programs/epro/ and https://www.parexel.com/solutions/informatics/clinical-outcome-assessments/epro/). Studies showed that use of health information technology may be associated with better outcomes (e.g., reductions in mortality, complications, and costs) [53]. Developed systems have become more affordable and feasible to implement [5]. Patients' and others stakeholders' integration into the development and implementation process is necessary and will lead to better acceptance of the systems [54].

The heterogeneity of systems allowing to document ePROMs becomes obvious from a cancer research review published in 2013. This paper identified at least 33 unique systems [41]. However, each of the systems differed in features and characteristics [41]. Considering publications on this topic, a similar number of systems is expectable in rheumatology. As evaluation data is not available for all systems, their number might even be underestimated in a meta-analyses.

ePROMs Application Systems and Device Aspects

Due to the rise in connectivity and the applicable devices, the range of times and locations where patients can complete assessments (e.g., at home, waiting room, or drug store/pharmacy kiosks, or use of their smartphone/tablet) has been enlarged [5]. There are different electronic devices that can assist gathering ePROMs: traditional computers, tablet PCs, smartphones, and online platforms.

Computer/Web-based documentation software-systems allow the collection and documentation of self-reported ePROMs data and/or physicians' clinical findings (e.g., http://www.raintreeinc.com/rheumatology-emr/ and http://dgrh.de/rheumaedv.html) [44]. Some German outpatient clinics and rheumatologists in private practices also use computer/Web-based documentation software-systems, such as ARDIS, DocuMed.rh, and RheumaDok, that allow linkage to EHRs and/or software systems in outpatient clinics and private practices [55]. Schacher et al. examined the usability of these three systems, concluding that they provide valid data with better data quality than the paper versions [56]. Additionally, documentation software systems bear the potential to support tight-control concepts.

There is an upcoming use of ePROMs and their related applications on *mobile electronic devices* such as tablet PCs or smartphones [35, 37, 57]. These devices are nowadays widely spread and highly valued by individuals, usually remain turned on and are kept with the owner during the whole day; hence, they offer the opportunity of using medical applications as electronic diaries in real-life contexts [58]. mHealth mobile software programs, known as applications ("apps") on smartphones and other wireless devices, rely on the advantages of being personal, intuitive, user friendly, and portable [57, 59]. Thus, ePROM assessment by mHealth apps can become more convenient to the technically equipped patients and liberate them from filling out questionnaires at the physician visit [17, 47]. This becomes even more important as today's digital natives will be the rheumatology patients of tomorrow, and consequently, it is important to start developments of such useful applications as soon as possible [57].

The use of mobile electronic devices, such as tablet PCs, simplifies data acquisition at the time and location of clinical decision making and its use has been evaluated positively in rheumatoid arthritis (RA), systemic lupus erythematosus (SLE), and spondyloarthritis (SpA) [33]. Thus, mobile-accessed ePROMs are a good and capable option in routine patient care [33]. Meanwhile, further supplementary apps running on tablet PCs also allow patients direct data entry in the waiting rooms (e.g., ScoreCheck® Rheuma, see https://www.grandcentrix.net/portfolio/roche-pharma-patientenberatung/). The linkage to existing patient documentation systems is enabled.

Smartphones also support mobile medical and public health practice and give great opportunities [57, 60]. Apps offer new forms of patient (self-)management [61]. For example, free-of-charge electronic diaries including ePROMs were developed for different devices (e.g., smartphones, tablet PCs) as well as for different operating systems (such as iOS, Android, and Windows) [62]. They allow remote ePROM documentation whenever wanted and in even more asynchrony with their patient visit to the caring physician and might lead to a fundamental change in patient–physician interaction and directly influence therapy [62]. Azevedo et al. give a current overview on smartphone apps for self-management of rheumatic diseases and related problems that at least partly include ePROMs [57].

Physical disability as a sequel of chronic rheumatic diseases might be considered as a handicap for the use of mobile devices. Nevertheless, RA patients use electronic diaries and self-report their symptoms, major restrictions were not yet reported [61–63]. Compliance with computerized diaries is said to be much higher than the compliance with paper diaries, and additionally computerized PRO assessment can increase patients' compliance [50, 64, 65].

Website-based systems permit the gathering of ePROMs [5, 49]. For example, the international METEOR Project (http://www.meteorfoundation.com/) developed a Web tool that allows registered user-restricted online documentation of PROs, physician-derived parameters, and an online access for patients to look in their electronic patient record [66]. Koevots et al. reported a high interest in online self-surveillance of the disease [67]. Although less than half of the patients used the system in their feasibility and acceptability study, the authors conclude that an autonomous online registry is feasible in daily clinical practice [67]. As a prerequisite for online data acquisition a cross-sectional study including ePROMs performed via a Web-portal showed that data assessed online is equivalent to paper-based data [68, 69]. As an initial example of a new approach to tight-control concepts, Walter et al. evaluated whether tightly controlled disease activity is possible with provided online PROMs [70].

However, collected ePROMs might be useless without being reviewed by physicians or other staff members. Thus, whenever ePROMs are incorporated in the care process, data should be shown to the physician during regular personal consultations. Alternatively, secure data transfer and exchange as well as remote reviewing should be provided to the stakeholders. Further research on the development and evaluation of applications are warranted [57, 59]. This includes remote ePROM documentation via apps integrated into the popular treat-to-target strategies and other new care management concepts. Other disciplines already have described that apps might improve treatment accessibility [59].

Concrete Examples of ePROMs Evaluation

Several studies have been performed on the large armamentarium of ePROMs available not only in rheumatology but also in other disciplines, such as cancer and neurology, that use similar PROMs as rheumatologists [41, 71, 72].

As disease-specific assessments are more common in RA and SpA, studies predominantly address these patient groups. Examples are briefly summarized in chronological order: Ryan et al. showed that 44 % of RA patients were more likely to skip a question or mark more than one answer to the given question in paper-based questionnaires when comparing a paper-based and an electronic version of the SF-36 General Health Questionnaire [36]. In patients with systemic lupus erythematosus and vasculitis, an electronic version of the SF-36 correlated well with the paper version [18]. Schaeren et al. validated the North American Spine Society outcome-assessment instrument for the lumbar spine (a valid and reliable tool for measuring the outcome in patients with low back pain) in a touchscreen format. The computerized version was as reliable as the paper–pencil version and nearly two-thirds of the patients preferred the computerized version [40]. Evaluations by Bent et al. not only showed a high degree of agreement between paper and computer-administered versions of the Quebec Scale, the Bath Ankylosing Spondylitis Disease Activity Index (BASDAI), the Bath Ankylosing Spondylitis Functional Index (BASFI), and the Bath AS Patient Global Score (BAS-G) on a computerized touchscreen system but also noticed small systematic differences for the Quebec Scale and in the BAS-G results [48].

A comparison of self-reported health status measures (pain, fatigue, and global health on visual analogue scales [VAS]; rheumatoid arthritis disease activity index; modified health assessment questionnaire; SF-36) of paper-based questionnaires and electronic versions on a personal digital assistant (PDA) in RA patients was published in 2005 [73]. The authors reported acceptable agreement between the scores and patients' preferences of the PDA version [73]. A study with touchscreen computers showed that assessment via computer was as fast as paper-based versions [32]. The authors investigated the Rheumatoid Arthritis Quality of Life Questionnaire (RAQol); the Stanford Health Assessment Questionnaire (HAQ); VAS for pain, fatigue, and global arthritis activity; as well as a joint assessment. Their touchscreen questionnaires produced similar results to the applied paper–pencil versions; age and computer experiences did not influence the results [32].

Thumboo et al. also reported that patients preferred computerized versions of the PROMs evaluated (EQ5D, the Health Utilities Index Mark 2 [HUI2] & 3 [HUI3], and the Family Functioning Measure [FFM]) [74]. They showed that differences in the mean scores (interviewer versus touchscreen) did not reach statistical significance with the exception of the EQ-VAS. The authors concluded that computerized PROMs may have great advantages for the conduction of clinical trials and cohort studies as they may lead to smaller sample size requirements as well as reductions in cost and recruitment time [74]. Richter et al. published data on the evaluation of the feasibility of electronic data capture of Hannover Functional Ability Questionnaire (FFbH)/HAQ, BASDAI, and SF-36 using a tablet PC connected to a patient documentation system [33]. The study showed no significant differences between the electronic and the paper-based assessments [33].

In patients from the DANBIO register, PROMs on a touchscreen were investigated. The ePROMs (BASDAI, BASFI, HAQ, and VAS for pain, fatigue, and global health) generated valid results in ankylosing spondylitis and rheumatoid arthritis patients [75]. Newman et al. successfully developed a touchscreen questionnaire and a Web-based dashboard (Patient Centric Electronic Redesign [PACER]) for the collection, scoring, storing, and presentation of PROs at the point of care [76]. Recently, again BASFI, BASDAI, and the Ankylosing Spondylitis Disease Activity Score assessment in a touchscreen system was feasible, well accepted by patients, and showed good data quality, reliability, and score agreement [77].

Although kids are nowadays digital natives, reports for pediatric rheumatology are scarce [78]. Having implemented and positively evaluated a Web-based application to monitor quality of life-related problems in pediatric rheumatology, the authors recommend implementation of ePROs in pediatric clinical practice [78].

Meanwhile, ePROMs in apps used on smartphones have been evaluated: Toruos et al. showed that patients with depressive disorders are able to use the Patient Health Questionnaire-9 (PHQ-9) in an app on their personal smartphones to self-assess their symptoms of depression and that app scores strongly correlated with traditionally administered PHQ-9 scores [63]. Recently, Richter et al. compared RA patients' mobile data entry of a set of PROs (FFbH/HAQ, RADAI) using an app on a smartphone to paper–pencil versions. The authors demonstrated that patients are able to complete ePROMs in a mobile medical app (mApp) on a smartphone and that scores obtained by patients direct data entry on the smartphone did not differ significantly from the paper–pencil scores [79]. Strengths and weaknesses of apps and mobile health in the routine rheumatology service have been summarized by El Miedany [80].

ePROMs in Telemedicine Applications

Telemedicine bridges a spatial distance and involves information technologies such as interactive audio and video communications, email, smartphone, and other forms of telecommunications technology [81]. Telemedicine respectively telemonitoring applications are complex innovations offering many evaluated opportunities: They showed positive effects on hospitalization, quality of life, and costs in other chronic diseases [82, 83]. Telemedicine developments are regarded as a healthcare alternative for patient remote monitoring even in more rural areas [84–86].

In 2012 "telerheumatology" was promoted as a solution to the national shortage of rheumatologists in Australia, which might serve as a model for other regions with shortages in manpower [85]. Additionally, a telemonitoring approach to self-managed kinesiotherapy sessions for the rehabilitation of hand function in patients with systemic sclerosis and RA has been evaluated positively [87]. In fibromyalgia, Salaffi et al. assessed an Internet-based home telemedical surveillance system. The system effectively evaluated pain and other health outcomes. The authors concluded that telemonitoring proved to be an easy to-use solution for patient-centered data acquisition [88]. From the patients' perspective, preliminary quality attributes important to telemedicine encounters have been published [89]. This underlines that telemedicine might provide further possibilities, but still needs further evaluation [82].

Design and Technical Aspects

Systems need to be user-friendly and intuitive and should pose minimal burden on the staff to reach successful integration and sustained use [41, 90]. Electronic PROMs questions can be depicted in different ways, for example, from one question to various questions per screen at a time, allowance of the "not applicable/unknown options," ticks, or radiobuttons. Software applications can be programmed differently, for example, they require an item response, represent missed items, and/or respect patients' rights to leave questions unanswered. The resulting varying design features may result in a different answering behavior and thus might affect ePROMs' results [41, 50]. Another biasing factor that needs to be considered is whether patients answer the ePROMs on their own or are assisted by relatives or support personnel; some PROMs offer even two different versions [91].

While most apps are developed without taking all stakeholders' needs and requirements into account, Herschman et al. published a methodology for developing a health app for patients with systemic lupus erythematosus to generate guidance to mobile app developers [92]. Besides well-known issues for software development (as easy navigation, informational content, etc.) aspects of gamification and options for customization were identified as being relevant in the development process [92]. As patient groups may have different technology comfort levels (e.g., of the graphical user interface) design needs to be evaluated by patients and adapted [51, 93]. In addition, as discussed for Internet sites that provide information on diseases, apps need to be flagged as high quality when their intended use is to enhance the interactions with the stakeholders [94, 95].

Technical and Data Security Aspects

Systems might handle missing data differently. This given situation is complicated by the fact that not all PROMs score algorithms comment on how to handle missing data. Thus, there may be errors in the calculation of the scores and this may have an effect on the clinical decision making. System validation studies are indispensible, as the user must be able to rely on correct score calculations.

Assessments of ePROMs implicate a large amount of infrastructure-related issues as data security, analytic, and practical issues. These issues may differ in the systems but include from the following: given IT infrastructure and related logistic issues at the clinic/private practice, link to patient health record or other data storage systems, data storage issues (databases locations and interactions, time periods, and copies), data access and user rights, pseudonymization issues, self-determinable data storage/withdrawal policies, and standardized analytic and reporting methods [93, 96]. Systems need to consider security issues: If ePROMs are presented to the patients on their own, secure log-ins need to be realized and levels of data encryption need to be determined as well as implemented [41]. Institutional support might influence ePRO assessment [93]. Computer-adaptive testing (CAT) allows less fixed-item testing and might improve data quality and collection efficiency [97].

IT solutions and applying stakeholders need to be aware of self-reported severe health problems: they need to be flagged by the system and/or at least reviewed and judged by qualified health personal (see earlier) and require feedback loops (e.g., for provision of personalized feedback and/or motivational support) that need to be defined as well as presented to all process participants. Systems' automatization processes vary [41]. For example, patients may complete PRO assessments when they want to, others rely on providers' selection of assessment frequency and topics. In addition, some systems alert patients, others do not, these different approaches result in specific education processes for all stakeholders [41].

Educational Tasks

Interactive educational work for patients about PROMs is required when the new terrain for health conversation is entered in rheumatology [98]. Patients might and will be unfamiliar with ePROMs scores depicted respectively communicated to them; thus, it is necessary to make resulting and represented scores intelligible and to inform on the consequences of the results and the minimal clinical important differences. In addition, explanation of the need for follow-ups and reminders is mandatory. (Online) education programs that need to be developed in cooperation with patient representatives might be of help and should consider European League Against Rheumatism (EULAR) recommendations for patient education [99]. The added value of the electronically generated data needs to be clarified to all stakeholders to achieve long-lasting beneficial effects on the treatment process. Other disciplines already have developed and evaluated programs for training clinicians to effectively use PRO data in routine practice [100]. However, training of the staff besides the physician and the patients is also mandatory, for example, nurses might play a key role in ePROMs' sustained implementation and utilization [20, 93].

Legal and Regulatory Aspects

When implementing ePROMs into IT solutions, complex licenses and legal aspects need to be considered [101]. "Copyleft" licensing has been proposed as a solution [101].

In addition to the legal aspects mentioned in the previous "*Technical and Data Security Aspects*" section of this chapter, patient's consent for electronic data transfer (e.g., via wireless/local area networks) and storage needs to be obtained regardless of the (mobile) IT solution. In general, data avoidance and minimization issues need to be taken into account, but the extent might change according to the underlying rheumatic disease and the responsible regulatory authorities [17, 102].

There is already a large number of medical apps on Apple's App Store and Google marketplace. Although many of them would probably need to be regarded as medical devices, they rarely carry, for example, the CE mark that signifies that the product conforms with all European Union (EU) directives or EU regulations that apply to it [103, 104]. One of the main intentions of these regulations is to prevent patients from the risks and potential harm that might overcome them from apps that are not running the way they are intended.

Various healthcare systems in the developed countries put a major focus on high quality of care that includes patients' perspectives and outcomes as "modern" quality of care indicators. Meanwhile regulatory authorities recommend PROMs assessments; even value-based reimbursements that rely on PROMs assessment in the physician office have been implemented [5, 105–107]. Software applications that integrate such quality indicators are capable to assist in monitoring and management as they might facilitate and improve the delivery process of the required information to the regulatory authorities and other key stakeholders [29]. To encourage the acceptance of ePROMs and IT solutions in rheumatology, it is necessary to actively promote the contribution of the use of technologies to outcomes and obligations to all stakeholders [108].

Conclusion

PROMs supply information on health-related topics patients know best. Electronic assessments of PROMs allow bringing the patient perspective into real-time clinical routine care and facilitate patients to participate in their healthcare process immediately. The implementation of new technological developments has become more feasible. Future systems will provide opportunities for automated integration of PROMs tailored to individual needs. The broad adoption of new applications on mobile devices and their connection to existing patient documentation systems might lead to more frequent and continuous documentation of the key outcome measures and thus to new possibilities for sustained implementation of treat to target and other patient management concepts. New business models need to be developed to reimburse ePROMs' assessments apart from the physician visit. However, all stakeholders need to align their interests and enhance their engagement in the multilateral partnership.

References

1. Sargious A, Lee SJ. Remote collection of questionnaires. Clin Exp Rheumatol. 2014;32:168–72.
2. El Miedany Y. Adopting patient-centered care in standard practice: PROMs moving toward disease-specific era. Clin Exp Rheumatol. 2014;32:S40–6.
3. Roy J. Why do we need new patient-reported outcomes? J Hand Ther. 2015;28:336. doi:10.1016/j.jht.2015.01.010.
4. Ayis S, Wellwood I, Rudd AG, McKevitt C, Parkin D, Wolfe CDA, et al. Variations in Health-Related Quality of Life (HRQoL) and survival 1 year after stroke: five European population-based registers. BMJ Open. 2015;5:e007101. doi:10.1136/bmjopen-2014-007101.

5. Jensen RE, Rothrock NE, DeWitt EM, Spiegel B, Tucker CA, Crane HM, et al. The role of technical advances in the adoption and integration of patient-reported outcomes in clinical care. Med Care. 2015;53:153–9. doi:10.1097/MLR.0000000000000289.
6. Calvert M, Blazeby J, Altman DG, Revicki DA, Moher D, Brundage MD. Reporting of patient-reported outcomes in randomized trials: the CONSORT PRO extension. JAMA. 2013;309:814–22. doi:10.1001/jama.2013.879.
7. El Miedany Y. PROMs in inflammatory arthritis: moving from static to dynamic. Clin Rheumatol. 2013;32:735–42. doi:10.1007/s10067-013-2228-0.
8. Snyder CF, Aaronson NK. Use of patient-reported outcomes in clinical practice. Lancet. 2009;374:369–70. doi:10.1016/S0140-6736(09)61400-8.
9. Valderas JM, Kotzeva A, Espallargues M, Guyatt G, Ferrans CE, Halyard MY, et al. The impact of measuring patient-reported outcomes in clinical practice: a systematic review of the literature. Qual Life Res. 2008;17:179–93. doi:10.1007/s11136-007-9295-0.
10. Eriksson JK, Askling J, Arkema EV. The Swedish Rheumatology Quality Register: optimisation of rheumatic disease assessments using register-enriched data. Clin Exp Rheumatol. 2014;32:S147–9.
11. Greene ME, Rolfson O, Gordon M, Garellick G, Nemes S. Standard Comorbidity Measures Do Not Predict Patient-reported Outcomes 1 Year After Total Hip Arthroplasty. Clin Orthop Relat Res. 2015;473(11):3370–9. doi:10.1007/s11999-015-4195-z.
12. Hetland ML. DANBIO—powerful research database and electronic patient record. Rheumatology. 2011;50:69–77. doi:10.1093/rheumatology/keq309.
13. Deutsch A, Smith L, Gage B, Kelleher C, Garfinkel D. Patient-reported outcomes (PROs) workshop # 1 July 30-31, 2012: workshop summary [Internet]. 2012. https://www.qualityforum.org/Calendar/2012/07/Patient-Reported_Outcomes--Workshop_-_2012-07-30.aspx. Accessed 24 Sep 2015.
14. Snyder CF, Jensen R, Courtin SO, Wu AW. PatientViewpoint: a website for patient-reported outcomes assessment. Qual Life Res. 2009;18:793–800. doi:10.1007/s11136-009-9497-8.
15. European Medical Agency. Committee for Medicinal Products for Human Use (CMHP). Reflection paper on the regulatory guidance for the use of health-related quality of life (HRQL) measures in the evaluation of medicinal products. Doc. Ref. EMEA/CHMP/EWP/139391/2004; 2005.
16. U.S. Department of Health and Human Services Food and Drug Administration. Guidance for industry: Patient-reported outcome measures: Use in medical product development to support labeling claims [Internet]. 2009. http://www.fda.gov/downloads/Drugs/…/Guidances/UCM193282.pdf. Accessed 21 Sep 2015.
17. Locklear T, Weinfurt KP, Abernethy A, Flynn KE, Riley W, Johnson LL. Patient-reported outcome [Internet]. http://sites.duke.edu/rethinkingclinicaltrials/patient-reported-outcomes/. Accessed 21 Sep 2015.
18. Wilson AS, Kitas GD, Carruthers DM, Reay C, Skan J, Harris S, et al. Computerized information-gathering in specialist rheumatology clinics: an initial evaluation of an electronic version of the Short Form 36. Rheumatology. 2002;41:268–73.
19. Bliven BD, Kaufman SE, Spertus JA. Electronic collection of health-related quality of life data: validity, time benefits, and patient preference. Qual Life Res. 2001;10:15–22.
20. Smith SK, Rowe K, Abernethy AP. Use of an electronic patient-reported outcome measurement system to improve distress management in oncology. Palliat Support Care. 2014;12:69–73. doi:10.1017/S1478951513000345.
21. Anderson J, Caplan L, Yazdany J, Robbins ML, Neogi T, Michaud K, et al. Rheumatoid arthritis disease activity measures: American College of Rheumatology recommendations for use in clinical practice. Arthritis Care Res. 2012;64:640–7. doi:10.1002/acr.21649.
22. Van Der Wees PJ, Nijhuis-Van Der Sanden MW, Ayanian JZ, Black N, Westert GP, Schneider EC. Integrating the use of patient-reported outcomes for both clinical practice and performance measurement: views of experts from 3 countries. Milbank Q. 2014;92:754–75. doi:10.1111/1468-0009.12091.
23. Gilek-Seibert K, Prescott K, Kazi S. Outcome assessments in rheumatoid arthritis. Curr Rheumatol Rep. 2013;15:370. doi:10.1007/s11926-013-0370-y.

24. Schoels M, Aletaha D, Smolen JS, Bijlsma JW, Burmester G, Breedveld FC, et al. Follow-up standards and treatment targets in rheumatoid arthritis: results of a questionnaire at the EULAR 2008. Ann Rheum Dis. 2010;69:575–8. doi:10.1136/ard.2009.108472.
25. Cush JJ, Curtis JR. Treat-to-target (T2T) and measuring outcomes in RA care: a 2014 longitudinal survey of US rheumatologists. Arthritis Rheumatol. 2014;66(11 Suppl):S48.
26. Ovretveit J, Keller C, Hvitfeldt Forsberg H, Essen A, Lindblad S, Brommels M. Continuous innovation: developing and using a clinical database with new technology for patient-centred care—the case of the Swedish quality register for arthritis. International J Qual Health Care. 2013;25:118–24. doi:10.1093/intqhc/mzt002.
27. Tran V, Harrington M, Montori VM, Barnes C, Wicks P, Ravaud P. Adaptation and validation of the Treatment Burden Questionnaire (TBQ) in English using an internet platform. BMC Med. 2014;12:109. doi:10.1186/1741-7015-12-109.
28. Rothman M, Gnanaskathy A, Wicks P, Papadopoulos EJ. Can we use social media to support content validity of patient-reported outcome instruments in medical product development? Value Health. 2015;18:1–4. doi:10.1016/j.jval.2014.10.001.
29. Bennett AV, Jensen RE, Basch E. Electronic patient-reported outcome systems in oncology clinical practice. CA Cancer J Clin. 2012;62:336–47. doi:10.3322/caac.21150.
30. Chung AE, Basch EM. Incorporating the patient's voice into electronic health records through patient-reported outcomes as the "review of systems". J Am Med Inform Assoc. 2015;22:914–6. doi:10.1093/jamia/ocu007.
31. McCall J. Mobile health (mHealth) and PROs [Internet]. 2014. http://sites.duke.edu/rethinkingclinicaltrials/2014/01/03/mhealth-presentations/. Accessed 21 Sep 2015.
32. Greenwood MC. Touch-screen computer systems in the rheumatology clinic offer a reliable and user-friendly means of collecting quality-of-life and outcome data from patients with rheumatoid arthritis. Rheumatology. 2006;45:66–71. doi:10.1093/rheumatology/kei100.
33. Richter JG, Becker A, Koch T, Nixdorf M, Willers R, Monser R, et al. Self-assessments of patients via Tablet PC in routine patient care: comparison with standardised paper questionnaires. Ann Rheum Dis. 2008;67:1739–41. doi:10.1136/ard.2008.090209.
34. Strong LE. The past, present, and future of patient-reported outcomes in oncology. Am Soc Clin Oncol Educ Book 2015:e616–20.
35. Buxton J, White M, Osoba D. Patients' experiences using a computerized program with a touch-sensitive video monitor for the assessment of health-related quality of life. Qual Life Res. 1998;7:513–9.
36. Ryan JM, Corry JR, Attewell R, Smithson MJ. A comparison of an electronic version of the SF-36 General Health Questionnaire to the standard paper version. Qual Life Res. 2002;11:19–26.
37. Sudano JJ, Kofford B, Wotman S. Using tablet PC's in dental practice research: technology, cost savings, and direct data entry "on the go". J Public Health Dent. 2005;65:244–5.
38. Snyder CF, Wu AW, Miller RS, Jensen RE, Bantug ET, Wolff AC. The role of informatics in promotingpatient-centeredcare.CancerJ.2011;17:211–8.doi:10.1097/PPO.0b013e318225ff89.
39. Desai SP, Yazdany J. Quality measurement and improvement in rheumatology: rheumatoid arthritis as a case study. Arthritis Rheum. 2011;63:3649–60. doi:10.1002/art.30605.
40. Schaeren S, Bischoff-Ferrari HA, Knupp M, Dick W, Huber JF, Theiler R. A computer touch-screen version of the North American Spine Society outcome assessment instrument for the lumbar spine. J Bone Joint Surg Br. 2005;87:201–4.
41. Jensen RE, Snyder CF, Abernethy AP, Basch E, Potosky AL, Roberts AC, et al. Review of electronic patient-reported outcomes systems used in cancer clinical care. J Oncol Pract. 2013;10:e215. doi:10.1200/JOP.2013.001067.
42. Glasgow RE, Kaplan RM, Ockene JK, Fisher EB, Emmons KM. Patient-reported measures of psychosocial issues and health behavior should be added to electronic health records. Health Aff (Millwood). 2012;31:497–504. doi:10.1377/hlthaff.2010.1295.
43. Stone AA, Shiffman S, Schwartz JE, Broderick JE, Hufford MR. Patient compliance with paper and electronic diaries. Control Clin Trials. 2003;24:182–99. doi:10.1016/S0197-2456(02)00320-3.

44. El Miedany Y, El Gaafary M, Palmer D. Assessment of the utility of visual feedback in the treatment of early rheumatoid arthritis patients: a pilot study. Rheumatol Int. 2012;32:3061–8. doi:10.1007/s00296-011-2098-1.
45. Newman ED, Lerch V, Billet J, Berger A, Kirchner HL. Improving the quality of care of patients with rheumatic disease using patient-centric Electronic Redesign Software. Arthritis Care Res. 2015;67:546–53. doi:10.1002/acr.22479.
46. Kirwan JR, Ahlmén M, de Wit M, Heiberg T, Hehir M, Hewlett S, et al. Progress since OMERACT 6 on including patient perspective in rheumatoid arthritis outcome assessment. J Rheumatol. 2005;32:2246–9.
47. Campbell N, Ali F, Finlay AY, Salek SS. Equivalence of electronic and paper-based patient-reported outcome measures. Qual Life Res. 2015;24:1949–61. doi:10.1007/s11136-015-0937-3.
48. Bent H, Ratzlaff CR, Goligher EC, Kopec JA, Gillies JH. Computer-administered bath ankylosing spondylitis and Quebec Scale outcome questionnaires for low back pain: agreement with traditional paper format. J Rheumatol. 2005;32:669–72.
49. Koevoets R, de Glas NA, Le Bourlout C, Huizinga TWJ, Allaart CF, Dougados M, et al. Autonomous online health assessment questionnaire registry in daily clinical practice. Rheumatology. 2013;52:883–7. doi:10.1093/rheumatology/kes389.
50. Gwaltney CJ, Shields AL, Shiffman S. Equivalence of electronic and paper-and-pencil administration of patient-reported outcome measures: a meta-analytic review. Value Health. 2008;11:322–33. doi:10.1111/j.1524-4733.2007.00231.x.
51. Kirwan JR, Hewlett SE, Heiberg T, Hughes RA, Carr M, Hehir M, et al. Incorporating the patient perspective into outcome assessment in rheumatoid arthritis-progress at OMERACT 7. J Rheumatol. 2005;32:2250–6.
52. Coons SJ, Gwaltney CJ, Hays RD, Lundy JJ, Sloan JA, Revicki DA, et al. Recommendations on evidence needed to support measurement equivalence between electronic and paper-based patient-reported outcome (PRO) measures: ISPOR ePRO Good Research Practices Task Force Report. Value Health. 2009;12:419–29. doi:10.1111/j.1524-4733.2008.00470.x.
53. Amarasingham R, Plantinga L, Diener-West M, Gaskin DJ, Powe NR. Clinical information technologies and inpatient outcomes: a multiple hospital study. Arch Intern Med. 2009;169:108–14. doi:10.1001/archinternmed.2008.520.
54. Hartzler A, McCarty CA, Rasmussen LV, Williams MS, Brilliant M, Bowton EA, et al. Stakeholder engagement: a key component of integrating genomic information into electronic health records. Genet Med. 2013;15:792–801. doi:10.1038/gim.2013.127.
55. Deutsche Gesellschaft für Rheumatologie. EDV Dokumentation online [Internet]. http://dgrh.de/rheumaedv.html. Accessed 20 Sep 2015.
56. Schacher et al. Projektförderung der AGRZ: Einsatz von IT-Dokumentationssystemen in der rheumatologischen Patientenversorgung—Anwendungserprobung und Usability-Vergleich der Softwaresysteme Ardis, Documed.rh und Rheumadok. Z Rheumatol. 2009:68(Suppl 1):34.
57. Azevedo AR, de Sousa HM, Monteiro JA, Lima AR. Future perspectives of Smartphone applications for rheumatic diseases self-management. Rheumatol Int. 2015;35:419–31. doi:10.1007/s00296-014-3117-9.
58. Dennison L, Morrison L, Conway G, Yardley L. Opportunities and challenges for smartphone applications in supporting health behavior change: qualitative study. J Med Internet Res. 2013;15:e86. doi:10.2196/jmir.2583.
59. Donker T, Petrie K, Proudfoot J, Clarke J, Birch M, Christensen H. Smartphones for smarter delivery of mental health programs: a systematic review. J Med Internet Res. 2013;15:e247. doi:10.2196/jmir.2791.
60. Martínez-Pérez B, de la Torre-Díez I, López-Coronado M. Mobile health applications for the most prevalent conditions by the World Health Organization: review and analysis. J Med Internet Res. 2013;15:e120. doi:10.2196/jmir.2600.
61. Heiberg T, Kvien TK, Dale Ø, Mowinckel P, Aanerud GJ, Songe-Møller AB, et al. Daily health status registration (patient diary) in patients with rheumatoid arthritis: a comparison between personal digital assistant and paper-pencil format. Arthritis Rheum. 2007;57:454–60. doi:10.1002/art.22613.

62. Luckmann R, Vidal A. Design of a handheld electronic pain, treatment and activity diary. J Biomed Inform. 2010;43:S32. doi:10.1016/j.jbi.2010.05.005.
63. Torous J, Staples P, Shanahan M, Lin C, Peck P, Keshavan M, et al. Utilizing a Personal Smartphone Custom App to assess the patient health questionnaire-9 (PHQ-9) depressive symptoms in patients with major depressive disorder. JMIR Mental Health. 2015;2:e8. doi:10.2196/mental.3889.
64. Hufford MR, Shields AL. Electronic diaries: applications and what works in the field. Appl Clin Trials. 2002;11(4):46–59.
65. Stone AA, Shiffman S, Schwartz JE, Broderick JE, Hufford MR. Patient non-compliance with paper diaries. BMJ. 2002;324:1193–4.
66. Gvozdenović E, Koevoets R, Wolterbeek R, van der Heijde D, Huizinga TW, Allaart CF, et al. Assessment of global disease activity in RA patients monitored in the METEOR database: the patient‘s versus the rheumatologist‘s opinion. Clin Rheumatol. 2014;33:461–6. doi:10.1007/s10067-013-2390-4.
67. Koevoets R, de Glas NA, Le Bourlout C, Huizinga TW, Allaart CF, Dougados M, et al. Autonomous online health assessment questionnaire registry in daily clinical practice. Rheumatology (Oxford). 2013;52:883–7. doi:10.1093/rheumatology/kes389.
68. Richter J, Muth T, Becker A, Koch T, Schneider M. Online data aquisition of medical outcome Studies Short Form (SF36) in female Systemic Lupus Erythematodes (SLE) patients. Ann Rheum Dis. 2009;68 (Suppl 3):356.
69. Richter J, Muth T, Becker A, Koch T, Schneider M. Is online data aquisition of medical outcome studies Short Form (SF36) feasible in female patients with Rheumatois Arthritis (RA) and delivering equivalent data compared to paper-based data acquisition? Ann Rheum Dis. 2010;69(Suppl3):650.
70. Walter MJ, Mohd Din SH, Hazes JM, Lesaffre E, Barendregt PJ, Luime JJ. Is tightly controlled disease activity possible with online patient-reported outcomes? J Rheumatol. 2014;41:640–7. doi:10.3899/jrheum.130174.
71. Kleinman L, Leidy NK, Crawley J, Bonomy A, Schoenfeld P. A comparative trial of paper-and-pencil versus computer administration of the Quality of Life in Reflux and Dyspepsia (QOLRAD) questionnaire. Med Care. 2001;39:181–9.
72. Velikova G, Wright EP, Smith AB, Cull A, Gould A, Forman D, et al. Automated collection of quality-of-life data: a comparison of paper and computer touch-screen questionnaires. J Clin Oncol. 1999;17:998–1007.
73. Kvien TK. Performance of health status measures with a pen based personal digital assistant. Ann Rheum Dis. 2005;64:1480–4. doi:10.1136/ard.2004.030437.
74. Thumboo J, Wee H, Cheung Y, Machin D, Luo N, Feeny D, et al. Computerized administration of health-related quality of life instruments compared to interviewer administration may reduce sample size requirements in clinical research: a pilot randomized controlled trial among rheumatology patients. Clin Exp Rheumatol. 2007;25:577–83.
75. Schefte DB, Hetland ML. An open-source, self-explanatory touch screen in routine care. Validity of filling in the Bath measures on Ankylosing Spondylitis Disease Activity Index, Function Index, the Health Assessment Questionnaire and Visual Analogue Scales in comparison with paper versions. Rheumatology. 2009;49:99–104. doi:10.1093/rheumatology/kep333.
76. Newman ED, Lerch V, Jones JB, Stewart W. Touchscreen questionnaire patient data collection in rheumatology practice: development of a highly successful system using process redesign. Arthritis Care Res. 2012;64:589–96. doi:10.1002/acr.21560.
77. Salaffi F, Gasparini S, Ciapetti A, Gutierrez M, Grassi W. Usability of an innovative and interactive electronic system for collection of patient-reported data in axial spondyloarthritis: comparison with the traditional paper-administered format. Rheumatology. 2013;52:2062–70. doi:10.1093/rheumatology/ket276.
78. Haverman L, van Rossum MA, van Veenendaal M, van den Berg JM, Dolman KM, Swart J, et al. Effectiveness of a web-based application to monitor health-related quality of life. Pediatrics. 2013;131:e533. doi:10.1542/peds.2012-0958.

79. Richter JG, Kampling C, Chehab G, Acar H, Becker A, Dieckert M, et al. Mobile medical documentation of patient-reported-outcome [abstract]. Arthritis Rheumatol. 2015;67:(Suppl 10). http://acrabstracts.org/abstract/mobile-medical-documentation-of-patient-reported-outcome/. Accessed 30 Sep 2015.
80. El Miedany Y. e-Rheumatology: are we ready? Clin Rheumatol. 2015;34:831–7. doi:10.1007/s10067-015-2897-y.
81. American Telemedicine Association. What is telemedicine? [Internet]. http://www.americantelemed.org/about-telemedicine/what-is-telemedicine#.VgeaJX0pXnl. Accessed 27 Sep 2015.
82. Ekeland AG, Bowes A, Flottorp S. Methodologies for assessing telemedicine: a systematic review of reviews. Int J Med Inform. 2012;81:1–11. doi:10.1016/j.ijmedinf.2011.10.009.
83. Inglis SC, Clark RA, McAlister FA, Ball J, Lewinter C, Cullington D, et al. Structured telephone support or telemonitoring programmes for patients with chronic heart failure. Cochrane Database Syst Rev. 2010:CD007228. doi:10.1002/14651858.CD007228.pub2.
84. Meade BJ, Dunbar JA. A virtual clinic: telemetric assessment and monitoring for rural and remote areas. 2004. http://www.rrh.org.au/articles/subviewnew.asp?ArticleID=296. Accessed 23 Sep 2015.
85. Roberts LJ, Lamont EG, Lim I, Sabesan S, Barrett C. Telerheumatology: an idea whose time has come. Intern Med J. 2012;42:1072–8. doi:10.1111/j.1445-5994.2012.02931.x.
86. Davis P, Howard R, Brockway P. Telehealth consultations in rheumatology: cost-effectiveness and user satisfaction. J Telemed Telecare. 2001;7 Suppl 1:10–1.
87. Piga M, Tradori I, Pani D, Barabino G, Dessì A, Raffo L, et al. Telemedicine applied to kinesiotherapy for hand dysfunction in patients with systemic sclerosis and rheumatoid arthritis: recovery of movement and telemonitoring technology. J Rheumatol. 2014;41:1324–33. doi:10.3899/jrheum.130912.
88. Salaffi F, Ciapetti A, Gasparini S, Atzeni F, Sarzi-Puttini P, Baroni M. Web/Internet-based telemonitoring of a randomized controlled trial evaluating the time-integrated effects of a 24-week multicomponent intervention on key health outcomes in patients with fibromyalgia. Clin Exp Rheumatol. 2015;33:S93–101.
89. LeRouge C, Garfield M, Hevner A. Patient perspectives of telemedicine quality. Patient Prefer Adherence. 2014;9:25–40. doi:10.2147/PPA.S67506.
90. Ennis L, Robotham D, Denis M, Pandit N, Newton D, Rose D, et al. Collaborative development of an electronic Personal Health Record for people with severe and enduring mental health problems. BMC Psychiatry. 2014;14:1477. doi:10.1186/s12888-014-0305-9.
91. Bullinger M, Kirchberger I. SF-36 Fragebogen zum Gesundheitszustand. Handanweisung. Göttingen: Hogrefe; 1998.
92. Herschman J, Kasenberg T, Levy D, Ruth N, Taberner C, Kaufman M, et al. Development of a smartphone app for adolescents with lupus: a collaborative meeting-based methodology inclusive of a wide range of stakeholders. Rev Panam Salud Publica. 2014;35:471–6.
93. Schick-Makaroff K, Molzahn A. Strategies to use tablet computers for collection of electronic patient-reported outcomes. Health Qual Life Outcomes. 2015;13:2. doi:10.1186/s12955-014-0205-1.
94. Richter JG, Becker A, Specker C, Monser R, Schneider M. Krankheitsbezogene Internetnutzung bei Patienten mit entzündlich-rheumatischen Systemerkrankungen. Z Rheumatol. 2004;63:216–22. doi:10.1007/s00393-004-0571-x.
95. Eysenbach G. Towards ethical guidelines for e-health: JMIR theme issue on eHealth ethics. J Med Internet Res. 2000;2:E7. doi:10.2196/jmir.2.1.e7.
96. Segal C, Holve E, Sabharwal R. Collecting and using patient-reported outcomes (PRO) for comparative effectiveness research (CER) and patient-centered outcomes research (PCOR): challenges and opportunities [Internet]. 2013. http://repository.academyhealth.org/edm_briefs/10. Accessed 27 Sep 2015.
97. Snyder CF, Jensen RE, Segal JB, Wu AW. Patient-reported outcomes (PROs): putting the patient perspective in patient-centered outcomes research. Med Care. 2013;51:S73–9. doi:10.1097/MLR.0b013e31829b1d84.

98. Baldwin M, Spong A, Doward L, Gnanasakthy A. Patient-reported outcomes, patient-reported information: from randomized controlled trials to the social web and beyond. Patient. 2011;4:11–7.
99. Zangi HA, Ndosi M, Adams J, Andersen L, Bode C, Boström C, et al. EULAR recommendations for patient education for people with inflammatory arthritis. Ann Rheum Dis. 2015;74:954–62. doi:10.1136/annrheumdis-2014-206807.
100. Santana MJ, Haverman L, Absolom K, Takeuchi E, Feeny D, Grootenhuis M, et al. Training clinicians in how to use patient-reported outcome measures in routine clinical practice. Qual Life Res. 2015;24:1707–18. doi:10.1007/s11136-014-0903-5.
101. Newman JC, Feldman R. Copyright and Open Access at the Bedside. N Engl J Med. 2011;365(26):2447–9.
102. German Federal Ministry of Justice and Consumer Protection. German Federal Data Protection Act [Internet]. 1990. http://www.gesetze-im-internet.de/bdsg_1990/. Accessed 22 Sep 2015.
103. European Parliament. Council Directive 93/42/EEC of 14 June 1993 concerning medical devices, OJ No L 169/1 of 1993-07-12 [Internet]. 1993. http://eur-lex.europa.eu/LexUriServ/LexUriServ.do?uri=CONSLEG:1993L0042:20071011:en:PDF. Accessed 27 Sep 2015.
104. U.S. Department of Health and Human Services Food and Drug Administration. Mobile medical applications: Guidance for Industry and Food and Drug Administration Staff Document [Internet]. http://www.fda.gov/downloads/MedicalDevices/DeviceRegulationandGuidance/GuidanceDocuments/UCM263366.pdf. 2015 Feb 9 [Accessed 27 Sep 2015].
105. Black N. Patient reported outcome measures could help transform healthcare. BMJ. 2013;346:f167. doi:10.1136/bmj.f167.
106. Devlin NJ, Parkin D, Browne J. Patient-reported outcome measures in the NHS: new methods for analysing and reporting EQ-5D data. Health Econ. 2010;19:886–905. doi:10.1002/hec.1608.
107. National Quality Forum. Patient reported outcomes (PROs) in performance measurement [Internet]. 2013. http://www.qualityforum.org/Publications/2012/12/Patient-Reported_Outcomes_in_Performance_Measurement.aspx. Accessed 27 Sep 2015.
108. Cox A, Illsley M, Knibb W, Lucas C, O'Driscoll M, Potter C, et al. The acceptability of e-technology to monitor and assess patient symptoms following palliative radiotherapy for lung cancer. Palliat Med. 2011;25:675–81. doi:10.1177/0269216311399489.

Chapter 16
PROMs and Patient Education

Deborah Palmer and Mwidimi Ndosi

Introduction

Inflammatory musculoskeletal conditions are complex in nature and have a negative impact on the individuals' physical, social, and psychological functioning [1]. This means that all aspects of the patient's life, and their caregivers or family members' lives, are affected. While the management of the disease is usually started in a specialist rheumatology unit, day-to-day management shifts from the health professionals to the patient and/or their caregivers who are expected to undertake self-management activities. Barlow et al. [2] has defined self-management as "the individual's ability to manage the symptoms and the consequences of living with a chronic condition, including treatment, physical, social, and lifestyle changes." To undertake self-management efficiently, patients and/or their caregivers require sufficient knowledge, skills, attitudes, and coping abilities, which can be provided through patient education that is timely and relevant to their needs [3, 4]. Patient education is regarded as an integral part of disease management of most rheumatic conditions. This has been specified in European League Against Rheumatism (EULAR) recommendations for patient education [5] as well as the treatment guidelines of most rheumatic diseases [6–12].

D. Palmer, Diploma Rheumatology Nursing (✉)
Department of Rheumatology, North Middlesex University Hospital, Wilbury Way, London N18 1BX, UK
e-mail: cnsdebsplamer@yahoo.co.uk

M. Ndosi, PhD, MSc, BSc (Hons), RN
School of Healthcare, University of Leeds, Baines Wing, Leeds, West Yorkshire LS2 9JT, UK
e-mail: m.e.ndosi@leeds.ac.uk

Y. El Miedany (ed.), *Patient Reported Outcome Measures in Rheumatic Diseases*,
DOI 10.1007/978-3-319-32851-5_16

The Changing Concepts of Patient Education

In the early years, physicians were regarded as the only authority and source (or "transmitters") of information while patients, playing a passive role, were expected to listen (or "receive") and comply by changing their behaviors. Hoving et al. [13] has described the development of patient education from the early 1960s to the twenty-first century. The major development has been identified as the patients have become more active participants in their care and are increasingly taking more responsibility for their health. It is now generally accepted that effective disease management requires a partnership between the patient and the treating healthcare professional. Shared decision-making helps combine the patient's experience of living with the disease, their values and preferences, together with the health professional's skills and knowledge of the best scientific evidence available [14]. This partnership in care enables effective disease management—targeting the common facets such as management of pain, flare-ups, fatigue, physical, and emotional disabilities, as well as medications—while taking into account the patient's values and needs. A shared decision-making approach is now incorporated in most disease management guidelines [8, 10, 11, 15–18].

The definition of patient education also has gone through many changes over the years. Although most definitions agree that patient education is a planned systematic process, initially the emphasis has focused on the patients' behavioral change or compliance to manage their disease [19, 20], whereas more recently they embrace a more collaborative, health-promoting, and well-being approach [5, 21, 22]. Recently, an international task force of health professionals and patients defined patient education as "a planned interactive learning process designed to support and enable people to manage their life with inflammatory arthritis and optimize their health and well-being" [5]. This definition includes a wide range of educational activities, such as provision of knowledge, written material, e-health, self-management programs, cognitive behavioral therapy (CBT), mindfulness, stress management, individual consultations with healthcare professionals, sharing experiences among patients, motivational discussions, exercise counseling, lifestyle change interventions, and self-help courses. This definition focuses on "supporting" and "enabling" the patients, which for some may lead to behavior change, whereas in others may equip and enable them to make choices that would help optimize their health.

The health-promoting approach is increasingly more relevant in the current management of inflammatory arthritis, which incorporates treat-to-target, time in remission, and management of comorbidities such as cardiovascular diseases. The current management of inflammatory arthritis is such that health professionals and patients need to think about prevention (or management) of comorbidities in addition to their rheumatic disease.

Education Tailored to the Patient's Needs

The Institute of Medicine [23] has defined patient-centered care as "providing care that is respectful of and responsive to individual patient preferences, needs, as well as values, and ensuring that patient values guide all clinical decisions." The underlying principle is similar to that of shared decision-making. This highlights the importance of assessing the patients' needs at the start of the education process. For an individual patient, this may mean assessing where they are in the disease trajectory, their immediate priorities, motivation, and expectations. This may provide an "intervention point," where the health professional may find an area to target patient education leading to an effect that is meaningful to the patient. Since rheumatic diseases have different effects on patients' lives, patients may indeed have different educational needs and priorities for which, if not taken into account, the provided education may not be relevant or meaningful to the patient. Studies of education needs have consistently revealed different levels of needs based on different patient characteristics. For example, in the Netherlands, younger patients with rheumatoid arthritis (RA) had higher levels of educational needs than older patients, especially in dealing with pain and feelings [24]. In the UK, the opposite was true; older patients had a higher level of needs [25]. In psoriatic arthritis (PsA), older patients had a higher level of needs than their younger counterparts in managing pain [26]. Country differences have also been observed. For example, while female patients with RA have been shown to have more educational needs than their male counterparts in the UK [25] and Austria [26], there were no gender differences in educational needs in the Netherlands [24]. This emphasizes the fact that needs may change from time to time and education should be planned to target individual priority needs.

Assessment of needs should culminate in a tailored plan of patient education and goal setting. This may mean, for example, that if a patient's priority need is returning to work, then education and support should be planned with an emphasis and focus on issues related to work; this may well include control of pain, pacing, and maximizing physical function amongst others. The goals of education should specify if patient education at this point is aimed at increasing knowledge, changing attitude, behavior, or all. The goals that constitute SMART [27] are: *S*pecific, *M*easurable, *A*chievable, *R*elevant, and *T*ime-bound. Furthermore, assessment of needs and goal setting will help later in the process of evaluation of the education, making the evaluation more relevant and sensitive to the intervention provided. Clarifying these aims will help both the patient and the clinician to assess the needs and to use effective delivery methods and the most appropriate measures to evaluate the effects. Seeing positive results is likely to motivate patients.

Patient Education: Challenges

Demonstrating the evidence for patient education has been problematic, especially in group-based education. This difficulty is partly contributed to by the use of generic health measures to evaluate the effects of educational programs, some of which did not have clear/specific goals and objectives [28]. Educational programs with more specific goals, such as those with a behavioral component or counseling, have shown superior effects compared to the information-only programs [29–31]. These findings were endorsed by a recent systematic review [5], which revealed that objectives of educational programs were not always clear. Generic measures such as disease activity score (DAS-28), which is unlikely to be directly affected by education, were used to evaluate the effects of patient education. While several biomedical measures are valid for assessing some aspects of disease activity, they are insensitive to most non-pharmacological interventions. Even measuring disease activity relies on composite measures, which take into account biomedical, clinical, as well as patient-reported outcome measures (PROMs). EULAR recommendations for patient education program have therefore specified that outcomes must reflect the objectives [5].

Outcomes of Patient Education

Outcomes of patient education can be categorized as increase in knowledge, improvement in psychosocial status, and change in behavior. Change in one or all of these aspects may translate into improvement of clinical symptoms. However, there is strong evidence to suggest that interventions that focus on change in knowledge only do not necessarily translate into improvement of health status. However, psycho-educational and behavioral interventions are more effective in improving health status [29–31]. While behavioral outcomes (such as adherence to therapy and exercise) can easily be measured using self-report or observation, validated PROMs are required to assess knowledge outcomes (e.g., patient knowledge, educational needs, and health literacy) as well as psycho-educational outcomes (e.g., as self-efficacy, coping, and patient activation). PROMs are more relevant than biomedical measures in evaluating outcomes of non-pharmacological interventions such as patient education. Therefore, it is important that specific PROMs validated for particular outcomes are used for assessment and evaluation in order to ensure that they accurately estimate the effects of patient education in a given domain.

Health professionals have used PROMs innovatively as part of intervention in the patients' care. A recent study revealed that sharing previous PROMs scores and goal setting had a significant impact on improving inflammatory arthritis patients' self-perceived health as well as their adherence to therapy [32]. These findings were endorsed by another work carried out using the Educational Needs Assessment Tool (ENAT) to derive needs-based education in the clinic. Results revealed improvement of patient's self-efficacy as well as other aspects of their health status [33]. However, whilst clinicians can easily deliver knowledge-related patient education [34–36], delivering psychosocial and behavioral-related education, such as cognitive behavior therapy, may require referral to other specialized professionals.

PROMs and Patient Education Programs

In standard clinical settings, two approaches to patient education and self-management have been adopted: the first is a condition/disease-specific self-management program, covering topics such as: managing flare-ups, pain, and fatigue; better use of medication; understanding the benefits of pacing; and action planning. The second approach is patient specific, adopting an individualized self-management program tailored to the patient's needs [5, 20–32, 37]. Recent reports [32, 37] revealed that patient-reported outcome measures can be used as a link between disease outcomes and patient education, as they enable the treating physician and the patient to identify the priority areas that need tackling. The integration of PROMs and patient education offered a new opportunity toward improving patient self-efficacy in disease management. Joint Fitness Program [38], a newly structured patient-derived education program, was recently published as an initiative for people suffering from inflammatory arthritis and/or joint pains. It showed how self-management can be tailored to match patients' needs as identified from the PROMs questionnaire. This represents a step forward in the management of patients suffering from chronic inflammatory musculoskeletal conditions as it integrates the education model into the routine clinical practice aiming at providing a care pathway matching the patient's needs. Thus the self-management/patient education program can be amended and tailored more than once to meet the patient's changing condition throughout their disease trajectory. Using PROMs for assessing and monitoring patient education also supports the patients in identifying their own health needs and responding to them by setting their own specific goals (knowledge/behavioral/psychosocial). Such an individualized need-based approach represents best practice and may help encourage patient motivation.

PROMs and Clinical Outcomes of Patient Education

The potential effect of patient education on disease outcome is of prime concern to both patients and treating clinicians. Quantitative evaluation of the impact of the educational intervention on the clinical outcomes, such as disease activity parameters as well as the patient outcomes including functional ability and quality of life, play an important role in the patient's day-to-day management. Furthermore, it helps to estimate the extent to which the educational goals translate to meaningful measures. Whilst there are specific tools to assess for the educational activity outcomes [33, 39, 40], these remain dedicated for research activities and cannot be implemented in standard clinical practice. A recent study [40] assessed the usability of the Educational Needs Assessment Tool (ENAT) in clinical practice, from a practitioner and patient perspective. Completing the ENAT, prior to clinical assessment, helped the patients to focus on what they needed to know from their visit on that day. However, this means the need for a dedicated session for educational needs assessment.

In contrast, in real life practice, time factor plays a vital role in the patients' assessment and management. Adopting an "all-in-one" service style is the most favorable for the majority of clinicians [41]. In a standard clinical setting, disease outcomes can be recognized as manifestations reflecting the underlying disease process (tender and swollen joints, acute phase response), measures of discomfort (pain, fatigue, patient global assessment, and duration of morning stiffness), measures of disability, quality of life, as well as comorbidity/comortality (such as cardiovascular risk, organ damage, and falls risks). PROMs questionnaires can be used as the link between outcomes and patient education. Identifying the patient's educational requirements from the PROMs questionnaire helps with setting up an educational program tailored to the patient's individual needs. Furthermore, PROMs were reported [42] to be malleable for guided education, meaning that the educational program can be devised to tackle the important components identified by the patient at this stage. As the patient's PROMs reveal improvement in response to the educational activity, other educational requirement may emerge. This would lead to re-stratifying a new self-management education activity adjusted to the patient's newly emerging needs.

PROMs and Cardiovascular Education in Arthritis Patients

While it is important to minimize the negative musculoskeletal aspects of arthritis, attention has been rising toward the other complications of the condition. Formulating an action plan to deal with associated comorbidities can enable patients to think positively and give them control of their situation. Recently, there has been a surge of interest in the assessment of cardiovascular outcomes in arthritic patients recommended by guidelines and highlighted by research studies. Earlier published data reported a cardiovascular risk in rheumatoid arthritis patients similar to that reported for diabetes mellitus [43, 44]. Therefore, it was recommended to include cardiovascular risk management, which comprises identification and treatment/prevention of these risk factors, in standard clinical practice [45, 46]. Recent PROMs questionnaires (Appendices 1 and 2) expanded the outcome measures assessed in a trial to give a comprehensive assessment of the patient's condition at this stage of his/her arthritis [37, 47–49]. This paved the way to include cardiovascular education as part of the disease management in patients with inflammatory arthritis. A recent systematic review of patient education in cardiac patients has supported the benefits of educational interventions in cardiac patients through increasing knowledge and promoting health behavioral change [50].

Visual Feedback and Patient Education

Visual feedback is a relatively new tool that enables the patient to visualize and monitor a real-time change of their disease activity parameters as well as the patient's reported outcome measures. Though research has shown that patient education can bring about improvements in health status [51], and many health professionals believe it to be the key to improved adherence, however, what appears to be consistent across studies of chronic diseases is the notion that patient education efforts alone are not sufficient to improve adherence. Treatment adherence is defined as the extent to which patients follow recommendations and take the medications prescribed by their physicians [52]. Another theoretical question also was raised regarding whether the statistically significant changes produced by the visual feedback intervention were clinically meaningful. In concordance with the note that "patients tend to forget," sharing with the patients their reported scores before and after self-management or therapeutic interventions was reported to have a positive impact on the patients' disease activity status as well as treatment. An earlier study [53] revealed that implementing patient education as part of the standard day-to-day practice and sharing the outcomes with the patients regularly had a positive and significant impact on the disease activity control. Results of another recent work [54] revealed that in early inflammatory arthritis patients the visual feedback provided a significant greater reduction in disease activity parameters as well as improvement of the patients' adherence to antirheumatic therapy. Also stopping the disease-modifying drug therapy because of intolerance was significantly less in the active group. Concern about the future was significantly less in the active group whereas inability to cope with daily life and disease stress were significantly greater among the control group. The improvement of disease activity parameters was associated with improvement in functional disability as well as quality of life scores. Adherence to medication was significantly correlated with changes in all measured disease parameters. The findings of this pilot study revealed that by incorporating the visual feedback approach into clinical practice a new experience can be created. Using visual feedback in the patients' management as well as patient education enabled the patients to see how they are doing regarding their disease activity and helps to optimize their adherence to their treatment.

Patient Activation Measure

"Patient activation" is a recently recognized concept that describes the knowledge, skills, and confidence a person has in managing their own health and healthcare [55]. People who have low activation levels are less likely to play an active role in remaining healthy. They are less good at seeking help when they need it, at following a doctor's advice, and at managing their health when they are no longer being treated. The Patient Activation Measure is a patient-reported measure that has been validated in the United Kingdom and was reported to be a powerful and reliable measure of patient activation [56]. Patient activation scores have been strongly demonstrated to predict a number of health behaviors. They are linked to clinical outcomes, patients' ratings of their experience, as well as the costs of healthcare. Highly activated patients are more likely to adopt healthy behavior, to have better clinical outcomes, to report higher levels of satisfaction with services, and lower rates of hospitalization. On the other hand, patients with low activation levels are more likely to attend accident and emergency departments, to be hospitalized, or to be re-admitted to hospital after being discharged. This is likely to lead to higher healthcare costs.

The Patient Activation Measure tool has been designed to assess an individual's knowledge, skill, and confidence for self-management. It was developed by Hibbard and colleagues in 2004 originally as a 22-item scale, the PAM 22, and subsequently as a 13-item short form [56, 57]. The PAM's 13-item scale asks people about their beliefs, knowledge, and confidence for engaging in a wide range of health behaviors and then assigns an activation score based on their responses to the 13-item scale. The tool was formulated in two versions targeted at people with or without chronic disease, with few reported semantic differences. The authors also reported that the measure has good psychometric properties, indicating that it can be used at the individual patient level to tailor interventions and assess changes. Hibbard and colleagues [56] identified four elements—knowledge, skills, confidence, and behaviors—that are critical for coping with a chronic illness, and suggested 4 stages of activation that patients go through on their way to becoming fully activated in managing their own health.

Positive changes in patient activation were reported as able to lead to positive self-management behavior changes in patients with chronic conditions [57]. Intervening to increase activation can improve a patient's engagement and health outcomes and is an important factor in helping patients to manage their health. Patient activation interventions have been developed for patients with cancer, diabetes, hypertension, obstetrical and gynecological issues, and end-stage renal disease, as well as osteoarthritis [58]. Improvements in patient activation scores have been seen for up to 18 months following intervention. In concordance, tailoring services provided to the patient's activation levels can maximize productivity and efficiency by safeguarding that the level of support provided is appropriate to the needs of the individual [59]. Therefore, patient activation measure provides a new insight into risk that goes beyond those attained using the traditional sociodemographic factors as it provides a unique measure of engagement and empowerment that can be used to appraise the effectiveness of interventions and to measure the performance of healthcare organizations in involving patients in their own care.

Conclusion

Whilst patients' assessment for their perceived needs/priorities is important, PROMs questionnaires can help clinicians identify their patients' educational requirements. In fact, PROMs can be the link between the needs-based and clinical-based patient education activity. PROMs also enable the treating healthcare professional to meet the expanding scope of patient education, which has gone beyond disease activity to include disability, quality of life, as well as disease-associated comorbidities. Routine use of PROMs has the potential to help transform arthritis treatment toward a targeted management approach tailored to the patient's needs.

Appendix 1: Multidimensional Questionnaire for Patient-Reported Outcome Measures: Arthritis

Reprinted with permission from El Miedany Y, El Gaafary M, Youssef SS, Palmer D. Incorporating patient-reported outcome measures in clinical practice: development and validation of a questionnaire for inflammatory arthritis. Clin Exp Rheumatol 2010; 28(5): 734–744.

Multi-Dimensional Questionnaire for Patient Reported Outcome Measures – Arthritis

This questionnaire includes information not available from blood tests, X-rays, or any source other than you. Please try to answer each question. There is **no right or wrong answer.** Please answer exactly as **YOU** think or feel.

1. We are interested in learning how your illness affects your ability to function in daily life. Please tick (√) the ONE best answer that describes your usual abilities OVER THE PAST WEEK:

Over the **LAST WEEK** were you able to	Without ANY Difficulty	With SOME Difficulty	With MUCH Difficulty	Unable TO DO	
1. Get on and off the toilet?	....	....	....	....	**Fn. Disability**
2. Use your grip strength; eg, open previously opened jars Or lift a saucepan during cooking?	....	....	....	....	
3. Dress yourself, including tying shoelaces & doing buttons?	....	....	....	....	**QoL**
4. Stand up from a chair without arms?	....	....	....	....	
5. Wait in a line for 15 minutes?	....	....	....	....	
6. Reach and get down a 5-pound object (such as a bag of sugar) from just above your head?	....	....	....	....	
7. Walk outdoors on flat ground?	....	....	....	....	
8. Go up 2 or more flights of stairs?	....	....	....	....	
9. Do housework/DIY jobs around the house?	....	....	....	....	
10. Move heavy objects?	....	....	....	....	
					Not Applicable
1. Get a good night's sleep?	....	....	....	....	....
2. Deal with the usual stresses of daily life?	....	....	....	....	....
3. Cope with social/family activities?	....	....	....	....	....
4. Deal with feelings of anxiety or being nervous?	....	....	....	....	....
5. Deal with feelings of low self-esteem or feeling blue?	....	....	....	....	....
6. Get going in the morning?	....	....	....	....	....
7. Do your work as you used to do?	....	....	....	....	....
8. Deal with any worries about your future?	....	....	....	....	....
9. Continue doing things you used to do, despite tiredness?	....	....	....	....	....
10. Continue your relationship with your partner (husband/wife)?	....	....	....	....	....

2. How much PAIN have you had because of your arthritis/joint or body aches OVER THE PAST WEEK? Please put a circle around the number that best indicates your level of pain: — Pain

NO PAIN — 0, 5, 10, 15, 20, 25, 30, 35, 40, 45, 50, 55, 60, 65, 70, 75, 80, 85, 90, 95, 100 — PAIN As Bad As It Could Be

3. Considering all the ways your arthritis/joint or body ache may be affecting you AT THIS TIME, Please put a circle around the number that best indicates how well you are doing: — PGA

VERY WELL — 0, 5, 10, 15, 20, 25, 30, 35, 40, 45, 50, 55, 60, 65, 70, 75, 80, 85, 90, 95, 100 — VERY POORLY

4. How much of a problem has UNUSUAL FATIGUE or tiredness been for you OVER THE PAST WEEK? (Please put a circle around the number that best indicates your fatigue) — Fatigue

FATIGUE No Problem — 0, 5, 10, 15, 20, 25, 30, 35, 40, 45, 50, 55, 60, 65, 70, 75, 80, 85, 90, 95, 100 — A MAJOR Problem

5. OVER THE LAST WEEK when you awakened in the morning, did you feel stiff? — MS

YES: ☐ Please indicate the number of minutes ...., or hours .... until you are as limber as you will be for the day.

NO: ☐

Clin Exp Rheumatol 2010; 28:734-744

6. Please place an (X) in the appropriate box to indicate in which of your joints you feel painful TODAY.

Alternatively you can put a figure 1, 2, or 3 to describe the severity of the pain you feel in any joint as follows:

1 = mild pain
2 = moderate pain
3 = severe pain

The section below is for official use. Please do not tick		
ESR:	CRP:	
SJC:	RF:	ACPA:
DAS-28:	BMI:	
B/P: /	Chol: HDL	

Shoulder
Elbow
Wrist
Knuckles/ Fingers
Hip
Knee
Ankle
Top Foot
Toes

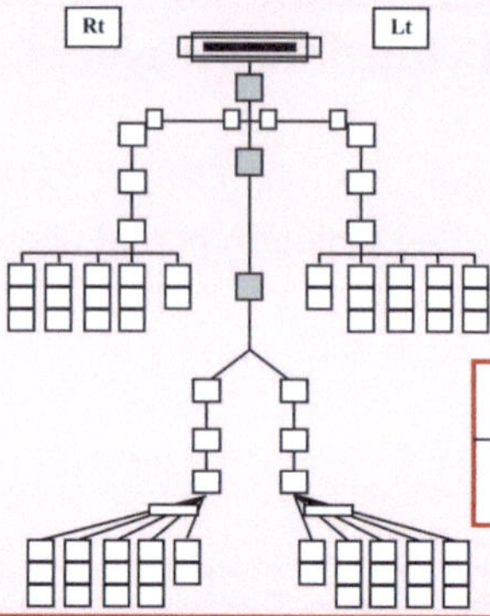

Neck
Shoulder Blade
Low Back

Tender Joint count	
Pt.	Phys.

7. Please tick (√) if you have experienced any of the following OVER THE LAST MONTH:

Fever		Dry eye		Gynecological problem		Cardiovascular Risk Assessment	
Weight loss (> 10 lbs)		Dry mouth		Short plans for having a baby		Age > 50 years old	
Loss of appetite		Other eye problems		Sexual relationship problems		High blood pressure	
Trouble swallowing		Headache		Problems with erection (for men)		High cholesterol	
Soreness in the mouth		Shortness of breath		I am registered disabled		Current smoker	
Bleeding/inflammation of the gum		Wheezing/asthma		Absent from work due to joint pain		Ischemic heart disease	
Psoriasis		Cough		> 3 alcoholic drinks per day		Stroke	
Unusual bruising or bleeding		Heartburn		Lost height		Irregular heart beats	
Numbness or tingling		Feeling sickly/Nausea		Had a recent fracture		Diabetes mellitus	
Loss of hair		Constipation		Falls Risk Assessment			
Swollen glands		Diarrhea		Loss of your balance		Take steroids > 5 mg/day	
Problems with hearing		Dark or bloody stools		Problems with your sight		Ulcer or stomach problem	
Thyroid Disease		Problems with urination		Weakness of your grip strength		Lung disease	
Diagnosed to have cancer		Kidney problems		> 1 fall in the last year		Admitted cos of infection	
Muscle pain, ache, or weakness		Pulmonary embolism/DVT		Change in gait/Slow walking speed		Liver disease	

8. The statements below concern your personal beliefs. Please circle the number that best describes how you feel about the statement. 0 = Not at all; 10 = Strongly Agree

RAI

1. My condition is controlling my life.	0 1 2 3 4 5 6 7 8 9 10
2. I would feel helpless if I could not rely on other people for help with my condition.	0 1 2 3 4 5 6 7 8 9 10
3. I am concerned that medicines cannot help me.	0 1 2 3 4 5 6 7 8 9 10
4. I've concerns regarding side effects of medications used to treat my condition.	0 1 2 3 4 5 6 7 8 9 10
5. I often do not take my medicines as directed.	0 1 2 3 4 5 6 7 8 9 10
6. No matter what I do, or how hard I try, I just cannot seem to get relief from my symptoms.	0 1 2 3 4 5 6 7 8 9 10
7. I am not coping effectively with my condition.	0 1 2 3 4 5 6 7 8 9 10
8. Sometimes I feel my condition is beyond both my and my doctor's control.	0 1 2 3 4 5 6 7 8 9 10
9. Sometimes my condition makes me feel like giving up.	0 1 2 3 4 5 6 7 8 9 10
10. Due to my condition, sometimes I feel I am a burden to those close to me.	0 1 2 3 4 5 6 7 8 9 10

Date: / /201_

□ I consent to my clinical data being used for research/audit.

Signature of the patient: ______________________

Patient:

D.O.B:

Appendix 2: Patient-Reported Outcome Measures for Spondyloarthritis (AS, Psoriasis, IBD)

Reprinted with permission from El Miedany Y, El Gaafary M, Youssef S, Palmer D. Towards a multidimensional patient-reported outcome measures assessment: development and validation of a questionnaire for patients with ankylosing spondylitis/spondyloarthritis. Joint Bone Spine 2010; 77(6): 575–581.

Patient Reported Outcome Measures for Spondyloarthritis (AS, Psoriasis, IBD)

This questionnaire includes information not available from blood tests, X-rays, or any source other than you. Please try to answer each question. There is **no right or wrong answer.** Please answer exactly as **YOU** think or feel.

1. We are interested in learning how your illness affects your ability to function in daily life. Please tick (√) the ONE best answer that describes your usual abilities OVER THE PAST WEEK:

Over the **LAST WEEK** were you able to	Without ANY Difficulty	With SOME Difficulty	With MUCH Difficulty	Unable TO DO	Not Applicable
1. Drink from a glass	....	....	....	....	
2. Dress yourself, including tying shoelaces & putting on socks	....	....	....	....	
3. Bend down to pick up object off the floor	....	....	....	....	
4. Sit for long periods of time; eg, working on flat-topped table or desk	....	....	....	....	
5. Walk outdoors on flat ground including crossing the road	....	....	....	....	
6. Go up 2 or more flights of stairs	....	....	....	....	
7. Play with/look after children	....	....	....	....	
8. Do outside work (such as DIY/gardening/lifting)	....	....	....	....	
9. Lie down/sleep on your back	....	....	....	....	
10. Turn your head whilst reversing your car or using the rear view mirror?	....	....	....	....	
1. Get a good night's sleep?	....	....	....	....	....
2. Deal with the usual stresses of daily life?	....	....	....	....	....
3. Cope with social/family activities?	....	....	....	....	....
4. Deal with feelings of anxiety or being nervous?	....	....	....	....	....
5. Deal with feelings of low self-esteem or feeling blue?	....	....	....	....	....
6. Get going in the morning?	....	....	....	....	....
7. Do your work as you used to do?	....	....	....	....	....
8. Deal with any worries about your future?	....	....	....	....	....
9. Continue doing things you used to do, despite tiredness?	....	....	....	....	....
10. Continue your relationship with your partner (husband/wife)?	....	....	....	....	....

Fn. Disability

QoL

2. How much SPINE PAIN have you had OVER THE PAST WEEK?

NO PAIN 0 0.5 1 1.5 2 2.5 3 3.5 4 4.5 5 5.5 6 6.5 7 7.5 8 8.5 9 9.5 10 SEVERE PAIN

3. How much JOINT PAIN have you had OVER THE PAST WEEK?

NO PAIN 0 0.5 1 1.5 2 2.5 3 3.5 4 4.5 5 5.5 6 6.5 7 7.5 8 8.5 9 9.5 10 SEVERE PAIN

Sp. Pain

J. Pain

4. Consider all the ways your Disease may be affecting you AT THIS TIME. Please put a circle around the number that best indicates how well you are doing.

Very Well 0 0.5 1 1.5 2 2.5 3 3.5 4 4.5 5 5.5 6 6.5 7 7.5 8 8.5 9 9.5 10 Very Poorly

5. How much of a problem has UNUSUAL FATIGUE or tiredness been for you OVER THE PAST WEEK? Please put a circle around the number that best indicates your fatigue.

Fatigue No Problem 0 0.5 1 1.5 2 2.5 3 3.5 4 4.5 5 5.5 6 6.5 7 7.5 8 8.5 9 9.5 10 A Major Problem

PGA

Fatigue

6. Over the Past Week, how much has your skin problem affected your life (felt embarrassed, influenced the clothes you wear, affected you doing a sport, caused problems with your partner or friends.

Not at all 0 0.5 1 1.5 2 2.5 3 3.5 4 4.5 5 5.5 6 6.5 7 7.5 8 8.5 9 9.5 10 Very much

7. How would you rate the severity of your psoriatic skin rash Over the Past Week:

I do not have Psoriasis: □ Please go to Q. 8

No Rash 0 0.5 1 1.5 2 2.5 3 3.5 4 4.5 5 5.5 6 6.5 7 7.5 8 8.5 9 9.5 10 Severe rash affecting my body & scalp

Ps. GA

Ps. QoL

8. OVER THE PAST WEEK how would you rate the severity of your morning stiffness?

NO STIFFNESS 0 5 10 15 20 25 30 35 40 45 50 55 60 65 70 75 80 85 90 95 100 SEVERE STIFFNESS

8. OVER THE PAST WEEK for how long (min./hours) did you feel stiff in the morning?

0 min 30 min 60 min 90 min ≥2h

0 1 2 3 4 5 6 7 8 9 10

MS

El Miedany et al, Joint Bone Spine 2010; 77(6):575

Right	Left
Upper Limb	
Tip of the Shoulder	Tip of the Shoulder
Outer side of the Arm	Outer side of the Arm
Outer/inner side of the Elbow	Outer/inner side of the Elbow
Lower Limb	
Outer Hip Area	Outer Hip Area
Front of the knee	Front of the knee
Back of the ankle	Back of the ankle
Heel	Heel
Jaw	
Jaw (Rt.)	Jaw (Lt.)
Trunk	
Neck	Chest
Upper Back	Abdomen
Lower Back	Other:

Please place (√) at the most painful area(s) over your body that you feel painful TODAY

Enthesitis score

Please place an (X) in the appropriate box to indicate in which of your joints you feel painful TODAY

Tender Joints

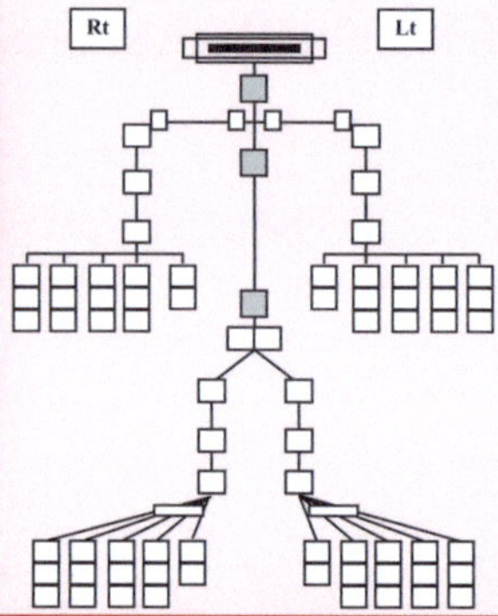

Neck
Shoulder
Shoulder Blade
Elbow
Wrist
Knuckles / Fingers
Low Back
Sacroiliac Joint
Hip
Knee
Ankle
Top Foot
Toes

Please tick (√) if you have experienced any of the following OVER THE LAST MONTH:

Fever	Dry eye	Vertebral fracture(s)	Cardiovascular Risk Assessment
Weight gain (> 10 lbs)	Dry mouth	Weakness/Paralysis of arms or legs	Age > 50 years old
Weight loss (>10 lbs)	Pain in the eye/photophobia	Numbness or tingling	High blood pressure
Night sweat	Headache	Muscle pain, ache, or cramps	High cholesterol
Loss of appetite	Wheezing in the chest	Problems with thiking/memory	Current smoker
Soreness in the mouth	Cough	Absent from work due to spine pain	Ischemic heart disease
Genital ulcers	Blood in your phlegm	Short plans for having a baby	Stroke
Skin rash	Shortness of breath	Sexual relationship problems	Irregular heart beats
Psoriasis	Heartburn	Problems with erection (for men)	Diabetes Mellitus
Painful swollen finger/toe	Dark or bloody stools	Falls Risk Assessment	
Change color/thickening of your nail	Feeling sickly/Nausea	> 1 fall in the last year	Take steroids > 5 mg/day
Inflammatory bowel disease	Constipation	Problems with your sight	Ulcer or stomach problem
Heart valve lesion	Diarrhea	Loss of your balance	Lung disease
Problems with hearing	Problems with urination	Change in gait/Walking speed	Admitted cos of infection
Ringing in the ears	> 3 alcoholic drinks per day	Weakness of your grip strength	Liver disease

The statements below concern your personal beliefs. Please circle the number that best describes how you feel about the statement. 0 = Not at all; 10 = Strongly Agree

mRAI

1. My condition is controlling my life.	0 1 2 3 4 5 6 7 8 9 10
2. I would feel helpless if I could not rely on other people for help with my condition.	0 1 2 3 4 5 6 7 8 9 10
3. I am concerned that medicines cannot help me.	0 1 2 3 4 5 6 7 8 9 10
4. I've concerns regarding side effects of medications used to treat my condition.	0 1 2 3 4 5 6 7 8 9 10
5. I often do not take my medicines as directed.	0 1 2 3 4 5 6 7 8 9 10
6. No matter what I do, or how hard I try, I just cannot seem to get relief from my symptoms.	0 1 2 3 4 5 6 7 8 9 10
7. I am not coping effectively with my condition.	0 1 2 3 4 5 6 7 8 9 10
8. Sometimes I feel my condition is beyond both my and my doctor's control.	0 1 2 3 4 5 6 7 8 9 10
9. Sometimes my condition makes me feel like giving up.	0 1 2 3 4 5 6 7 8 9 10
10. Due to my condition, sometimes I feel I am a burden to those close to me.	0 1 2 3 4 5 6 7 8 9 10

Date: / /201_

□ I consent to my clinical data being used for research/audit.

Signature of the patient: ____________________

Patient:

D.O.B:

References

1. Ryan S, Carr A. Applying the biopsychosocial model to the management of rheumatic disease. Rheumatology: evidence-based practice for physiotherapists and occupational therapists. London: Elsevier Health Sciences; 2010.
2. Barlow J, Wright C, Sheasby J, Turner A, Hainsworth J. Self-management approaches for people with chronic conditions: a review. Patient Educ Couns. 2002;48(2):177–87.
3. Bishop P, Kirwan J, Windsor K. The arc patient literature evaluation project: brief report. Chesterfield: Arthritis and Rheumatism Council for Research; 1997.
4. Koehn CL, Esdaile JM. Patient education and self-management of musculoskeletal diseases. Best Pract Res Clin Rheumatol. 2008;22(3):395–405.
5. Zangi HA, Ndosi M, Adams J, Andersen L, Bode C, Bostrom C, et al. Eular recommendations for patient education for people with inflammatory arthritis. Ann Rheum Dis. 2015;74:954–62.
6. Combe B, Landewé R, Lukas C, Bolosiu HD, Breedveld F, Dougados M, et al. Eular recommendations for the management of early arthritis: report of a task force of the european standing committee for international clinical studies including therapeutics (escisit). Ann Rheum Dis. 2007;66(1):34–45.
7. Khanna D, Fitzgerald JD, Khanna PP, Bae S, Singh MK, Neogi T, et al. 2012 american college of rheumatology guidelines for management of gout. Part 1: systematic nonpharmacologic and pharmacologic therapeutic approaches to hyperuricemia. Arthritis Care Res. 2012;64(10):1431–46.
8. NICE. Rheumatoid arthritis: the management of rheumatoid arthritis in adults. London: Royal College of Physicians; 2009 [cited 29 Jan 2015]. http://www.nice.org.uk/guidance/CG79
9. Bertsias GK, Ioannidis JP, Aringer M, Bollen E, Bombardieri S, Bruce IN, et al. Eular recommendations for the management of systemic lupus erythematosus with neuropsychiatric manifestations: report of a task force of the eular standing committee for clinical affairs. Ann Rheum Dis. 2010;69(12):2074–82.
10. Braun J, van den Berg R, Baraliakos X, Boehm H, Burgos-Vargas R, Collantes-Estevez E, et al. 2010 update of the asas/eular recommendations for the management of ankylosing spondylitis. Ann Rheum Dis [Consensus Development Conference]. 2011;70(6):896–904.
11. Smolen JS, Aletaha D, Bijlsma JW, Breedveld FC, Boumpas D, Burmester G, et al. Treating rheumatoid arthritis to target: recommendations of an international task force. Ann Rheum Dis. [Consensus Development Conference Practice Guideline Research Support, Non-U.S. Gov't]. 2010;69(4):631–7.
12. Fernandes L, Hagen KB, Bijlsma JW, Andreassen O, Christensen P, Conaghan PG, et al. Eular recommendations for the non-pharmacological core management of hip and knee osteoarthritis. Ann Rheum Dis. 2013;72(7):1125–35.
13. Hoving C, Visser A, Mullen PD, van den Borne B. A history of patient education by health professionals in Europe and north America: from authority to shared decision making education. Patient Educ Couns. [Historical Article Review]. 2010;78(3):275–81.
14. Chewning B, Bylund CL, Shah B, Arora NK, Gueguen JA, Makoul G. Patient preferences for shared decisions: a systematic review. Patient Educ Couns. 2012;86(1):9–18.
15. Smolen JS, Landewe R, Breedveld FC, Buch M, Burmester G, Dougados M, et al. Eular recommendations for the management of rheumatoid arthritis with synthetic and biological disease-modifying antirheumatic drugs: 2013 update. Ann Rheum Dis. 2014;73(3):492–509.
16. Luqmani R, Hennell S, Estrach C, Birrell F, Bosworth A, Davenport G, et al. British society for rheumatology and british health professionals in rheumatology guideline for the management of rheumatoid arthritis (the first two years). Rheumatology. 2006;45(9):1167–9.
17. Scottish Intercollegiate Guidelines Network (SIGN). Management of early rheumatoid arthritis—a national clinical guideline. Edinburgh: SIGN; 2011.
18. Peters M, Symmons D, McCarey D, Dijkmans B, Nicola P, Kvien T, et al. Eular evidence-based recommendations for cardiovascular risk management in patients with rheumatoid arthritis and other forms of inflammatory arthritis. Ann Rheum Dis. 2010;69(2):325–31.

19. Green LW, Kreuter MW, Deeds SG, Partridge KB, Bartlett E. Health education planning: a diagnostic approach. Mountain View: Mayfield; 1980.
20. Lorig K, Visser A. Arthritis patient education standards: a model for the future. Patient Educ Couns. 1994;24(1):3–7.
21. Dreeben-Irimia O. Patient education in rehabilitation. Sudbury: Jones & Bartlett Publishers; 2010.
22. Bastable SB. Nurse as educator. Sudbury: Jones & Bartlett Publishers; 2008.
23. Anonymous. Crossing the quality chasm: a new health system for the 21st century. Washington, DC: National Academy Press; 2001.
24. Meesters JJ, Vliet Vlieland T, Hill J, Ndosi M. Measuring educational needs among patients with rheumatoid arthritis using the dutch version of the educational needs assessment tool (denat). Ann Rheum Dis. 2009;68 Suppl 3:773.
25. Ndosi M, Hill J, Hale C, Hardware B. Educational needs of patients with 6 rheumatic diseases. Rheumatology. [Meeting Abstract]. 2009;48:I160–1.
26. Dragoi RG, Ndosi M, Sadlonova M, Hill J, Duer M, Graninger W, et al. Patient education, disease activity and physical function: can we be more targeted? A cross sectional study among people with rheumatoid arthritis, psoriatic arthritis and hand osteoarthritis. Arthritis Res Ther. 2013;15(5):R156.
27. Barnes MP, Ward AB, Barnes MPTorm. Oxford handbook of rehabilitation medicine. New ed. Oxford: Oxford University Press; 2005.
28. Li LC. If knowledge is power, why don't rheumatoid arthritis education programs show better outcomes? J Rheumatol. 2007;34(8):1645–6.
29. Niedermann K, Fransen J, Knols R, Uebelhart D. Gap between short- and long-term effects of patient education in rheumatoid arthritis patients: a systematic review. Arthritis Care Res. 2004;51(3):388–98.
30. Riemsma RP, Taal E, Kirwan JR, Rasker JJ. Systematic review of rheumatoid arthritis patient education. Arthritis Care Res. 2004;51(6):1045–59.
31. Warsi A, LaValley MP, Wang PS, Avorn J, Solomon DH. Arthritis self management education programs: a meta analysis of the effect on pain and disability. Arthritis Rheum. 2003;48(8): 2207–13.
32. El Miedany Y, El Gaafary M, El Arousy N, Ahmed I, Youssef S, Palmer D. Arthritis education: the integration of patient-reported outcome measures and patient self-management. Clin Exp Rheumatol. 2012;30(6):899–904.
33. Ndosi M, Johnson D, Hardware B, Young T, Hill J, Hale C, et al. Effects of needs-based education on self-efficacy and health outcomes in people with rheumatoid arthritis: a multicentre, single blind, randomised controlled trial. Ann Rheum Dis. 2015. doi:10.1136/annrheumdis-2014-207171.
34. Ndosi M, Vinall K, Hale C, Bird H, Hill J. The effectiveness of nurse-led care in people with rheumatoid arthritis: a systematic review. Int J Nurs Stud. 2011;48(5):642–54.
35. Gronning K, Rannestad T, Skomsvoll JF, Rygg LO, Steinsbekk A. Long-term effects of a nurse-led group and individual patient education programme for patients with chronic inflammatory polyarthritis—a randomised controlled trial. J Clin Nurs. 2014;23(7–8):1005–17.
36. Gronning K, Skomsvoll JF, Rannestad T, Steinsbekk A. The effect of an educational programme consisting of group and individual arthritis education for patients with polyarthritis—a randomised controlled trial. Patient Educ Couns. 2012;88(1):113–20.
37. El Miedany Y, El Gaafary M, Youssef S, Palmer D. Incorporating patient reported outcome measures in clinical practice: development and validation of a questionnaire for inflammatory arthritis. Clin Exp Rheumatol. 2009;28(5):734–44.
38. El Miedany Miedany YE. Joint fitness program for arthritic patients—the value of patient-reported outcome measures in designing a tailored approach to patient education. 2012 [August 28, 2015]. www.touchmusculoskeletal.com
39. Ndosi M, Tennant A, Bergsten U, Kukkurainen ML, Machado P, de la Torre-Aboki J, et al. Cross-cultural validation of the educational needs assessment tool in RA in 7 European countries. BMC Musculoskelet Disord. 2011;12:110.

40. Ndosi M, Bremander A, Hamnes B, Horton M, Kukkurainen ML, Machado P, et al. Validation of the educational needs assessment tool as a generic instrument for rheumatic diseases in seven european countries. Ann Rheum Dis. 2014;73(12):2122–9.
41. Hardware BJD, Hale C, Ndosi M, Adebajo A. Patients and nursing staff views of using the education needs assessment tool in rheumatology clinics: a qualitative study. J Clin Nurs. 2015;24(7–8):1048–58.
42. Palmer D, El Miedany Y. Proms: a novel approach to arthritis self-management. Br J Nurs. 2012;21(10):601–2, 605–7.
43. Palmer D, El Miedany Y. From guidelines to clinical practice: cardiovascular risk management in inflammatory arthritis patients. Br J Community Nurs. 2013;18(9):424–8.
44. Desai SS, Myles JD, Kaplan MJ. Suboptimal cardiovascular risk factor identification and management in patients with rheumatoid arthritis: a cohort analysis. Arthritis Res Ther. 2012;14(6):R270.
45. Pincus T, Gibofsky A, Weinblatt ME. Urgent care and tight control of rheumatoid arthritis as in diabetes and hypertension: better treatments but a shortage of rheumatologists. Arthritis Rheum. 2002;46(4):851–4.
46. Smolen JS, Landewé R, Breedveld FC, Buch M, Burmester G, Dougados M, et al. Eular recommendations for the management of rheumatoid arthritis with synthetic and biological disease-modifying antirheumatic drugs: 2013 update. Ann Rheum Dis. 2013;69(6):964–75.
47. El Miedany Y, El Gaafary M, Youssef S, Palmer D. Towards a multidimensional patient reported outcome measures assessment: development and validation of a questionnaire for patients with ankylosing spondylitis/spondyloarthritis. Joint Bone Spine. 2010;77(6):575–81.
48. El Miedany YEGM, El Yassaki A, Ahmed I, Youssef S, Hegazi M, Palmer D. Incorporating patient reported outcome measures in clinical practice: development and validation of a proms questionnaire for sle. Ann Rheum Dis. 2013;72 Suppl 3:484.
49. El Miedany Y, El Gaafary M, El Aroussi A, Ahmed I, Youssef S, Palmer D. Towards a multidimentional assessment: development and validation of a questionnaire for patients with fibromyalgia. Ann Rheum Dis. 2013;72 Suppl 3:719.
50. Ghisi GL, Abdallah F, Grace SL, Thomas S, Oh P. A systematic review of patient education in cardiac patients: do they increase knowledge and promote health behavior change? Patient Educ Couns. [Review]. 2014;95(2):160–174.
51. Lorig K, Konkol L, Gonzalez V. Arthritis patient education: a review of the literature. Patient Educ Couns. 1987;10(3):207–52.
52. Hirano PC, Laurent DD, Lorig K. Arthritis patient education studies, 1987–1991: a review of the literature. Patient Educ Couns. 1994;24(1):9–54.
53. Cramer JA, Roy A, Burrell A, Fairchild CJ, Fuldeore MJ, Ollendorf DA, et al. Medication compliance and persistence: terminology and definitions. Value Health. 2008;11(1):44–7.
54. El Miedany Y, El Gaafary M, Palmer D. Assessment of the utility of visual feedback in the treatment of early rheumatoid arthritis patients: a pilot study. Rheumatol Int. [Randomized Controlled Trial]. 2012;32(10):3061–8.
55. Hibbard JH, Mahoney ER, Stockard J, Tusler M. Development and testing of a short form of the patient activation measure. Health Serv Res. 2005;40(6 Pt 1):1918–30.
56. Hibbard JH, Stockard J, Mahoney ER, Tusler M. Development of the patient activation measure (PAM): conceptualizing and measuring activation in patients and consumers. Health Serv Res. 2004;39(4 Pt 1):1005–26.
57. Hibbard JH, Mahoney ER, Stock R, Tusler M. Do increases in patient activation result in improved self-management behaviors? Health Serv Res. 2007;42(4):1443–63.
58. Alegría M, Sribney W, Perez D, Laderman M, Keefe K. The role of patient activation on patient–provider communication and quality of care for us and foreign born latino patients. J Gen Intern Med. 2009;24(3):534–41.
59. Mosen DM, Schmittdiel J, Hibbard J, Sobel D, Remmers C, Bellows J. Is patient activation associated with outcomes of care for adults with chronic conditions? J Ambul Care Manage. 2007;30(1):21–9.

Chapter 17
PROMs vs. PREMs (Patient-Reported Experience Measures)

Marwan Bukhari

Patient-Reported Outcome Measures (PROMs) Versus Patient-Reported Experience Measures (PREMs)

Capturing the patient's perspective of their condition and treatment is a core element in the management of chronic conditions such as rheumatoid arthritis. Overarching objectives for engaging with and actively seeking patient input in disease management is to improve the quality of care and to monitor outcomes of the treatment approach selected.

Patient-reported outcome measures (PROMs) provide an assessment of the patient's health status or health-related quality of life (HRQoL) at a single time point. Importantly, PROMs collect information directly from the patient without interpretation by clinicians or others and therefore should reflect health issues most relevant to the patients themselves. Examples of PROMs include measures of symptoms, activities, and limitations. More recently, PROMs have also been used in clinical trials to address issues of patient satisfaction, compliance with treatment, and treatment preferences [1]. An important distinction between measures of satisfaction and PROMs such as HRQoL is that they address the *process* of treatment rather than its outcome [2].

While patient satisfaction surveys are increasingly used to gauge performance, they differ from patient-reported experience measures (PREMs). Unlike general satisfaction surveys, PREMs aim to enhance the patient experience of care and

M. Bukhari, M.B.B.S., M.Sc., Ph.D., F.R.C.P. (✉)
Department of Rheumatology, Royal Lancaster Infirmary,
Ashton Road, Lancaster, Lancashire LA1 4RP, UK
e-mail: Marwan.Bukhari@mbht.nhs.uk

Y. El Miedany (ed.), *Patient Reported Outcome Measures in Rheumatic Diseases*,
DOI 10.1007/978-3-319-32851-5_17

incorporate questions about specific aspects of organization and delivery of care that impact quality. In a study of 4573 patients in 27 practices across 9 primary care trusts in England, measures of patients' experiences discriminated more effectively between practices than did measures of satisfaction [3]. In addition, patients can describe high levels of satisfaction at the same time as describing experiences that are suboptimal [4, 5]. Thus it has been suggested that for continuous quality improvement it would be more fruitful to look at the underlying components of the concept of satisfaction, namely expectations and experiences [6].

Much work has been done on PROMs in a range of diseases, countries, and care settings [1, 7–15]. Similar work was carried out in rheumatology [16–19] where PROMs have proven to be a useful tool for patient management [20]. The US National Institutes of Health Patient-Reported Outcomes Measurement Information System (PROMIS) allows assessment of the impact of chronic conditions on HRQoL across diseases. Using this tool demonstrated that chronic diseases are associated with poorer HRQoL relative to the general US population [21]. PROMIS has also demonstrated validity and reliability in osteoarthritis [22]. The potential benefit of adopting a more dynamic role for PROMs in disease management has been discussed, with potential benefits including modification of disease impact through improved patient adherence to treatment as patients monitor their response to therapy [23]. The development of more holistic tools that captures both PROMs and patient experience has also been proposed [8].

A recent meta-analysis [24] identified 42 PROMs in rheumatoid arthritis (RA), showing that differing groups have felt the need to address this in different ways and that PROMs measure different aspects of the patients' disease experiences. The European League Against Rheumatism (EULAR) has dedicated a special Website for patient-reported outcome measures available for different rheumatic diseases in different languages (http://oml.eular.org). The Website aims at providing a comprehensive database of validated patient-reported instruments (indices, questionnaires, scales, or others) used in rheumatology. The database includes a detailed description of each instrument, including: the instrument itself, description of the population(s) or settings where it has been validated, recommendations and rules for use (data collection and scoring method), guideline for interpretation of the results in clinical practice or in research, references, and validated translated versions in the European Union (EU) languages, with download if possible or link to an access page as well as information on how validation aspects were tested.

However, even with existing PROMs in rheumatology, there is a need to ensure that the PROMs are truly from the patient perspective and reflect outcomes that are a priority for the patient rather than those that are perceived as a priority by healthcare professionals [25, 26]. It has been suggested that a more comprehensive approach capturing personal life impact measures (PLIMs) would take into account the broader impact of living with the disease and its consequences [25]. In contrast to the wealth of information available on PROMs, relatively little published information is available for PREMs in general or PREMs in rheumatology specifically.

The Patient Experience and Quality of Care

The importance of incorporating the patient perspective and experience in assessments of quality of healthcare has long been recognized internationally by organizations such as the World Health Organization (WHO) [27] and the Organization for Economic Cooperation and Development [28]. In the US, the Consumer Assessment of Healthcare Providers and Systems (CAHPS) survey tool aims to facilitate consumer (patient) choice and to offer guidance to healthcare providers on how to improve service [29]. The Picker Institute's hospital survey (PPE-15) is one of the most widely used tools internationally for measuring patients' hospital experiences in order to benchmark quality of care [5]. PPE-15 comprises a basic set of 15 questions that are designed to be applicable in all hospitals, and relevant to all patients. In a review of US and UK patient experience initiatives, the need to measure detailed patient experiences instead of general patient satisfaction, to introduce an integrated system, and to standardize questionnaires and methods has been highlighted [29].

In the UK, several government reports and initiatives have emphasized the importance of incorporating the patient experience into the delivery of quality care [30–34]. The government's white paper "Equity and Excellence, Liberating the NHS" puts the patient experience and patient outcomes as the metrics for quality improvements in healthcare [34]. In addition, the annual Quality Account produced by National Health Service (NHS) trusts incorporates three principles of safety, effectiveness, and patient experience. The 2012/2013 NHS Operating Framework requires frequent patient surveys and engagement with patients to enable quality. Furthermore, the new Quality Standard and guidance on patient experience in adult NHS services, published by the National Institute for Health and Care Excellence (NICE) in February 2012, incorporates 14 quality statements central to patient experience of care [33]. More recently, in May 2013, the Healthcare Quality Improvement Partnership (HQIP) announced the award of a national clinical audit of rheumatoid and early inflammatory arthritis [35]. The audit aims to capture patient-reported outcomes and experience data (where appropriate) for all patients presenting from the 1 October 2013 to the end of September 2015. The importance of patient experience has also been highlighted within commissioning. The UK Department of Health's World Class Commissioning outlines 11 competencies required of commissioners [36]. Competency 3 requires Primary Care Trusts (PCTs) to "proactively build continuous and meaningful engagement with the public and patients to shape services and improve health" [36].

The NHS Outcomes Framework has been developed to drive these improvements in quality. The Framework identifies long-term conditions and patient's experience of care as two of its five domains [37]. The latest version of the Outcomes Framework now incorporates two additional indicators within the patient experience domain. The first is the "Friends and Family" test, which asks patients whether they would recommend the hospital where they received their treatment and care to a family member or friend. The second focuses on improving experience of integrated care, following recommendations from the NHS Future Forum. From April

2013, the NHS Outcomes Framework will form part of the way in which the Secretary of State will hold the new NHS Commissioning Board to account for the commissioning system in the English NHS.

Several studies have reported improvements following systematic gathering of patient feedback by hospitals [38–45]. A report by the Picker Institute Europe on trends from 26 national patient surveys, carried out under the auspices of the NHS patient survey program in England between 2002 and 2007 to assess the quality of NHS care through patients' eyes, has explored the experience of care of nearly one and a half million NHS patients [46]. The report indicates that despite improvements over the time period, the service as a whole is still far from patient-centered. The most significant problem highlighted was the failure of clinical staff to provide active support for patient engagement. This demonstrates that further improvement and the routine incorporation of patient experience into NHS services is required.

Importance of PREMs in Chronic Diseases: The Diabetes Experience

The management of chronic diseases necessitates a high degree of self-management requiring patient concordance and understanding of their condition. In addition effective self-management is facilitated by patients having confidence in the advice and strategies proposed by their healthcare team and a positive experience of care. A US study of 51,129 patients with a chronic disease (asthma, diabetes, and cardiovascular disease) used patient surveys to assess the relationship between clinical care metrics and patient experiences of care among patients with chronic disease. In this study, performance on patient experiences of care measures was highest for the quality of clinical interactions (88.5) and lowest for delivery of self-management support (68.8; scale 0–100) [47]. PREMs are in development for a variety of chronic diseases including: chronic obstructive pulmonary disease [48] and chronic heart failure [49]. Currently the most advanced PREMs have been developed for diabetes for both adult and younger patients.

The Diabetes Patient Experience Project (DPEP) has developed PREMs tools to assess experiences of adult patients with diabetes about their continuing care and inpatient stays [50]. Using either a postal or online questionnaire, patients are asked about the planning and provision of their diabetes care. With regard to planning, the tools include questions that cover: whether during appointments patients were able to discuss their ideas for managing their condition and their goals; whether they were given dietary and physical activity advice; whether a printed copy of their care plan was made available; whether they were listened to and had things explained clearly; and whether the appointments made them feel more confident about managing their diabetes. With regard to provision of care, the tools include questions that cover: whether they received conflicting information; whether they had to repeat important information provided previously; whether they had a contact number to call if concerned;

whether they had had blood and urine tests in the past 12 months and understood the purpose and results of these tests; knowledge and understanding of the medications prescribed and treatment options; and whether they felt clinic staff were aware of the latest treatments. The questionnaire also collected basic demographic data about the type of diabetes, gender, age, postcode, and ethnic group.

A separate tool has been developed for pediatric patients [51]. This tool includes questions that cover: whether appointments are delayed; whether they have enough time with the relevant healthcare professional to discuss any questions or concerns; timely access to advice; adequate information and knowledge for managing their condition; access to information about specific technologies; whether written information was understandable; appropriateness of dietary advice; respect for cultural and/or religious beliefs; the availability of an interpreter; and whether they would recommend the clinic to others.

Patient Assessment of Chronic Illness Care (PACIC) is a tool used to evaluate the chronic care experiences of patients. A study examining the PACIC to improve and validate its potential to measure the experience of diabetes patients in daily chronic care practice revealed that the reliability of the PACIC and the extended PACIC (PACIC+), which also includes team functioning, reliably measures chronic care experience of patients with diabetes [52]. The results with PACIC+ are of particular note given the importance of effective multidisciplinary team functioning in chronic care management.

PREMs in Rheumatoid Arthritis

Patient experience is not currently routinely measured in RA and there is no standard method of capturing data on the patient experience of care, despite increasing awareness of its potential value in improving quality of care. Studies have tended to focus on PROMs [16–18, 20, 53, 54] or patient experience of educational services for RA [55–57] rather than on the patient experience of care.

Data from one study in nine women who had RA for ≥3 years, and had received inpatient treatment for ≥5 days within the previous 2 years, revealed that the experiences of patients focused on five themes: uncertainty during first admission, becoming an experienced patient, the positive and negative effects of other patients, the experience and knowledge of staff, and the loss of privacy [58].

A PREM questionnaire was developed for 94 patients with RA [59] (Appendix 1), this was centered around five categories including: (1) journey to diagnosis, (2) impact of the disease on the patient's everyday life, (3) knowledge about the disease, (4) care in the hospital, and (5) patient education and aftercare (including what to do in case of flare). It correlated with disease activity, which would indicate it also had an element of activity measured. It was retested in 184 other patients but no external validation was performed on the data.

A further PREM questionnaire was developed in a larger cohort of patients with RA [60]. This was developed after focus group discussions and piloted on 524 patients in different UK settings (Appendix 2).

Effective Use of PREMs for Improving Services: A UK Perspective

The UK Department of Health has produced a practical guide to aid use of patient experience to improve service quality: "Understanding What Matters: A Guide to Using Patient Feedback to Transform Services" [61]. The guide includes an experience feedback cycle that describes the process of collecting and analyzing patient experience data to design and implement service improvements. There are several issues that may impact routine incorporation and translation of patient experience into service improvements. For example, the optimal method for delivery of PREMs—postal versus online—remains to be established [49]. It is likely to be a combination that allows the greatest patient choice to maximize patient engagement and involvement. Another consideration is the use of multimedia technology to enable capture of information from patients with limited literacy skills [62]. One study suggests that computer touchscreen questionnaires were well accepted by RA patients, with good data quality, reliability, and score agreement when compared with standardized paper questionnaires [63]. The potential impact of literacy on patient experience for diseases with a large element of self-management such as RA should also be considered [64].

For data analysis, it may be relevant to adjust measures of patient experience for case mix in order to correct for differences in patient characteristics not under the control of providers. This would facilitate fair comparison among healthcare providers by estimating the scores providers would have received if serving a common population [65]. Data analysis should also consider the link between expectations and experience: What people expect from their healthcare, compared with their experiences of it in practice, may influence their satisfaction with their care. There is some evidence that patients who receive the healthcare they expect are likely to recover better than patients who do not. An expectations questionnaire may provide a useful tool to benchmark the extent to which expectations are being met and to identify the types of expectations that are and are not being met, thus potentially informing treatment policy and practices [66].

Patient interactions with staff who provide healthcare services will impact patient experience of care, therefore staff training may be appropriate. A national survey of training courses provided by higher education providers and healthcare organizations in England was administered to all 180 providers of higher education to student/qualified doctors, nurses, and allied health professionals, and all 390 National Health Service trusts in England, as a single question to the NHS 2010 Staff Survey ($n=306{,}000$) relating to the training staff had received to deliver a good patient experience. Results suggest that specific training with regard to the physical needs and comfort of patients, and how patient experiences can be measured and used to improve services, should be introduced. The report further suggested that future developments should also focus, firstly, on involving a wider range of patients in planning and delivering courses and, secondly, evaluating whether courses impact on the attitudes and behaviors of different professional groups and might therefore contribute to improved patient experiences [67]. Another study to evaluate the effectiveness of patient-led teaching compared with doctor-led teaching, regarding the impact of RA suggests that the patient was at least as good as a doctor at teaching about the impact of chronic disease on patients and that students appreciated the personal insight that a patient can offer [68]. Therefore a potential role for patients in the training and teaching of healthcare professionals could be further explored.

Conclusion

The traditional view of the user as a passive recipient of a product or service has begun to give way to the new view of users as integral to the improvement and innovation process [43]. The challenge now is to effectively use patient experience to drive improvements in service. A US study, aimed at understanding factors affecting the use of patient survey data in quality improvement, highlighted that effective use of patient survey data may require a more concerted effort than for other clinical data. Organizations may need to develop cultures that support patient-centered care, quality improvement capacity, and to align professional receptiveness and leadership with technical expertise with the data [40]. Feedback on patients' experiences of healthcare is essential in order to determine priorities for quality improvement and should be seen as an important element of performance assessment.

Appendix 1: Patient-Reported Experience Measures

Reprinted with permission from El Miedany Y, El Gaafary M, Youssef S, Ahmed I, Palmer D. The arthritic patients' perspective of measuring treatment efficacy: Patient-Reported Experience Measures (PREMs) as a quality tool. Clin Exp Rheumatol. 2014 Jul-Aug;32(4):547–52.

Patient Reported Experience Measures

We would like to know how you feel about your experience and treatment that you received at the place where you were given this survey. Your views are very important to us to help find out how satisfied you are with the service provided. This would help us to continue providing an efficient service for our patients as well as how we can make them better. It is up to you whether you want to take part in this survey – you do not have to. All responses will be kept confidential. Thank you for your time.

Your Age: ....years.
Your Sex: Male: ❑ Female: ❑
Your Diagnosis: ....

I. Arthritis & your life:

-How does your Arthritis affect ability to carry out your daily tasks?
Always: ❑ Usually ❑ At times: ❑
occasionally: ❑ Not at all: ❑

-How would you rate the severity of your Arthritis?
Very Severe: ❑ Severe: ❑ Moderate:❑ Mild: ❑

-Have you changed your life style to address your Arthritis? I have made:
No change: ❑ Few changes:❑ Some changes: ❑
Many changes: ❑ Altered my lifestyle: ❑

II. Your Arthritis Management:

-Were you given the opportunity to discuss your health concerns, preferences of management& potential consequences?
Yes: ❑ No: ❑

-Were you given the opportunity to choose, accept or decline medical treatment?
Yes: ❑ No: ❑

-Have you been treated with respect, dignity and compassion?
Yes: ❑ No: ❑

In the next section, Please circle the number which reflects your experience in the following areas, please note that:
1= Poor, 2= Fair, 3= OK, 4= Good, 5- Excellent

III. Journey to Diagnosis:

• Diagnosis & Ease of getting care:
How would you rate your experience with
Time taken to be referred by your GP to the clinic: 1 2 3 4 5
Time taken from being referred by your GP to being seen in the hospital: 1 2 3 4 5
Time taken to start your treatment: 1 2 3 4 5
Helpline facility : 1 2 3 4 5
Not Applicable: ❑

• Waiting: How would you rate your experience with
Time in waiting area: 1 2 3 4 5
Time in exam room: 1 2 3 4 5
Waiting for X-rays: 1 2 3 4 5
Waiting for Blood tests:1 2 3 4 5

IV: Care in the hospital: Staff:
Has the treating Dr. / Rheumatology Nurse
Listened to you: 1 2 3 4 5
Taken enough time with you: 1 2 3 4 5
Explained your condition: 1 2 3 4 5
Given you advice and treatment: 1 2 3 4 5
Answered your questions: 1 2 3 4 5

Clinic Nurse: Was the Nurse
Friendly and helpful to you: 1 2 3 4 5
Answered your questions: 1 2 3 4 5

Others (e.g. Receptionists/Assistants):Were they
Friendly and helpful to you: 1 2 3 4 5
Answered your questions: 1 2 3 4 5

• Questionnaire regarding your Arthritis:
-No Questionnaire was given: ❑
-Did you find the questionnaire given to you today of relevance to your condition?
Yes: ❑ No: ❑
-To enable us to monitor your disease activity & provide appropriate treatment are you happy to complete the arthritis questionnaire in your next clinic visit?
Yes: ❑ No: ❑

• How would you rate the explanation of any procedures carried out & their findings:
Ultrasound: 1 2 3 4 5
Nerve conduction testing: 1 2 3 4 5
Interpretation of X-rays/MRI: 1 2 3 4 5
Joint / Soft tissue injection: 1 2 3 4 5
No Procedure was carried out ❑

V: Patient Education and Aftercare:

• Aftercare: Please rate your satisfaction with
Length of time till your next appointment date: 1 2 3 4 5
Ease of obtaining advise between appointments: 1 2 3 4 5
Would you recommend this clinic to your friends and relatives: 1 2 3 4 5

• Patient education: Information leaflets
Not given: ❑
If given, it was:
-Clear and informative: 1 2 3 4 5
-Answer your queries: 1 2 3 4 5
-Patient friendly: 1 2 3 4 5

You are welcome to put any further comments/ suggestion on the back of the page. Thank you

Appendix 2: Rheumatology Care: Patient Questionnaire

Reprinted with permission from the National Rheumatoid Arthritis Society. CQRA PREMs Non-RA Rheumatic Conditions. http://www.nras.org.uk/commissioning-for-quality-in-rheumatoid-arthritis-cqra.

CQRA Commissioning for Quality in Rheumatoid Arthritis

Rheumatology care: patient questionnaire

Section	Statement	Strongly agree	Agree	Neither agree nor disagree	Disagree	Strongly disagree	Not applicable
1. Your needs and preferences	a) Whenever I attended a clinic, I felt that I was treated respectfully as an individual	○	○	○	○	○	
	b) I was involved as much as I wanted to be in decisions about my treatment and care	○	○	○	○	○	
	c) My personal circumstances (see note 1 below) and preferences were taken into account when planning and deciding on my treatment and care	○	○	○	○	○	
	d) I was given information in a way that I could understand	○	○	○	○	○	
	e) I was given enough information to help me make decisions about my treatment	○	○	○	○	○	
2. Co-ordination of care and communication Care across departments	a) I was made aware that there is a team of health professionals (see note 2 below) looking after me	○	○	○	○	○	○
	b) When I needed help I was able to access different members of my health team	○	○	○	○	○	○
	c) There is a member of my health team who can help me to see other specialists in the team if I need to	○	○	○	○	○	○
	d) I feel that the people I see at the clinic are fully up to date with my current situation	○	○	○	○	○	
3. Information, education and self-care	a) I feel that I was given information at the time I needed it	○	○	○	○	○	
	b) I feel that I have a good understanding of the treatments I am on or being offered	○	○	○	○	○	
	c) I have been told about patient organisations or groups that can help me	○	○	○	○	○	
	d) I have been offered an opportunity to attend a self-management programme suitable to my needs	○	○	○	○	○	○

Note 1: Examples of 'personal circumstances' could be whether you work or have carer responsibilities. Note 2: The type of health professionals in the team will vary from region to region but should include a consultant, a nurse specialist, an occupational therapist and a physiotherapist, as well as access to a podiatrist.

Page 1 of 3

Section	Statement	Strongly agree	Agree	Neither agree nor disagree	Disagree	Strongly disagree	Not applicable
4. Daily living and physical comfort	a) I feel that my rheumatic condition is being controlled enough to let me get on with my daily life and usual activities	○	○	○	○	○	
	b) If I have had a 'flare' (when my symptoms get much worse), I have been able to get help quickly	○	○	○	○	○	○
5. Emotional support	a) I feel able to approach a member of my health team to discuss any worries about my condition and my treatment or their effect on my life	○	○	○	○	○	
	b) I feel able to discuss personal or intimate issues about relationships with my health team if I want to	○	○	○	○	○	
6. Family and friends	a) I feel able to take members of my family to outpatient appointments to become involved in decisions about my care if I want to	○	○	○	○	○	
7. Access to care	a) At appointments, I feel that I have enough time with the healthcare professional to cover everything I want to discuss	○	○	○	○	○	
	b) I have had clinic appointments cancelled unexpectedly	○ Yes	○ No				
	c) If yes, how long have you had to wait for a new appointment?	○ *Up to 1 week*	○ *1 to 3 weeks*	○ *4 to 6 weeks*	○ *7 to 12 weeks*	○ *More than 12 weeks*	
	d) I have needed extra treatment or a change of treatment (between routine clinic appointments)	○ Yes	○ No				
	e) If yes, how long did it take for this to happen?	○ *Up to 1 week*	○ *1 to 3 weeks*	○ *4 to 6 weeks*	○ *7 to 12 weeks*	○ *More than 12 weeks*	
8. Overall experience of care	a) Overall in the past year, I have had a good experience of care for my rheumatic condition	○	○	○	○	○	

Page 2 of 3

Your rheumatic condition, the length of time you have had the condition, your age, sex and ethnic background may affect the kind of care you have experienced and affect your answers to the questions. To help us fully understand your answers, please fill in the section below.				
9. What rheumatic condition(s) do you attend the rheumatology clinic for?				
Rheumatoid arthritis O	Sjögren's syndrome O	Fibromyalgia O	SLE / lupus O	Adult with juvenile idiopathic arthritis O
Gout O	Polymyalgia rheumatic O	Chronic back pain O	Osteoarthritis O	Don't know O
Inflammatory polyarthritis O	Ankylosing spondylitis O	Psoriatic arthritis O	Scleroderma O	Other (please specify) ....

10. How long have you had this rheumatic condition?
O Less than 2 years O Between 2 and 5 years O Between 6 and 10 years O More than 10 years

11. How old are you?

18 to 24 O	25 to 34 O	35 to 44 O	45 to 54 O	55 to 64 O	65 to 74 O	75 to 84 O	85 and over O

12. Are you:
O male? O female?

13. What is your ethnic group?

White O British, Irish, Other White background	Mixed O White and Black Caribbean, White and Black African, White and Asian, Other Mixed background	Asian or Asian British O Indian, Pakistani, Bangladeshi, Other Asian background	Black or Black British O Caribbean, African, Other Black background	Chinese or Other Ethnic Group O Chinese, Other ethnic group	Prefer not to say O

Page 3 of 3

References

1. McKenna SP. Measuring patient-reported outcomes: moving beyond misplaced common sense to hard science. BMC Med. 2011;9:86.
2. Doward LC, McKenna SP. Defining patient-reported outcomes. Value Health. 2004;7 Suppl 1:S4–8.
3. Salisbury C, Wallace M, Montgomery AA. Patients' experience and satisfaction in primary care: secondary analysis using multilevel modelling. BMJ. 2010;341:c5004.
4. Jenkinson C, Coulter A, Bruster S, et al. Patients' experiences and satisfaction with health care: results of a questionnaire study of specific aspects of care. Qual Saf Health Care. 2002;11:335–9.
5. Jenkinson C, Coulter A, Bruster S. The Picker Patient Experience Questionnaire: development and validation using data from in-patient surveys in five countries. Int J Qual Health Care. 2002;14(5):353–8.
6. Sixma HJ, Kerssens JJ, Campen CV, Peters L. Quality of care from the patients' perspective: from theoretical concept to a new measuring instrument. Health Expect. 1998;1:82–95.
7. Brod M, Skovlund SE, Wittrup-Jensen KU. Measuring the impact of diabetes through patient report of treatment satisfaction, productivity and symptom experience. Qual Life Res. 2006;15(3):481–91.
8. Somner JE, Sii F, Bourne RR, et al. Moving from PROMs to POEMs for glaucoma care: a qualitative scoping exercise. Invest Ophthalmol Vis Sci. 2012;53(9):5940–7.
9. Ramaswami U, Stull DE, Parini R, et al. Measuring patient experiences in Fabry disease: validation of the Fabry-specific Pediatric Health and Pain Questionnaire (FPHPQ). Health Qual Life Outcomes. 2012;10:116.
10. Kleinman L, Mannix S, Yuan Y, et al. Review of patient-reported outcome measures in chronic hepatitis C. Health Qual Life Outcomes. 2012;10:92.
11. Abetz L, Rajagopalan K, Mertzanis P, et al. Development and validation of the impact of dry eye on everyday life (IDEEL) questionnaire, a patient-reported outcomes (PRO) measure for the assessment of the burden of dry eye on patients. Health Qual Life Outcomes. 2011;9:111.
12. Bateman E, Keefe D. Patient-reported outcomes in supportive care. Semin Oncol. 2011;38(3):358–61.
13. Haywood KL, Staniszewska S, Chapman S. Quality and acceptability of patient-reported outcome measures used in chronic fatigue syndrome/myalgic encephalomyelitis (CFS/ME): a systematic review. Qual Life Res. 2012;21(1):35–52.

14. Flythe JE, Powell JD, Poulton CJ, Westreich KD, Handler L, Reeve BB, Carey TS. Patient-Reported Outcome Instruments for physical symptoms among patients receiving maintenance dialysis: a systematic review. Am J Kidney Dis. 2015.;66(6):1033-46. pii: S0272-6386(15)00849-5. doi:10.1053/j.ajkd.2015.05.020.
15. Højmark K, Støttrup C, Carreon L, Andersen MO. Patient-reported outcome measures unbiased by loss of follow-up. Single-center study based on DaneSpine, the Danish spine surgery registry. Eur Spine J. 2016;25(1):282–6. PMID: 620893.
16. Kirwan JR, Fries JF, Hewlett SE, et al. Patient perspective workshop: moving towards OMERACT guidelines for choosing or developing instruments to measure patient-reported outcomes. J Rheumatol. 2011;38(8):1711–5.
17. Khanna D, Krishnan E, Dewitt EM, et al. Patient-Reported Outcomes Measurement Information System (PROMIS®)—the future of measuring patient reported outcomes in rheumatology. Arthritis Care Res (Hoboken). 2011;63(S11):S486–90.
18. Her M, Kavanaugh A. Patient-reported outcomes in rheumatoid arthritis. Curr Opin Rheumatol. 2012;24(3):327–34.
19. Doganay Erdogan B, Leung YY, Pohl C, Tennant A, Conaghan PG. Minimal clinically important difference as applied in rheumatology: an OMERACT Rasch Working Group Systematic Review and Critique. J Rheumatol. 2016;43(1):194–202. pii:jrheum.141150.
20. Amaya-Amaya J, Botello-Corzo D, Calixto OJ, et al. Usefulness of patients-reported outcomes in rheumatoid arthritis focus group. Arthritis. 2012;2012:935187.
21. Rothrock NE, Hays RD, Spritzer K, et al. Relative to the general US population, chronic diseases are associated with poorer health-related quality of life as measured by the Patient-Reported Outcomes Measurement Information System (PROMIS). J Clin Epidemiol. 2010;63(11):1195–204.
22. Broderick JE, Schneider S, Junghaenel DU, et al. Validity and reliability of patient-reported outcomes measurement information system (PROMIS) instruments in osteoarthritis. Arthritis Care Res (Hoboken). 2013;65(10):1625–33. doi:10.1002/acr.22025.
23. El Miedany Y. PROMs in inflammatory arthritis: moving from static to dynamic. Clin Rheumatol. 2013;32(6):735–42.
24. Dür M, Coenen M, Stoffer MA, Fialka-Moser V, Kautzky-Willer A, Kjeken I, Drăgoi RG, Mattsson M, Boström C, Smolen J, Stamm TA. Do patient-reported outcome measures cover personal factors important to people with rheumatoid arthritis? A mixed methods design using the International Classification of Functioning, Disability and Health as frame of reference. Health Qual Life Outcomes. 2015;13:27. doi:10.1186/s12955-015-0214-8.
25. Sanderson T, Kirwan J. Patient-reported outcomes for arthritis: time to focus on personal life impact measures? Arthritis Rheum. 2009;61(1):1–3. doi:10.1002/art.24270.
26. Taylor PC. The importance of the patients' experience of RA compared with clinical measures of disease activity. Clin Exp Rheumatol. 2010;28(3 Suppl 59):S28–31.
27. Murray CJ, Frenk J. A framework for assessing the performance of health systems. Bull World Health Organ. 2000;78(6):717–31.
28. Hurst J, Jee-Hughes M. Performance measurement and performance management in OECD Health Systems. In: OECD labour market and social policy occasional papers no. 47. OECD Publishing; 2001. doi:10.1787/788224073713.
29. Delnoij DM. Measuring patient experiences in Europe: what can we learn from the experiences in the USA and England? Eur J Public Health. 2009;19(4):354–6.
30. NHS NPEF. NHS Patient Experience Framework. 2012. www.dh.gov.uk/health/2012/02/patient-experience-framework/. Accessed July 2014.
31. NICE clinical guideline 138. Patient experience in adult NHS services: improving the experience of care for people using adult NHS services. Issued February 2012. guidance.nice.org.uk/cg138. Accessed Mar 2013.
32. NICE Clinical Guideline 79: the management of rheumatoid arthritis in adults. http://www.nice.org.uk/CG79. Accessed Mar 2013.

33. NICE QS15: Quality standard for patient experience in adult NHS services. 2012. www.guidance.nice.org.uk/QS15. Accessed July 2014.
34. Equity and excellence: liberating the NHS. 2010. http://www.official-documents.gov.uk/document/cm78/7881/7881.pdf. Accessed Feb 2013.
35. HQIP RA Audit. Healthcare Quality Improvement Partnership (HQIP) National clinical audit for rheumatoid and early inflammatory arthritis. http://www.rheumatology.org.uk/resources/audits/national_ra_audit/information_pack.aspx. Patient data collection form—follow up at 3 months. Accessed July 2014.
36. How to Achieve World Class Commissioning Competencies. Practical tips for NHS Commissioners. Published October 2008. http://webarchive.nationalarchives.gov.uk/20130107105354/http://www.dh.gov.uk/prod_consum_dh/groups/dh_digitalassets/documents/digitalasset/dh_089019.pdf. Accessed Mar 2013.
37. The NHS Outcomes Framework 2013/14. https://www.wp.dh.gov.uk/publications/files/2012/11/121109-NHS-Outcomes-Framework-2013-14.pdf. Accessed Feb 2013.
38. Draper M, Cohen P, Buchan H, et al. Seeking consumer views: what use are results of hospital patient satisfaction surveys? International J Qual Health Care. 2001;13(6):463–8.
39. Crawford MJ, Rutter D, Manley C, et al. Systematic review of involving patients in the planning and development of health care. Br Med J. 2002;325(7375):1263.
40. Davies E, Cleary PD. Hearing the patient's voice? Factors affecting the use of patient survey data in quality improvement. Qual Saf Health Care. 2005;14(6):428–32.
41. Richards N, Coulter A. Is the NHS becoming more patient-centred? Trends from the national surveys of NHS patients in England 2002-07. Published September 2007. http://www.fundsis.org/docs_act/99_Trends_2007_final%5B1%5D.pdf. Accessed March 2013.
42. Davies E, Shaller D, Edgman-Levitan S, et al. Evaluating the use of a modified CAHPS survey to support improvements in patient-centred care: lessons from a quality improvement collaborative. Health Expect. 2008;11(2):160–76.
43. Bate P, Robert G. Experience-based design: from redesigning the system around the patient to co-designing services with the patient. Qual Saf Health Care. 2006;15(5):307–10.
44. Forbat L, Cayless S, Knighting K, et al. Engaging patients in health care: an empirical study of the role of engagement on attitudes and action. Patient Educ Couns. 2009;74(1):84–90.
45. Land L, Hathorn E, Ross JD. Using patient experience to measure the quality of HIV care. Int J STD AIDS. 2011;22(7):366–7.
46. Richards N, Coulter A. Is the NHS becoming more patient-centred? Trends from the national surveys of NHS patients in England 2002–07. Oxford: Picker Institute Europe; 2007.
47. Sequist TD, Von Glahn T, Li A, et al. Measuring chronic care delivery: patient experiences and clinical performance. Int J Qual Health Care. 2012;24(3):206–13.
48. Developing a patient reported experience measure for chronic obstructive pulmonary disease (PREM-COPD). Final report. http://www.rcplondon.ac.uk/sites/default/files/developing_a_patient_reported_experience_measure_for_chronic_obstructive_pulmonary_disease_2.pdf. Accessed Feb 2013
49. Lagha E, Noble A, Smith A, et al. Patient reported experience measures (PREMs) in chronic heart failure. J R Coll Physicians Edinb. 2012;42(4):301–5.
50. Diabetes Patient Experience Project (DPEP). www.diabetes.nhs.uk/information_and_data/. Accessed Mar 2013.
51. Christie D. Developing the National Paediatric Diabetes Audit Patient Reported Experience Measure. Diabetes Care Child Young People. 2012;1(2):47–8.
52. Drewes HW, de Jong-van Til JT, Struijs JN, Baan CA, Tekle FB, Meijboom BR, Westert GP. Measuring chronic care management experience of patients with diabetes: PACIC and PACIC+ validation. Int J Integrated Care 2012;12:1–11.
53. Sokka T, Rannio T, Khan NA. Disease activity assessment and patient-reported outcomes in patients with early rheumatoid arthritis. Rheum Dis Clin North Am. 2012;38(2):299–310.
54. Dougados M, Brault Y, Logeart I, et al. Defining cut-off values for disease activity states and improvement scores for patient-reported outcomes: the example of the Rheumatoid Arthritis Impact of Disease (RAID). Arthritis Res Ther. 2012;14(3):R129.

55. Firth J. Rheumatoid arthritis: diagnosis and multidisciplinary management. Br J Nurs. 2011;20(18):1179–80, 1182, 1184–5.
56. Rademakers J, Delnoij D, Nijman J, et al. Educational inequalities in patient-centred care: patients' preferences and experiences. BMC Health Serv Res. 2012;12:261.
57. John H, Hale ED, Treharne GJ, et al. A randomized controlled trial of a cognitive behavioural patient education intervention vs a traditional information leaflet to address the cardiovascular aspects of rheumatoid disease. Rheumatology (Oxford). 2013;52(1):81–90.
58. Carter M. The experiences of patients with rheumatoid arthritis admitted to hospital focused on 5 interrelated themes. Evid Based Nurs. 2002;5(2):63.
59. El Miedany Y, El Gaafary M, Youssef S, Ahmed I, Palmer D. The arthritic patients' perspective of measuring treatment efficacy: patient reported experience measures (PREMs) as a quality tool. Clin Exp Rheumatol. 2014;32(4):547–52. Epub 2014 Jun 30.
60. Bosworth A, Cox M, O'Brien A, Jones P, Sargeant I, Elliott A, Bukhari M. Development and validation of a Patient Reported Experience Measure (PREM) for patients with rheumatoid arthritis (RA) and other rheumatic conditions. Curr Rheumatol Rev. 2015 May 21.
61. Understanding what matters: a guide to using patient feedback to transform services. 2009. http://www.dh.gov.uk/en/Publicationsandstatistics/Publications/PublicationsPolicyAndGuidance/DH_099780. Accessed Feb 2013.
62. Hahn EA, Cella D, Dobrez D, et al. The talking touchscreen: a new approach to outcomes assessment in low literacy. Psychooncology. 2004;13(2):86–95.
63. Salaffi F, Gasparini S, Grassi W. The use of computer touch-screen technology for the collection of patient-reported outcome data in rheumatoid arthritis: comparison with standardized paper questionnaires. Clin Exp Rheumatol. 2009;27(3):459–68.
64. Wallace AS, Carlson JR, Malone RM, et al. The influence of literacy on patient-reported experiences of diabetes self-management support. Nurs Res. 2010;59(5):356–63.
65. Paddison C, Elliott M, Parker R, et al. Should measures of patient experience in primary care be adjusted for case mix? Evidence from the English General Practice Patient Survey. BMJ Qual Saf. 2012;21(8):634–40.
66. Bowling A, Rowe G, Lambert N, et al. The measurement of patients' expectations for health care: a review and psychometric testing of a measure of patients' expectations. Health Technol Assess. 2012;16(30):i–xii, 1–509.
67. Robert G, Waite R, Cornwell J, et al. Understanding and improving patient experience: a national survey of training courses provided by higher education providers and healthcare organizations in England. Nurse Educ Today. 2014;34(1):112–20. pii:S0260-6917(12)00364-4.
68. Phillpotts C, Creamer P, Andrews T. Teaching medical students about chronic disease: patient-led teaching in rheumatoid arthritis. Musculoskeletal Care. 2010;8(1):55–60.

Chapter 18
PROMs and Musculoskeletal Ultrasonography

Jacqueline Uson and Yasser El Miedany

Introduction

Over the past decade, musculoskeletal ultrasound's (MSUS) role for the assessment and management of musculoskeletal disorders has grown rapidly. In contrast to conventional radiography, MSUS is able to provide multi-planner images of bone, cartilage, synovial membrane, fluid collection, muscles, ligament, and nerves, as well as vasculature. Furthermore, owing to its good resolution, it can depict even minute bone surface abnormalities. Thus destructive and/or hypertrophic or reparative changes on the bone surface could be seen before they appear on plain X-rays or even magnetic resonance imaging (MRI). Newer ultrasound (US) techniques and several research studies have demonstrated validity, reliability, and responsiveness of the MSUS in several rheumatic diseases [1, 2]. This gave MSUS its description of being the physician's extended finger and booked its place as the cornerstone in today's standard rheumatology practice for the articular as well as periarticular imaging. However, some apprehensions were raised regarding its reproducibility, and interpretations made. This may be attributed to the fact that MSUS is an operator-dependent imaging modality which, in turn, would reflect on the intrinsic

J. Uson, M.D. (✉)
Department of Rheumatology, Hospital Universitario de Móstoles, Madrid, Spain
e-mail: jusonjaeger@gmail.com

Y. El Miedany, M.D., F.R.C.P. (UK)
Honorary Senior Clinical Lecturer, King's College London, London, UK

Professor of Rheumatology and Rehabilitation, Ain Shams University, Cairo, Egypt

Department of Rheumatology, Darent Valley Hospital, Gravesend, Kent, UK
e-mail: drelmiedany@rheumatology4u.com

Y. El Miedany (ed.), *Patient Reported Outcome Measures in Rheumatic Diseases*,
DOI 10.1007/978-3-319-32851-5_18

real time taken for image acquisition as well as proficiency; both items require a rather long learning curve. Therefore, specific curriculum and training programs have been designed to ensure standardized joint scanning technique as well as recognition and usage for normal and pathologic sonographic definitions [3–6].

The Concept of Ultrasound-Detected Inflammatory and Structural Damage

Morphologic Inflammatory Damage

In the "window of opportunity" era, MSUS has gained the prestige as an adjuvant method for the diagnosis and monitoring of rheumatoid arthritis. Pathologically, MSUS joint imaging has shown that "*morphologic inflammation*" can be detected before structural damage occurs and that it is reversible on management. Therefore, it has been suggested as a predictor of poorer functional outcome in early chronic inflammatory arthritic conditions such as rheumatoid arthritis (RA) [7]. The three principle European League Against Rheumatism (EULAR) MSUS joint recommendations for the clinical management of RA stated that joint ultrasonography should be considered for accurate evaluation of joint inflammation, for monitoring disease activity, as well as subclinical inflammation assessment [8]. MSUS depicts three articular morpho-functional features including joint, tendon sheath, and synovitis: *effusion* defined on grayscale (GS) US as an anechogenic or hypoechogenic compressible material that denotes the exudative aspect of the synovia; *synovial hypertrophy* defined on grayscale US as hypoechogenic noncompressible material that represents its proliferative characteristic; and *abnormal synovial vascularization* assessed with power or color Doppler US and defined as the presence of Doppler signal in the synovia that indicates the invasive nature of the synovia [5]. The presence of Doppler signal is considered an important marker of *active inflammatory status* at joint and patient level, given that it correlates with ongoing joint destruction and disease activity [9].

To monitor treatment in rheumatoid arthritis, a precise measure of the disease activity should be obtained by both clinical and para-clinical parameters. The disease activity of a joint is correlated with the synovial vascularization [9]. Therefore quantitative assessment of synovial vascularization plays an important role in monitoring the disease activity status and response to therapy. There are several synovitis grayscale and Doppler scoring systems for joint synovitis, yet the more widely used is a semiquantitative system proposed by OMERACT (Outcome Measures in Rheumatology), which was reported easy to learn, valid, as well as reliable [10]. The approach features the use of 0–3 scale, in which 0 entails no synovitis, 1 = mild, 2 = moderate, and 3 = severe synovitis [4]. Synovial Doppler signal is scored as 0 = no signal, 1 = single vessel signal, 2 = confluent vessels less than 50 % of the joint area, and 3 = more than 50 % of the joint area. OMERACT score called GLOSS is a global synovitis scoring system that combines grayscale synovial hypertrophy and power Doppler (PD) in one. Its responsiveness has been tested in one international multicenter open-label medication trial. It has the advantage that it can be performed *á la carte* [11].

Although tenosynovitis is a common manifestation in RA and was reported to be an early marker of the disease, it received much less attention by the scientific community than joint synovitis [12]. There is evidence that MSUS-detected tenosynovitis is more sensitive than physical examination [13], it is responsive to effective treatment [14, 15], and that its persistence, namely extensor carpi ulnaris tenosynovitis, predicts structural bone damage [16]. Tenosynovitis is defined as a hypoechoic or anechoic thickened tissue with or without fluid within the tendon sheath, which is seen in two perpendicular plains and that may exhibit Doppler signal [5]. Quantitative assessment of tenosynovitis in RA patients was studied by the single multi-expert-examiner consensus exercise [17]. Results revealed a good reproducibility using a semiquantitative scoring system based on the extension of Doppler signal within the widened synovial sheath (excluding the feeding blood supply Doppler signal). The scoring system rated from: 0 = no Doppler signal, 1 = peritendinous focal signal within the widened synovial sheath, 2 = peritendinous multifocal signal within the widened synovial sheath, and 3 = peritendinous diffuse signal within the widened synovial sheath. If abnormal intra-tendinous signal existed in two perpendicular planes, then grades 1 and 2 are increased by one point.

Structural Damage

Structural MSUS joint disorders include intra-articular erosions, synovial-tendon damage, as well as cartilage changes. Bone erosions are a destructive consequence of synovitis and osteitis. A MSUS-detected erosion is defined as a cortical break seen in two perpendicular planes [5]. When compared with radiography, MSUS detects more erosions in the hand, shoulder, and feet [18–21]. This is attributed to the fact that MSUS examination is multi-planer whereas radiography is two-dimensional. However, MSUS-detected erosion is determined by the size of the acoustic window. In routine clinical practice, MSUS-erosions are searched for diagnostic purposes and ongoing damage at specific sites in RA (distal ulna, second to fifth metacarpophalangeal [MCP] head, and fifth metatarsophalangeal [MTP] head) [22]. Doppler signal within an erosion probably signifies ongoing bone damage [23] and is often called a hot or active erosion. MSUS-erosions ≥ 2.5 mm are highly sensitive and more specific for RA than those ≤ 2 mm that may be visualized in normal individuals or in degenerative joint disorders [22]. Currently there is no recommended erosion scoring system.

The natural history of synovial-tendon damage in RA is unclear. It has been suggested that synovitis produces internal tendon damage leading to partial and ultimately complete tendon tear. Unfortunately, physical examination is unable to detect tendon structural damage until the tendon is totally torn exhibiting loss of function. The sonopathologic features of MSUS-detected synovial-tendon damage range from loss of the normal fibrillar echotexture, irregularity of the tendon margin, hypoechoic areas within the tendon, and discontinuity of the tendon [24]. In the clinical setting, MSUS assessment of synovial-tendon damage may be used to identify and follow tendons that are prone to rupture. To date the available grading system proposed by OMERACT has been tested in one expert multiobserver study [17]. They defined synovial-tendon damage on GS as internal and/or peripheral focal tendon defect (i.e., absence of fibers) in the region enclosed by the tendon sheath, seen in two perpendicular planes. The grade of damage assessed in both longitudinal and transverse planes compasses three semiquantitative scores: grade 0 = normal, grade 1 = partial tendon rupture, and grade 2 = complete tendon rupture. The most reliable tendons were the extensor carpialis ularis and tibialis posterior—probably because both tendons are thick straight-running and do not split.

As far as the articular cartilage, MSUS is able to depict several hyaline cartilage abnormalities; however, its clinical use in RA is hampered because there are no longitudinal studies aimed to identify cartilage damage progression. In fact, only few MSUS studies in RA have included descriptions of cartilage abnormalities [25, 26]. Recently, it has been demonstrated that MSUS measures of metacarpal cartilage is closely related to anatomical cartilage thickness in anatomic specimens and that both radiographic joint space widening and joint space narrowing represents cartilage thickness in patients with RA [27]. These authors suggested that MSUS metacarpal cartilage thickness measurement could be used when radiographs are not available or when joint malalignment exists. The qualitative MSUS cartilage-changes include loss of sharpness of the superficial margin, focal or diffuse cartilage thinning, and loss of sharpness of the deep margin that represents subchondral bone involvement secondary to cartilage attached inflamed synovial tissue in RA [25, 28]. A study was carried out to assess the reproducibility of the proposed cartilage scoring system. Results depicted a moderate to good interobserver reproducibility of a semiquantitative scoring system based on the qualitative morphological cartilage damage in RA [29].

The Synovio-Entheseal Complex and Synovitis

The "synovio-entheseal complex" represents the close anatomical integration between the enthesis and synovium. According to this scenario, the enthesis fibrocartilages that are located next to synovium (in joint, bursae, or tendons) rely on the synovium for lubrication, oxygenation, and removal of microdebris. Being fibrocartilagenous, the enthesis insertion is avascular. Therefore, derangements in the enthesis are expected to trigger an inflammatory response in the adjacent vascular synovium [30].

In spondyloarthropathies (SpA), enthesitis has been considered the pathologic hallmark and have been reported early in the disease course before irreversible lesions develop. In contrast to both clinical and radiographic assessments of enthesitis, which have been shown to be inaccurate, MSUS has the advantage of being able to directly visualize disorders of the enthesis as well as entheseal-related structures. This may appear as hypoechogenic thickening of the enthesis with or without Doppler signal, enthesial erosion, entesophytes, calcifications, cortical irregularities, or bursitis and tendonitis [31]. These inflammatory and structural disorders have been encompassed, years ago, in the OMERACT ultrasound definition of *entesopathy* [5]. A definition of *active enthesitis* should denote potentially reversible MSUS disorders and perhaps ongoing disease severity, analogous to active synovitis in rheumatoid arthritis. Recently OMERACT reported the first consensus-based US definition of enthesitis and its elementary components to ensure a higher degree of homogeneity and comparability [32]. There was agreement on the inclusion of hypoechogenicity, increased thickness at the tendon insertion, calcifications, enthesophytes, erosions, and Doppler activity as elementary lesions of enthesitis. Whereas, there was no agreement obtained regarding the inclusion of bursitis or tendonitis. Furthermore, the consensus delineated signs of active inflammation from signs of structural damage at the enthesis site, where hypo-echogenicity, thickening, and Doppler signal represent the main signs of *active enthesitis.*

Subclinical enthesitis was reported in earlier MSUS studies, which revealed a high frequency of abnormalities in asymptomatic patients with psoriasis without musculoskeletal clinical signs or symptoms [33, 34]. In concordance, it was also reported in both early [35–37] and established SpA including psoriatic arthritis [31, 38–40]. Recently EULAR published the first recommendation of MSUS-imaging in the diagnosis and management of SpA in clinical practice based on the best available evidence and clinical expertise supported by an international panel of experts [41]. When peripheral SpA is suspected, MSUS is advised to detect peripheral enthesitis, which may support the diagnosis of SpA. It also recommends the use of US to monitor disease activity (particularly synovitis and enthesitis) in peripheral SpA, providing additional information on top of clinical and biochemical assessments.

Several MSUS enthesitis assessment tools have been developed in SpA cohorts for diagnosis and classification as well as for monitoring response to treatment [39, 42–44]. The Glasgow Ultrasound Enthesitis Scoring System (GUESS) tool is a semiquantitative GS 5 enthesial site scoring system (Achilles, quadriceps, superior and inferior patellar tendons, and plantar fascia) [42]. The Madrid Sonographic Enthesitis Index (MASEI) is a semiquantitative GS and PD 6 enthesial site scoring system (triceps, Achilles, quadriceps, superior and inferior patellar tendons, and plantar fascia) [39]. MASEI scores bone erosions, power Doppler signal, and severe enthesophytes higher than tendon thickening, hypo-echogenicity, or small enthesophytes. MASEI performed well for diagnosis and classification [41]. Both scoring systems have shown good reproducibility [45].

While the role of the enthesis is fully appreciated in SpA, there are some recent findings pointing toward similar novel mechanisms of synovitis and joint damage in osteoarthritis that have previously been unacknowledged [46, 47]. Normal enthesis fibrocartilage shows age-related changes similar to osteoarthritis, including fissuring, fibrillation, and degeneration. Therefore, the term "enthesopathy" is recommended for use to describe the changes in osteoarthritis as these changes appear to be less inflammatory. The role of the enthesis organ in bone erosion formation in rheumatoid arthritis has recently been described [48]. Specifically, early rheumatoid arthritis erosion formation occurs immediately adjacent to the small joint collateral ligament insertions as a result of enthesis-associated compression of bone at these sites. These findings moved enthesitis, from being a "second-class citizen" in SpA, to the center stage as a structure responsible for morphologic changes in both inflammatory and degenerative arthritic diseases.

Table 18.1 depicts the joint sonopathologic definitions together with its corresponding MSUS images (Figs. 18.1, 18.2, 18.3, 18.4, 18.5, 18.6, 18.7, 18.8, 18.9, 18.10, 18.11, and 18.12).

Musculoskeletal Ultrasound and Patient Reported Outcome Measures

The new concept redefining health outcomes has gone beyond disease activity control and status of remission to include other parameters that are also vital in the disease management process. This includes patient-reported as well as structural outcomes. The correlation of joint ultrasonographic findings and clinical assessment has been studied thoroughly over the past years and US was reported to be a more reliable measure of disease activity than clinical evaluation in patients with inflammatory arthritis. Furthermore, sonographic outcomes have shown a better discriminatory capacity in both early and late stages of the disease process [49, 50]. In contrast, both US and patient reported outcomes demonstrated similar predictive validity with regard to disease progression as well as joint damage. Taking into account the differences in quantification schemes used to assess both tools (visual analogue scale in patient reported outcome measures versus graded semiquantitative synovitis assessment in joint ultrasonography), the persistence of such relation early in the disease course, during disease activity, as well as in remission, has added a potential value for patient reported outcome measures in standard clinical practice. Though there was no direct studies linking sonographic findings to individual patient reported disease activity parameters, such correlations were evident as secondary outcomes in different studies.

Ultrasound Versus Functional Disability

The outcome of inflammatory arthritis relies mainly on the severity of joint damage, the patient's physical ability status, psychological health, and the presence of associated comorbid illness such as cardiovascular disease or infection. Functional disability has been reported to be a biomarker for inflammatory arthritis [51]. Its

Table 18.1 MSUS joint sonopathologic definitions and examples

Synovial fluid (effusion) (2005 OMERACT)	Abnormal hypoechoic or anechoic intra-articular material that is displaceable and compressible but does not exhibit Doppler signal
Synovial hypertrophy (2005 OMERACT)	Abnormal hypoechoic intra-articular tissue that is non-displaceable and poorly compressible and which may exhibit Doppler signal
Tenosynovitis (2005 OMERACT)	Hypoechoic or anechoic thickened tissue with or without fluid within the tendon sheath, which is seen in two perpendicular planes and which may exhibit Doppler signal. And may be accompanied by structural tendon lesions
Intra-articular erosion (2005 OMERACT)	An intra-articular discontinuity of the bone surface that is visible in two perpendicular planes
Cartilage damage (2005 OMERACT)	Loss of normal anechoic echostructure, and/or loss of sharpness of at least one margin, and/or irregularity of the superficial margin, and/or thinning of the cartilage layer
Enthesopathy (2005 OMERACT)	Abnormally hypoechoic and/or thickened tendon or ligament at its bony attachment (may occasionally contain hyperechoic foci consistent with calcification), seen in two perpendicular planes that may exhibit Doppler signal and/or bony changes including enthesophytes, erosions, or irregularity
Enthesial hypoechogenicity (2014 OMERACT)	Lack of the homogeneous fibrillar pattern with loss of the tightly packed echogenic lines after correcting for anisotropy
Enthesial increased thickness (2014 OMERACT)	Increased thickness of the tendon/ligament/capsule insertion into the bone, as compared to the body of the tendon/ligament/capsule, with or without blurring of the tendon/ligament/capsule margins
Enthesophyte (2014 OMERACT)	A step up of bony prominence at the end of the normal bone contour, seen in two perpendicular planes, with or without acoustic shadow
Enthesial calcifications	Hyperechoic (bright) foci consistent with calcific deposits, with or without acoustic shadow, seen in two perpendicular planes, detected at the tendon insertion into the bone
Enthesial erosion	Cortical breakage with a step down contour defect, seen in two perpendicular planes, at the insertion of the enthesis to the bone
Enthesial Doppler signal	Doppler activity approximately < 2 mm near the bony cortex. The Doppler signal must be at the enthesis, different from reflecting surface artifact or nutrition vessel signal, with or without cortical irregularities, erosions, or entesophytes

validity was depicted in patients presenting with early inflammatory arthritis where progression of the patient's functional disability over a short period of time was predictive of persistent inflammatory arthritis status [52]. Similarly, deterioration of the patient's functional disability correlated significantly with the progression of the patient's joint damage [53]. Moreover, functional disability has been used to evaluate response to therapies and is a prerequisite for proving that a drug has disease-controlling capacity [54, 55]. In concordance, several other studies revealed that US

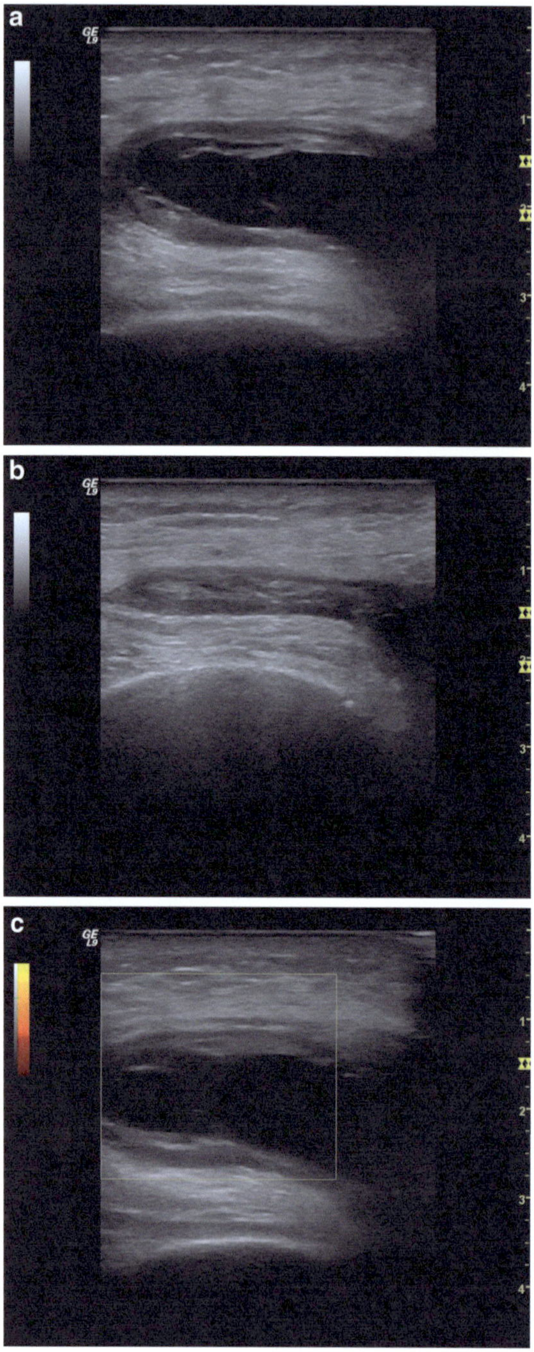

Fig. 18.1 Transverse image of the medial knee parapatellar recess. (**a**) Anechogenic synovial fluid. (**b**) Compressible. (**c**) No power Doppler signal

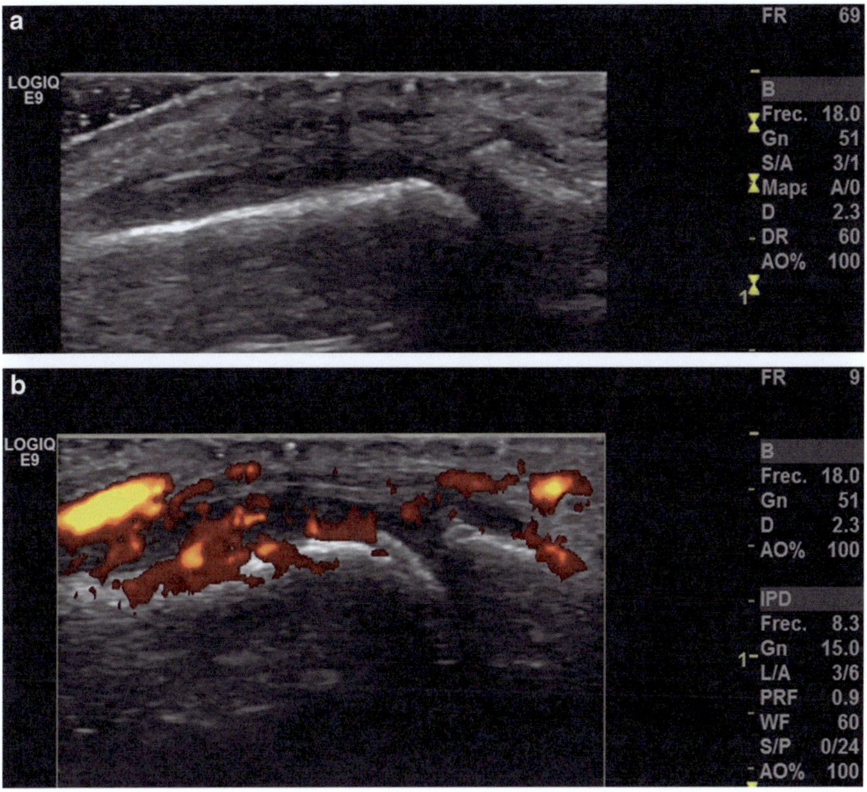

Fig. 18.2 Longitudinal dorsal image of a PIP joint with (**a**) GS and (**b**) PD synovitis

has the ability to detect early synovial hypertrophy and effusion as well as active inflammatory arthritic status [13, 56–59]. Similarly, it is relevant in predicting the course of the disease as well as the radiographic progression [23]. This agreement between US and functional disability measurements was supported by the findings of the study carried out by Gartner et al. [60] on 90 patients known to have inflammatory arthritis for a mean of 9.4 years (SD 8.9). Results revealed that RA patients having a high-grade PD signal (PD grade 3) showed a doubling of the Health Assessment Questionnaire-Disability Index (HAQ-DI) values (mean ± SD HAQ-DI score 0.45 ± 0.62) compared to patients whose PD grades were lower (PD grade ≤ 2) where HAQ-DI score (mean ± SD) was 0.24 ± 0.41 and in patient with any PD grade, the HAQ DI score was 0.20 ± 0.35. These findings are also in agreement with those reported in another recent study [50], which included 480 patients suffering from early inflammatory arthritis (mean disease duration was 6.3 ± 2.1 months). Results revealed that changes in functional disability scores were significantly correlated with changes in power Doppler scores. Similarly, flare up of the disease was associated with poor baseline functional disability measures as well as US-Grayscale score/PD score ≥ 2.

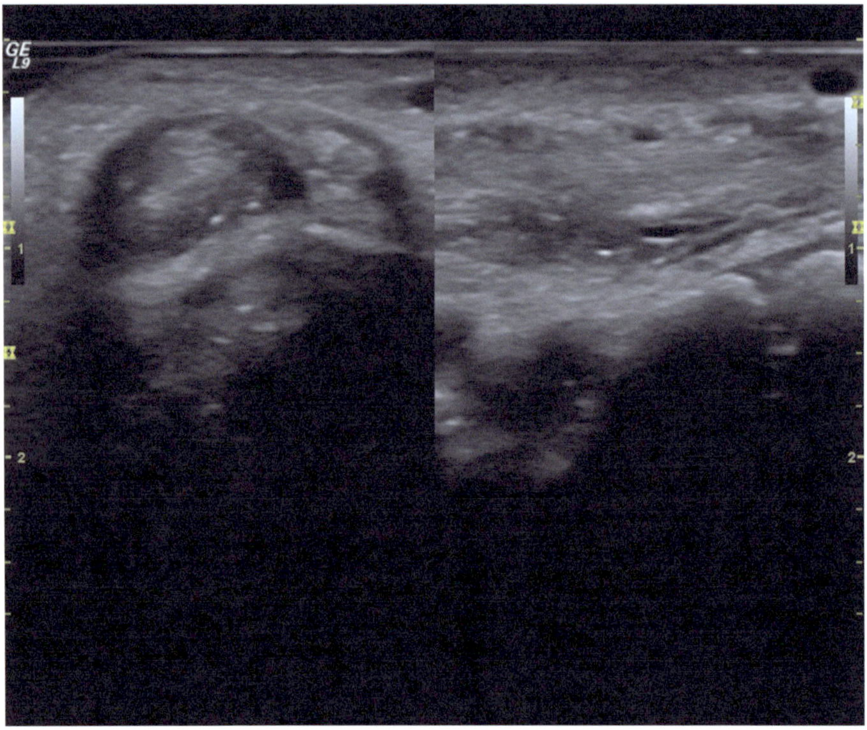

Fig. 18.3 Longitudinal and transverse image of tenosynovitis of the second extensor wrist compartment. Note the tendon margin irregularities

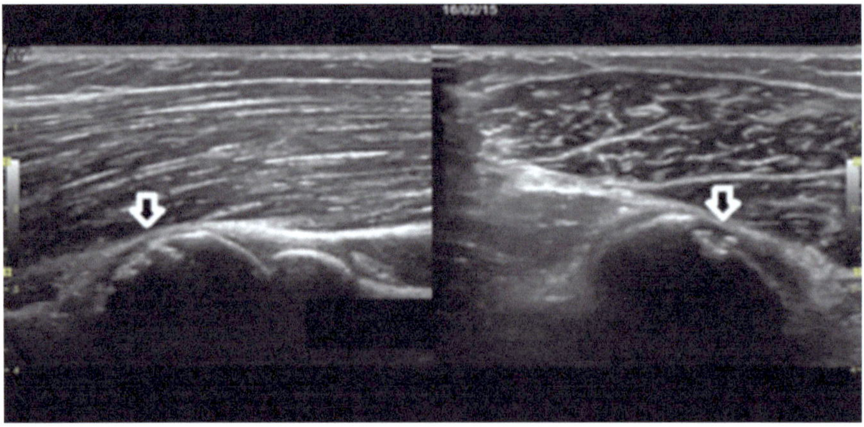

Fig. 18.4 Longitudinal and transverse image of a humeral condyle erosion of the elbow joint

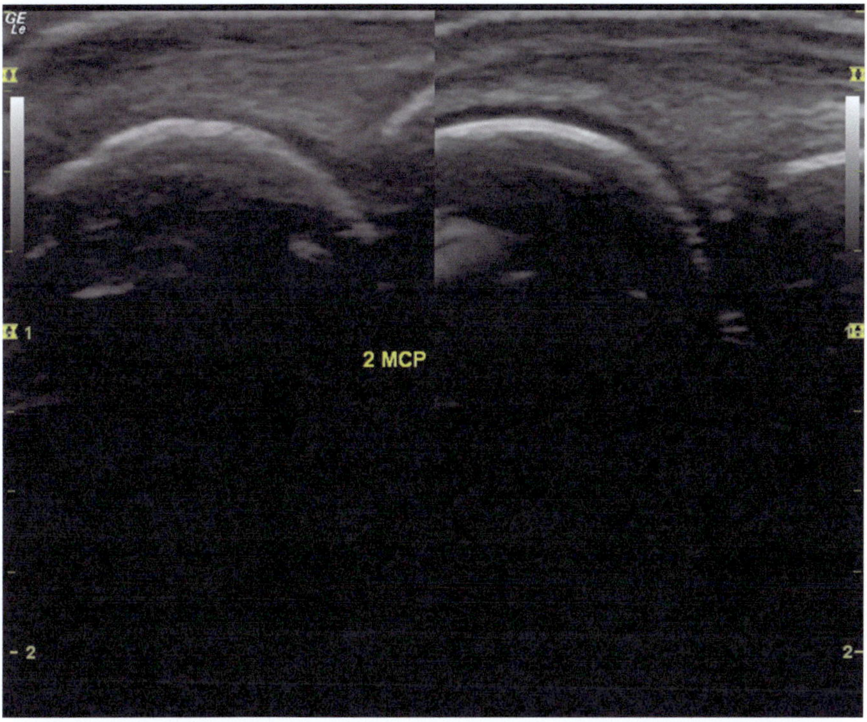

Fig. 18.5 Longitudinal MCP cartilage. Left severe abnormalities and right normal cartilage

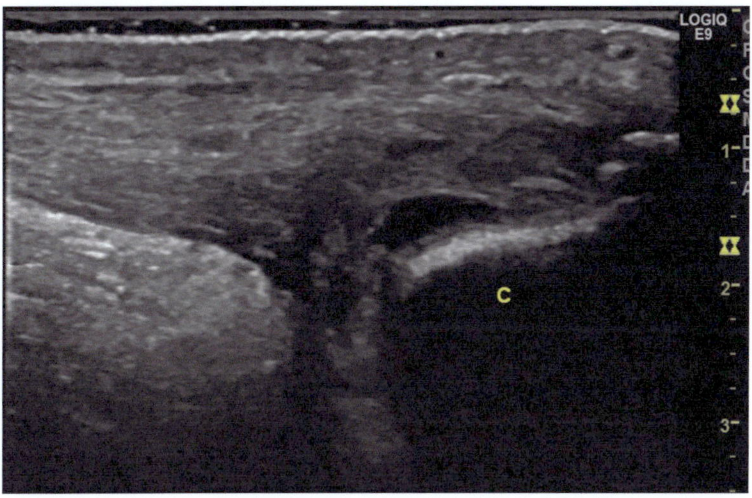

Fig. 18.6 Longitudinal Aquillies tendon insertion showing enthesial thickening, retro-Aquilles bursitis and calcifications

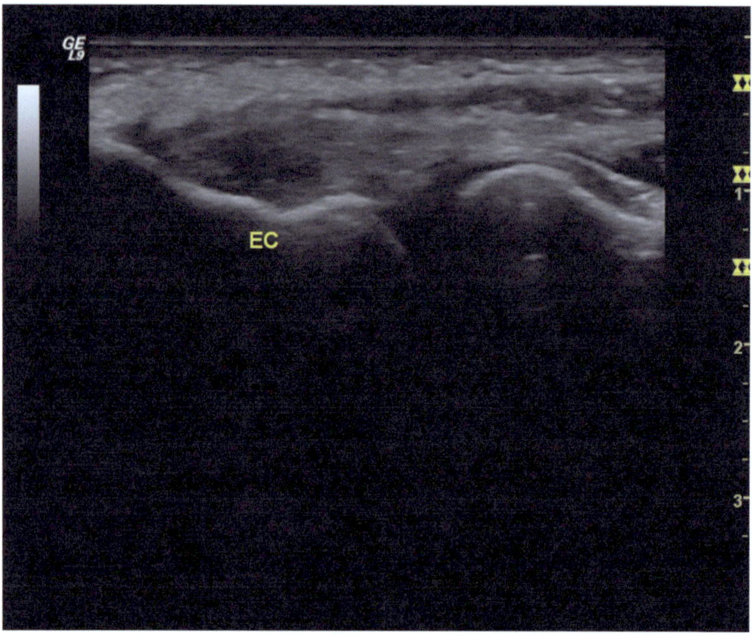

Fig. 18.7 Longitudinal image of a hypoechoic common extensor tendon insertion

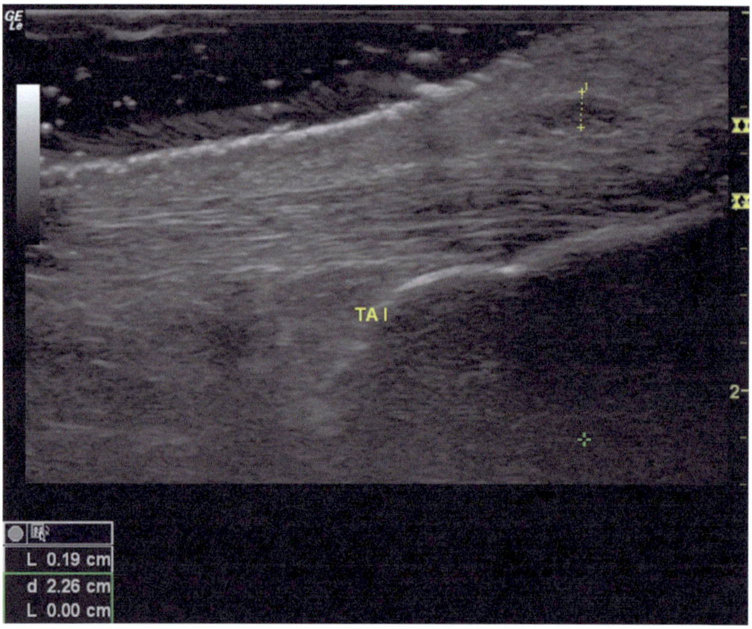

Fig. 18.8 Longitudinal image of an increased hypoechogenic Achilles tendon insertion. Calipers show a pre-Achilles bursitis

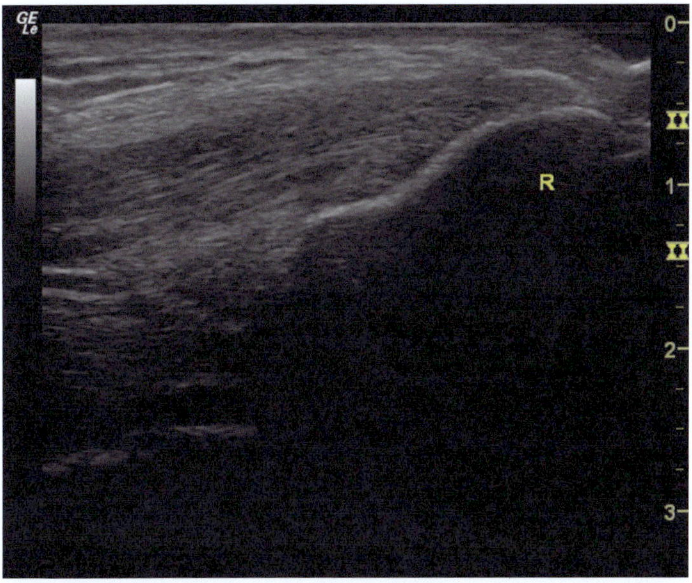

Fig. 18.9 Longitudinal image of a patellar entesophyte

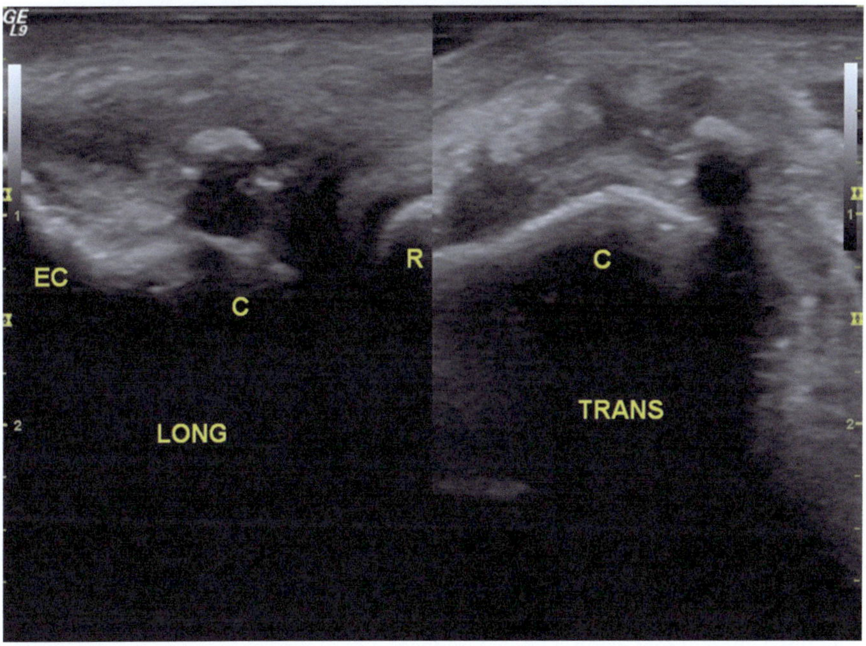

Fig. 18.10 Longitudinal and transverse image of calcifications within the common extensor tendon

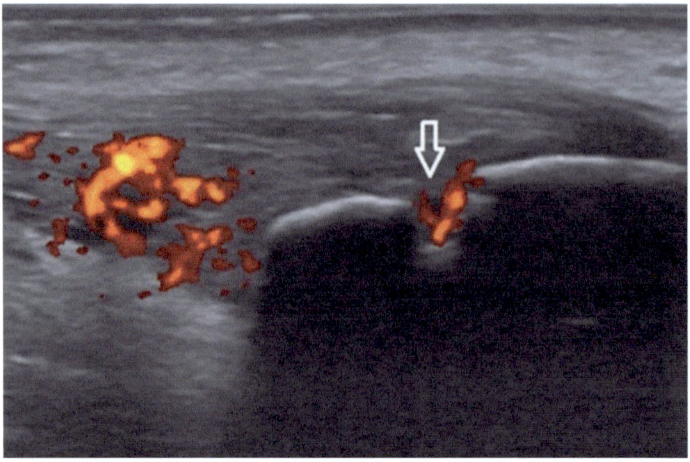

Fig. 18.11 Longitudinal image of a bone erosion with PD signal of the calcaneous

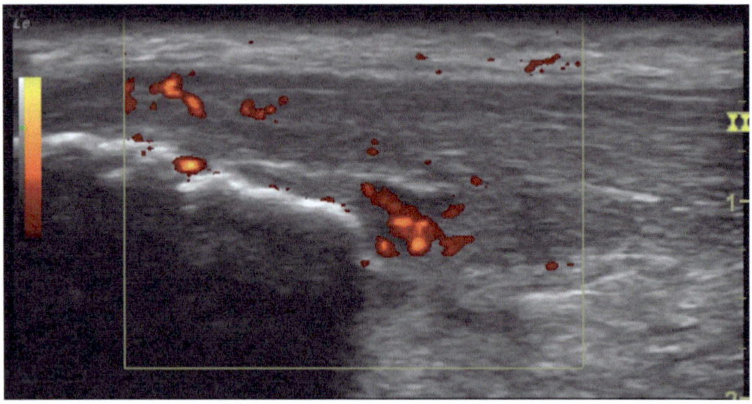

Fig. 18.12 Longitudinal image of a hypoechoic thickened common extensor tendon insertion with PD signal

Ultrasound Versus Tender Joints

Tender and swollen joints are the corner stone for the clinical disease activity assessment, as they enable the treating rheumatologist to detect and quantify synovitis in RA patients [61]. Furthermore, joint counts help steer treatment decisions to achieve the aimed clinical remission, which composes a vital part of the overarching "treating to target" principle [62]. Due to the importance of joint counts in disease activity assessment, and the fact that formal joint counts are not routinely performed by the rheumatologists in the standard clinical practice, possibly limited by constraints of resources and time [63], there is renewed interest in examining the role of patient-reported tender and swollen joint counts [64–66], which may be helpful in monitoring disease activity between clinic visits. A study carried out by Cheung et al. [67] to evaluate the relationship between patient-reported tender and swollen joints with active inflammation assessed by power Doppler and whether this relationship is affected by significant joint damage. The study included RA patients with long-standing disease (median disease duration of 15 years) and moderate Disease Activity Score (median DAS-28: 3.5). Results revealed that the joints showing significant active inflammation (e.g., grade 3 on PD assessment), RA patients identified 75 % as tender and 63 % as swollen. Swollen joints showed strong association at the joint level with active synovitis when there was no significant radiographic damage (LR 2.54, 95 % CI 1.93–3.34). Swollen joint counts were statistically correlated with PDUS-DAS28 and CRP, but not PDUS score.

Sensitivity analysis revealed better agreement of tender and swollen joints with active synovitis when DAS28 was ≤3.2 and when patient global pain was <50 mm on visual analogue scale. These results are in agreement with the findings of another work done by El Miedany et al. [68] which included 121 RA patients who have achieved remission and were monitored on a 3-monthly basis. The aim of the study was to assess US imaging as an outcome measure in monitoring the RA patients' response to therapy and its impact on the patients' management. Also to identify which joints should be US scanned in the standard clinical practice. Results revealed that in comparison to clinical examination, US showed significantly more joints with effusion (mean 14.2) and synovitis (mean 16.1) than clinical examination (mean 10.2, $p<0.05$). A significant correlation was found between patient self-reported joint tenderness and both US-PD and total US scores. The study concluded that in standard clinical practice, patient self-reported joint tenderness is the best marker to identify joints that need to be US scanned. However, such significant correlation between patient reported tender joints and joint ultrasonography was not reported in patients suffering from significant joint damage, deformities, or long-standing chronic synovitis [67]. A study by Janta et al. [69] compared disease activity assessed by the patient, the physician, and musculoskeletal US in patients with RA in clinical remission. Results revealed that patient-assessed and physician-assessed overall RA activity showed acceptable agreement, and that at the patient level, physician-assessed joint swelling showed an acceptable concordance with Doppler US synovitis.

Ultrasound Versus Other Reported Clinical Outcomes

Today's therapeutic target in RA patients is achievement of disease remission or low disease activity, whereby the term remission comprises lack of clinical disease activity, halt of joint damage progression, and normalization or maximal improvement of patient global assessment as well as physical function [70]. Patient global assessment is included in both the DAS28 score assessment and the American

College of Radiology (ACR) response criteria. Morphologic assessment of painful sites using MSUS would help to identify whether the cause of pain is either synovitis, tenosynovitis, or enthesitis. This would help avoid overestimation of patients/physicians global assessment, meanwhile it will help in setting a treatment program tailored to the patient's underlying pathology. Recently it was reported to show significant correlation with disease activity better than the physician global assessment particularly in RA patients presenting with moderate-high disease activity [71]. The relation between US and variable patient reported outcome measures was depicted as secondary outcomes of earlier published studies. In a study carried out on established RA patients to compare clinically active joints to sonographically active joints in RA patients, results revealed significant correlations between sonographic findings (Grayscale score ≥ 2, PD score ≥ 2) and other clinical measures, such as laboratory results, VAS score for pain, patient's global assessment of disease activity, physician global assessment of disease activity, as well as duration of morning stiffness [60]. In concordance, similar findings were reported in another study, which included early inflammatory arthritis patients who were treated to target and monitored for 52 weeks [50]. Results revealed that changes in the functional disability scores and duration of morning stiffness were significantly correlated to changes in PD scores. These findings show that, indeed, the differences between sonographic and patient reported outcome measures are considerably low in particular when higher cutoff points for defining an active joint in sonography is used.

Ultrasound and Adherence to Therapy

Whilst several studies depicted the value of US in the management of inflammatory arthritis and its ability to detect subclinical synovitis, assess joint damage, and guide joint aspiration as well as injection [71–75], there is little published data regarding its use in patient education or as a tool to improve adherence/compliance to medication. Humans possess an innate cognitive preference for visually presented information [76, 77]. It is therefore not surprising to find that the use of pictorial aids was associated with improved medication instruction recall, comprehension, and adherence, especially when combined with supportive written or verbal information [78]. This was supported by the findings of earlier studies that revealed that health interventions containing visual elements and simple comprehensible information were effective at improving patient understanding of the condition and treatment [79, 80].

Musculoskeletal US can be a valuable patient education tool [81] as it enables the treating clinician to enhance patient understanding through "real-time" visual demonstration of joint structures, synovial inflammation, and articular damage. The ability to navigate around the site of interest on the patient's own anatomy may improve patient understanding more than the traditional static images, especially when combined with clinician–patient interaction at close quarters. Furthermore, the recognition of structural damage with MSUS—such as erosions, tendon damage, and cartilage abnormalities—would help the patients understand the need for medical or surgical management and the reasons behind changing their medication type or dose. In addition, the visualization of severity of the disease activity or joint damage using musculoskeletal US would have a positive impact on patient-centered outcomes such as belief in the necessity of medication, activation (i.e., engagement with therapy), and medication adherence in patients with RA. This was assessed recently in a study [82] that included 18 patients with active RA (DAS-28 > 2.6) who require increased immunosuppression. At baseline, 3 and 10 days post US every patient completed three different questionnaires including: (1) Beliefs about Medicines Questionnaire (BMQ) to measure the cost-benefit analysis made by patients regarding the necessity versus concern of medication; (2) Patient Activation Measure (PAM-13) to assess patient activation; and (3) Compliance Questionnaire-Rheumatology (CQR) to measure medication adherence. In addition, every patient was assessed clinically and patient reported outcome measures were recording for physical function, pain, and global status. Results revealed that showing the patients "real-time" US images of their clinically inflamed joints on one occasion reduced patient concerns regarding escalation of immunosuppression, while maintaining a positive and stable belief in the necessity of medication as assessed by the Beliefs about Medicines Questionnaire. This resulted in patients' cost-benefit analyses shifting in favor of the benefits (or necessities) of pharmacotherapy. Stable disease activity score and patient outcome measures during the study suggested that the observed change in the Beliefs about Medicines Questionnaire scores was not due to fluctuation in disease severity. The authors concluded that it is heartening that a simple intervention of one 20-min US session with the treating rheumatologist appeared to be an effective patient educational tool that was associated with a reduction in patient concerns about medication. This is particularly important in RA as patient levels of concern are high and associated with medication non-adherence and helplessness [83]. Table 18.2 includes the main studies carried out to assess the relation between MSUS-synovitis assessment and patient reported outcome measures in rheumatoid arthritis patients at different disease stages [50, 60, 67, 68, 82].

Ultrasound-Guided Procedures and Patient Reported Outcome Measures

US offers a real-time visual aid helping to carry out a quick, safe, and precise intra-articular or soft tissue procedures. Furthermore, US enables the treating health care professional to see beneath the skin's surface, make immediate care decisions, and avoid or minimize complications. In some cases, this added information has changed the course of action or treatment completely. Several studies were carried out comparing the accuracy of blind versus US-guided procedures and systematic meta-analysis studies repeatedly gave the privilege to US-guided procedures [84–87]. However, outcomes of any interventional procedure is mainly "patient" based,

Table 18.2 The relation between MSUS-synovitis assessment and patient reported outcome measures in rheumatoid arthritis patients at different disease stages

US parameter	PROMs parameter	Study	Number of patients	Disease duration (mean ± SD)	Significance
PD ≥ grade 2	Functional disability	• Gartner et al. [60]	• 90	• 9.4 ± 8.9 year	• *P*-value: 0.019
		• El Miedany et al. [50]	• 480	• 6.3 ± 2.1 month	• *P* < 0.01
PD ≥ grade 2	Tender Joint count	• Cheung et al. [67]	• 50	• 15-years (median) range: 10–21 year	• Positive LR (95 % CI): 1.89 (1.52–2.35)
		• El Miedany [68]	• 121	• 6.3 + 1.2 months	• *P* < 0.01
PD ≥ grade 2	Swollen Joint count	• Cheung et al. [67]	• 50	• 15-years (median)	• Positive LR (95 % CI): 2.54 (1.93–3.34)
Grayscale ≥ grade 2	Patient Global Assessment	• El Miedany et al. [50]	• 480	• 6.3 ± 201 month	• *P* < 0.01
	Pain Score				
	Morning Stiffness				
Grayscale	Adherence to therapy	• Joplin et al. [82]	• 18	• 49.2 ± 58.8 months	• *P* < 0.01

hence the role of patient reported outcome measures. PROMs facilitate quantitative assessment of the patient's response to the US-guided procedure. Four main patient reported parameters have been included in previous studies as primary or secondary outcomes, namely: (1) pain; (2) functional ability; (3) quality of life, such as sleep and ability to work; as well as (4) patient global assessment [88, 89]. Results revealed that the patients who underwent US-guided injections had statistically significant greater improvement in joint pain and function at 6 weeks after injection, and also had less adverse events in comparison to blinded injections. In a systematic meta-analysis, which included 12 randomized controlled trials [90], assessing the effectiveness of US guidance on intra- and periarticular joint injections, results revealed that US-guided intra-articular and periarticular joint injections were more accurate than the landmark-guided injections. Ultrasound-guided procedures significantly decreased the visual analogue scale scores for pain, patient global assessment, and functional ability, as well as quality of life at both 2 and 6 weeks after injection. The meta-analysis conclusion recommended routine ultrasound guidance for intra-articular and periarticular injections. Subsequently, PROMs is advised for use in standard clinical practice as it would enable the treating doctor to quantitate and record the response to management.

Conclusion

MSUS has emerged as a powerful adjunctive clinical imaging tool for assessment of inflammatory as well as noninflammatory arthritic conditions. It is more sensitive than clinical assessment as it has the ability to detect synovial hypertrophy and effusion through Grayscale ultrasonography as well as active inflammation through Doppler mode. Several studies depicted the relationship of patient reported outcomes such as functional disability, patient reported tender and swollen joint counts, pain score, patient global assessment, and morning stiffness with the MSUS, which detected morphologic inflammatory/structural changes. In addition, MSUS plays an important role to improve patients' adherence to therapy, identify the underlying cause of joint pain, and helping to set up a treatment program tailored to the patient's needs as well as patient education. There is a potential role for linking PROMs and MSUS outcomes in the setting of a minimal to low disease activity without erosive changes.

References

1. Keen HI, Wakefield R, Conaghan PG. Optimising ultrasonography in rheumatology. Clin Exp Rheumatol. 2014;32(5 Suppl 85):S-13–6.
2. Naredo E. Ultrasound in rheumatology: two decades of rapid development and evolving implementation. Med Ultrason. 2015;17(1):3–4.

3. Naredo E, Bijlsma JWJ, Conaghan PG, Acebes C, Balint P, Berner-Hammer H, et al. Recommendations for the content and conduct of European League Against Rheumatism (EULAR) musculoskeletal ultrasound courses. Ann Rheum Dis. 2008;67(7):1017–22.
4. Terslev L, Hammer H, Torp-Pedersen S, Szkudlarek M, Iagnocco A, D'Agostino M, Schmidt W, et al. EFSUMB minimum training requirements for rheumatologists performing musculoskeletal ultrasound. Ultraschall Med. 2013;24(5):475–7.
5. Wakefield RJ, Balint PV, Szkudlarek M, Filippucci E, Agostino MD, Sanchez EN, et al. Musculoskeletal ultrasound including definitions for ultrasonographic pathology. J Rheumatol. 2005;32(12):2485–7.
6. Schmidt WA, Schmidt H, Schicke B, Gromnica-Ihle E. Standard reference values for musculoskeletal ultrasonography. Ann Rheum Dis. 2004;63(8):988–94.
7. Fukae J, Isobe M, Kitano A, Henmi M, Sakamoto F, Narita A, et al. Structural deterioration of finger joints with ultrasonographic synovitis in rheumatoid arthritis patients with clinical low disease activity. Rheumatology. 2014;53(9):1608–12.
8. Colebatch AN, Edwards CJ, Østergaard M, van der Heijde D, Balint PV, D'Agostino M-A, et al. EULAR recommendations for the use of imaging of the joints in the clinical management of rheumatoid arthritis. Ann Rheum Dis. 2013;72(6):804–14.
9. Fukae J, Tanimura K, Atsumi T, Koike T. Sonographic synovial vascularity of synovitis in rheumatoid arthritis. Rheumatology. 2014;53(4):586–91.
10. Mandl P, Naredo E, Wakefield R, Conaghan P, D'Agostino M, et al. A systematic literature review analysis of ultrasound joint count and scoring systems to assess synovitis in rheumatoid arthritis according to the OMERACT filter. J Rheumatol. 2011;38(9):2055–62.
11. D´Agostino M, Wakefield R, Berner-Hammer H, Vittecoq O,Filippou G et al. Value of ultrasonography as a marker of early response to abatacept in patients with rheumatoid arthritis and an inadequate response to methotrexate:results from the APPRAISE study. Ann Rheum Dis 2015; doi 10.1136.
12. Filer A, Cader M, Abhishek A. Ultrasound defined tenosynovitis improves the prediction of rheumatoid arthritis and persistent disease in patients with very early synovitis. Ann Rheum Dis. 2013;71:506–7.
13. Naredo E, Bonilla G, Gamero F, Uson J, Carmona L, Laffon A. Assessment of inflammatory activity in rheumatoid arthritis: a comparative study of clinical evaluation with grey scale and power Doppler ultrasonography. Ann Rheum Dis. 2005;64(3):375–81.
14. Uson J, Morcillo M, Naredo E, Collado P, Palop M, Muñoz P, Bustabad S. Estudio ecografico de la inflamación de los tendones de la muñeca y mano en pacientes con artritis reumatoide en terapia anti-TNF. Reum Clin. 2006;2:80:154.
15. Hammer HB, Kvien TK. Ultrasonography shows significant improvement in wrist and ankle tenosynovitis in rheumatoid arthritis patients treated with adalimumab. Scand J Rheumatol. 2011;40(3):178–82.
16. Lillegraven S, Boyesen P, Hammer HB, Ostergaard M, Uhlig T, Sesseng S, et al. Tenosynovitis of the extensor carpi ulnaris tendon predicts erosive progression in early rheumatoid arthritis. Ann Rheum Dis. 2011;70(11):2049–50.
17. Bruyn GA, Hanova P, Iagnocco A, d'Agostino M-A, Möller I, Terslev L, et al. Ultrasound definition of tendon damage in patients with rheumatoid arthritis. Results of a OMERACT consensus-based ultrasound score focussing on the diagnostic reliability. Ann Rheum Dis 2014;73(11):1929–34.
18. Szkudlarek M, Narvestad E, Klarlund M, Court-Payen M, Thomsen HS, Østergaard M. Ultrasonography of the metatarsophalangeal joints in rheumatoid arthritis: comparison with magnetic resonance imaging, conventional radiography, and clinical examination. Arthritis Rheum. 2004;50(7):2103–12.
19. Wakefield RJ, Gibbon WW, Conaghan PG, Connor PO, Gonagle DMC, Pease C, et al. The value of sonography in the detection of bone erosions in patients with rheumatoid arthritis a comparison with conventional radiography. Arthritis Rheum. 2000;43(12):2762–70.

20. Hermann K-G, Backhaus M, Schneider U, Labs K, Loreck D, Zühlsdorf S, et al. Rheumatoid arthritis of the shoulder joint: comparison of conventional radiography, ultrasound, and dynamic contrast-enhanced magnetic resonance imaging. Arthritis Rheum. 2003;48(12):3338–49.
21. Grassi W, Filippucci E, Farina A, Sala FY, Cervini C. Ultrasonography in the evaluation of bone erosions. Ann Rheum Dis. 2001;60:98–103.
22. Zayat AS, Ellegaard K, Conaghan PG, Terslev L, Hensor EM, Freeston JE, et al. The specificity of ultrasound-detected bone erosions for rheumatoid arthritis. Ann Rheum Dis. 2015;74(5):897–903.
23. Brown AK, Conaghan PG, Karim Z, Quinn MA, Ikeda K, Peterfy CG, et al. An explanation for the apparent dissociation between clinical remission and continued structural deterioration in rheumatoid arthritis. Arthritis Rheum. 2008;58(10):2958–67.
24. Grassi W, Filippucci E, Farina A, Cervini C. Sonographic imaging of tendons. Arthritis Rheum. 2000;43(5):969–76.
25. Grassi W, Tittarelli E, Pirani O, Avaltroni D, Cervini C. Ultrasound examination of metacarpophalangeal joints in rheumatoid arthritis. Scand J Rheumatol. 1993;22(5):243–7.
26. Möller B, Bonel H, Rotzetter M, Villiger PM, Ziswiler HR. Measuring finger joint cartilage by ultrasound as a promising alternative to conventional radiograph imaging. Arthritis Care Res. 2009;61(4):435–41.
27. Mandl P, Supp G, Baksa G, Radner H, Studenic P, Gyebnar J, et al. Relationship between radiographic joint space narrowing, sonographic cartilage thickness and anatomy in rheumatoid arthritis and control joints. Ann Rheum Dis. 2015;74(11):2022–7. doi:10.1136/annrheumdis-2014-205585.
28. Grassi W, Lamanna G, Farina A, Cervini C. Sonographic imaging of normal and osteoarthritic cartilage. Semin Arthritis Rheum. 1999;28(6):398–403.
29. Filippucci E, da Luz KR, Di Geso L, Salaffi F, Tardella M, Carotti M, et al. Interobserver reliability of ultrasonography in the assessment of cartilage damage in rheumatoid arthritis. Ann Rheum Dis. 2010;69(10):1845–8.
30. McGonagle D, Lories RJU, Tan AL, Benjamin M. The concept of a "synovio-entheseal complex" and its implications for understanding joint inflammation and damage in psoriatic arthritis and beyond. Arthritis Rheum. 2007;56(8):2482–91.
31. Balint PV, D'Agostino MA. Spondyloarthritis: a journey within and around the joint. Rheumatology. 2012;51:13–7.
32. Terslev L, Naredo E, Iagnocco A, Balint PV, Wakefield RJ, Aegerter P, et al. Defining enthesitis in spondyloarthritis by ultrasound: results of a Delphi process and of a reliability reading exercise. Arthritis Care Res. 2014;66(5):741–8.
33. Gutierrez M, Filippucci E, De Angelis R, Salaffi F, Filosa G, Ruta S, et al. Subclinical entheseal involvement in patients with psoriasis: an ultrasound study. Semin Arthritis Rheum. 2011;40(5):407–12.
34. Naredo E, Möller I, de Miguel E, Batlle-Gualda E, Acebes C, Brito E, et al. High prevalence of ultrasonographic synovitis and enthesopathy in patients with psoriasis without psoriatic arthritis: a prospective case-control study. Rheumatology. 2011;50(10):1838–48.
35. D'Agostino MA. Ultrasound imaging in spondyloarthropathies. Best Pract Res Clin Rheumatol. 2010;24(5):693–700.
36. El Miedany Y, El Gaafary M, Youssef S, Ahmed I, Nasr A. Tailored approach to early psoriatic arthritis patients: clinical and ultrasonographic predictors for structural joint damage. Clin Rheumatol. 2015;34(2):307–13.
37. Freeston JE, Coates LC, Helliwell PS, Hensor EM, Wakefield RJ, Emery P, et al. Is there subclinical enthesitis in early psoriatic arthritis? A clinical comparison with power doppler ultrasound. Arthritis Care Res. 2012;64(10):1617–21.
38. D'Agostino M. Role of ultrasound in the diagnostic work-up of spondyloarthritis. Curr Opin Rheumatol. 2012;24(4):374–739.
39. De Miguel E, Cobo T, Muñoz-Fernández S, Naredo E, Usón J, Acebes JC, et al. Validity of enthesis ultrasound assessment in spondyloarthropathy. Ann Rheum Dis. 2009;68(2):169–74.

40. Ventura-Ríos L, Navarro-Compan V, Aliste M, Linares MA, Areny R, Audisio M, et al. Is entheses ultrasound reliable? A reading Latin American exercise. Clin Rheumatol 2015. s10067-015-3007-x.
41. Mandl P, Navarro-Compan V, Terslev L, Aegerter P, van der Heijde D, D'Agostino MA, et al. EULAR recommendations for the use of imaging in the diagnosis and management of spondyloarthritis in clinical practice. Ann Rheum Dis. 2015;74(7):1327–39.
42. Balint PV, Kane D, Wilson H, McInnes IB, Sturrock RD. Ultrasonography of entheseal insertions in the lower limb in spondyloarthropathy. Ann Rheum Dis. 2002;61(10):905–10.
43. Alcalde M, Acebes JC, Cruz M, González-Hombrado L, Herrero-Beaumont G, Sánchez-Pernaute O. A sonographic enthesitic index of lower limbs is a valuable tool in the assessment of ankylosing spondylitis. Ann Rheum Dis. 2007;66(8):1015–9.
44. D'Agostino MA, Aegerter P, Bechara K, Salliot C, Judet O, Chimenti MS, et al. How to diagnose spondyloarthritis early? Accuracy of peripheral enthesitis detection by power Doppler ultrasonography. Ann Rheum Dis. 2011;70(8):1433–40.
45. Eder L, Barzilai M, Peled N, Gladman DD, Zisman D. The use of ultrasound for the assessment of enthesitis in patients with spondyloarthritis. Clin Radiol. 2013;68(3):219–23.
46. Tan AL, Grainger AJ, Tanner SF, Shelley DM, Pease C, Emery P, et al. High-resolution magnetic resonance imaging for the assessment of hand osteoarthritis. Arthritis Rheum. 2005;52(8):2355–65.
47. Benjamin M, McGonagle D. Histopathologic changes at "synovio-entheseal complexes" suggesting a novel mechanism for synovitis in osteoarthritis and spondylarthritis. Arthritis Rheum. 2007;56(11):3601–9.
48. McGonagle D, Tan AL, Døhn UM, Østergaard M, Benjamin M. Microanatomic studies to define predictive factors for the topography of periarticular erosion formation in inflammatory arthritis. Arthritis Rheum. 2009;60(4):1042–51.
49. El Miedany Y, Youssef S, Mehanna AN, El Gaafary M. Development of a scoring system for assessment of outcome of early undifferentiated inflammatory synovitis. Joint Bone Spine. 2008;75(2):155–62.
50. El Miedany YE, Gaafary ME, Ahmed I, Youssef S, Nasr A. US guided treat-to-target approach in early RA: implications for uncoupling of disease activity and structural joint damage. Curr Rheumatol Rev. 2015;11(1):18–27.
51. Felson DT, Anderson JJ, Boers A, et al. The American College of Rheumatology preliminary core set of disease activity measures for rheumatoid arthritis clinical trials. Arthritis Rheum. 1993;36:729–40.
52. Russak SM, Croft JD, Furst D, et al. The use of rheumatoid arthritis health-related quality of life patient questionnaires in clinical practice: lessons learned. Arthritis Care Res. 2003; 49:574–84.
53. Pincus T, Strand V, Koch G, et al. A n index of the three core data set patient questionnaire measures distinguishes efficacy of active treatment from placebo as effectively as the American College of Rheumatology 20% response criteria (ACR20) or the disease activity score (DAS) in a rheumatoid arthritis clinical trial. Arthritis Rheum. 2003;48:625–30.
54. Pincus T, Sokka T, Kava N. Quantitative documentation of benefit/risk of new therapies for rheumatoid arthritis: patient questionnaires as an optimal measure in standard care. Clin Exp Rheumatol. 2004;22 Suppl 35:S26–33.
55. Wolfe F. Which HAQ is best? A comparison of the HAQ, MHAQ and RA-HAQ, a difficult 8 item HAQ/DHAQ, and a rescored 20 item HAQ (HAQ20): analyses in 2491 rheumatoid arthritis patients following leflunomide initiation. J Rheumatol 2001;28:982–9.
56. Wakefield RJ, Green MJ, Marzo-Ortega H, et al. Should oligoarthritis be reclassified? Ultrasound reveals a high prevalence of subclinical disease. Ann Rheum Dis. 2004;63:382–5.
57. Salaffi F, Fillippucci E, Carrotti E, et al. Inter-observer agreement of standard joint counts in early rheumatoid arthritis: a comparison with grey scale ultrasonography—a preliminary study. Rheumatology (Oxford). 2008;47:54–8.
58. Dopazo Gonzalez N, Ten Cate DF, SwenN WA, et al. The most reliable position in the ultrasonographic examination of the wrist in rheumatoid arthritis. Clin Exp Rheumatol. 2012;30:566–9.

59. Seymour M, Petavy F, Chiesa F, et al. Ultrasonographic measures of synovitis in an early phase clinical trial: a double-blind, randomised, placebo and comparator controlled phase IIa trial of GW274150 (a selective inducible nitric oxide synthase inhibitor) in rheumatoid arthritis. Clin Exp Rheumatol. 2012;30:254–61.
60. Gartner M, Mandl P, Radner H, et al. Sonographic joint assessment in rheumatoid arthritis associations with clinical joint assessment during a state of remission. Arthritis Rheum. 2013;65(8):2005–14.
61. Scott DL, Antoni C, Choy EH, et al. Joint counts in routine practice. Rheumatology (Oxford). 2003;42:919–23.
62. Smolen JS, Aletaha D, Bijlsma JW, et al. Treating rheumatoid arthritis to target: recommendations of an international task force. Ann Rheum Dis. 2010;69:631–7.
63. Pincus T, Segurado OG. Most visits of most patients with rheumatoid arthritis to most rheumatologists do not include a formal quantitative joint count. Ann Rheum Dis. 2006;65:820–2.
64. Radner H, Grisar J, Smolen JS, Stamm T, Aletaha D. Value of self-performed joint counts in rheumatoid arthritis patients near remission. Arthritis Res Ther. 2012;14:R61.
65. Kavanaugh A, Lee SJ, Weng HH, et al. Patient-derived joint counts are a potential alternative for determining disease activity score. J Rheumatol. 2010;37:1035–41.
66. Riazzoli J, Nilsson JA, Teleman A, et al. Patient-reported 28 swollen and tender joint counts accurately represent RA disease activity and can be used to assess therapy responses at the group level. Rheumatology (Oxford). 2010;49:2098–103.
67. Cheung P, Gossec L, Ruyssen-Witrand A, Le Bourlout C, et al. The relationship of patient-reported joints with active synovitis detected by power Doppler ultrasonography in rheumatoid arthritis. Clin Exp Rheumatol. 2013;31:490–7.
68. El Miedany Y, El Gaafary M, Palmer D, Youssef S. Imaging as an outcome measure in early inflammatory arthritis: monitoring disease activity and patients' response to therapy using ultrasonography. Arthritis Rheum. 2011;63(10 Suppl):S319.
69. Janta I, Naredo E, Martínez-Estupiñán L, Nieto JC, et al. Patient self-assessment and physician's assessment of rheumatoid arthritis activity: which is more realistic in remission status? A comparison with ultrasonography. Rheumatology (Oxford). 2013;52(12):2243–50.
70. Felson D. Defining remission in rheumatoid arthritis. Ann Rheum Dis 2012;71 Suppl 2:ii86–8.
71. El Miedany Y, El Gaafary M, Youssef S, Palmer D. Physician versus patient global assessment in early rheumatoid arthritis: putting the cart before the horse. Ann Rheum Dis. 2014;73 Suppl 2:616–7. doi:10.1136/annrheumdis-2014-eular.1408.
72. Naredo E, Collado P, Cruz A, et al. Longitudinal power Doppler ultrasonographic assessment of joint inflammatory activity in early rheumatoid arthritis: predictive value in disease activity and radiologic progression. Arthritis Rheum. 2007;57:116–24.
73. Ogasawara M, Murayama G, Yamada Y, et al. Auto feedback from ultrasound images provides rapid improvement in palpation skills for identifying joint swelling in rheumatoid arthritis. J Rheumatol. 2012;39:1207–14.
74. Wright SA, Bell AL. Enhancement of undergraduate rheumatology teaching through the use of musculoskeletal ultrasound. Rheumatology (Oxford). 2008;47:1564–6.
75. Van Den Bemt BJ, Van Den Hoogen FH, Benraad B, Hekster YA, Van Riel PL, Van Lankveld W. Adherence rates and associations with nonadherence in patients with rheumatoid arthritis using disease modifying antirheumatic drugs. J Rheumatol. 2009;36:2164–70.
76. Paivio A, Rogers TB, Smythe PC. Why are pictures easier to recall than words? Psychon Sci. 1968;11:137–8.
77. Elliott RA. Poor adherence to medication in adults with rheumatoid arthritis: reasons and solutions. Dis Manag Health Outcomes. 2008;16:13–29.
78. Katz MG, Kripalani S, Weiss BD. Use of pictorial aids in medication instructions: a review of the literature. Am J Health Syst Pharm. 2006;63:2391–7.
79. Houts PS, Doak CC, Doak LG, Loscalzo MJ. The role of pictures in improving health communication: a review of research on attention, comprehension, recall, and adherence. Patient Educ Couns. 2006;61:173–90.

80. Horne R, Weinman J. Patients' beliefs about prescribed medicines and their role in adherence to treatment in chronic physical illness. J Psychosom Res. 1999;47:555–67.
81. Joshua F. Ultrasound applications for the practicing rheumatologist. Best Pract Res Clin Rheumatol. 2012;26:853–67.
82. Joplin K, van der Zwan R, Bagga H, Joshua F. Pilot study assessing the novel use of musculoskeletal ultrasound in patients with rheumatoid arthritis to improve patient attitudes and adherence to medication. Int J Rheum Dis 2014. doi:10.1111/1756-185X.12402.
83. Neame R, Hammond A. Beliefs about medications: a questionnaire survey of people with rheumatoid arthritis. Rheumatology (Oxford). 2005;44:762–7.
84. Sibbitt Jr WL, Peisajovich A, Michael AA, Park KS, Sibbitt RR, Band PA, Bankhurst AD. Does sonographic needle guidance affect the clinical outcome of intraarticular injections? J Rheumatol. 2009;36:1892–902.
85. Eustace JA, Brophy DP, Gibney RP, Bresnihan B, FitzGerald O. Comparison of the accuracy of steroid placement with clinical outcome in patients with shoulder symptoms. Ann Rheum Dis. 1997;56:59–63.
86. Yi TI, Kim ST, Kim DH, Kim JS, Park JS, Lee JH. Comparison of blind technique and ultrasonography guided technique of intraarticular injection of the shoulder. J Korean Acad Rehabil Med. 2006;30:45–50.
87. Hasiuchi T, Sakurai G, Sakamoto Y, Takakura Y, Tanaka Y. Comparative survey of pain-alleviating effects between ultrasound-guided injection and blind injection of lidocaine alone in patients with painful shoulder. Arch Orthop Trauma Surg. 2010;130:847–52.
88. Buchbinder R, Green S, Youd JM. Corticosteroid injections for shoulder pain. Cochrane Database Syst Rev. 2003;1, CD004016.
89. Soh E, Li W, Ong K, Chen W, Bautista D. Image-guided versus blind corticosteroid injections in adults with shoulder pain: a systematic review. BMC Musculoskelet Disord. 2011;12:137.
90. Huang Z, Du S, Qi Y, Chen G, Yan W. Effectiveness of ultrasound guidance on intraarticular and periarticular joint injections: systematic review and meta-analysis of randomized trials. Am J Phys Med Rehabil. 2015;94(10):775–83.
91. Filer A, DePablo P, Allen G, et al. Utility of ultrasound joint counts in the prediction of rheumatoid arthritis in patients with very early synovitis. Ann Rheum Dis. 2011;70:500–7.
92. Saleem B, Brown AK, Keen H, et al. Should imaging be a component of rheumatoid arthritis remission criteria? A comparison between traditional and modified composite remission scores and imaging assessments. Ann Rheum Dis. 2011;70:792–8.

Index

Y. El Miedany (ed.), *Patient Reported Outcome Measures in Rheumatic Diseases*,
DOI 10.1007/978-3-319-32851-5

MIX
Papier aus verantwortungsvollen Quellen
Paper from responsible sources
FSC® C105338

If you have any concerns about our products,
you can contact us on
ProductSafety@springernature.com

In case Publisher is established outside the EU,
the EU authorized representative is:
Springer Nature Customer Service Center GmbH
Europaplatz 3, 69115 Heidelberg, Germany

Printed by Libri Plureos GmbH
in Hamburg, Germany